Data Analytics and Applications of the Wearable Sensors in Healthcare

Special Issue Editors

Shabbir Syed-Abdul
Taipei Medical University
Taiwan

Luis Fernandez Luque Qatar
Computing Research Institute
Qatar

Pei-Yun Sabrina Hsueh
IBM Thomas J. Watson Research Center
USA

Juan M. García-Gomez
Universitat Politecnica de Valencia
Spain

Begoña Garcia-Zapirain
University of Deusto Spain

Editorial Office
MDPI
St. Alban-Anlage 66
4052 Basel, Switzerland

This is a reprint of articles from the Special Issue published online in the open access journal *Sensors* (ISSN 1424-8220) (available at: https://www.mdpi.com/journal/sensors/special_issues/Wearable_Sensors_in_the_Healthcare).

For citation purposes, cite each article independently as indicated on the article page online and as indicated below:

LastName, A.A.; LastName, B.B.; LastName, C.C. Article Title. *Journal Name* **Year**, *Article Number*, Page Range.

ISBN 978-3-03936-350-6 (Pbk)
ISBN 978-3-03936-351-3 (PDF)

© 2020 by the authors. Articles in this book are Open Access and distributed under the Creative Commons Attribution (CC BY) license, which allows users to download, copy and build upon published articles, as long as the author and publisher are properly credited, which ensures maximum dissemination and a wider impact of our publications.

The book as a whole is distributed by MDPI under the terms and conditions of the Creative Commons license CC BY-NC-ND.

Data Analytics and Applications of the Wearable Sensors in Healthcare

Special Issue Editors

Shabbir Syed-Abdul
Luis Fernandez Luque
Pei-Yun Sabrina Hsueh
Juan M. García-Gomez
Begoña Garcia-Zapirain

MDPI • Basel • Beijing • Wuhan • Barcelona • Belgrade • Manchester • Tokyo • Cluj • Tianjin

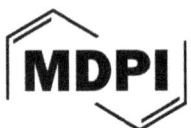

Contents

About the Special Issue Editors ix

Mohy Uddin and Shabbir Syed-Abdul
Data Analytics and Applications of the Wearable Sensors in Healthcare: An Overview
Reprinted from: *Sensors* 2020, *20*, 1379, doi:10.3390/s20051379 1

Jose-Luis Bayo-Monton, Antonio Martinez-Millana, Weisi Han, Carlos Fernandez-Llatas and Vicente Traver
Wearable Sensors Integrated with Internet of Things for Advancing eHealth Care
Reprinted from: *Sensors* 2018, *18*, 1851, doi:10.3390/s18061851 7

Saurabh Singh Thakur, Shabbir Syed-Abdul, Hsiao-Yean (Shannon) Chiu, Ram Babu Roy, Po-Yu Huang, Shwetambara Malwade, Aldilas Achmad Nursetyo and Yu-Chuan (Jack) Li
Artificial-Intelligence-Based Prediction of Clinical Events among Hemodialysis Patients Using Non-Contact Sensor Data
Reprinted from: *Sensors* 2018, *18*, 2833, doi:10.3390/s18092833 25

Rob Argent, Patrick Slevin, Antonio Bevilacqua, Maurice Neligan, Ailish Daly and Brian Caulfield
Wearable Sensor-Based Exercise Biofeedback for Orthopaedic Rehabilitation: A Mixed Methods User Evaluation of a Prototype System
Reprinted from: *Sensors* 2019, *19*, 432, doi:10.3390/s19020432 41

Miguel Enrique Iglesias Martínez, Juan M. García-Gomez, Carlos Sáez, Pedro Fernández de Córdoba and J. Alberto Conejero
Feature Extraction and Similarity of Movement Detection during Sleep, Based on Higher Order Spectra and Entropy of the Actigraphy Signal: Results of the Hispanic Community Health Study/Study of Latinos
Reprinted from: *Sensors* 2018, *18*, 4310, doi:10.3390/s18124310 55

Shih-Sung Lin, Chien-Wu Lan, Hao-Yen Hsu and Sheng-Tao Chen
Data Analytics of a Wearable Device for Heat Stroke Detection
Reprinted from: *Sensors* 2018, *18*, 4347, doi:10.3390/s18124347 73

Francisco Luna-Perejón, Manuel Jesús Domínguez-Morales and Anton Civit-Balcells
Wearable Fall Detector Using Recurrent Neural Networks
Reprinted from: *Sensors* 2019, *19*, 4885, doi:10.3390/s19224885 97

Katharina Stollenwerk, Jonas Müller, André Hinkenjann and Björn Krüger
Analyzing Spinal Shape Changes During Posture Training Using a Wearable Device
Reprinted from: *Sensors* 2019, *19*, 3625, doi:10.3390/s19163625 117

Mario Vega-Barbas, Jose A. Diaz-Olivares, Ke Lu, Mikael Forsman, Fernando Seoane and Farhad Abtahi
P-Ergonomics Platform: Toward Precise, Pervasive, and Personalized Ergonomics using Wearable Sensors and Edge Computing
Reprinted from: *Sensors* 2019, *19*, 1225, doi:10.3390/s19051225 139

Wen-Yen Lin, Hong-Lin Ke, Wen-Cheng Chou, Po-Cheng Chang, Tsai-Hsuan Tsai and Ming-Yih Lee
Realization and Technology Acceptance Test of a Wearable Cardiac Health Monitoring and Early Warning System with Multi-Channel MCGs and ECG
Reprinted from: *Sensors* 2018, *18*, 3538, doi:10.3390/s18103538 157

Se-Min Lim, Hyeong-Cheol Oh, Jaein Kim, Juwon Lee and Jooyoung Park
LSTM-Guided Coaching Assistant for Table Tennis Practice
Reprinted from: *Sensors* 2018, *18*, 4112, doi:10.3390/s18124112 179

Ke Lu, Liyun Yang, Fernando Seoane, Farhad Abtahi, Mikael Forsman and Kaj Lindecrantz
Fusion of Heart Rate, Respiration and Motion Measurements from a Wearable Sensor System to Enhance Energy Expenditure Estimation
Reprinted from: *Sensors* 2018, *18*, 3092, doi:10.3390/s18093092 193

Andreas Ejupi and Carlo Menon
Detection of Talking in Respiratory Signals: A Feasibility Study Using Machine Learning and Wearable Textile-Based Sensors
Reprinted from: *Sensors* 2018, *18*, 2474, doi:10.3390/s18082474 205

Ambra Cesareo, Ylenia Previtali, Emilia Biffi and Andrea Aliverti
Assessment of Breathing Parameters Using an Inertial Measurement Unit (IMU)-Based System
Reprinted from: *Sensors* 2019, *19*, 88, doi:10.3390/s19010088 217

Jose Manjarres, Pedro Narvaez, Kelly Gasser, Winston Percybrooks and Mauricio Pardo
Physical Workload Tracking Using Human Activity Recognition with Wearable Devices
Reprinted from: *Sensors* 2020, *20*, 39, doi:10.3390/s20010039 241

Hyung Seok Nam, Woo Hyung Lee, Han Gil Seo, Yoon Jae Kim, Moon Suk Bang and Sungwan Kim
Inertial Measurement Unit Based Upper Extremity Motion Characterization for Action Research Arm Test and Activities of Daily Living
Reprinted from: *Sensors* 2019, *19*, 1782, doi:10.3390/s19081782 259

Wei Zhang, Michael Schwenk, Sabato Mellone, Anisoara Paraschiv-Ionescu, Beatrix Vereijken, Mirjam Pijnappels, A. Stefanie Mikolaizak, Elisabeth Boulton, Nini H. Jonkman, Andrea B. Maier, Jochen Klenk, Jorunn Helbostad, Kristin Taraldsen and Kamiar Aminian
Complexity of Daily Physical Activity Is More Sensitive Than Conventional Metrics to Assess Functional Change in Younger Older Adults
Reprinted from: *Sensors* 2018, *18*, 2032, doi:10.3390/s18072032 269

Chien-Chin Hsu, Bor-Shing Lin, Ke-Yi He and Bor-Shyh Lin
Design of a Wearable 12-Lead Noncontact Electrocardiogram Monitoring System
Reprinted from: *Sensors* 2019, *19*, 1509, doi:10.3390/s19071509 281

Udeni Jayasinghe and William S. Harwin, Faustina Hwang
Comparing Clothing-Mounted Sensors with Wearable Sensors for Movement Analysis and Activity Classification
Reprinted from: *Sensors* 2020, *20*, 82, doi:10.3390/s20010082 295

Hoda Allahbakhshi, Lindsey Conrow, Babak Naimi and Robert Weibel
Using Accelerometer and GPS Data for Real-Life Physical Activity Type Detection
Reprinted from: *Sensors* 2020, *20*, 588, doi:10.3390/s20030588 309

Ying Kuen Cheung, Pei-Yun Sabrina Hsueh, Ipek Ensari, Joshua Z. Willey and Keith M. Diaz
Quantile Coarsening Analysis of High-Volume Wearable Activity Data in a Longitudinal Observational Study
Reprinted from: *Sensors* **2018**, *18*, 3056, doi:10.3390/s18093056 . . . . **331**

Yashodhan Athavale and Sridhar Krishnan
A Device-Independent Efficient Actigraphy Signal-Encoding System for Applications in Monitoring Daily Human Activities and Health
Reprinted from: *Sensors* **2018**, *18*, 2966, doi:10.3390/s18092966 . . . . **343**

Luis A. Trejo and Ari Yair Barrera-Animas
Towards an Efficient One-Class Classifier for Mobile Devices and Wearable Sensors on the Context of Personal Risk Detection
Reprinted from: *Sensors* **2018**, *18*, 2857, doi:10.3390/s18092857 . . . . **359**

Aras Yurtman, Billur Barshan,* and Barış Fidan
Activity Recognition Invariant to Wearable Sensor Unit OrientationUsing Differential Rotational Transformations Represented by Quaternions
Reprinted from: *Sensors* **2018**, *18*, 2725, doi:10.3390/s18082725 . . . . **379**

Arindam Dutta, Owen Ma, Meynard Toledo, Alberto Florez Pregonero,
Barbara E. Ainsworth, Matthew P. Buman and Daniel W. Bliss
Identifying Free-Living Physical Activities Using Lab-Based Models with Wearable Accelerometers
Reprinted from: *Sensors* **2018**, *18*, 3893, doi:10.3390/s18113893 . . . . **407**

Samanta Rosati, Gabriella Balestra and Marco Knaflitz
Comparison of Different Sets of Features for Human Activity Recognition by Wearable Sensors
Reprinted from: *Sensors* **2018**, *18*, 4189, doi:10.3390/s18124189 . . . . **421**

Davide Morelli, Alessio Rossi, Massimo Cairo and David A. Clifton
Analysis of the Impact of Interpolation Methods of Missing RR-Intervals Caused by Motion Artifacts on HRV Features Estimations
Reprinted from: *Sensors* **2019**, *19*, 3163, doi:10.3390/s19143163 . . . . **437**

Alexis Fortin-Côté, Jean-Sébastien Roy, Laurent Bouyer, Philip Jackson and
Alexandre Campeau-Lecours
Allumo: Preprocessing and Calibration Software for Wearable Accelerometers Used in Posture Tracking
Reprinted from: **2020**, *20*, 229, doi:10.3390/s20010229 . . . . **451**

Robert W. Broadley, Jochen Klenk, Sibylle B. Thies, Laurence P. J. Kenney and
Malcolm H. Granat
Methods for the Real-World Evaluation of Fall Detection Technology: AScoping Review
Reprinted from: *Sensors* **2018**, *18*, 2060, doi:10.3390/s18072060 . . . . **459**

About the Special Issue Editors

Shabbir Syed-Abdul M.D., M.S., Ph.D., Associate Professor at Taipei Medical University. Dr. Shabbir Syed-Abdul is an associate professor at the Institute of Biomedical Informatics, a leading researcher and a principal investigator at the International Center for Health Information Technology, Taipei, Taiwan. He is an educator for MOOCs on FutureLearn, one of his renowned courses is on the Internet of Things for active aging. Shabbir's major research interests are long-term care with wearable technologies, mHealth, big data analysis and visualization, artificial intelligence, personal health records, social network in healthcare, and hospital information systems. He wants to empower care providers and improve patient engagement. He feels one of the methods to achieve this goal is to focus on the management and flow of the health and medical information among health care providers and seekers.

Dr. Shabbir's previous experiences working as a physician, researcher, and principal investigator both in the developed and developing world makes him an ideal candidate for this post leading advance global knowledge on the factors that impact on the development of sustainable healthcare, in particular focusing on innovation and ageing populations.

Luis Fernandez Luque, Ph.D. eHealth|Researcher at QCRI|Co-founder at Salumedia (Seville, Spain). Qatar Computing Research Institute, HBKU, Qatar Foundation, University of Tromsø (UiT).

Luis is committed to identifying how technology can support people to live healthier. His passions are health, computing, and improving reality, which led him to a career in eHealth, both as a researcher and as anentrepreneur. Luis Fernandex is currently an eHeath researcher at the Qatar Computing Research Institute—Qatar Foundation. He is also the co-founder and advisor in the digital health start-up Salumedia.

Pei-Yun Sabrina Hsueh received her B.S. from the National Taiwan University, M.S. from University of California at Berkeley, and Ph.D. from the University of Edinburgh. She is currently an IBM Academy of Technology Member and Research Staff Member in the Center for Computational Health at IBM Watson Research Center, Yorktown Heights, NY. Currently, she is leading the efforts toward computational health behavioral understanding with applications in care management and health decision support (using patient-generated health data from wearable sensors, mobile devices, and patient-reported outcomes). She is a pioneer in the area of consumer and pervasive health informatics, and is a serial winner of IBM Inventor Plateau awards, Manager Choice Awards, Eminence and Excellence, and Research Achievement Award. She has authored 20+ patents, 50+ technical papers, and 3 textbook chapters. She co-chairs the IBM Health Informatics professional interest community and is actively serving on various scientific program committees in ACM, IEEE, AMIA, and IMIA. She was elected as the Chair of Consumer and Pervasive Health Informatics Work Group of American Medical Informatics Association in 2017 for the term of 2018–2022. Her expertise on emerging health informatics topics makes her a sought-after speaker and consultant in science-driven industry solutions. Prior to IBM, she worked in the EU FP6 an FP7 Augmented Multiparty Interaction project with 22 partner sites across 7 countries and has been selected as European Google Anita Borg Scholar.

Juan M. García-Gomez, Ph.D. in Computer Engineering (2009) is Senior Lecturer at UPV, a leader of the research group in data-driven approaches to improving healthcare at the ITACA Institute, and has been the advisor of 6 Ph.D. theses about clinical decision support systems applied to brain tumors, breast cancer and biomedical data quality assessment. In 2007, he was visiting researcher at ESAT-KU Leuven. In 2016, he was involved at IHI-ULC as a visiting researcher. His research interests mainly focus on machine learning techniques for developing clinical decision support systems (CDSS), the definition of data quality metrics for assessing biomedical repositories, and the design of medical applications based on big data technologies. He is author of more than 40 articles published in specialized journals (including *JAMIA*, *Nucleic Acids Research*, *PLoS ONE*, and *Bioinformatics* among others). His work on an HL7-CDA wrapper for facilitating semantic interoperability to rule-based Clinical Decision Support Systems (doi:10.1016/j.cmpb.2012.10.003) was selected as the best of the medical informatics papers published in 2013, sub-field of Health Information Systems by the International Medical Informatics Association (IMIA) for the IMIA Yearbook 2014. He has coordinated the pattern recognition WP of the FP6 EU eTUMOUR project (LSHC-CT-2004- 503094), the predictive analysis of the HealthAgents Project (IST-2004-27214), and WP leader in the FP7 European project Help4Mood (FP7-ICT-2009-4; 248765).

Begoña Garcia-Zapirain, Ph.D. graduated in communications engineering, specializing in telematics at the Basque Country University, Bilbao (Spain) in 1994. In 2003, she defended her doctoral thesis in the pathological speech digital processing field. After many years of working for ZIV Company, in 1997, Dr. García joined the University of Deusto faculty as a lecturer in signal theory and electronics. She has been the head of the Telecommunication Department at the University of Deusto since 2002. In 2001, she created the e-Life research group at the same university, playing the role of lead researcher. She has participated in more than 80 research projects on international, national, and regional levels; published more than 35 papers in international scientific journals; and presented more than 160 papers in international and national scientific conferences.

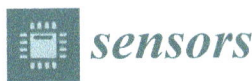

Editorial

Data Analytics and Applications of the Wearable Sensors in Healthcare: An Overview

Mohy Uddin [1] and Shabbir Syed-Abdul [2],*

[1] Executive Office, King Abdullah International Medical Research Center, King Saud bin Abdulaziz University for Health Sciences, King Abdulaziz Medical City, Ministry of National Guard—Health Affairs, Riyadh 11426, Saudi Arabia; drmohyuddin@yahoo.com
[2] Graduate Institute of Biomedical Informatics, Taipei Medical University, Taipei 10675, Taiwan
* Correspondence: drshabbir@tmu.edu.tw; Tel.: +886-2-6638-2736 (ext. 1514); Fax: +886-2-6638-0233

Received: 26 February 2020; Accepted: 29 February 2020; Published: 3 March 2020

1. Introduction

Improving health and lives of people is undoubtedly one of the prime goals of healthcare organizations, policy-makers, and leaders around the world. The need of ageing, disability, long-term care, and palliative care in our current society pose formidable challenges for disease burden and healthcare systems that must be addressed [1]. In order to tackle the leading causes of morbidity and mortality that may result from infections to chronic conditions especially in older adults and ageing population, the accessibility and provision of long-term care and palliative care, when and where needed by them, is crucial. With the continuous challenges and rising demands of the elderly, remote and home-based care, the technological innovations in the fields of digital health and health information and communication technologies, such as mobile health, wearable technologies, telemedicine and personalized medicine have transformed the ways of practice and delivery of healthcare in the recent decades [2]. Wearable technologies have been extensively used in the healthcare sector with multi-purpose applications ranging from patient care to personal health. In clinical and remote care, the applications of wearable devices/sensors, mobile applications, and tracking technologies are of immense importance for the diagnosis, prevention, monitoring, and management of chronic diseases and conditions [3]. The data generated from the wearable devices/sensors are a cornerstone for healthcare data analytics, especially when it is utilized by latest technologies, such as Artificial Intelligence (AI), Machine Learning (ML), Big Data Intelligence, and Internet of Things (IoT) Systems. The literature has many successful examples of utilization of these data in various branches of medicine, such as oncology, radiology, surgery, geriatrics, rheumatology, neurology, hematology, and cardiology. With the regular ongoing updates, the outcomes of data analytics and their applications are already making a huge impact in transforming and revolutionizing the healthcare industry.

In this special issue, we aim to provide new insights on research data analytics and applications of wearable devices/sensors in healthcare by covering wide range of related topics. This issue represents the latest research that spans across 19 countries, 37 institutions and is covered by a total of 28 articles. To make better understanding of the research articles, we have arranged them in an order to show various covered aspects in this field, such as technology integration research, prediction systems, rehabilitation studies, prototype systems, community health studies, detection systems, ergonomics studies, technology acceptance studies, monitoring systems, warning systems, sports studies, clinical systems, feasibility studies, parameters measurement systems, design studies, location based systems, tracking systems, observational studies, risk assessment studies, activity recognition systems, impact measurement systems and systematic review.

2. Summary of Special Issue Papers

In order to provide a basic overview, we will go through and provide brief summary of all the articles of wearable devices/sensors covered in this issue one by one. Bayo-Monton et al. [4] provided an implementation of new portable system for remote management of chronic diseases by presenting and evaluating an embedded and scalable distributed system using wearable sensors for the connection of cheap health devices based on prototyping eHealth platforms. The results of their analysis showed that portable devices ($p \ll 0.01$) are suitable for supporting the transmission and analysis of biometric signals into scalable telemedicine systems. In an observational study, Thakur et al. [5] presented a supervised ML-based model for predicting the clinical events during dialysis sessions using data from a non-contact sensor device. The authors found the findings and performance of the ML model quite encouraging and suggested the use of non-contact sensors in clinical settings for monitoring patients' vital parameters and in early warning solutions for predicting the clinical events. In a study involving patients that recently had knee replacement surgery, Argent et al. [6] explored and evaluated the feasibility, usability, impact and user experience of an exemplar exercise biofeedback system for orthopedic rehabilitation at home. In order to maximize the engagement and impact, the study incorporated user-centered design approaches by incorporating participants' evaluation during the design of the system. The findings of the study support the ongoing development and evaluation of sensor-based biofeedback systems, and authors found the system highly usable and effective for patient support and engagement. In a community health study, Martinez et al. [7] developed a new unsupervised exploratory method for characterizing feature extraction and detecting movement similarity in sleep by using actigraphy signals. The results of statistical analysis showed the potentials of this method for sleep disorders and their link with other conditions. The authors suggested the possible application of proposed approach for the extraction and comparison of sleep movements' patterns in the field of medicine. Based on a previous work of a Wearable Heat stroke Detection Device (WHDD) [8] that was used for heat stroke prediction capability for any activity or exercise. Lin et al. [9] investigated the detailed information analysis and performed static and dynamic experiments for verifying the availability and effectiveness of WHDD experimental subjects. The results of their work demonstrated the superior applicability of the WHDD for predicting the occurrence of heat stroke effectively and ensuring the safety of runners. Using recurrent neural networks (RNNs)-based deep learning models, Luna-Perejon [10] presented a feasibility study of implementing a wearable system for the detection of falls and its associated risks/hazards in real time through accelerometer signals. Based on the results of the study, the authors recommended RNNs models as an effective method for creation of autonomous wearable fall detection systems in real time. Using a large real-world database of posture data, Stollenwerk et al. [11] analyzed the postural changes that are induced under postural training in three different positions, sitting, standing, and hip hinging, and compared the snapshots of unguided-guided posture pair based on features resulted from 2D spine curve geometry. The results showed the novelty of the work in the field of wearable-sensor-based evaluation of spine curves. Vega-Barbas et al. [12] proposed a precise and pervasive ergonomic platform for accurate assessment of continuous risk and personalized automated coaching by utilizing in-house developed garments and a mobile application. The results of the study demonstrating a good usability score proved the acceptable usability of the platform. The authors expected that wearable technology in the field of ergonomics can have cost effective risk assessment and economical solutions in the future. The study from Lin et al. [13] presented the design of a wearable cardiac health monitoring platform, implemented it as wearable smart clothing system with multi-channel mechanocardiograms and electrocardiograms measurements, and evaluated the usability of the system using technology acceptance model. The analysis and the results of the study showed the positive attitude of subjects for using this wearable system in providing early risk warnings. Based on deep learning, Lim et al. [14] presented a coaching assistant method to provide useful information for table tennis practice, and used long short-term memory (LSTM) recurrent neural networks (RNNs) with deep state space model and probabilistic inference to support practice. The promising results provided by this method showed its capability in characterizing high-dimensional time series patterns and providing useful information with wearable sensors in table tennis coaching. Lu et al. [15] developed and tested a new method that combined information from heart rate, respiration, and accelerations measurements to estimate energy expenditure. These data measurements were taken from wearable sensor system and were integrated by neural network based model. The results of the proposed method showed improved accuracy over two existing established methods. The authors suggested that this model along with wearable system could be utilized in both occupational as well as general health applications. Ejupi [16] investigated the feasibility of wearable textile-based sensors to accurately monitor breathing patterns, develop algorithm to detect talking using ML algorithm, and evaluate the model's performance with the study participants. The evaluation showed random forest classifier as the best performer in the dataset. The authors suggested that this approach could be used to quantify talking through social interaction and prevent social isolation and loneliness. Using a previously developed inertial measurement unit device based on three sensor [17], Cesareo et al. [18] presented an automatic and position-independent algorithm to derive the respiration-induced movement and determine the respiratory rate accurately. The results showed that principal component analysis (PCA) fusion method obtained overall highest performance in terms of breathing frequency estimation, in both supine as well as seated position. The authors suggested that PAC fusion, as dimension-reduction method, can be used to analyze further data in the future. Using wearable technology and ML algorithms, Manjarres et al. [19] developed a smart physical workload tracking system in real time for simultaneous remote monitoring of people. The established framework was based on the concept of ergonomics to facilitate the work of health professionals and fitness experts. The results of two case studies in real time showed good accuracy and reliability of the system. The authors recommended the future developments by combining ergonomics and ML to predict the physical effort of activities and for injury prevention environments. Nam et al. [20] used an inertial measurement unit-based motion capture and analysis system to access arm movements. The study provided an important database on the dimensions of workspace and range of motions for arm movements. The validation results showed high accuracy and reliability of the system and emphasized on the importance of designing new exoskeletons for neurorehabilitation purposes. Zhang et al. [21] examined the relevance of different conventional physical activity metrics and complexity in the assessment of functional change after exercise intervention in younger and older adults. The findings of the study demonstrated the potential and usefulness of physical activity complexity metrics as compared to conventional metrics in assessment of functional changes for younger and older adults, and recommended them for the feasibility and effectiveness of risk identification and interventions. Hsu et al. [22] proposed a wearable 12-lead electrocardiogram monitoring system to measure the electrocardiogram (ECG) signals of patients with myocardial ischemia and arrhythmia. The experimental results of the study provided a good ECG signal quality even while walking and detected ECG features of the mentioned patients. The authors suggested the possible usefulness of the proposed system in future mobile ECG monitoring applications. Jayasinghe et al. [23] investigated and quantified the data received from sensors in different types of clothing in order to characterize the activities as compared to the body worn sensors' data. The case study analysis indicated that clothing sensors data correlated well with the body worn sensors data, and classification results from clothing sensors were also promising compared to body-worn sensors. The results of the study showed potentials of this approach in daily monitoring. Allahbakhshi et al. [24] examined the role of Global Positioning System (GPS) sensors data for detection of physical activity in semi-structured and real-life protocols using participants with wearable devices in a study. The results provided insights in assisting physical activity for future study designs and guidance related to detection of posture and transport related motion activities. Cheung et al. [25] proposed a novel quantile coarsening analysis (QCA) for reducing the dimension of data from wearable devices and demonstrated the feasibility of this approach in a small cohort of relatively healthy individuals. Because of the versatility of the QCA approach, the authors suggested that it can provide useful analytical tools for data in multi-modal monitoring. By explaining the role of actigraphs in personalized health, fitness monitoring and Internet of Medical Things (IoMT) paradigm, Athavale [26] presented a study utilizing wearable devices to capture and analyze physiological data at home-based health monitoring in an IoMT environment, and proposed a low level encoding scheme to improve actigraphy analysis. In order to ensure that there was no loss of information in encoding process, ML approach was used for the study validation. Based on the dataset Personal RIsk DEtection (PRIDE) [27], a study by Trejo [28] first explored the impact of using dimension reduction techniques and frequency domain features for personal risk detection through correlation matrix and principal component analysis, and then efficiently accelerated the training and classification process of a given classifier for mobile devices. The results of the study were encouraging for timely detection of risk prone situations that can threaten a person's physical integrity. Yurtman et al. [29] proposed a methodology to transform the recorded motion sensor sequences to sensor unit orientation unchangeably and incorporated it in pre-processing stage of the standard activity recognition scheme. The results from comparative evaluation of proposed method with the existing state-of-the-art classifiers showed its substantially better output in classifying stationary activities and hence its possible application in various wearable systems. Dutta et al. [30] used a novel framework to classify and model the physical activities performed by different participants in a supervised lab-based protocol and then utilized it to identify the physical activities in a free-living setting using the data from wrist worn accelerometers. The positive results of the study demonstrated its application for estimating physical activities in future cohort or intervention studies. In a study, Rosati et al. [31] compared two different feature sets for real-time human activity recognition (HAR) applications; one comprising time, frequency, and time-frequency related parameters used in the literature and the other containing only time-related variables linked with biomechanical meaning of acquired signals. The results showed that both set of features can reach high accuracy with support vector machine (SVM) classifier, but the new proposed variables can be easily interpreted and employed for better understanding of the alterations of biomechanical behavior in complex situations. In a study focusing on healthy subjects having normal heart activity, Morelli et al. [32] investigated the effects of interpolation on time and duration with increasing missing values to assess the interpolation strategy for better results during the estimation of heart rate variability (HRV) features. The results concluded that interpolation in time is the most favorable method for producing better HRV features estimation as compared to interpolation on duration. Fortin-Cote et al. [33] presented a graphical software for the visualization and preprocessing of raw data received from accelerometer for human posture tracking and assessment. This tool was aimed to provide support for calibration of orientation estimate of inertial measurement units (IMUs) that are used for joint angle measurement. Two case studies were used to demonstrate the usefulness of this open source software. Broadley et al. [34] presented a systematic review to assess existing methods of evaluating fall detection systems, identify their limitations, and propose improved evaluation methods in the literature. The search results of articles that met the inclusion criteria identified few issues, such as use of small population datasets and inconsistency for performance quantification for these systems. Sensitivity, precision, and F-measures were derived as the most appropriate and robust measures for their realistic performance evaluation.

Conflicts of Interest: The authors declare no conflict of interest.

References

1. The, L. Global elderly care in crisis. *Lancet* **2014**, *383*, 927. [CrossRef]
2. Malwade, S.; Abdul, S.S.; Uddin, M.; Nursetyo, A.A.; Fernandez-Luque, L.; Zhu, X.; Cilliers, L.; Wong, C.-P.; Bamidis, P.; Li, Y.-C. Mobile and wearable technologies in healthcare for the ageing population. *Comput. Methods Programs Biomed.* **2018**, *161*, 233–237. [CrossRef] [PubMed]
3. Sim, I. Mobile Devices and Health. *N. Engl. J. Med.* **2019**, *381*, 956–968. [CrossRef] [PubMed]
4. Bayo-Monton, J.-L.; Martinez-Millana, A.; Han, W.; Fernandez-Llatas, C.; Sun, Y.; Traver, V. Wearable Sensors Integrated with Internet of Things for Advancing eHealth Care. *Sensors* **2018**, *18*, 1851. [CrossRef]

5. Thakur, S.S.; Abdul, S.S.; Chiu, H.-Y.; Roy, R.B.; Huang, P.-Y.; Malwade, S.; Nursetyo, A.A.; Li, Y.-C. Artificial-Intelligence-Based Prediction of Clinical Events among Hemodialysis Patients Using Non-Contact Sensor Data. *Sensors* **2018**, *18*, 2833. [CrossRef]

6. Argent, R.; Slevin, P.; Bevilacqua, A.; Neligan, M.; Daly, A.; Caulfield, B. Wearable Sensor-Based Exercise Biofeedback for Orthopaedic Rehabilitation: A Mixed Methods User Evaluation of a Prototype System. *Sensors* **2019**, *19*, 432. [CrossRef]

7. Iglesias Martínez, M.E.; García-Gomez, J.M.; Sáez, C.; Fernández de Córdoba, P.; Alberto Conejero, J. Feature Extraction and Similarity of Movement Detection during Sleep, Based on Higher Order Spectra and Entropy of the Actigraphy Signal: Results of the Hispanic Community Health Study/Study of Latinos. *Sensors* **2018**, *18*, 4310. [CrossRef]

8. Chen, S.T.; Lin, S.S.; Lan, C.W.; Hsu, H.Y. Design and Development of a Wearable Device for Heat Stroke Detection. *Sensors* **2017**, *18*, 17. [CrossRef]

9. Lin, S.-S.; Lan, C.-W.; Hsu, H.-Y.; Chen, S.-T. Data Analytics of a Wearable Device for Heat Stroke Detection. *Sensors* **2018**, *18*, 4347. [CrossRef]

10. Luna-Perejón, F.; Domínguez-Morales, M.J.; Civit-Balcells, A. Wearable Fall Detector Using Recurrent Neural Networks. *Sensors* **2019**, *19*, 4885. [CrossRef]

11. Stollenwerk, K.; Müller, J.; Hinkenjann, A.; Krüger, B. Analyzing Spinal Shape Changes During Posture Training Using a Wearable Device. *Sensors* **2019**, *19*, 3625. [CrossRef] [PubMed]

12. Vega-Barbas, M.; Diaz-Olivares, J.A.; Lu, K.; Forsman, M.; Seoane, F.; Abtahi, F. P-Ergonomics Platform: Toward Precise, Pervasive, and Personalized Ergonomics using Wearable Sensors and Edge Computing. *Sensors* **2019**, *19*, 1225. [CrossRef] [PubMed]

13. Lin, W.-Y.; Ke, H.-L.; Chou, W.-C.; Chang, P.-C.; Tsai, T.-H.; Lee, M.-Y. Realization and Technology Acceptance Test of a Wearable Cardiac Health Monitoring and Early Warning System with Multi-Channel MCGs and ECG. *Sensors* **2018**, *18*, 3538. [CrossRef] [PubMed]

14. Lim, S.-M.; Oh, H.-C.; Kim, J.; Lee, J.; Park, J. LSTM-Guided Coaching Assistant for Table Tennis Practice. *Sensors* **2018**, *18*, 4112. [CrossRef] [PubMed]

15. Lu, K.; Yang, L.; Seoane, F.; Abtahi, F.; Forsman, M.; Lindecrantz, K. Fusion of Heart Rate, Respiration and Motion Measurements from a Wearable Sensor System to Enhance Energy Expenditure Estimation. *Sensors* **2018**, *18*, 3092. [CrossRef]

16. Ejupi, A.; Menon, C. Detection of Talking in Respiratory Signals: A Feasibility Study Using Machine Learning and Wearable Textile-Based Sensors. *Sensors* **2018**, *18*, 2474. [CrossRef]

17. Cesareo, A.; Gandolfi, S.; Pini, I.; Biffi, E.; Reni, G.; Aliverti, A. A novel, low cost, wearable contact-based device for breathing frequency monitoring. In Proceedings of the 2017 39th Annual International Conference of the IEEE Engineering in Medicine and Biology Society (EMBC), Seogwipo, Korea, 11–15 July 2017; pp. 2402–2405.

18. Cesareo, A.; Previtali, Y.; Biffi, E.; Aliverti, A. Assessment of Breathing Parameters Using an Inertial Measurement Unit (IMU)-Based System. *Sensors* **2018**, *19*, 88. [CrossRef]

19. Manjarres, J.; Narvaez, P.; Gasser, K.; Percybrooks, W.; Pardo, M. Physical Workload Tracking Using Human Activity Recognition with Wearable Devices. *Sensors* **2019**, *20*, 39. [CrossRef]

20. Nam, H.S.; Lee, W.H.; Seo, H.G.; Kim, Y.J.; Bang, M.S.; Kim, S. Inertial Measurement Unit Based Upper Extremity Motion Characterization for Action Research Arm Test and Activities of Daily Living. *Sensors* **2019**, *19*, 1782. [CrossRef]

21. Zhang, W.; Schwenk, M.; Mellone, S.; Paraschiv-Ionescu, A.; Vereijken, B.; Pijnappels, M.; Mikolaizak, A.S.; Boulton, E.; Jonkman, N.H.; Maier, A.B.; et al. Complexity of Daily Physical Activity Is More Sensitive Than Conventional Metrics to Assess Functional Change in Younger Older Adults. *Sensors* **2018**, *18*, 2032. [CrossRef]

22. Hsu, C.-C.; Lin, B.-S.; He, K.-Y.; Lin, B.-S. Design of a Wearable 12-Lead Noncontact Electrocardiogram Monitoring System. *Sensors* **2019**, *19*, 1509. [CrossRef]

23. Jayasinghe, U.; Harwin, W.S.; Hwang, F. Comparing Clothing-Mounted Sensors with Wearable Sensors for Movement Analysis and Activity Classification. *Sensors* **2019**, *20*, 82. [CrossRef] [PubMed]

24. Allahbakhshi, H.; Conrow, L.; Naimi, B.; Weibel, R. Using Accelerometer and GPS Data for Real-Life Physical Activity Type Detection. *Sensors* **2020**, *20*, 588. [CrossRef] [PubMed]

25. Cheung, Y.K.; Hsueh, P.-Y.S.; Ensari, I.; Willey, J.Z.; Diaz, K.M. Quantile Coarsening Analysis of High-Volume Wearable Activity Data in a Longitudinal Observational Study. *Sensors* **2018**, *18*, 3056. [CrossRef] [PubMed]
26. Athavale, Y.; Krishnan, S. A Device-Independent Efficient Actigraphy Signal-Encoding System for Applications in Monitoring Daily Human Activities and Health. *Sensors* **2018**, *18*, 2966. [CrossRef]
27. Barrera-Animas, A.Y.; Trejo, L.A.; Medina-Pérez, M.A.; Monroy, R.; Camiña, J.B.; Godínez, F. Online personal risk detection based on behavioural and physiological patterns. *Inf. Sci.* **2017**, *384*, 281–297. [CrossRef]
28. Trejo, L.A.; Barrera-Animas, A.Y. Towards an Efficient One-Class Classifier for Mobile Devices and Wearable Sensors on the Context of Personal Risk Detection. *Sensors* **2018**, *18*, 2857. [CrossRef]
29. Yurtman, A.; Barshan, B.; Fidan, B. Activity Recognition Invariant to Wearable Sensor Unit Orientation Using Differential Rotational Transformations Represented by Quaternions. *Sensors* **2018**, *18*, 2725. [CrossRef]
30. Dutta, A.; Ma, O.; Toledo, M.; Pregonero, A.F.; Ainsworth, B.E.; Buman, M.P.; Bliss, D.W. Identifying Free-Living Physical Activities Using Lab-Based Models with Wearable Accelerometers. *Sensors* **2018**, *18*, 3893. [CrossRef]
31. Rosati, S.; Balestra, G.; Knaflitz, M. Comparison of Different Sets of Features for Human Activity Recognition by Wearable Sensors. *Sensors* **2018**, *18*, 4189. [CrossRef]
32. Morelli, D.; Rossi, A.; Cairo, M.; Clifton, D.A. Analysis of the Impact of Interpolation Methods of Missing RR-intervals Caused by Motion Artifacts on HRV Features Estimations. *Sensors* **2019**, *19*, 3163. [CrossRef] [PubMed]
33. Fortin-Côté, A.; Roy, J.-S.; Bouyer, L.; Jackson, P.; Campeau-Lecours, A. Allumo: Preprocessing and Calibration Software for Wearable Accelerometers Used in Posture Tracking. *Sensors* **2019**, *20*, 229. [CrossRef] [PubMed]
34. Broadley, R.W.; Klenk, J.; Thies, S.B.; Kenney, L.P.J.; Granat, M.H. Methods for the Real-World Evaluation of Fall Detection Technology: A Scoping Review. *Sensors* **2018**, *18*, 2060. [CrossRef] [PubMed]

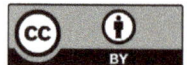

© 2020 by the authors. Licensee MDPI, Basel, Switzerland. This article is an open access article distributed under the terms and conditions of the Creative Commons Attribution (CC BY) license (http://creativecommons.org/licenses/by/4.0/).

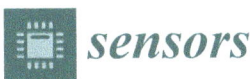

Article

Wearable Sensors Integrated with Internet of Things for Advancing eHealth Care

Jose-Luis Bayo-Monton [1],*, Antonio Martinez-Millana [1], Weisi Han [2], Carlos Fernandez-Llatas [1,3], Yan Sun [2] and Vicente Traver [1,3]

- [1] Instituto Universitario de Investigación de Aplicaciones de las Tecnologías de la Información y de las Comunicaciones Avanzadas (ITACA), Universitat Politècnica de València, Camino de Vera S/N, Valencia 46022, Spain; anmarmil@itaca.upv.es (A.M.-M.); cfllatas@itaca.upv.es (C.F.-L.); vtraver@itaca.upv.es (V.T.)
- [2] School of Electronic Engineering and Computer Science, Queen Mary University of London, London E1 4NS, UK; w.han@se13.qmul.ac.uk (W.H.); yan.sun@qmul.ac.uk (Y.S.)
- [3] Unidad Mixta de Reingeniería de Procesos Sociosanitarios (eRPSS), Instituto de Investigación Sanitaria del Hospital Universitario y Politecnico La Fe, Bulevar Sur S/N, Valencia 46026, Spain
- * Correspondence: jobamon@itaca.upv.es; Tel.: +34-963-877606

Received: 15 May 2018; Accepted: 4 June 2018; Published: 6 June 2018

Abstract: Health and sociological indicators alert that life expectancy is increasing, hence so are the years that patients have to live with chronic diseases and co-morbidities. With the advancement in ICT, new tools and paradigms are been explored to provide effective and efficient health care. Telemedicine and health sensors stand as indispensable tools for promoting patient engagement, self-management of diseases and assist doctors to remotely follow up patients. In this paper, we evaluate a rapid prototyping solution for information merging based on five health sensors and two low-cost ubiquitous computing components: Arduino and Raspberry Pi. Our study, which is entirely described with the purpose of reproducibility, aimed to evaluate the extent to which portable technologies are capable of integrating wearable sensors by comparing two deployment scenarios: Raspberry Pi 3 and Personal Computer. The integration is implemented using a choreography engine to transmit data from sensors to a display unit using web services and a simple communication protocol with two modes of data retrieval. Performance of the two set-ups is compared by means of the latency in the wearable data transmission and data loss. PC has a delay of 0.051 ± 0.0035 s (max = 0.2504 s), whereas the Raspberry Pi yields a delay of 0.0175 ± 0.149 s (max = 0.294 s) for N = 300. Our analysis confirms that portable devices ($p \ll 0.01$) are suitable to support the transmission and analysis of biometric signals into scalable telemedicine systems.

Keywords: eHealth; wearable; monitoring; services; integration; IoT; Telemedicine

1. Introduction

Internet of Things (IoT) is a framework in which sensors, devices and actuators can be managed in an ubiquitous and distributed way [1]. The health sector is not outside of the IoT revolution and there already exist multiple applications and services for improving health care quality [2].

Within this context, telemedicine is an ideal scenario for the expansion and improvement of health IoT technologies [3]. Remote monitoring using accessible and easy-to-use sensors are the avant-garde of the application of these type of technologies [4].

Distributed systems for remote monitoring have been presented elsewhere [5,6] describing two main types of architectures. On the one hand, the first type of system allows storing biometric, behavior and context variables from commercial sensors into devices (mobile phones, tablets and computers) thereafter to generate comprehensive reports to support health-related decision making [7].

On the other hand, the second type of systems automatically forwards the acquired data (without storing it) with Bluetooth or WiFi wireless transmissions [8,9].

To date, one of the largest systems for remote monitoring was deployed and piloted in the *Whole System Demonstrator Programme* (WSD) [10]. This program was promoted by the National Health System of the United Kingdom to stimulate the adoption of telecare. The main purpose was to provide more than 6000 patients with tools to manage their chronic conditions with a tight supervision of clinical staff (up to 238 physicians) through the use of sensors for monitoring physiological signals integrated into a complex communication system. The WSD consisted of three deployments with different technological choices, but the architecture was the same: a base unit to visualize data and questionnaires and peripheral health monitoring devices. Each deployment site used different protocols for allocating sensors: a pulse-oximeter, a glucometer, weighing scales, etc. Data were transmitted from the base unit to a monitoring centre via a secure server Internet connection. These sensors were capable of monitoring very important variables such as blood glucose, body weight, blood oxygenation, pulse and blood pressure, among others, However, these were not integrated with the base unit and mobile devices in every case. The interim results report pilot study was able to show some improvements, but the final report concluded that the intervention group was not benefiting from the use of remote care [11].

Authors of WSD suggest that the impact of remote care interventions are dependent on the architecture and the performance of the system, as other authors confirmed recently [12]. There are qualitative and quantitative tools to measure the user response to a telemedicine system [13]; however, more details about the technical implementation and the technical assessment should be reported to put the results into a context of significance. Clinical outcomes may be distorted by transmission errors, data duplication and missing data due to timeouts.

The Personal Connected Health Alliance (PCHA) (http://www.pchalliance.org/continua/) has gathered more than 200 manufacturers of health sensors and software companies to boost inter-operable eHealth devices and build fully integrated solutions. PCHA was established as a non-profit organization to promote the adoption of medical devices (hardware or software) standards as a way to build complex solutions based on the IoT paradigm. The International Standard Organization (ISO) and the Institute of Electrical and Electronic Engineers (IEEE) launched the 11,073 Communication Standard compendium which describes the behavior, information exchange, nomenclature and connection rules for the health and wellness devices to be integrated into different operational scenarios: from Body Area Networks to location-distributed systems.

However, the complexity of this standard has limited the widespread adoption in the wearable and medical device ecosystem [14]. PCHA certified products are often more expensive than the same product without the communication standard, and, moreover, the adoption of it into commercial sensors is testimonial [15].

Connecting health sensors into the IoT paradigm could be an easy and fast way to deploy complex telemedicine intervention, as these do not need implementing complex connection rules and deep nomenclatures and they put a special focus on the simplicity, interoperability and traceability as the basement for the integration of sensors into a health management system. Health Level 7 Association (HL7) has recently launched Fast Health Interoperability Resources (FHIR) protocol [16], a lite version of HL7 Control Protocol and the Reference Information model aiming to attract developers to build efficient inter-operable solutions [17]. Bluetooth Low Energy (BLE) defines a special profile for Health and Fitness devices, but it has shown several implementation constraints that may reduce BLE performance in a real scenario, in comparison with the theoretically expected [18,19].

Considering the contributions from BLE and FHIR, main shortcomings for prototyping new eHealth solutions under the IoT paradigm are the unnecessary overload of data exchange and difficulties to build demonstration scenarios [20]. At the sensor–device communication level (for instance, electrocardiography sensor to a mobile device), there are a huge amount of headers and data descriptors which are only useful for high communication layers. Although messages should be controlled by standard quality metrics and procedures, adding unnecessary data to wireless physical interfaces may cause more problems than what they actually tend to solve. Moreover, when moving towards a real user case in which patients and health professionals exchange data, there are needs of deploying a Graphical User Interface (GUI), for instance a webpage running on a specific webserver (or even a mobile application), which adds hurdles to the potential and strengths of the interconnection of distributed systems.

In this paper, we present and evaluate an embedded distributed system with a custom lite protocol for the connection of cheap health devices based on prototyping eHealth solutions (Arduino, Raspberry Pi, and biosignals kit). All components are interconnected using the process choreography paradigm [21,22]. To evaluate the extent to which portable devices can be compared with fix systems, the overall deployment has been configured into two different deployment scenarios: (1) Desktop Computer with Windows 10 Operating System; and (2) Raspberry Pi with Windows 10 Core IoT Operating System. The same functionalities for requesting and retrieving data from health sensors and hosting an HTLM5 webpage were embedded into the two systems to compare a key performance indicator: the time delay between acquiring and displaying the bio-signal. Our experiments confirm the expected hypothesis, that is: portable components have an increased latency in the communications, but this latency is negligible. Portable devices are suitable to support the transmission and analysis of biometric signals into scalable telemedicine systems. Our conclusion is that portable computing fosters new opportunities to expand the use of wearables in health care research. Strengths of the proposed system are the open specification of the protocol, the open-communications method using standard communication structures (based on XML) and choreography, and the direct connection to open-source hardware components. These results make it possible to enhance the system for other domains, such as Ambient Assisted Living (AAL) and smart-home sensors.

2. Material and Methods

In this section, we describe the materials and methodology we used to test the two deployment scenarios for a remote health management system. We first describe the hardware to sense biometric signals using the eHealth Sensors kit and Arduino. Second, we describe the integration paradigm based on service choreography. Third, we describe the communication protocol. Finally, we describe the experimental setup.

2.1. eHealth Sensors Kit

Arduino is an open-specification platform based on an ATmega328P micro-controller with the minimum capacity to execute simple programs (sketches). Arduino provides an easy but effective hardware to connect and use many electronic components with a wide variety of applications [23,24]. The official website of Arduino [25] has a comprehensive collection of information, downloads, tutorials and examples about how to use the platform.

Arduino provides an excellent platform to test and prototype solutions by adding supplemental modules (Bluetooth, WiFi boards, LEDs, and servo-motors) and other hardware. In this research, we have set up the eHealth Biometric Sensor Platform created by Libelium [26]. This kit allows users to acquire a set of physiological signals such as ECG, EMG, breathing rate, surface temperature, GSR, blood glucose and SpO2 (Table 1). eHealth kit has been used in wearable sensors research [27,28].

The Libelium kit is not a certified medical device. We used this platform as a virtual medical device because it implements the same physical interfaces and monitoring circuits as certified and commercial sensors do. Moreover, it prevents us from developing manufacturer protocols to retrieve raw physiological signals to test our principal hypothesis.

Table 1. eHealth sensors.

Sensor Name	Description
Temperature Sensor	Body temperature depends upon the place in the body in which the measurement is made, and the time of day and the level of activity of the subject. Different parts of the body have different temperatures.
	Discrete data
Airflow Sensor	Respiratory rate is a broad indicator of major physiological instability. The sensor measures the breathing flow of a person in the up airways (nose). Airflow sensor can also provide an early warning of hypoxemia and apnea.
	Continuous data
Galvanic Skin Response Sensor (GSR)	It can be used to measure the electrical conductance of the skin, which varies with its moisture level. Skin conductance is used as an indication of psychological or physiological arousal. GSR measures the electrical conductance between 2 points, and is essentially a type of ohmmeter.
	Continuous data
Electrocardiography Sensor (ECG)	A diagnostic tool that is routinely used to assess the electrical and muscular functions of the heart. ECG has grown to be one of the most commonly used medical tests in modern medicine. Some diseases have no modifications on ECG waveform.
	Continuous data
Electromyogram Sensor (EMG)	It can be used as a diagnostic tool to evaluate and record the electrical activity produced by skeletal muscles by measuring the electrical activity of muscles at rest and during contraction. EMG is used for identifying neuromuscular diseases, assessing low-back pain, kinesiology, and disorders of motor control.
	Continuous data

The whole sensing information detection part for biometric information relies on the Arduino eHealth Sensor Kit (Figure 1).

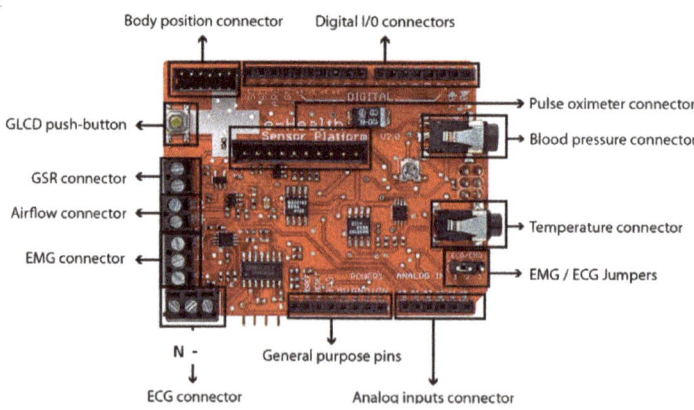

Figure 1. eHealth shield input/output pins [26].

These sensors can be used as diagnostic tools in clinical settings and also used to remotely monitor the state of a patient in real time. Some of the sensors which use the electro-physiological techniques (e.g., ECG, EMG, and GSR) require a time series to make a sense of them. All biometric sensors should be integrated on one Arduino board to collect comprehensive biometric information at the same time.

2.2. Choreography Integration

One of the objectives to improve health care services is to provide reliable remote access to the data retrieved by the sensors of the eHealth kit. A Service Oriented Architecture (SOA) involves the use of weakly coupled services to support such processes in a high inter-operable way. In an SOA environment, network resources are available through services which can be accessed through standard methods. Masking such resources with services allows accessing them without the needs of knowing how they were implemented internally.

The software enabling communication between the sensors and the displaying interfaces was implemented using a choreography engine [12], a semantic engine capable of connecting registered services and functions. The Choreographer dispatches messages among the modules using a specific eXtensible Markup Language (XML) message protocol called eXtensible MeSsaGe (XMSG) [21]. XMSG is based on the Foundation for Intelligent Physical Agents (FIPA) recommendations [29] and Simple Object Access Protocol (SOAP) [30] headers to route and characterize messages. The XMSG protocol allows broad-/multi-cast, as well as Peer to Peer (P2P) message calls, using custom symbols in the destination address. XMSG can be serialized and transmitted over any transport protocol such as REST and HTTP.

Services are designed to fit into three categories: serial communication, data translation and web-client. The client part is defined as a web service to deliver an interactive interface in a web browser. Serial communication service establishes the connection with the Arduino hardware to read data from wearable sensors. The translator service verifies data packets and translates information according to a predefined communication protocol. After extracting data from the packets, a new message is generated and sent to the client service to be displayed in web interface. These services also allow controlling the sensors (turn on/off, change sampling frequency, etc.). Figure 2 draws the information flow between the hardware and the interactive interface. Figure 3 shows a schema of the physical connection of the components, enhancing the information flow of Figure 2. In this schema, we show how the wearable sensors are connected to the Arduino + eHealth shield and how this component enables the communication to the Choreographer software (blue cross) in the Raspberry and other applications in the Pebble smart watch. In this paper, we have analyzed the flow of information through the serial communication port to the Choreographer, and then, from the Choreographer to the webpage by using WiFi interface. The webpage is a front-end which can be executed in a browser on any computer/tablet.

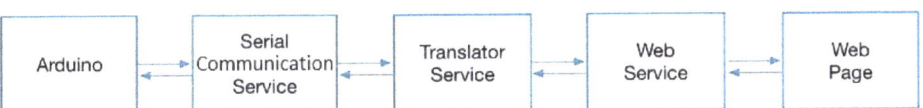

Figure 2. Choreography integration.

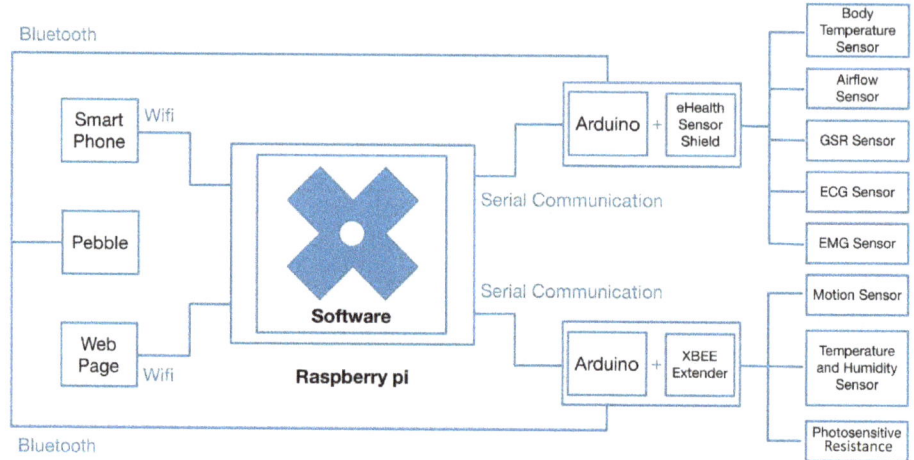

Figure 3. System architecture including health wearable sensors.

2.3. Communication Protocol

Once the sensors have been connected to the eHealth shield, the most important issue is to define a communication protocol to ensure correct data transmission. As illustrated in Figure 3, information should be handled between the webpage and the Arduino board through a distributed system (Sensors + Arduino in Location A and the Webpage in Location B). This type of information involves sensor data (type of measurement, value, units, time stamp, etc.) and the control commands that manage the sensors. Besides, error detection mechanism should also be added since the messages may be corrupted during the transmission.

Two operational modes are defined for operating with sensors. This first is the Active mode, through which sensors can automatically collect and send measurements to the software at every time interval according to their individual settings. Thus, data from all sensors can be displayed in real-time. The second is the passive mode, which implies that users can send different commands from the webpage to a specific sensor to request its data or change acquisition parameters. Users should be capable of interacting and operating with sensors: to request the current value of a sensor, to stop data retrieval, to set the time interval, etc. The structure of the commands is described in Tables 2 and 3. Therefore, the protocol should consider the following descriptors: **Kit Type**: Type of the sensor kit used for extensions to other type of sensing environments such as smart homes. **Destination**: Name of the sensor which identifies the destination of the command. **Command**: Different commands which can be used to ask for the sensor data or change some default settings. **Parameter**: This field corresponds to the Command field for changing some settings (e.g. transmit the parameter of the time interval in active mode). **Checksum**: The checksum field is the 16 bit sum of all bytes of the command packet. It can be used to detect command error which might be introduced during the transmission. **Sensor Type**: Name of the sensor which sends data or response. **Response To**: This field indicates which command the sensor is responding to, so the communication can be asynchronous. **Data**: This is the data part measured by the sensors or the answer of the command. **Unit**: This field corresponds to the Data field and it is the unit of the data.

Table 2. Text-based Command format.

Header		Data		Tail
Kit Type	Destination	Command	Parameter	Checksum
		Field Delimiter	'|'	

The format of the sensor data packet and response packet is shown in Table 3.

Table 3. Sensor data and response format.

Header		Data			Tail
Kit Type	Sensor Type	Response To	Data	Unit	Checksum
		Field Delimiter	'|'		

2.4. Portable Embedded System

Raspberry Pi was introduced in 2012 [31] and has been extensively used in home monitoring environments [32,33]. It integrates a computer board with support for many input and output peripherals through standard interfaces (Serial, Bluetooth and Wi-Fi) and allows the installation of several operative systems. Dimensions of the device are 85.60 mm × 53.98 mm × 17 mm, with a weight of approximately 45 grams. The device is cased and mounted inside a plastic box with a 7 inch touchscreen and powered with a battery. Raspberry Pi 3 is a platform suitable for embedding high level applications which allow the interaction with different devices and users in a wide range of applications. In this study, we used the Raspberry Pi 3 with the operating system from Microsoft Windows 10 IoT Core [34]. Windows 10 IoT Core is an optimized version of Windows 10 for small portable ARM and ×86/×64 devices. One of the aims of this paper is to evaluate the extent to which portable systems are ready to substitute computers in the way they connect and process information coming from several eHealth sensors. To this end, we will evaluate the Raspberry Pi 3 in comparison to a desktop computer.

2.5. Design of Experiments

The proposed system must provide a record track of the executed services, their results, time stamp and other audit information. A track component should be in charge of recording the trace of all the activities that take place during the performance of the system. The records must be standardized (or even normalized), understandable and ready to be parsed and mined. Therefore, this component will record all interaction events among the modules and components.

The experiments assessed the communication delay between distributed physical components among service request and service response for all integrated sensors. The main key performance indicator is the latency, which is defined as the difference of time between the start of the transmission of the first message and the end of the correct reception of the last message [18]. The latency was measured and compared in two environments using the same choreography software:

- Raspberry Pi 3 device with a Windows 10 IoT Core Operating System. Processor ARMv8 at 1.2 GHz and 1 GB of RAM.
- Desktop computer with a Windows 10 Operating System. Processor Dual Core at 2.6 GHz and 4 GB of RAM.

Due to the skewed distribution of the latency parameters, a Wilcoxon signed-rank test at 95% C.I. was used to assess the independence of intra and inter schema differences. Significance was assumed for $p < 0.05$. Statistical and graphical analysis was done using Matlab 2016R version using Academic License.

3. Results

The choreography engine uses SOA and implements a Windows Presentation Foundation GUI [35] application with several services declared and running in the background. Each service represents a specific functionality and different services interact with each other by passing messages.

3.1. Choreographer Functions to Manage eHealth Sensors

The services for accessing eHealth sensors are managed by the choreography engine (Table 4). As shown in Section 2.2, the Arduino board communicates with the serial communication service, and, analogously, users interacts with the web dashboard to request data from sensors. The translator service performs as a middleware by connecting the web service and serial communication service while data are exchanged between entities. Figures 4 and 5 show the sequence diagram of the three services.

Table 4. Classification and list of services in the Serial Communication and the RS232 Communication components.

Serial Communication Service	RS232 Communication Service
Translator Services	Airflow Translator Body Temperature Translator ECG Translator EMG Translator GSR Conductance Translator GSR Resistance Translator GSR Conductance Voltage Translator
Web Services	Airflow Web Service Body Temperature Web Service ECG Web Service EMG Web Service GSR Conductance Web Service GSR Resistance Web Service GSR Conductance Voltage Web Service

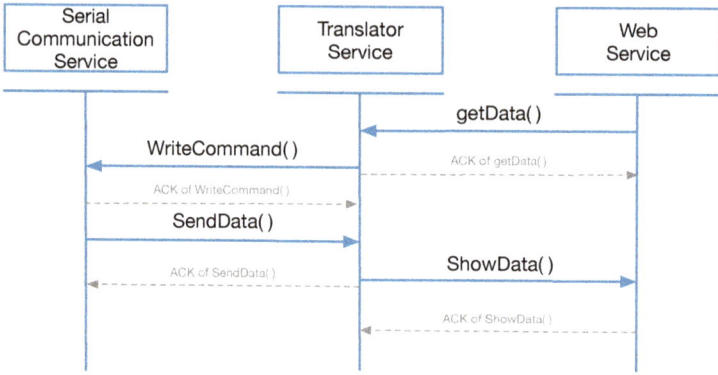

Figure 4. Passive mode.

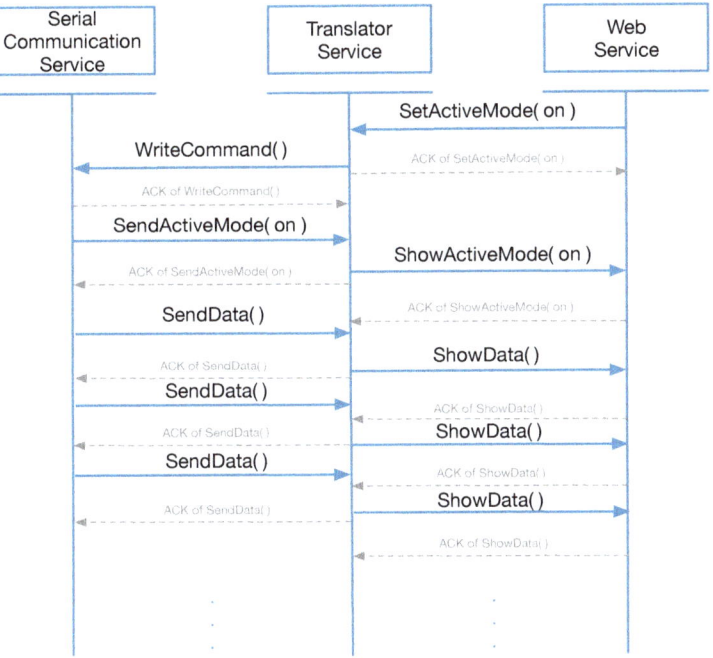

Figure 5. Active mode.

Illustrated by the sequential diagram in Figure 5 and Table 5, the translator service is one of the most crucial parts of the overall architecture since it is the only service which implements the communication protocol. Each sensor has one translator and different methods are used to parse the information coming from the serial communication service or encapsulate various commands received from web service into command packets.

Table 5. Methods implemented for the information exchange between the communication services and their description.

Web Service → Serial Communication Service	
getData()	Request for the sensor data one real-time.
SetActiveMode(onOff)	If the parameter is *on*, start active mode of the target sensor and request for the continuous data. If the parameter is *off*, stop active mode.
ChecksumCalculate(command)	Calculate the checksum of the full command and append it at the end of the packet.
Serial Communication Service → Service	
sendData(figure, unit)	Send the sensor data and unit
sendActiveMode(figure)	Send the response of the SetActiveMode command
ChecksumCheck(old_cks, new_cks) packet and compared it with the one in the packet.	Calculate the checksum of the received data

Each sensor has an individual webpage to control and display biometric signals. Therefore, for passive mode, once a user taps a button on the webpage to request data or set up operational modes, the web service sends a command to the corresponding translator. The translator service identifies the intent of the request and translates it into the predefined format, adding header and checksum to the command, and then sends the restructured new message to serial communication service. When the Arduino board receives the message from serial communication service, it retrieves *Destination* and *Command* information to effectively execute the command (e.g., read ECG).

After executing the command, the Arduino board generates a response packet for answering the request. The serial communication service transmits the packet to all translator services and each translator has to verify and parse it if it is a valid message. Translator service is able to distinguish which request this packet answers by means of *Response To* field. The *Data* part and *Units* part are then extracted and transmitted to the target web service by referring to *Sensor Type* part of the packet. Finally, data are shown on the webpage using a time series chart.

To illustrate the operation in detail, we can take body temperature data request as an example. When the user clicks the button on the webpage to request body temperature, the Body Temperature Web Service calls *getData* method in Body Temperature Translator Service and the translator starts to construct a command packet. It sets the *Kit Type* field as *EHEALTH*, *Destination* field as *BODYTEMPERATURE*, *Command* field as *GETDATA*, no *Parameter* and uses delimiter '|' to concatenate each individual field. After calculating the checksum of the whole command, it is appended as the tail of the packet and the resulting command packet stands as "*EHEALTH|BODYTEMPERATURE|GETDATA||2657*".

Similarly, when the Arduino board finishes reading the command, it creates a data packet and sends it to the serial communication service. The data packet could look like "*EHEALTH|BODYTEMPERATURE|GETDATA |36.5|C|3052*". Later, it will be transmitted to Body Temperature Translator Service, where the checksum of this packet will be calculated again and compared with the original one. If there is a match, the packet is validated.

For the active mode, the web service should send a *setActiveMode* command with parameter *on*. Once the active mode has been configured, the Arduino board will send the specific sensor data at a predefined rate. This behavior will not stop until another *setActiveMode off* command is triggered. When it comes to sensors such as the ECG, Airflow and GSR, the active mode can be extremely important. These continuous data are collected and utilized to generate a biometric signal for real-time monitoring.

3.2. Track Component

The Choreographer included a service to keep track of all the exchanged messages across components. As the limitations on the time resolution deserved special attention and open a brand new study field, all the interactions on the webpage were recorded in a special format and placed in a basic Comma-Separated Values file (to make easy the access for the information). A file named *choreo_track* was automatically generated upon first launch of the system (see Figure 6). A main class controlled the interaction events during a session and tracked them in that file. Each interaction event was written in a line with the following format:

<Timestamp>, <sender>, <receiver>, <message>

- Time stamp: dd/mm/yyyy hh:mm:ss.sssss.
- Sender: The module who triggered or controlled the action (see Figure 2).
- Destination: The module who was receiving the service request.
- Method: To indicate whether it was a request or an inform method.
- Message: The data exchanged, for instance the packets described in previous sections.

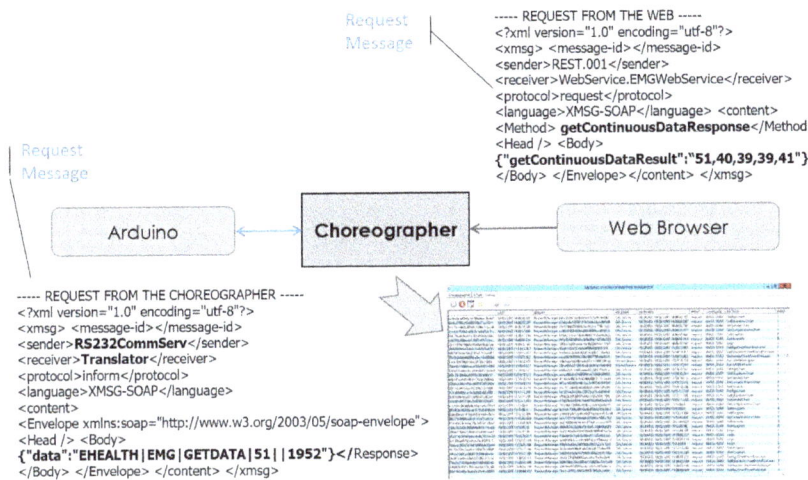

Figure 6. Choreographer track service.

3.3. Raspberry Pi for Hosting and Serving a Webpage

Web service representation for both scenarios are based on RESTful (Representational State Transfer) service. A service in the Choreographer is in charge of serving a webpage based on JavaScript and HTML5. The implementation is based on the .NET v4.5 framework for webservers and implementation of RESTful services. As Figure 7 shows, in the case of the computer implementation, libraries are directly used from Windows Communication Foundation (WCF), whereas, for the Raspberry, the use of RESTUP libraries was needed [36]. RESTUP maps web service libraries from WCF to be compatible with Windows 10 IoT Core operating system. Other studies have shown good results by implementing this architecture based on Apache Server [37].

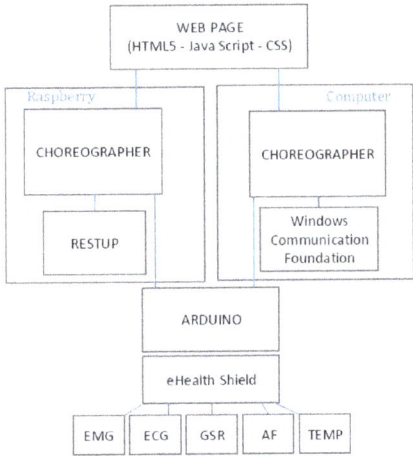

Figure 7. Services for hosting and serving the webpage. The schema shows how the Choreographer is connected to the sensors through the Arduino module and the needed libraries to self host and serve the webpage, which is based on HTML5 + Java Script + CSS.

3.4. Deployment

Figure 8 illustrates the final system. The picture shows the first term the Arduino Uno mounted with the eHealth shield and the health sensors kit. Different sensors should be connected to the eHealth shield. The EMG sensor and the ECG cannot work simultaneously since a jumper should be switched in the board to use one adaptation circuit or another. The Arduino is connected through a USB interface to the Raspberry Pi or the PC, in which an instance of the Choreographer is installed.

The computer screen shows the welcome page of the web application, which shows access to analyze data from the five sensors (the three buttons are for the three variables of the GSR sensor). After clicking on each button, the user can access individual pages for each sensor where different operations can be executed. For sensors such as ECG, EMG, GSR and Airflow sensor, single datum seems meaningless, thus users can start active mode to monitor and graph real-time sensor data. Besides, it is also feasible for users to set a time interval to retrieve past values from the sensors. Once these values are prepared, a chart would be plotted for each different set of data. The chart is real-time updated (see time delays in Figures 9 and 10), and it is refreshed every 250 ms. For body temperature sensor, apart from the above functions, users can access current body temperature data by clicking *GETDATA* button.

The Raspberry Pi (below the screen) shows the control Graphical User Interface of the Choreographer. The Choreographer was created similar to a tab in our window, containing graphical services which can be used to manage the five sensors in the system. By doing so, users can interact with the sensors without the needs of accessing the webpage.

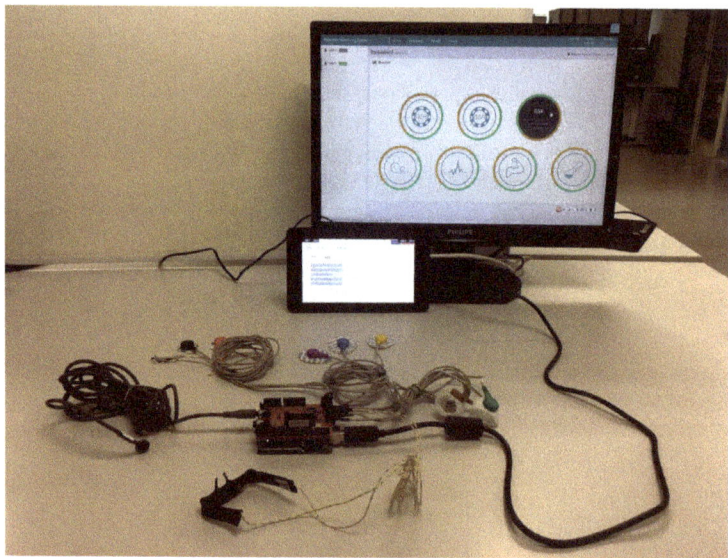

Figure 8. Sensor deployment.

3.5. Experiments

Sensors that support the active mode (ECG, EMG, Airflow and GSR) have a default sampling rate set to 20 Hz (20 Samples per second); this means that the interval between two samples is 50 ms for both PC and Raspberry Pi. Besides, the webpage is set to request data every 250 ms. The experiment shows that the PC deployment generated less latency in the communication segment between the Arduino and the Choreographer (Figure 9). Our measurements correspond to the theoretical sample period, which is 50 ms. Nonetheless, we do not see this behavior in the Raspberry Pi: The mean value of the time delay is around 50 ms, but the standard deviation is greater than the standard deviation of the PC. These points are distributed sparsely but showed the pattern of an arithmetic series. The gap between two corresponding points is approximately 10 ms to 20 ms.

The communication of the active mode between Choreographer and webpage (Figure 10) shows a similar situation. The PC shows a good result with all the measurements concentrated around 250 ms. We see a different pattern in the Raspberry PI with all the measurements with a fixed interval (mean value is 250 ms and the gap is about 10 ms to 20 ms).

We compared the communication segment between the Arduino and the Choreographer for the two deployments (Raspberry and PC). This segment is composed of the Serial Communication Service and the Translator service. Results show that Raspberry Pi has a statistically significant increased delay ($p \ll 0.01$) for all the five sensors, whereas, for the segment between the Choreographer and the web service, all sensors except ECG showed a not statistically significant increased delay (for ECG $p \ll 0.01$, and $p > 0.5$ for the rest).

Figures 9 and 10 show the cumulative scatter plots for the delays tracked with the tracker component (Figure 6). Even though the results are scattered, it is notorious that the delay experimented for the Raspberry Pi shows a clear pattern (especially for ECG, EMG and GSR in Figure 10). This pattern may be caused by the internal delay of the Arduino for acquiring measurements (10 ms–20 ms), and the reason of not having it on the PC may depend of the communication stack, which is bigger in the PC. In this case, the Choreographer can fill the memory stack with more measurements which will be delivered faster to the web interface.

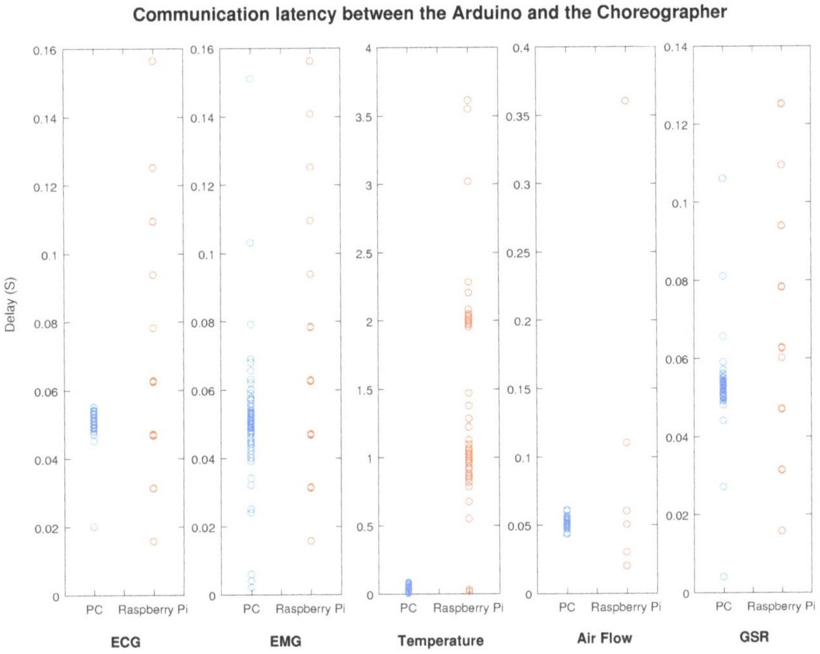

Figure 9. Comparison of the delay in the communications for the system deployed on a desktop computer and a Raspberry Pi for the segment between the Arduino and the Choreographer for the active communication mode.

Another finding involves the precision of time intervals. The PC shows a bigger reliability by means of a lower standard deviation and a lower range. As an example, for the EMG communication between the Arduino and the Choreographer (Figure 9), the PC has a delay of 0.051 ± 0.0035 s and a range of 0.2504 s (N = 300), whereas the Raspberry has a delay of 0.0175 ± 0.149 s and a range of 0.294 s (N = 300). Therefore, the Choreographer achieves a higher reliability for acquiring measurements if deployed in a PC.

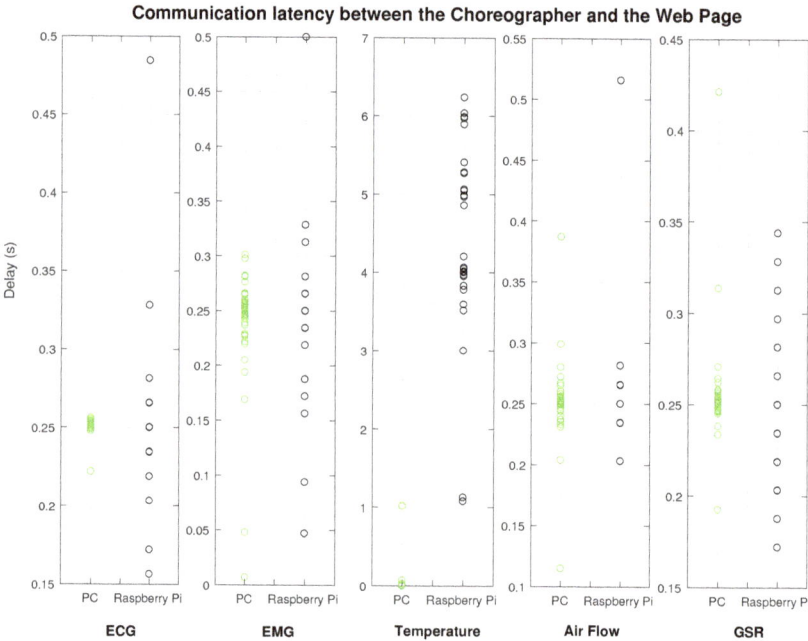

Figure 10. Comparison of the delay in the communications for the system deployed on a desktop computer and a Raspberry Pi for the segment between the Choreographer and the webpage with the active communication mode.

4. Discussion

In this paper, we present an integration of two innovative paradigms: Health Sensors and IoT focused on simple deployments. These two streams, which are widely accepted by the scientific community, are seen as the future of how information and communication technologies can make health care system sustainable. Moreover, the connection of these two paradigms with new ubiquitous computing and artificial intelligence models can promote the crucial step-forward for the adoption and spread use of health sensors for the management of chronic conditions.

In this context, forecasts on the increment of the population over 60 years old in developed countries and the pandemic dimension some diseases are reaching deserves special attention. Health care systems are not prepared to sustain these numbers and there is increased demand for better and personalized care services. This is the main reason that pushes us to propose cheap and scalable solutions that allow users to plug and play them without the need of understanding complex standards or programming frameworks.

One of the flagship projects on the evaluation of remote care presented in Section 1 (Whole System Demonstrator Programme) has demonstrated favorable results on the management of patients with chronic conditions, but stating that the technology is not yet ready for scaling-up [11]. The system proposed and evaluated in this study is based on a Service Oriented Architecture with a central component (Choreographer). The Choreographer works as a message dispatcher that allows connecting different modules (health sensors, webpages, etc.). The simplicity of the Choreographer prevents us from using another type of complex integration solutions like Enterprise Serial Bus (ESB), which provides a gain on the performance of its execution and fault tolerance [20].

The Choreographer relies on existing libraries and communication stacks of Microsoft .NET v4.5 framework, a key element for ensuring its reutilization and the compatibility with legacy systems in hospitals and health care infrastructures. The Choreographer implements a protocol based on a custom formatting message exchange language, XMGS. XMSG is based on SOAP and not REST to achieve a minimum level of standardization of information exchange across the system. Nevertheless, as reported in Section 3, REST stands as a proper methodology for describing the interfaces of the system by simply serializing XSMG. The proposed architecture can be adapted to a RESTful architecture with JSON messages, but due to the complexity of the distributed system, the number of sensors and client applications, it is needed to ensure a minimum set of information into the exchanged messages.

The eHealth sensing platform has been built on purpose using the Arduino Libellium kit, a low-cost solution that allows the integration of a wide range of physiological sensors. Even though these sensors are for prototyping, they are useful to work with on the design, development and evaluation of possible solutions to record, store and transmit biometric signals (ECG, EMG, Airflow, etc.). This technology was chosen over other commercial health sensors because of the cost as well as the integration simplicity: Arduino provides serial communication over wired and wireless physical interfaces, whereas the majority of sensors only provide wired communication, and, most of the time, the protocols to retrieve measurements are not available for third parties or are based on complex standards as the ISO/IEEE 11073 [14].

The proposed system is capable of hosting and serving a website as a regular web service. This is an extremely important feature that allows certifying the system as plug-and-play. With the proposed architecture of communications, health sensors may be configured to be subscribed to a specific website to perform a real-time broadcasting of the measurements, at the same time that these measurements may be stored in cloud services or analyzed by complex algorithms.

The deployment of this system is feasible on either a PC or a Raspberry Pi. According to our experiments (Figures 9 and 10), there is a statistically significant increased delay on the Raspberry Pi with respect the PC, which is understandable considering the unbalanced set of computational resources. However, for some specific cases, this delay is not relevant for the medical and monitoring purpose; (in the case of ECG, latency difference is below 0.030 s).

The significantly increased delay of Raspberry Pi may be related to the processor technical features, which has fewer capabilities than the personal Computer processor (ARMv8 @1.2 GHz and 1 GB RAM versus Dual Core @2.6 GHz and 4 GB RAM). Future work should consider experimental verification of the causes of the delay. Our results show that the latency experimented from side-to-side (meaning from sensors to the webpage) has not a big difference (even though significant), and the delay introduced by the Raspberry Pi is assumable. The low costs and requirements of a Raspberry Pi are not comparable with the high costs and requirements of a personal computer. Therefore, our experiments suggest that the new architectures for monitoring bio-signals could rely on the implementation of networks based on the Raspberry Pi without compromising the latency.

5. Conclusions

In this manuscript, we present and evaluate a scalable system based on five wearable sensors that allow the plug-and-play deployment on different use scenarios (on Raspberry and desktop computer). Raspberry pi yields a significant increased delay with respect to the same implementation in a personal computer. However, the measured delay is negligible and acceptable in real-time remote monitoring. Implementation of health web sensor node as a part of the Internet of Things using a Raspberry Pi has benefits with respect the use of a desktop computer, which paves the way to the implementation of new portable systems for remote management of chronic conditions. Future work will pursue on this line, finding out the percent of missing packets and the throughput in terms of other KPIs, such as the error rate, memory use, power consumption and influence of the network load (4 G/5 G). Moreover, future research should implement large amounts of traffic (several users and longer periods) to reflect the performance differences in commercial environments.

Author Contributions: J.-L.B.-M. and A.M.-M. conceived and designed the experiments; W.H. performed the experiments; A.M.-M., J.-L.B.-M. and W.H. analyzed the data; C.F.-L., Y.S. and V.T. contributed to materials and analysis tools; and J.-L.B.-M.and A.M.-M. wrote the paper.

Funding: This research received no external funding.

Acknowledgments: The authors would like to acknowledge *Cátedra Telefónica* at the Universitat Politècnica de València for supporting the acquisition of the materials used in the research herein presented.

Conflicts of Interest: The authors declare no conflict of interest. The founding sponsors had no role in the design of the study; in the collection, analyses, or interpretation of data; in the writing of the manuscript, and in the decision to publish the results.

Abbreviations

The following abbreviations are used in this manuscript:

AF	Air Flow
ECG	ElectroCardioGraphy
EMG	ElectroMioGraphy
GSR	Galvanic Skin Response
HL7	Health Level 7
PCHA	Personal Connected Health Alliance
SOA	Service Oriented Architecture

References

1. Wortmann, F.; Fluchter, K. Internet of things. *Bus. Inf. Syst. Eng.* **2015**, *57*, 221–224. [CrossRef]
2. Whitmore, A.; Agarwal, A.; Da Xu, L. The Internet of Things—A survey of topics and trends. *Inf. Syst. Front.* **2015**, *17*, 261–274. [CrossRef]
3. Warren, S. Beyond telemedicine: Infrastructures for intelligent home care technology. In Proceedings of the Pre-ICADI Workshop on Technology for Aging, Disability, and Independence, London, UK, 26–27 June 2003.
4. Weinstein, R.S.; Lopez, A.M.; Joseph, B.A.; Erps, K.A.; Holcomb, M.; Barker, G.P.; Krupinski, E.A. Telemedicine, telehealth, and mobile health applications that work: Opportunities and barriers. *Am. J. Med.* **2014**, *127*, 183–187. [CrossRef] [PubMed]
5. Lin, C.H.; Young, S.T.; Kuo, T.S. A remote data access architecture for home-monitoring health-care applications. *Med. Eng. Phys.* **2007**, *29*, 199–204. [CrossRef] [PubMed]
6. Meneu, T.; Martínez-Romero, Á.; Martínez-Millana, A.; Guillén, S. An integrated advanced communication and coaching platform for enabling personalized management of chronic cardiovascular diseases. In Proceedings of the 2011 Annual International Conference of the IEEE, Engineering in Medicine and Biology Society, EMBC, Boston, MA, USA, 30 August–3 September 2011; pp. 1563–1566.
7. Patel, M.S.; Asch, D.A.; Volpp, K.G. Wearable devices as facilitators, not drivers, of health behavior change. *JAMA* **2015**, *313*, 459–460. [CrossRef] [PubMed]
8. Orwat, C.; Graefe, A.; Faulwasser, T. Towards pervasive computing in health care—A literature review. *BMC Med. Inf. Decis. Mak.* **2008**, *8*, 26. [CrossRef] [PubMed]
9. Rashvand, H.F.; Salcedo, V.T.; Sanchez, E.M.; Iliescu, D. Ubiquitous wireless telemedicine. *IET Commun.* **2008**, *2*, 237–254. [CrossRef]
10. Bower, P.; Cartwright, M.; Hirani, S.P.; Barlow, J.; Hendy, J.; Knapp, M.; Henderson, C.; Rogers, A.; Sanders, C.; Bardsley, M.; et al. A comprehensive evaluation of the impact of telemonitoring in patients with long-term conditions and social care needs: Protocol for the whole systems demonstrator cluster randomised trial. *BMC Health Services Res.* **2011**, *11*, 184. doi:10.1186/1472-6963-11-184. [CrossRef] [PubMed]

11. Cartwright, M.; Hirani, S.P.; Rixon, L.; Beynon, M.; Doll, H.; Bower, P.; Bardsley, M.; Steventon, A.; Knapp, M.; Henderson, C.; et al. Effect of telehealth on quality of life and psychological outcomes over 12 months (Whole Systems Demonstrator telehealth questionnaire study): Nested study of patient reported outcomes in a pragmatic, cluster randomised controlled trial. *BMJ* **2013**, *346*, f653. [CrossRef] [PubMed]
12. Martinez-Millana, A.; Fico, G.; Fernández-Llatas, C.; Traver, V. Performance assessment of a closed-loop system for diabetes management. *Med. Biol. Eng. Comput.* **2015**, *53*, 1295–1303. [CrossRef] [PubMed]
13. Van der Weegen, S.; Verwey, R.; Spreeuwenberg, M.; Tange, H.; van der Weijden, T.; de Witte, L. The development of a mobile monitoring and feedback tool to stimulate physical activity of people with a chronic disease in primary care: A user-centered design. *JMIR mHealth uHealth* **2013**, *1*, e8. [CrossRef] [PubMed]
14. Fioravanti, A.; Fico, G.; Arredondo, M.; Salvi, D.; Villalar, J. Integration of heterogeneous biomedical sensors into an ISO/IEEE 11073 compliant application. In Proceedings of the 2010 Annual International Conference of the IEEE, Engineering in Medicine and Biology Society (EMBC), Buenos Aires, Argentina, 31 August–4 September 2010; pp. 1049–1052.
15. Sagahyroon, A. Remote patients monitoring: Challenges. In Proceedings of the 2017 IEEE 7th Annual Conference on Computing and Communication Workshop and Conference (CCWC), Las Vegas, NV, USA, 9–11 January 2017; pp. 1–4.
16. Bender, D.; Sartipi, K. HL7 FHIR: An Agile and RESTful approach to healthcare information exchange. In Proceedings of the 2013 IEEE 26th International Symposium on Computer-Based Medical Systems (CBMS), Porto, Portugal, 20–22 June 2013; pp. 326–331.
17. Oh, A.S. A study on standardized healthcare system based on HL7. *J. Korea Inst. Inf. Commun. Eng.* **2013**, *17*, 656–664. [CrossRef]
18. Gomez, C.; Oller, J.; Paradells, J. Overview and Evaluation of Bluetooth Low Energy: An Emerging Low-Power Wireless Technology. *Sensors* **2012**, *12*, 11734–11753, doi:10.3390/s120911734. [CrossRef]
19. Chang, K.M.; Liu, S.H.; Wu, X.H. A wireless sEMG recording system and its application to muscle fatigue detection. *Sensors* **2012**, *12*, 489–499. [CrossRef] [PubMed]
20. Hassanalieragh, M.; Page, A.; Soyata, T.; Sharma, G.; Aktas, M.; Mateos, G.; Kantarci, B.; Andreescu, S. Health monitoring and management using Internet-of-Things (IoT) sensing with cloud-based processing: Opportunities and challenges. In Proceedings of the 2015 IEEE International Conference on Services Computing (SCC), New York, NY, USA, 27 June–2 July 2015; pp. 285–292.
21. Fernández-Llatas, C.; Mocholi, J.B.; Sanchez, C.; Sala, P.; Naranjo, J.C. Process choreography for Interaction simulation in Ambient Assisted Living environments. In Proceedings of the XII Mediterranean Conference on Medical and Biological Engineering and Computing, Chalkidiki, Greece, 27–30 May 2010.
22. Fernández-Llatas, C.; Mocholí, J.B.; Moyano, A.; Meneu, T. Semantic Process Choreography for Distributed Sensor Management. In Proceedings of the International Workshop on Semantic Sensor Web, in Conjunction with IC3K 2010, Valencia, Spain, 27–28 October 2010; pp. 32–37.
23. Buechley, L.; Eisenberg, M.; Catchen, J.; Crockett, A. The LilyPad Arduino: Using computational textiles to investigate engagement, aesthetics, and diversity in computer science education. In Proceedings of the SIGCHI Conference on Human Factors in Computing Systems, Florence, Italy, 5–10 April 2008; pp. 423–432.
24. Banzi, M.; Shiloh, M. *Getting Started with Arduino: The Open Source Electronics Prototyping Platform*; Maker Media, Inc.: San Francisco, CA, USA, 2014.
25. Arduino Website. 2017. Available online: http://www.arduino.org (accessed on 10 April 2018).
26. eHeatlh Website. 2017. Available online: https://www.cooking-hacks.com/documentation/tutorials/ehealth-biometric-sensor-platform-arduino-raspberry-pi-medical (accessed on 10 April 2018).
27. Saleem, K.; Abbas, H.; Al-Muhtadi, J.; Orgun, M.A.; Shankaran, R.; Zhang, G. Empirical Studies of ECG Multiple Fiducial-Points Based Binary Sequence Generation (MFBSG) Algorithm in E-Health Sensor Platform. In Proceedings of the 2016 IEEE 41st Conference on Local Computer Networks Workshops (LCN Workshops), Dubai, United Arab Emirates, 7–10 November 2016; pp. 236–240.
28. Petrellis, N.; Birbas, M.K.; Gioulekas, F. The Front End Design of a Health Monitoring System. In Proceedings of the 7th International Conference on Information and Communication Technologies in Agriculture, Food and Environment (HAICTA 2015), Kavala, Greece, 17–20 September 2015; pp. 426–436.
29. OBrien, P.D.; Nicol, R.C. FIPA Towards a Standard for Software Agents. *BT Technol. J.* **1998**, *16*, 51–59, doi:10.1023/a:1009621729979. [CrossRef]

30. Gudgin, M.; Hadley, M.; Mendelsohn, N.; Moreau, J.J.; Nielsen, H.F.; Karmarkar, A.; Lafon, Y. SOAP Version 1.2 Part 1: Messaging Framework (Second Edition). W3C Recommendation 27 April 2007. Available online: https://www.w3.org/TR/soap12-part1/ (accessed on 5 June 2018)
31. Schmidt, M. *Raspberry Pi*; Pragmatic Bookshelf: Raleigh, NC, USA, 2014.
32. Vujovic, V.; Maksimovic, M. Raspberry Pi as a wireless sensor node: Performances and constraints. In Proceedings of the 2014 37th International Convention on Information and Communication Technology, Electronics and Microelectronics (MIPRO), Opatija, Croatia, 26–30 May 2014; pp. 1013–1018.
33. Sahani, M.; Nanda, C.; Sahu, A.K.; Pattnaik, B. Web-based online embedded door access control and home security system based on face recognition. In Proceedings of the 2015 International Conference on Circuit, Power and Computing Technologies (ICCPCT), Nagercoil, India, 19–20 March 2015; pp. 1–6.
34. Windows Core IoT Website. 2017. Available online: https://developer.microsoft.com/en-us/windows/iot (accessed on 11 April 2018).
35. WPF Website. 2017. Available online: https://msdn.microsoft.com/en-us/library/ms754130.aspx (accessed on 11 April 2018).
36. RESTUP. Webserver for Universal Windows Platform (UWP) Apps. 2017. Available online: https://github.com/tomkuijsten/restup (accessed on 13 April 2018).
37. Vujović, V.; Maksimović, M. Raspberry Pi as a Sensor Web node for home automation. *Comput. Electr. Eng.* **2015**, *44*, 153–171.10.1016/j.compeleceng.2015.01.019. [CrossRef]

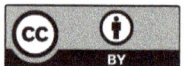

© 2018 by the authors. Licensee MDPI, Basel, Switzerland. This article is an open access article distributed under the terms and conditions of the Creative Commons Attribution (CC BY) license (http://creativecommons.org/licenses/by/4.0/).

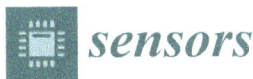

Article

Artificial-Intelligence-Based Prediction of Clinical Events among Hemodialysis Patients Using Non-Contact Sensor Data

Saurabh Singh Thakur [1], Shabbir Syed-Abdul [2,3,*], Hsiao-Yean (Shannon) Chiu [4,5], Ram Babu Roy [1], Po-Yu Huang [6], Shwetambara Malwade [3], Aldilas Achmad Nursetyo [2,3] and Yu-Chuan (Jack) Li [2,3,7]

[1] Rajendra Mishra School of Engineering Entrepreneurship, Indian Institute of Technology Kharagpur, Kharagpur 721302, India; saurabhjan07@gmail.com (S.S.T.); rambabu@see.iitkgp.ac.in (R.B.R.)
[2] Graduate Institute of Biomedical Informatics, Taipei Medical University, Taipei 110, Taiwan; mail.aldilas@gmail.com (A.A.N.); jaak88@gmail.com (Y.-C.L.)
[3] International Center for Health Information Technology (ICHIT), Taipei Medical University, Taipei 110, Taiwan; sv14kekade@tmu.edu.tw
[4] School of Nursing, College of Nursing, Taipei Medical University, Taipei 110, Taiwan; hychiu0315@tmu.edu.tw
[5] School of Medicine, Research Center of Sleep Medicine, Taipei Medical University, Taipei 110, Taiwan
[6] School of Medicine, Taipei Medical University, Taipei 110, Taiwan; b101100089@tmu.edu.tw
[7] TMU Research Center of Cancer Translational Medicine, Taipei Medical University, Taipei 110, Taiwan
* Correspondence: drshabbir@tmu.edu.tw; Tel.: +886-2-6638-2736 (ext. 1514)

Received: 3 July 2018; Accepted: 23 August 2018; Published: 27 August 2018

Abstract: Non-contact sensors are gaining popularity in clinical settings to monitor the vital parameters of patients. In this study, we used a non-contact sensor device to monitor vital parameters like the heart rate, respiration rate, and heart rate variability of hemodialysis (HD) patients for a period of 23 weeks during their HD sessions. During these 23 weeks, a total number of 3237 HD sessions were observed. Out of 109 patients enrolled in the study, 78 patients reported clinical events such as muscle spasms, inpatient stays, emergency visits or even death during the study period. We analyzed the sensor data of these two groups of patients, namely an event and no-event group. We found a statistically significant difference in the heart rates, respiration rates, and some heart rate variability parameters among the two groups of patients when their means were compared using an independent sample t-test. We further developed a supervised machine-learning-based prediction model to predict event or no-event based on the sensor data and demographic information. A mean area under curve (ROC AUC) of 90.16% with 96.21% mean precision, and 88.47% mean recall was achieved. Our findings point towards the novel use of non-contact sensors in clinical settings to monitor the vital parameters of patients and the further development of early warning solutions using artificial intelligence (AI) for the prediction of clinical events. These models could assist healthcare professionals in taking decisions and designing better care plans for patients by early detecting changes to vital parameters.

Keywords: artificial intelligence; supervised machine learning; predictive analytics; hemodialysis; non-contact sensor; heart rate; respiration rate; heart rate variability

1. Introduction

Hemodialysis (HD) has been one treatment of choice for renal replacement therapy among patients with possible renal dysfunction [1]. Hemodialysis uses an apparatus to filter blood that can be carried out either in a dialysis center or at home. By doing so, it replaces the natural function of the kidneys to remove waste and maintain blood pressure among renal failure patients [2]. Hemodialysis has proved to prolong survival of end-stage renal disease patients aged more than 75 with multiple comorbidities [3]. Typically, HD consists of three sessions per week and each session lasts around 4 h [4,5].

Despite its function in terms of prolonging patients' life expectancy and increasing the quality of life, patients may undergo several clinical events during HD. Among them are infection, cardiovascular events, muscle spasm, and even death [6]. Research by Han [7] successfully predicted cardiovascular events using echocardiographic parameters, but not other non-cardiovascular and cerebrovascular events. Similarly, some studies have been conducted to predict cardiovascular events in liver transplant patients [8,9].

Ambient intelligence (AmI) is an evolving research area that attempts to bring intelligence to our environment and make it much sensitive to our day-to-day life [10]. Various technologies like sensors, sensor networks, pervasive computing, and artificial intelligence (AI) are used in AmI to make our environment more sensitive to living. AmI attempts to make our life easier and safer and is being deployed in many areas that affect human life. It is becoming more significant in healthcare in both clinical and non-clinical settings like telemedicine, home automation, health behavior informatics and patient monitoring [11–17]. For instance, AmI interacts with humans (e.g., patients) using sensors and might be able to predict upcoming events before they occur.

Research has been done in the past into which sensors can be used to monitor or detect some health conditions or parameters. However, the use of artificial intelligence using sensor data to predict an upcoming event is rarely found. Research has been carried out by Tereul et al. [18] utilizing an ultrasonic sensor to measure blood flow during dialysis sessions. Trebbels et al. [19] measured hematocrit levels by designing impedance-spectroscopy-based sensors for dialysis apparatus. Yi-Chun Du et al. [20] proposed a wearable device to monitor blood leakage during HD using an array sensing patch. However, these studies did not embed the technology with an artificial intelligence feature. Artificial intelligence has been used to improve anemia management during dialysis treatment [21].

Methods or devices using physical contact with patients during their clinical care do not offer round-the-clock monitoring of their vital signs. On the other hand, data on vital signs, like blood pressure, heart rate, respiration rate, and body temperature are very important factors when a decision is being taken by the physician and healthcare professional. Nowadays, non-contact sensor devices are available that offer round-the-clock monitoring of the various vital signs of patients [22,23]. Further, this data can also be useful in predicting clinical events in patients for several clinical processes like HD, liver transplants, kidney transplants, etc. Various studies predicting cardiovascular events in liver transplant patients have been carried out in the past using contact or non-contact sensor data. However, there have been very few studies conducted to predict clinical events in HD patients using non-contact sensors.

In this study, a prediction model was developed based on supervised machine learning (ML) algorithms to predict clinical events during dialysis sessions. We used the data from a non-contact sensor device [24] that records vital signs like the heart rate, respiration rate, and heart rate variability. In the following sections, we present our methodology, results, discussion, limitations and conclusion.

2. Materials and Methods

2.1. Study Details

In this observational study, we included 109 patients who were undergoing HD at Taipei Medical University (TMU) hospital, Taipei, Taiwan. To conduct this study, ethical clearance was taken from the Joint Institutional Review Board (JIRB) of Taipei Medical University, Taipei, Taiwan (JIRB No. N201512031). During the period of HD, some patients experienced clinical events of certain types and a few patients did not report any clinical event. A clinical event can be defined as any medical problem experienced and reported by the patient. The clinical events suffered by the patients and considered in this study were sudden death (SD), emergency visit (ER), muscle spasm (MS), inpatient (IP), emergency visit and inpatient (ERIP).

2.2. Data Collection

Patient data were collected using a piezo-electric non-contact sensor system that measured respiration rate (RR), heart rate (HR), and body movement data (MD). These vital parameters of the patients were captured during the HD sessions for a period of 23 weeks from March 2016 to August 2016. The sensor unit was placed under the mattress and had no direct contact with the patient. The sensor system used in this study was developed by EarlySense Ltd., Ramat Gan, Israel [24]. When this sensor is kept under the mattress, a force is applied to the sensor that comes from three sources. These sources are gross body movement, chest wall movement, and recoil of the body due to the cardio-ballistic effect. The latter two are related to respiration effort and stroke volume. The signals generated by the sensor can be separated into motion, respiration and ballistocardiogram (BCG) waveforms, from which MD, RR and HR can be obtained, respectively [24]. The sensor system for patient monitoring in hospital settings has been validated and used in many clinical studies [22,25–27]. Similarly, the heart rate variability parameters like high frequency (HF), low frequency (LF), the ratio of HF–LF (HF/LF), and very low frequency (VLF) were also obtained from the raw BCG waveforms [28,29]. The heart rate variability (HRV) parameters including HR, RR, and MD were processed from the raw data and provided to us by a data scientist from EarlySense Ltd. The final dataset we received contained the mean of every 30 s for HR, RR, MD, and all the HRV parameters along with the date and patient ID (without revealing the personal identity of the patient). The demographic data like gender, age, height, and weight of the patients was also obtained during the study using a predesigned form.

2.3. Data Cleaning and Feature Extraction

There were some errors, missing values, and duplicate data files in the raw dataset. The raw data was cleaned to remove all the errors, missing values, and duplicate data files. This was done programmatically in the Python programming language and using the library *pandas*. The errors were the presence of the values 0 and −1 or missing values in some data fields. The entire row was deleted if it had either of these errors in any of its data fields. In the case of duplicate data files for the same HD session, the file which had the lesser number of data readings was ignored and that with data readings was selected. We had the following data variables after data cleaning and arranging the data from different files into a single data file:

Patient ID, date of session, RR, MD, HR, and HRV parameters like HF, LF, HF/LF, VLF, and (VLF+LF)/HF. We also had demographic details of the patients like the gender, age, height, and weight of the patients.

Since HRV parameters will be accurate only when the patient is relaxed and stable, we considered only those data samples in the analysis when the patient was in a stable and non-moving condition [30]. Therefore, we utilized the body movement data and further shortlisted only those data samples where the value of MD was less than a threshold of 30 amplitudes. Further, we extracted data samples for the vital parameters from the first five minutes (FFM) and last five minutes (LFM) of HD sessions. The reason for extracting FFM and LFM was to see the change in the vital parameters as the HD session progresses. The FFM data was extracted from the early period of the HD session and LFM was extracted from the end period of the session, since the short-term recording (5 min) of HRV is sufficient for monitoring the autonomic nervous system [31]. Therefore, in this study, instead of considering HRV and other recorded vital parameters for a complete length of the HD session, only 5 min of data samples from the beginning and end of the HD session were considered. We also extracted the total number of HD sessions a patient had attended and the total number of clinical events reported by a patient. In addition, the body mass index (BMI) of each patient was calculated from the height, weight and gender data information of the patient. Finally, we had the following variables:

Patient ID, Number of Sessions, Number of Events, Time_FFM, HR_FFM, RR_FFM, MD_FFM, HF_FFM, LF_FFM, HF/LF_FFM, VLF_FFM, (VLF+LF)/HF_FFM, Time_LFM, HR_LFM, RR_LFM, MD_LFM, HF_LFM, LF_LFM, HF/LF_LFM, VLF_LFM, (VLF+LF)/HF_LFM, Gender, Age, Weight, Height, BMI, and Class. Here, the variable "Class" represents the two categories of patients, one in which the patient had reported any of the five mentioned clinical events and the other in which patient had not reported any clinical event. We selected a subset of features from the above-mentioned features as input variables. The backward elimination method was used to select an optimal subset of features.

2.4. Model Development

In this work, we developed three predictive models. In each model, we tested five supervised machine-learning-based classification algorithms. We will call these classification algorithms classifiers. The classifiers used in each model were logistic regression (LR) [32,33], k-nearest neighbor (kNN) [34,35], adaptive boosting (AdaBoost) [36,37], random forest (RF) [38,39], and support vector machine (SVM) [40]. The results of the performance of the various classifiers are reported in the next section. To develop these classifiers, we used the Python distribution *Anaconda* of version 5.1.0 and various libraries of *scikit-learn 0.19.1* [41]. Each parameter recorded was sampled at the period of 30 s i.e., and for each 30 s we have one reading for all the vital parameters recorded by sensor. The basic difference between the three models being discussed in this study is the number of samples selected in each model. In model 1, we considered all the data samples selected for FFM and LFM. For each five-minute data we had 10 readings of all the vital parameters at the rate of 30 s. In model 2, we considered one sample for each HD session from each patient. The considered sample was the mean of all samples of FFM and LFM for that HD session. In this model, we also added more input features. These features are the variance of FFM and LFM of all the vital parameters. In model 3, we considered only one data sample corresponding to each patient by further taking out the mean of all the input features present in model 2. A block diagram of the predictive model is shown in Figure 1.

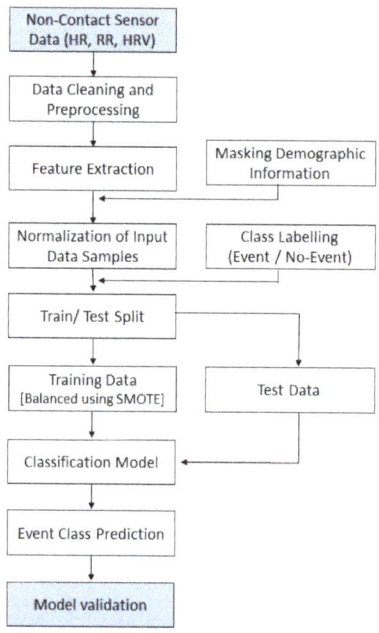

Figure 1. Prediction model for event class prediction. HR: Heart Rate; RR: Respiration Rate; HRV: Heart Rate Variability; SMOTE: Synthetic Minority Oversampling Technique.

The models developed in this study are being trained and tested on two datasets. Since, the number of HD sessions undergone by each patient was different, there were chances of overfitting the classifiers. As some patients had a greater number of HD sessions, they had more data samples in comparison with other patients. Therefore, we selected data samples from 15 recent HD sessions for each patient. In this process, data samples of 105 patients who had undergone at least 15 HD sessions were selected and we discarded the data samples of the remaining four patients. Of these 105 patients, 76 had reported an event during the study period and 29 had not reported any event. In this way, we separated two datasets, one with data samples from all the HD sessions for all the patients and one with data samples taken only from the most-recent 15 HD sessions.

The dataset in which data samples from all HD sessions was considered had 109 patients who underwent a total number of 3237 HD sessions. Therefore, for this dataset, model 1 had a total number of 32,370 data samples. Model 2 had 3237 data samples and model 3 had 109 data samples. The data set in which data samples from the 15 recent HD sessions were selected had a total number of 105 patients with 1575 HD sessions. Therefore, model 1 had 15,750 data samples, model 2 had 1575 data samples and model 3 had 105 data samples.

2.5. Model Validation

There is unequal representation of the two classes because the number of patients from the event class is much higher than the number of patients from the no event class. To overcome this imbalance in the data we used the synthetic minority over-sampling technique (SMOTE) [42]. In this technique, the minority class is over-sampled to balance the representation of both the classes. This is done by "taking each minority class data point and introducing synthetic examples along the line segments joining any or all of the k-minority class nearest neighbors" [43]. The process is repeated until the representation of both classes becomes approximately equal. This approach can be implemented in several open-source software (e.g., the R Programming Language, Python, and Weka). More information on SMOTE is available in reference [42]. In this study, SMOTE was applied only to the training dataset and the testing dataset was left unchanged. To validate the model, we used the stratified *k*-fold cross-validation method [44]. In stratified cross-validation, the folds are selected such that the percentage of samples is preserved for each class. In each fold of the validation, the testing dataset was first balanced using SMOTE and then the classifier was trained.

In this study, the precision, recall, accuracy and receiver operating characteristic area under curve (ROC AUC) were used as evaluation measures to evaluate the performance of the various classifiers being developed [45]. A brief description of all these measures are given below:

2.5.1. Precision

Precision (P) is the fraction of true positives (TP) predicted to the total predicted positives i.e., true positives plus false positives (FP). In some scenarios, it is also called as confidence. Precision is defined as:

$$P = \frac{TP}{TP + FP}. \qquad (1)$$

2.5.2. Recall

The recall is the fraction of TP predicted from the total of real positives i.e., true positive plus false negatives. It is also sometimes referred to as sensitivity. The recall is an important measure in the context of medical or clinical studies because it identifies all real positive cases. It is also important in ROC analysis in which it is referred to as the true positive rate. It is defined as:

$$R = \frac{TP}{TP + FN}. \qquad (2)$$

2.5.3. Accuracy

Accuracy is one of the most intuitive and basic performance measures for any ML model. It is not a good criterion by which to evaluate any model when the dataset is imbalanced. However, it is a good measure for a balanced dataset where all the classes to be classified are equally represented. It can be defined as:

$$\text{Accuracy} = \frac{TP + TN}{TP + FP + TN + FN}. \quad (3)$$

2.5.4. Receiver Operating Characteristic

This is one of the most important and widely accepted evaluation criteria. It compares the true positive rate (TPR) and the false positive rate (FPR). It is created by plotting the TPR against the FPR. TPR i.e., sensitivity or recall is already defined above and FPR can be defined as follows:

$$\text{FPR} = \frac{FP}{FP + TN}. \quad (4)$$

2.5.5. Descriptive Analyses and Independent t-Test

We used SPSS 22.0 (IBM, Armonk, NY, USA) to carry out basic statistical analyses of the data. Descriptive analyses were used to examine the baseline characteristics. Differences in the HR, RR and HRV parameters between the event and no-event groups were examined using the independent samples t-test. The P value is described in terms of rejecting the null hypothesis when it is true. The null hypothesis is usually a hypothesis of no difference (i.e., no difference in a variable among the two groups). The term alpha refers to a pre-chosen probability and the term "p value" is the calculated probability. The choice of the significance level at which the null hypothesis can be rejected is subjective. Conventionally, the 5%, 1% and 0.1% ($p < 0.05$, 0.01 and 0.001) levels have been used.

In this study, the statistical significance (alpha) was set at $p < 0.05$. We selected the level of significance i.e., alpha = 0.05 so that the probability of making a wrong decision is at most 5% when the null hypothesis is true and also to balance the tradeoff between type 1 and type 2 errors. It also keeps the type 2 errors within acceptable limit and does not reject a null hypothesis (even if there is a significant difference when it is false). A type I error is the false rejection of the null hypothesis and a type II error is the false acceptance of the null hypothesis. While testing the hypothesis on the difference in mean for the event and no-event samples, we had two samples (for the event and no-event group) with different sizes. However, the differences in sample size have been accounted for in the computation of t-statistics (that is, in the estimation of the standard error of difference) for the hypothesis testing.

2.6. Sample Size

Since this study is in the medical domain, we have inherent limitations on our sample size due to problems associated with data collection from patients. We validated the sample size requirements for this study statistically. We determined the sample size requirement based on our assumption of a 50% prevalence rate and an error margin of 10% at the 95% confidence level. The required sample size turned out to be, $n = 96$. We used the standard formula for sample size determination used in cross-sectional studies [46].

3. Results

The baseline characteristics of the data used in this study are presented in Table 1. The values are presented for both the datasets considered in the study, namely the one that had 109 patients with data for all HD sessions and the other which had 105 patients with data from the most recent 15 HD sessions. Of 109 patients, 78 patients suffered from clinical event(s) and 31 patients did not report any clinical event during the whole period of HD. The total number of clinical events reported by patients during the study period was 166 and the frequency of events reported per patient ranged from 1–9. The distribution of different types of events is presented in Table 2. Patients were 30–89 years old with mean age 66.3 and standard deviation (std.) ± 12.2. There were 58 (53.2%) male and 51 (46.8%) female patients in the study. The BMI of patients ranged from 17.4 to 42.3, with a mean of 24.1 and std. ± 12.2.

A descriptive analysis was carried out in which the mean of all the variables was compared between the event group and the no-event group and are shown in Table 3. This was carried out on data samples selected from 15 recent HD sessions. A total number of $n = 11,400$ data samples were from the event group of patients and $n = 4350$ were from the no-event group of patients. We found that the mean heart rate, respiration rate and some HRV parameters were significantly different between the two groups. The mean heart rate and respiration rate of both the first five minutes and the last five minutes were different in the two groups with $p < 0.0001$. The mean heart rate of the first five minutes and last five minutes in the event group were found to be higher than those in the non-event group (FFM: 75.58 vs. 70.56 and LFM: 75.85 vs 70.61). Similarly, the respiration rate was also observed to be different among the two groups. It is also higher in the event group as compared to the no-event group (FFM: 17.80 vs. 16.48 and LFM: 17.49 vs. 16.11).

A statistically significant difference was found in the mean values of the vital parameters among event and no-event patients. Therefore, it became the basis for proceeding with further data analytics. As mentioned in the previous section, three predictive models were developed to predict the clinical event. The models were validated using the stratified k-fold cross validation method where $k = 10$. In model 1 and model 2, the dataset was divided into a training and validation set in each fold at the observation level, and at the patient level in model 3. In models 1 and 2, a single patient had many data samples, i.e., observations, therefore data splitting in these models occurred at observation level. However, each patient had a single corresponding data sample in model 3, therefore the data splitting occurred at the patient level in this model.

Table 1. Baseline characteristics of the study data (n = number of patients).

Characteristics	Values (n = 109, All HD Sessions)	Values (n = 105, 15 HD Sessions)
Number of Male participants (%)	58 (53.2)	54 (51.4)
Number of Female participants (%)	51 (46.8)	51(48.6)
Age Range	30–89	30–89
Mean Age (±std.)	66.3 (±12.2)	66.4 (±12.2)
BMI Range	17.4–42.3	17.4–42.3
Mean BMI (±std.)	24.1 (± 3.6)	24.1 (±3.6)
Total Number of Hemodialysis Sessions	3237	1575
HD Sessions Range	7–52	15
Average No. of Sessions (±std.)	29.69 (±9.97)	15

HD: Hemodialysis; BMI: Body Mass Index.

Table 2. Details of events reported during study period.

Event Details	Values
Number of different events	5
Number of sessions with events	166
Number of patients reporting the event	78
Number of patients who did not report the event	31
Number of patients with sudden death	6
Number of patients reporting an ER visit	33
Number of patients reporting inpatient (IP)	32
Number of patients reporting ERIP	28
Number of patients reporting muscle spasm	45

ER: Emergency Room visit; ERIP: Emergency Room visit and Inpatient.

Table 3. Comparison of mean values of various parameters between the event and no-event class.

Features	Event (n = 11,400)		No Event (n = 4350)		p Values
	Mean	(SD)	Mean	(SD)	
HR_FFM	75.58	11.84	70.56	11.96	<0.0001
HR_LFM	75.86	12.33	70.62	12.01	<0.0001
RR_FFM	17.80	4.28	16.49	3.72	<0.0001
RR_LFM	17.50	4.35	16.12	3.49	<0.0001
HF_FFM	0.42	0.23	0.41	0.22	0.0035
HF_LFM	0.41	0.22	0.40	0.21	0.0803
LF_FFM	0.39	0.16	0.40	0.16	<0.0001
LF_LFM	0.39	0.15	0.40	0.15	<0.0001
LF/HF_FFM	1.30	1.16	1.36	1.23	0.0053
LF/HF_LFM	1.33	1.15	1.38	1.27	0.0187
VLF_FFM	0.35	0.19	0.35	0.17	0.0297
VLF_LFM	0.36	0.18	0.35	0.17	<0.0001
(VLF+LF)/HF_FFM	2.28	1.56	2.31	1.52	0.2177
(VLF+LF)/HF_LFM	2.34	1.55	2.32	1.51	0.4651
Age	66.18	12.45	67.10	11.33	<0.0001
BMI	24.14	3.91	24.32	2.78	0.0056

In each model, we tried and tested various classification methods like kNN, AdaBoost, SVM, RF and logistic regression (LR). When these classifiers were trained using the dataset in which data samples from all the HD sessions of patients were considered, the performance of the AdaBoost classifier which is an ensemble ML technique, was found to be better in all the models. kNN and SVM also performed well in model 1 and model 2. In model 1, a mean accuracy of 89.48% was achieved using kNN with 96.21% mean precision and 88.47% mean recall. The mean area under curve (AUC) was 90.16% in kNN classifier of model 1. Similarily, in AdaBoost the mean accuracy of 83.81% was achieved with mean precision, recall and AUC at 94.07%, 82.09%, and 83.81% respectively. In model 1, the mean accuracy of SVM was 76.94% with mean precision and mean recall of 90.19% and 75.28%, respectively, whereas in random forest and logistic regression the classifier recall was 62.84% and 59.76%, respectively. A decent accuracy with high precision, recall and area under ROC curve were obtained through the AdaBoost, kNN and SVM classifiers in model 1 and AdaBoost further performed better in model 2 and model 3 among other classifiers.

When we used data samples from recent 15 HD sessions to train the models, the performance of the classifiers was in line with those reported using data samples from all HD sessions. The mean accuracy of the kNN classifier was observed to be 87.95% with 89.01% AUC, 96.35% precision and 86.64% recall. The performance of the AdaBoost classifier in model 1, when this dataset was used, was also similar. A mean AUC of 85.38% with 81.86% recall and 95.09% precision was observed. The comparison of all the classifiers under each model considering various evaluation criteria was shown in Table 4, when data samples from all the HD sessions were considered in developing the model. In Table 5, evaluations of all the classifiers are shown when the models were developed using only the data samples from the 15 recent HD sessions. The ROC AUC plots of all the models depicting the mean area under the curve is presented in Figures 2–7. The ROC AUC plots of each classifier under each model when the data samples from all the HD sessions were considered are shown in Figures 2–4, respectively, and the ROC AUC plots when data samples from the 15 recent HD session were considered are shown in Figures 5–7, respectively.

Table 4. Validation results of classifiers using stratified 10-fold cross-validation when data samples from all HD sessions were considered.

Model	Classifier	Mean Precision (±Std.)	Mean Recall (±Std.)	Mean Accuracy (±Std.)	Mean AUC (±Std.)
Model-1	AdaBoost	0.9407 (0.011)	0.8209 (0.015)	0.8381 (0.011)	0.8497 (0.013)
	kNN	0.9621 (0.004)	0.8847 (0.007)	0.8948 (0.004)	0.9016 (0.004)
	SVM	0.9019 (0.006)	0.7528 (0.011)	0.7694 (0.008)	0.7805 (0.007)
	RF	0.8352 (0.009)	0.6284 (0.014)	0.6528 (0.011)	0.6691 (0.012)
	LR	0.7908 (0.008)	0.5976 (0.008)	0.6073 (0.008)	0.6138 (0.009)
Model-2	AdaBoost	0.9047 (0.021)	0.8073 (0.026)	0.8051 (0.022)	0.8036 (0.026)
	kNN	0.8914 (0.019)	0.7178 (0.022)	0.7408 (0.019)	0.7562 (0.022)
	SVM	0.8711 (0.014)	0.7443 (0.025)	0.7436 (0.020)	0.7431 (0.020)
	RF	0.8665 (0.026)	0.6235 (0.047)	0.6688 (0.037)	0.6992 (0.035)
	LR	0.7928 (0.021)	0.6028 (0.038)	0.6114 (0.030)	0.6172 (0.028)
Model-3	AdaBoost	0.9417 (0.077)	0.8750 (0.125)	0.8618 (0.085)	0.8542 (0.101)
	kNN	0.8237 (0.136)	0.5875 (0.194)	0.6147 (0.165)	0.6354 (0.167)
	SVM	0.8821 (0.107)	0.6375 (0.221)	0.6594 (0.124)	0.6813 (0.109)
	RF	0.8639 (0.104)	0.8482 (0.093)	0.7897 (0.124)	0.7449 (0.167)
	LR	0.9437 (0.095)	0.8232 (0.139)	0.8362 (0.140)	0.8491 (0.155)

kNN: k-nearest neighbor; AdaBoost: adaptive boosting; LR: logistic regression; RF: random forest; SVM: support vector machine.

Table 5. Validation results of classifiers using stratified 10-fold cross-validation when data samples from the 15 recent HD sessions were considered.

Model	Classifier	Mean Precision (±Std.)	Mean Recall (±Std.)	Mean Accuracy (±Std.)	Mean AUC (±Std.)
Model-1	AdaBoost	0.9509 (0.012)	0.8186 (0.018)	0.8380 (0.016)	0.8538 (0.017)
	kNN	0.9635 (0.006)	0.8664 (0.010)	0.8795 (0.009)	0.8901 (0.009)
	SVM	0.8982 (0.008)	0.7622 (0.014)	0.7653 (0.012)	0.7679 (0.013)
	RF	0.8462 (0.021)	0.7196 (0.019)	0.7021 (0.022)	0.6879 (0.030)
	LR	0.8212 (0.012)	0.6216 (0.013)	0.6281 (0.014)	0.6334 (0.016)

Table 5. *Cont.*

Model	Classifier	Mean Precision (±Std.)	Mean Recall (±Std.)	Mean Accuracy (±Std.)	Mean AUC (±Std.)
Model-2	AdaBoost	0.8809 (0.023)	0.7886 (0.028)	0.7695 (0.027)	0.7541 (0.033)
	kNN	0.8889 (0.029)	0.7035 (0.042)	0.7213 (0.033)	0.7357 (0.036)
	SVM	0.8625 (0.043)	0.7404 (0.046)	0.7251 (0.042)	0.7127 (0.059)
	RF	0.8295 (0.038)	0.6982 (0.057)	0.6762 (0.039)	0.6583 (0.048)
	LR	0.8188 (0.046)	0.6202 (0.028)	0.6248 (0.042)	0.6285 (0.060)
Model-3	AdaBoost	0.7171 (0.094)	0.7464 (0.162)	0.6044 (0.143)	0.4899 (0.164)
	kNN	0.7733 (0.131)	0.4054 (0.136)	0.4824 (0.121)	0.5443 (0.127)
	SVM	0.7423 (0.117)	0.6071 (0.223)	0.5461 (0.139)	0.4869 (0.146)
	RF	0.6680 (0.143)	0.5393 (0.204)	0.4663 (0.152)	0.4113 (0.168)
	LR	0.7183 (0.073)	0.5893 (0.088)	0.5308 (0.069)	0.4780 (0.100)

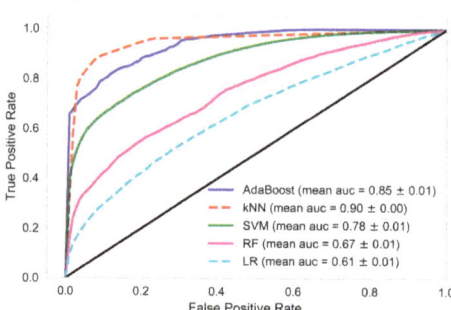

Figure 2. Receiver Operating Characteristics plot showing mean area under curve of all the classifiers of Model-1 when all HD sessions were considered.

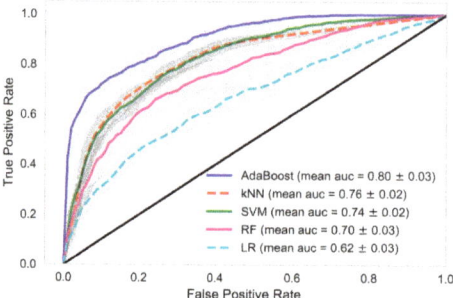

Figure 3. Receiver Operating Characteristics plot showing mean area under curve of all the classifiers of Model-2 when all HD sessions were considered.

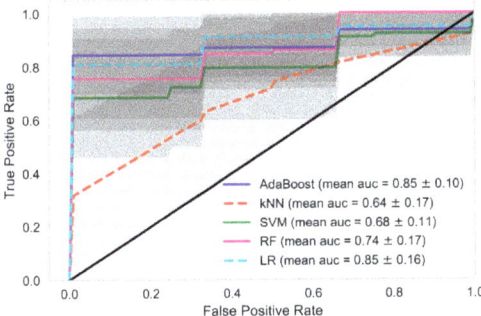

Figure 4. Receiver Operating Characteristics plot showing mean area under curve of all the classifiers of Model 3 when all HD sessions were considered.

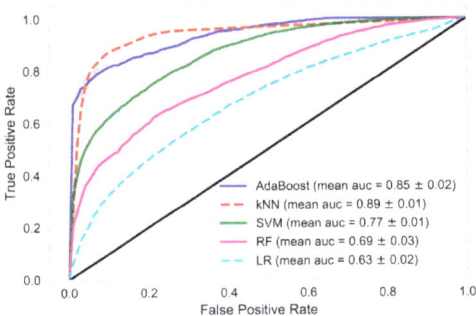

Figure 5. Receiver Operating Characteristics plot showing mean area under curve of all the classifiers of Model 1 when the 15 recent HD sessions were considered.

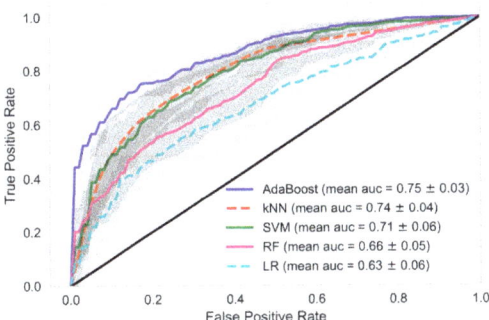

Figure 6. Receiver Operating Characteristics plot showing mean area under curve of all the classifiers of Model 2 when the 15 recent HD sessions were considered.

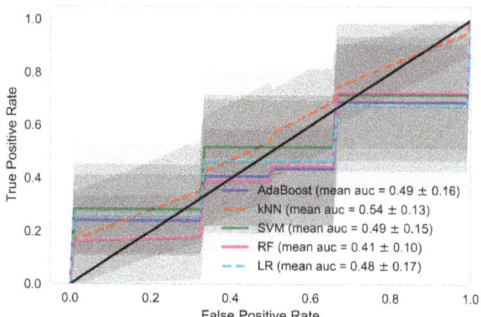

Figure 7. Receiver Operating Characteristics plot showing mean area under curve of all the classifiers of Model 3 when the 15 recent HD sessions were considered.

4. Discussion

In this study, we presented the novel use of non-contact sensor data in clinical settings during the process of HD of 109 patients. Hemodialysis is a procedure to purify the blood when the kidneys stop functioning normally. Hemodialysis may cause certain complications like cardiovascular, non-cardiovascular, and cerebrovascular issues, and even sudden death. During the 3237 HD sessions and 23 weeks of this study, we found that 78 patients reported 166 episodes of clinical events. We compared the differences among the group of patients who reported clinical events to those who did not report any clinical event. We found a statistically significant difference in the heart rates and respiration rates ($p < 0.0001$) recorded by the non-contact sensors among the two groups of patients. Various HRV parameters also showed significant differences, like high frequency and low frequency. The heart rate in both the first five minutes and last five minutes was found to be higher in the event group of patients compared to the no-event group of patients by an almost five-point basis. A similar pattern was observed for the respiration rate. Our findings suggest that an increased heart rate and respiration rate indicates the unwellness of the patient and that some kind of clinical event may happen in the near future that needs attention and care in advance.

It is further observed that the mean heart rate values of the last five minutes (HR_LFM) were slightly higher than the heart rate values for the first five minutes (HR_FFM). Various studies conducted in the past also point towards an increase in heart rate during HD [47–50]. This phenomenon is observed across both groups of patients. It is generally observed that the heart rate increases during HD because of the removal of excess body water, which triggers a significant increase in the heart rate. This finding is consistent with those reported in the literature. The mean values of all vital parameters are shown in Table 3. The basic statistical analysis shows differences in the values of most of the vital parameters among the two groups of patients that were also found to be statistically significant.

The performance of the developed predictive models was also in line with the statistical findings. We obtained very high accuracy for our ML-based predictive models. In this study, we demonstrated the use of non-contact sensors to monitor the vital parameters of patients during HD and in the early prediction of any clinical event that may occur during the period of hemodialysis-based treatment. The results of our study show the possibility of accurately and precisely predicting chances in a clinical event. Although we were dealing with a smaller dataset, the model we developed still performed extremely well. If we evaluate our dataset in terms of the frequency of data points, we had a reasonable number of data samples, namely 32,370. However, if we evaluate our dataset in terms of individual patients, we had only 109 data points, which is very few to train a ML model. Model 1 exploited the large frequency of our dataset, whereas model 3 relied on the individual patients. In model 1, we achieved 90.16% ROC with a recall rate of 88.47% with a kNN classifier and ROC of 84.97%, with a recall of 82.09% in the AdaBoost classifier. In model 2, we achieved 80.36% ROC with a recall rate of 80.73% with an AdaBoost classifier. Recall or sensitivity analysis was an important measure in the context of our study. It tells us the rate of predicting true positives. A high recall rate was achieved in this study, which validates the practicality of an early warning system based predictive analytics using non-contact sensor data in hospital settings. This type of system can alert the healthcare provider, physicians, and healthcare professionals so that they provide extra care to the patient and the patient can be saved from any forthcoming life-threatening clinical events.

In our model, we selected a subset of variables from the available variables. We used heart rate and respiration rate, two features that had HF and LF from the HRV along with age, gender and BMI as input features in our models. The rest of the available variables were not considered as input features for the models. The notion behind selecting HR and RR is that they are the two main vital parameters used for continuous patient monitoring. The objective of this study was to understand whether we can make early predictions of clinical events by monitoring these vital parameters. The HRV parameters are basically variables derived from the heart rate. HRV is related to the autonomic nervous system. High frequency is linked to the parasympathetic nervous system (PSNS) and LF is linked to the sympathetic nervous system (SNS), as reported in the literature [51]. The other HRV variables were not considered as input features because they did not have enough influence on the outcome of the classifiers. Therefore, we considered these variables as important markers for the prediction of the physiological health of patients. Further, there are various methods for deciding the best subset of features [52] reported in the literature, namely the filter method, wrapper method, and embedded method. We used the backward elimination technique of the wrapper method for feature selection, which showed optimum performance for the predictive models developed in this study.

We found that under real circumstances the use of non-contact sensors is highly beneficial in two ways. Firstly, it provides the continuous monitoring of the vital parameters of the patient during the HD session. It can help the physician or the care provider to take a decision in providing better care and comfort to the patients. Secondly, this data can be used for analyses and the prediction of any clinical emergency. It could predict event occurrences based on the increased heart rate and respiration rate during HD. Although it would be early to say that the proposed supervised ML-based predictive model could be used in real life, on the basis of the obtained results we suggest that more such studies are conducted using non-contact sensors in clinical settings. These proposed studies could validate the findings of this study and further be useful in the development of a more robust predictive application to predict clinical events in advance.

5. Limitations of This Study

We had certain limitations in this study in terms of the clinical variables available for analysis. We had only three critical parameters in our dataset to build our model, i.e., heart rate, respiration rate, and HRV parameters. The inclusion of other vital parameters like blood pressure and patient's medical history could add more weight to such predictive modeling approaches. One of the major issues observed in HD is the sudden death of patients, including various other events like ER visits or inpatient stays due to cardiovascular problems, infection, renal problems, etc. During this study, six people suffered sudden death. It was one of our objectives to develop a multi-class prediction model that is able to predict chances of different events occurring in advance. We had details of the medical issues reported during the clinical event in the form of International Classification of Diseases (ICD) codes, but the number of cases reported was very low. Therefore, in this study we limited our analysis to a binary classification model instead of building a multi-class classification model.

6. Conclusions

The initial findings and the performance of the predictive model developed using this data are highly encouraging. It is also a novel application for non-contact sensors in clinical settings, especially for HD patients. The authors found very few studies that used AI for the prediction of events in liver transplant patients, but could not find any study using AI on sensor data to predict clinical events in

HD patients. On the basis of our findings, we recommend further studies using non-contact sensors to monitor the vital parameters of chronic kidney disease (CKD) patients during HD. This can be utilized to predict the possibility of medical problems in HD patients in advance. In addition, as a part of future work, we are further interested in analyzing this data more specifically using the available ICD code information reported during clinical events. This will enable us to identify whether there is any difference in the recordings when the event is reported as compared to when it is not reported. Furthermore, a patient might have reported several issues during the reporting of clinical events. It will be intriguing to learn whether there is any association between the different types of medical issues reported by the patients and the trends between different patients as far as the association of different medical issues are concerned. We also plan to check the importance of each feature variable used in the ML models. It will be intriguing to learn which feature variable has greater impact on the efficiency of the developed predictive ML models.

Author Contributions: Conceptualization: S.S.A.; Data curation: P.-Y.H; Formal analysis: S.S.T and H.-Y.C; Investigation: S.S.T.; Methodology: S.S.T.; Supervision, S.S.A., R.B.R. and Y.-C.L.; Validation: S.S.T., R.B.R.; Visualization, S.S.T.; Writing—original draft, S.S.T.; Writing—review & editing: S.S.T., S.S.A., R.B.R., S.M., A.A.N.

Funding: This research is funded by the Ministry of Science and Technology (MOST) under grant MOST 106-2221-E-038-005 and the Tatung Medical and Healthcare Technologies under grant number A-105-010. This project has been sponsored in part by MOST under grant 106-2923-E-038-001-MY2, 107-2923-E-038 -001 -MY2, Taipei Medical University under grant number 106-3805-004-111 and Wanfang hospital under grant number 106TMU-WFH-01-4.

Acknowledgments: We are thankful to the Ministry of Science and Technology (MOST), Tatung Medical and Healthcare Technologies, and Taipei Medical University for providing the necessary funding to carry out this research work. We are thankful to Taipei Medical University Hospital for facilitating the data collection on HD patients. We are also thankful to EarlySense Ltd., Israel for providing us with the non-contact sensor and raw HRV data. We also acknowledge Rajendra Mishra School of Engineering Entrepreneurship, Indian Institute of Technology Kharagpur, India for this collaboration and enabling student exchange with partial financial support to facilitate this research work.

Conflicts of Interest: The authors declare no conflicts of interest.

References

1. Villa, G.; Ricci, Z.; Ronco, C. Renal Replacement Therapy. *Crit. Care Clin.* **2015**, *31*, 839–848. [CrossRef] [PubMed]
2. NIDDK. Choosing a Treatment for Kidney Failure | NIDDK. National Institute of Diabetes and Digestive and Kidney Diseases, 2016. Available online: https://www.niddk.nih.gov/health-information/kidney-disease/kidney-failure/choosing-treatment (accessed on 10 June 2018).
3. Lin, Y.C.; Hsu, C.Y.; Kao, C.C.; Chen, T.W.; Chen, H.H.; Hsu, C.C.; Wu, M.S. Incidence and Prevalence of ESRD in Taiwan Renal Registry Data System (TWRDS): 2005–2012. *Acta Nephrol.* **2014**, *28*, 65–68.
4. Shafiee, M.A.; Chamanian, P.; Shaker, P.; Shahideh, Y.; Broumand, B. The Impact of Hemodialysis Frequency and Duration on Blood Pressure Management and Quality of Life in End-Stage Renal Disease Patients. *Healthcare* **2017**, *5*, 52. [CrossRef] [PubMed]
5. Susantitaphong, P.; Koulouridis, I.; Balk, E.M.; Madias, N.E.; Jaber, B.L. Effect of Frequent or Extended Hemodialysis on Cardiovascular Parameters: A Meta-analysis. *Am. J. Kidney Dis.* **2012**, *59*, 689–699. [CrossRef] [PubMed]
6. Ravani, P.; Palmer, S.C.; Oliver, M.J.; Quinn, R.R.; MacRae, J.M.; Tai, D.J.; Pannu, N.I.; Thomas, C.; Hemmelgarn, B.R.; Craig, J.C.; et al. Associations between Hemodialysis Access Type and Clinical Outcomes: A Systematic Review. *J. Am. Soc. Nephrol.* **2013**, *24*, 465–473. [CrossRef] [PubMed]
7. Han, S.S.; Cho, G.Y.; Park, Y.S.; Baek, S.H.; Ahn, S.Y.; Kim, S.; Chin, H.J.; Chae, D.W.; Na, K.Y. Predictive value of echocardiographic parameters for clinical events in patients starting hemodialysis. *J. Korean Med. Sci.* **2015**, *30*, 44–53. [CrossRef] [PubMed]
8. Raszeja-Wyszomirska, J.; Glowczynska, R.; Kostrzewa, K.; Janik, M.; Zygmunt, M.; Zborowska, H.; Krawczyk, M.; Niewinski, G.; Galas, M.; Krawczyk, M.; et al. Evaluation of liver graft recipient work-up in predicting of early cardiovascular events during liver transplantation—A single-center experience. *Transplant. Proc.* **2018**, in press. [CrossRef]

9. Gallegos-Orozco, J.F.; Charlton, M.R. Predictors of Cardiovascular Events After Liver Transplantation. *Clin. Liver Dis.* **2017**, *21*, 367–379. [CrossRef] [PubMed]
10. Cook, D.J.; Augusto, J.C.; Jakkula, V.R. Ambient intelligence: Technologies, applications, and opportunities. *Pervasive Mob. Comput.* **2009**, *5*, 277–298. [CrossRef]
11. Barsocchi, P.; Cimino, M.G.C.A.; Ferro, E.; Lazzeri, A.; Palumbo, F.; Vaglini, G. Monitoring elderly behavior via indoor position-based stigmergy. *Pervasive Mob. Comput.* **2015**, *23*, 26–42. [CrossRef]
12. Chan, M.; Estève, D.; Fourniols, J.-Y.; Escriba, C.; Campo, E. Smart wearable systems: Current status and future challenges. *Artif. Intell. Med.* **2012**, *56*, 137–156. [CrossRef] [PubMed]
13. Dobbins, C.; Rawassizadeh, R.; Momeni, E. Detecting physical activity within lifelogs towards preventing obesity and aiding ambient assisted living. *Neurocomputing* **2016**, *230*, 110–132. [CrossRef]
14. Pavel, M.; Jimison, H.; Spring, B. Behavioral Informatics: Dynamical Models for Measuring and Assessing Behaviors for Precision Interventions. In Proceedings of the 2016 38th Annual International Conference of the IEEE Engineering in Medicine and Biology Society (EMBC), Orlando, FL, USA, 16–20 August 2016; pp. 190–193.
15. Yang, J.J.; Li, J.; Mulder, J.; Wang, Y.; Chen, S.; Wu, H.; Wang, Q.; Pan, H. Emerging information technologies for enhanced healthcare. *Comput. Ind.* **2015**, *69*, 3–11. [CrossRef]
16. Liu, L.; Stroulia, E.; Nikolaidis, I.; Miguel-Cruz, A.; Rincon, A.R. Smart homes and home health monitoring technologies for older adults: A systematic review. *Int. J. Med. Inform.* **2016**, *91*, 44–59. [CrossRef] [PubMed]
17. Chan, M.; Estève, D.; Escriba, C.; Campo, E. A review of smart homes—Present state and future challenges. *Comput. Methods Programs Biomed.* **2008**, *91*, 55–81. [PubMed]
18. Teruel, J.L.; Lucas, M.F.; Marcen, R.; Rodriguez, J.R.; Sánchez, J.L.; Rivera, M.; Liano, F.; Ortuno, J. Differences between Blood Flow as Indicated by the Hemodialysis Blood Roller Pump and Blood Flow Measured by an Ultrasonic Sensor. *Nephron* **2000**, *85*, 142–147. [CrossRef] [PubMed]
19. Trebbels, D.; Hradetzky, D.; Zengerle, R. Capacitive on-line hematocrit sensor design based on impedance spectroscopy for use in hemodialysis machines. *Ann. Int. Conf. IEEE Eng. Med. Biol. Soc.* **2009**, *2009*, 1208–1211.
20. Du, Y.-C.; Lim, B.-Y.; Ciou, W.-S.; Wu, M.-J. Novel Wearable Device for Blood Leakage Detection during Hemodialysis Using an Array Sensing Patch. *Sensors* **2016**, *16*, 849. [CrossRef] [PubMed]
21. Barbieri, C.; Molina, M.; Ponce, P.; Tothova, M.; Cattinelli, I.; Titapiccolo, J.I.; Mari, F.; Amato, C.; Leipold, F.; Wehmeyer, W.; et al. An international observational study suggests that artificial intelligence for clinical decision support optimizes anemia management in hemodialysis patients. *Kidney Int.* **2016**, *90*, 422–429. [CrossRef] [PubMed]
22. Tal, A.; Shinar, Z.; Shaki, D.; Codish, S.; Goldbart, A. Validation of Contact-Free Sleep Monitoring Device with Comparison to Polysomnography. *J. Clin. Sleep Med.* **2017**, *13*, 517–522. [CrossRef] [PubMed]
23. Hall, T.; Lie, D.Y.; Nguyen, T.Q.; Mayeda, J.C.; Lie, P.E.; Lopez, J.; Banister, R.E. Non-Contact Sensor for Long-Term Continuous Vital Signs Monitoring: A Review on Intelligent Phased-Array Doppler Sensor Design. *Sensors* **2017**, *17*, 2632. [CrossRef] [PubMed]
24. Klap, T.; Shinar, Z. Using piezoelectric sensor for continuous-contact-free monitoring of heart and respiration rates in real-life hospital settings. In Proceedings of the Computing in Cardiology Conference (CinC), Zaragoza, Spain, 22–25 September 2013.
25. Zimlichman, E.; Szyper-Kravitz, M.; Shinar, Z.; Klap, T.; Levkovich, S.; Unterman, A.; Rozenblum, R.; Rothschild, J.M.; Amital, H.; Shoenfeld, Y. Early recognition of acutely deteriorating patients in non-intensive care units: Assessment of an innovative monitoring technology. *J. Hosp. Med.* **2012**, *7*, 628–633. [CrossRef] [PubMed]
26. Ben-Ari, J.; Zimlichman, E.; Adi, N.; Sorkine, P. Contactless respiratory and heart rate monitoring: Validation of an innovative tool. *J. Med. Eng. Technol.* **2010**, *34*, 393–398. [CrossRef] [PubMed]
27. Davidovich, M.L.Y.; Karasik, R.; Tal, A.; Shinar, Z. Sleep Apnea Screening with a Contact-Free Under-the-Mattress Sensor. In Proceedings of the Computing in Cardiology Conference (CinC), Vancouver, BC, Canada, 11–14 September 2016.
28. Lahdenoja, O.; Hurnanen, T.; Tadi, M.J.; Pänkäälä, M.; Koivisto, T. Heart Rate Variability Estimation with Joint Accelerometer and Gyroscope Sensing. In Proceedings of the 2016 Computing in Cardiology Conference (CinC), Vancouver, BC, Canada, 11–14 September 2016.

29. Malik, M.; Bigger, J.T.; Camm, A.J.; Kleiger, R.E.; Malliani, A.; Moss, A.J.; Schwartz, P.J. Heart rate variability: Standards of measurement, physiological interpretation, and clinical use. *Eur. Heart J.* **1996**, *17*, 354–381. [CrossRef]
30. Sinnreich, R.; Kark, J.D.; Friedlander, Y.; Sapoznikov, D.; Luria, M.H. Five minutes recordings of heart rate variability for population studies: Repeatability and age-sex characteristics. *Heart* **1998**, *80*, 156–162. [CrossRef] [PubMed]
31. Min, K.B.; Min, J.-Y.; Paek, D.; Cho, S.-I.; Son, M. Is 5-minute heart rate variability a useful measure for monitoring the autonomic nervous system of workers? *Int. Heart J.* **2008**, *49*, 175–181. [CrossRef] [PubMed]
32. Cox, D.R. The Regression Analysis of Binary Sequences. *J. R. Stat. Soc. Ser. B Methodol.* **1958**, *20*, 215–242.
33. Walker, S.H.; Duncan, D.B. Estimation of the Probability of an Event as a Function of Several Independent Variables. *Biometrika* **1967**, *54*, 167. [CrossRef] [PubMed]
34. Altman, N.S. An Introduction to Kernel and Nearest-Neighbor Nonparametric Regression. *Am. Stat.* **1992**, *46*, 175–185.
35. Burba, F.; Ferraty, F.; Vieu, P. k-Nearest Neighbour method in functional nonparametric regression. *J. Nonparametr. Stat.* **2009**, *21*, 453–469. [CrossRef]
36. Freund, Y.; Schapire, R.E. A Short Introduction to Boosting. *J. Jpn. Soc. Artif. Intell.* **1999**, *14*, 771–780.
37. Freund, Y.; Schapire, R.E. A Decision-Theoretic Generalization of On-Line Learning and an Application to Boosting. *J. Comput. Syst. Sci.* **1997**, *55*, 119–139. [CrossRef]
38. Hastie, T.; Tibshirani, R.; Friedman, J. Random Forests. In *The Elements of Statistical Learning: Data Mining, Inference, and Prediction*; Springer: New York, NY, USA, 2009; pp. 587–604.
39. Hastie, T.; Tibshirani, R.; Friedman, J. *The Elements of Statistical Learning*; Springer: New York, NY, USA, 2009.
40. Cristianini, N.; Shawe-Taylor, J. *An Introduction to Support Vector Machines: And Other Kernel-Based Learning Methods*; Cambridge University Press: Cambridge, UK, 2000.
41. Pedregosa, F.; Varoquaux, G.; Gramfort, A.; Michel, V.; Thirion, B.; Grisel, O.; Blondel, M.; Prettenhofer, P.; Weiss, R.; Dubourg, V.; et al. Scikit-learn: Machine Learning in Python. *J. Mach. Learn. Res.* **2011**, *12*, 2825–2830.
42. Chawla, N.V.; Bowyer, K.W.; Hall, L.O.; Kegelmeyer, W.P. SMOTE: Synthetic Minority Over-sampling Technique. *J. Artif. Intell. Res.* **2002**, *16*, 321–357. [CrossRef]
43. Das, B.; Krishnan, N.C.; Cook, D.J. RACOG and wRACOG: Two Probabilistic Oversampling Techniques. *IEEE Trans. Knowl. Data Eng.* **2015**, *27*, 222–234. [CrossRef] [PubMed]
44. Arlot, S.; Celisse, A. A survey of cross-validation procedures for model selection. *Stat. Surv.* **2010**, *4*, 40–79. [CrossRef]
45. Powers, D.M. Evaluation: from precision, recall and F-measure to ROC, informedness, markedness correlation. *J. Mach. Learn. Technol. ISSN* **2011**, *2*, 2229–3981.
46. Charan, J.; Biswas, T. How to calculate sample size for different study designs in medical research? *Indian J. Psychol. Med.* **2013**, *35*, 121–126. [CrossRef] [PubMed]
47. Severi, S.; Cavalcanti, S.; Mancini, E.; Santoro, A. Heart rate response to hemodialysis-induced changes in potassium and calcium levels. *J. Nephrol.* **2001**, *14*, 488–496. [PubMed]
48. Lertdumrongluk, P.; Streja, E.; Rhee, C.M.; Sim, J.J.; Gillen, D.; Kovesdy, C.P.; Kalantar-Zadeh, K. Changes in pulse pressure during hemodialysis treatment and survival in maintenance dialysis patients. *Clin. J. Am. Soc. Nephrol.* **2015**, *10*, 1179–1191. [CrossRef] [PubMed]
49. Iseki, K.; Nakai, S.; Yamagata, K.; Tsubakihara, Y. Tachycardia as a predictor of poor survival in chronic haemodialysis patients. *Nephrol. Dial. Transplant.* **2011**, *26*, 963–969. [CrossRef] [PubMed]
50. Chan, C.T.; Chertow, G.M.; Daugirdas, J.T.; Greene, T.H.; Kotanko, P.; Larive, B.; Pierratos, A.; Stokes, J.B. Effects of daily hemodialysis on heart rate variability: Results from the Frequent Hemodialysis Network (FHN) Daily Trial. *Nephrol. Dial. Transplant.* **2014**, *29*, 168–178. [CrossRef] [PubMed]
51. Billman, G.E. The LF/HF ratio does not accurately measure cardiac sympatho-vagal balance. *Front. Physiol.* **2013**, *4*, 26. [CrossRef] [PubMed]
52. Guyon, I.; Andre, E. An Introduction to Variable and Feature Selection. *J. Mach. Learn. Res.* **2003**, *3*, 1157–1182.

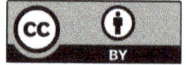

© 2018 by the authors. Licensee MDPI, Basel, Switzerland. This article is an open access article distributed under the terms and conditions of the Creative Commons Attribution (CC BY) license (http://creativecommons.org/licenses/by/4.0/).

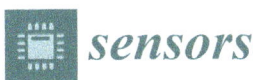

Article

Wearable Sensor-Based Exercise Biofeedback for Orthopaedic Rehabilitation: A Mixed Methods User Evaluation of a Prototype System

Rob Argent [1,2,3,*], Patrick Slevin [2,3], Antonio Bevilacqua [2], Maurice Neligan [1], Ailish Daly [1] and Brian Caulfield [2,3]

1. Beacon Hospital, Sandyford, Dublin 18, Ireland; maurice.neligan@beaconhospital.ie (M.N.); ailish.daly@beaconhospital.ie (A.D.)
2. Insight Centre for Data Analytics, University College Dublin, Dublin 4, Ireland; patrick.slevin@insight-centre.org (P.S.); antonio.bevilacqua@insight-centre.org (A.B.); b.caulfield@ucd.ie (B.C.)
3. School of Public Health, Physiotherapy and Sport Science, University College Dublin, Dublin 4, Ireland
* Correspondence: rob.argent@insight-centre.org; Tel.: +353-(0)-1-650-4646

Received: 12 December 2018; Accepted: 18 January 2019; Published: 21 January 2019

Abstract: The majority of wearable sensor-based biofeedback systems used in exercise rehabilitation lack end-user evaluation as part of the development process. This study sought to evaluate an exemplar sensor-based biofeedback system, investigating the feasibility, usability, perceived impact and user experience of using the platform. Fifteen patients participated in the study having recently undergone knee replacement surgery. Participants were provided with the system for two weeks at home, completing a semi-structured interview alongside the System Usability Scale (SUS) and user version of the Mobile Application Rating Scale (uMARS). The analysis from the SUS (mean = 90.8 [SD = 7.8]) suggests a high degree of usability, supported by qualitative findings. The mean adherence rate was 79% with participants reporting a largely positive user experience, suggesting it offers additional support with the rehabilitation regime. Overall quality from the mean uMARS score was 4.1 out of 5 (SD = 0.39), however a number of bugs and inaccuracies were highlighted along with suggestions for additional features to enhance engagement. This study has shown that patients perceive value in the use of wearable sensor-based biofeedback systems and has highlighted the benefit of user-evaluation during the design process, illustrated the need for real-world accuracy validation, and supports the ongoing development of such systems.

Keywords: biofeedback; biomedical technology; exercise therapy; orthopedics; mobile health; qualitative; human factors; wearables; inertial measurement unit

1. Introduction

In response to changing global health economics, connected health solutions have the potential to improve the outcomes and accessibility of healthcare [1]. Within rehabilitation, remotely collating and aggregating data from patients has been suggested to have numerous benefits in terms of cost, clinical outcome and patient satisfaction, and can encourage self-management of long-term conditions [2,3]. These connected health solutions can include a biofeedback system which not only gathers data, but also offers the user meaningful information in real-time that is otherwise unavailable to them. This can consist of measurements from the neuromuscular system, or biomechanical variances such as strength or exercise technique [4]. This has led to the development of a number of biofeedback systems utilising a variety of technologies including cameras and wearable sensors [5–8]. The use of wearable inertial measurement units (IMUs) is one such method of measuring biomechanical variance during exercise and providing feedback to the patient [4,9,10]. The portability of IMUs means that they provide an easy and cost-effective method of capturing human movement data [4,11], and they have been shown to be an accurate method of assessing exercise technique in numerous rehabilitation exercises [11–14].

IMU based biofeedback systems are particularly suited to the orthopaedic rehabilitation pathway, with an increasing prevalence of surgery and a clearly defined rehabilitation regime. The demand for primary total knee replacement (TKR) for example is estimated to grow 673% in the United States between 2005 to 2030, to almost 3.5 million procedures performed annually [15]. Exercise rehabilitation is the cornerstone of the post-acute recovery process, yet patients report a lack of confidence and vulnerability in the post-operative period [16]. Combine this with the advancement of value-based care, and there is a clear need for interventions to support self-management whilst maximising clinical and cost effectiveness.

Usability is one of the main barriers to widespread uptake of most connected health interventions [17], however there is a distinct lack of both technical and usability validation of sensor-based systems in the peer-reviewed literature [10,18]. To encourage engagement, it is important that the design of biofeedback systems adopts a user-centred iterative process [19], where developers consult end-users to evaluate the system, identify their usability criteria, and understand the perceived benefits and challenges of its implementation in the real-world [20]. To further promote user-engagement, it is also possible to include interventions aiming to increase adherence to exercise within the design of these solutions [21,22].

Thus, this study sought to explore the feasibility, usability, perceived impact, and user experience of an exemplar exercise biofeedback system for orthopaedic rehabilitation in the home. In addition, it was desirable to incorporate user-centred design approaches by encouraging participants to highlight potential refinements or issues in implementation, and to express the criteria they would require in order to maximise engagement and impact.

2. Materials and Methods

2.1. Participants

A total of 15 patients volunteered to participate in the study (nine females, six males; age: 63 [standard deviation (SD): 8.32]). Participants were recruited from a private hospital in Dublin, Ireland and had recently undergone knee replacement surgery (TKR or unicompartmental knee replacement (UKR)). Participants were required to live within 30 km of the hospital, have no history of cognitive dysfunction, and no difficulty understanding English. The study received ethical approval from the Beacon Hospital Research Ethics Committee (BEA0065), and written informed consent was obtained from all participants prior to commencing the study.

The participants were split into two groups for pragmatic reasons. Group 1 consisted of five participants (Post-Acute) who had all undergone knee replacement surgery at least six weeks previously, and were approaching the end of the acute rehabilitation regime. This group were tested first in order to establish any significant shortcomings in the system that may increase risk of harm to the acute patient group. The second group of 10 participants (Acute) were introduced to the study prior to surgery and then recruited directly from the ward between 2 to 3 days following the operation. This group represents the target user for such a system designed to be implemented in support of discharge home from hospital.

2.2. Prototype Exercise Biofeedback System

The prototype system evaluated by all participants consisted of a single wearable IMU (Shimmer, Dublin, Ireland) [9], and a tablet computer with a custom-built Android application. The Shimmer3 IMU, utilising a tri-axial low-noise accelerometer (±2 g) and tri-axial gyroscope (500 °/s) configured to sample at 102.4 Hz, was placed at the midpoint of the anterior aspect of the shin in a neoprene sleeve, and streamed data via Bluetooth to the tablet whilst the user was guided through their exercises (Figure 1). An avatar mirrored the movements of the user in real-time, the repetitions were counted (Figure 2), and at the end of each exercise, the user was given advice on their technique based on supervised machine learning.

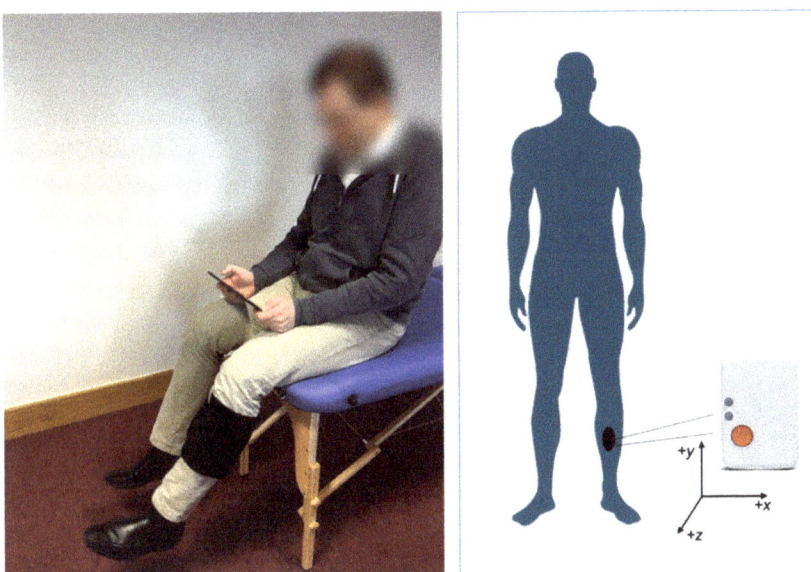

Figure 1. User setup and IMU orientation of the biofeedback system consisting of a single IMU and associated Android tablet application (figure adapted from [23]).

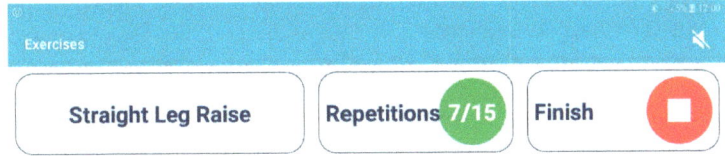

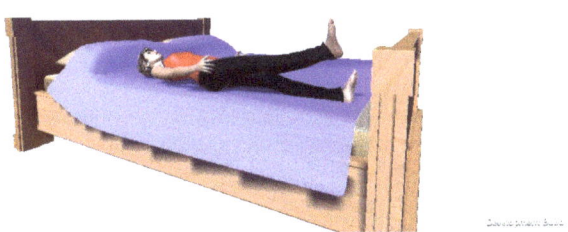

Figure 2. Screenshot of the Android tablet application during the straight leg raise exercise.

These methods allow for segmentation and classification of sensor data using support vector machine and random forest techniques described in further detail elsewhere [11,14]. The application also captures patient reported outcomes such as pain and perceived exercise difficulty, and provides all the relevant educational material from the healthcare provider in interactive formats. The user is able to track their progress by viewing their adherence statistics and results of previous patient reported outcome measures such as the Oxford Knee Score or the Western Ontario and McMaster Universities osteoarthritis index [24]. A video of the system can be viewed in the Supplementary Materials (Supplementary File 1).

2.3. Experimental Procedure

A mixed methods approach consisting of both quantitative and qualitative data was collected to provide greater insight into the performance of the system, and reduce the weaknesses in using each method in isolation [17,25]. Once signed informed consent was provided, the investigator met participants in their home or at the hospital, whichever was more convenient. Demographic data including age, gender, education, and ownership of mobile technology devices were first collected by self-report. Participants then partook in a user-training session of the biofeedback system lasting approximately 30 minutes, which included completing a full set of the rehabilitation exercises as prescribed in the post-operative protocol. They were then provided with the system and asked to use it at home for the following two weeks to complete the exercises as prescribed by their Physiotherapist.

The investigator met each participant on two additional occasions in their own home during the testing period. During each session, the participant completed a set of the rehabilitation exercises using the biofeedback system, with the investigator observing and making notes on system crashes or user-errors as the participant used the system. After the final session, a semi-structured interview was completed with each participant. Open ended questions were used to establish the perceived impact, usability and user experience of the system, and to explore their opinions on how the prototype could be improved. A Dictaphone was used to record all interview data, and to ensure consistency in questioning, an interview topic guide was constructed based on the aims of the study and the main research questions [26] (Supplementary File 2).

Prior to the final interview, and to provide quantitative data to support the system evaluation, participants also completed two questionnaires; the System Usability Scale (SUS) [27] and the "user version of the Mobile Application Rating Scale" (uMARS) [28]. The SUS is a 10-item questionnaire that has been used to quickly and reliably assess the usability of a system across a number of sectors [27,29]. The output from each user is a score out of 100 which can be used to compare to a growing body of literature to find percentile rankings of a system's usability performance [30].

The uMARS is designed to be completed by the end-user of mobile applications, rather than the more expert-driven "Mobile Application Ratings Scale" [31]. The application is assessed under the categories of aesthetics, functionality, engagement and information to produce a score out of 5, as well as separate measures to assess the perceived impact of the system and subjective app quality. Similar to previous work [25], this perceived impact section was tailored to identify the perceived impact of the person "exercising with their best technique".

2.4. Data Analysis

All audio data from interviews was transcribed and anonymised. The transcripts were analysed thematically with a grounded theory approach [26]. An early coding template was created based on the interview topic guide which was refined and finalised as themes emerged throughout the analysis [32] by RA (research physiotherapist) and PS (anthropologist). Regular cross-checking was undertaken in a constant-comparison approach ensuring correlation between researchers and reliability of sub-themes [33]. Discrepancies were discussed until agreement was reached, and data saturation was agreed when no further themes and no new data were occurring [26].

The SUS and uMARS scores were calculated following the standard scoring procedure, with the SUS mean and standard deviation (SD) of scores across all participants calculated [27,28,30]. For each participant, a uMARS score out of 5 was calculated under the sections of engagement, functionality, aesthetics and information. The mean of these scores produced an overall score for each participant, perceived impact and subjective app quality were also calculated out of 5 for each user. The means and SDs for the uMARS scores were then calculated across all participants. Estimated adherence rates were also calculated for each user in the acute group. The number of times each participant finished an exercise session was logged within the system and compared with the prescribed number, in order to provide an understanding of the participant's compliance to the exercise programme.

3. Results

All 15 participants completed the semi-structured interview and surveys following two-weeks of using the exemplar biofeedback system. Table 1 illustrates the demographics of participants, including their current access to mobile technology. A summary of the results from interview data are reported in this section, with additional quotations available in Supplementary File 3.

Table 1. Participant demographics and technology ownership.

Demographic Details	n = 15	
Marital Status	Married	86.6%
	Single	0%
	Widowed	6.6%
	Other	6.6%
Lives with	Spouse	46.6%
	Family	40%
	Alone	13.3%
Education	Degree Educated	73.3%
	Completed Secondary	20%
	Completed Primary	6.6%
Technology Ownership	Mobile Phone	100%
	Smart Phone	86.6%
	Tablet	66.6%
	WiFi	93.3%
	Health/Fitness App	26.6%

3.1. Usability, Functionality and User Experience

The system achieved a mean SUS score of 90.8 (SD 7.8). This places the system above the 95th percentile when compared with published results using this scale [29]. Table 2 displays the results from the uMARS scores, subjective app quality and perceived impact. The results from the functionality section of this survey support this high usability rating with a mean score of 4.2 out of 5 (SD 0.34).

Table 2. Results from the user version of the Mobile Application Rating Scale (uMARS). Overall uMARS quality score shown in bold.

uMARS Section (score out of five)	Mean (SD)
Engagement	3.5 (0.69)
Functionality	4.2 (0.34)
Aesthetics	4.2 (0.45)
Information	4.4 (0.34)
Overall Quality	**4.1 (0.39)**
Perceived Impact	4.4 (0.83)
Subjective App Quality	4.2 (0.86)

Whilst these scores suggest a high degree of usability for the system evaluated, the qualitative data from interview transcripts provided a greater context and support as to the reason that participants scored the system this way. Specifically, almost all participants commented on how they found the system easy to use, regardless of their perceived literacy with technology:

It's very simple to use, very simple. And it flows through on a good progression. [Acute 2]

Initially I said to you I wasn't very computer literate but it's very simple to use. Once you do it once or twice you can do it with your eyes closed essentially. [Acute 9]

Participants reported positively on their user experience, finding that the system gave them an added incentive to complete their exercises, and provided them with support once they were at home:

I think it set me on a routine very, very quickly and a routine that I actually got to enjoy in a certain way. It was not like holding a sheet of paper . . . you became involved in it and so user friendly that I really think it was a great aid to me. [Acute 5]

It's very helpful, it's much better than leafing through static illustrations. It's 3D real time. It made what are otherwise boring exercises more interesting. [Acute 9]

Some usability issues were highlighted by participants however, with many reporting inconsistencies in the repetition counter and the technique feedback. Participants also noted that the information presented in the progress section was not displayed intuitively and, on a number of occasions, a bug led to the exercises not being recorded correctly:

There is a bit of problem with the counting in it . . . Yeah sometimes it misses a few you do . . . it just runs away with itself. [Post-Acute 1]

Some of the technique feedback seems to be quite inconsistent. [Acute 9]

On the graph I don't know what the interpretation is supposed to be. [Acute 6]

We had just the one where it says unusual behaviour, unexpected behaviour, please repeat the exercise. I think I was saying to you that on two occasions I actually repeated the exercise . . . I just said there was a glitch and it didn't really bother me. [Acute 5]

These issues consequently had a negative impact on user experience. Despite the above participant saying it did not trouble them, other users reported frustration with this, as the exercises are not easy to do and therefore this bug reduced their trust in the system.

It's just very frustrating as I say it's on the three that are really painful to do, and you struggle through them and you think well I think I have done them fairly well and then it says unexplained behaviour do them again and you just can't. [Post-Acute 4]

3.2. Perceived Impact

Almost all participants made a reference to the system improving their adherence to the rehabilitation programme, whether that was in the quantity of exercises performed, or the quality with which they completed them:

It kept me doing physio when I might not have done it at home, especially with various things that have been happening at home. So it kept me doing physio and made sure I did it every day. [Post-Acute 3]

Well I can 100% tell you that I had a previous knee operation and I didn't have an app and I did the exercises as diligently and frequently as I could, but I certainly didn't do them with the thoroughness and regularity that I've done them this time [Acute 3]

One of the main reasons reported for this perceived improvement in adherence largely related to the monitoring provided by such a system provides, be that self-monitoring via the progress graphs or remote monitoring by the clinician:

I found it, I have to say, it made me do the exercises when I didn't really want to do them, knowing I was being monitored, I do think it helped me a lot. [Acute 2]

I kind of felt that that app now made me do my exercises, the three times a day, and secondly at least it was recording it and you could see, that's what I liked, you could see the progress from, I'm sure you have the record there of the beginning ones weren't great. [Acute 4]

Participants reported a motivation for using the system, whether as a result of the monitoring aspect, or from the enjoyment they achieved from using it and improving their self-efficacy:

Oh yes it made a huge difference, that was a great motivation ... It just meant that I was in control of my situation and I didn't feel the days were endless. I was looking forward to doing it to see how well I was doing. [Acute 7]

A huge incentive and even if you try it and say, I'm too tired tonight and then you say no, no I have to do it and I have to try and improve on it. [Acute 6]

Users were keen to point out the importance of the technique classification and felt this was an integral part of the support the system provided:

That's the important bit about it that it tells you straight away, you need feedback, there is no point in having the app if it doesn't give you feedback ... Because if you are waiting for someone to come in and check it out for you, that's two to three weeks, but it's two to three weeks of doing it wrong. [Post-Acute 2]

It's ideal for somebody that's coming straight out of hospital and they have to do the exercises on their own, because if you are not doing it correctly why are you bothering doing them in the first place. So that as a tool in itself is worth a hell of a lot. [Post-Acute 3]

Only one participant responded negatively when asked about their overall experience of using such a system. Whilst many others summed up their experience positively, reporting benefits to their confidence and their health literacy regarding the procedure and rehabilitation:

Yes first couple of days that was very interesting and I liked the idea of looking at the little cartoon. But after 2 or 3 days it was for me, I thought it was unnecessary ... I have no interest because I know very well if I'm doing better or not. So I find it unnecessary. [Acute 1]

I think the fact that I was almost keen for the next session, it led to a regularity and I think that has paid huge dividends in the exercises and in the result of the exercises on the leg. I really think it was extremely beneficial. [Acute 5]

It was so positive. It was just brilliant. It just meant that I was in control whereas normally I would be coming home and in the hospital it would be altogether different because there's so much support there, but when you come home its gone except that I had that. [Acute 7]

These comments were supported by the quantitative findings listed in Table 1. Specifically, the high result seen within the perceived impact subsection of the uMARS (4.4/5), which focused on the change in awareness, knowledge and behaviour regarding exercising with the best technique. The subjective app quality scored 4.2/5, with particularly high ratings for when participants were asked if they would recommend the system to others who might benefit (4.6).

3.3. Refinements

Participants offered a number of suggestions for refinements or additional features they would like to see to further maximise potential impact in such a system. A large number of participants ($n = 9$) requested that additional exercises were included in the system, including progressions beyond the basic regime:

I think if you gave me progression on the exercises, well done, try this one now, I'd like that. [Post-Acute 5]

Participants also felt that given the specific outcomes and targets following knee replacement surgery, a measurement of their joint angle would be beneficial:

This is probably not possible, but to get the angle of that knee bend, if you knew that ... for me that is where I'm really stuck so just to know that ... I know it counts it and it said you did it right, but I'm not sure what the angle of the bend is, and I'm rather obsessed with that. [Post-Acute 4]

The other one thing that I'd love to be able to see is you know when you do the knee bends, I'd love to be able to see what angle you got ... Now it just you know then the way at least you could say well I've gone from a 50 to a 75 rather than just ok it looks like I am doing it ok. [Acute 4]

Other suggestions were based on some of the usability issues discussed previously, with requests for greater clarity in the progress reports, a quality score after each exercise session and improving the graphical interfaces within the system:

And you know the way your Fitbit would have the circle that you have to fill the circle and obviously this system is basic bar charts ... Yes that (the Fitbit) does make more sense. [Post-Acute 3]

It would be very difficult to rate it from the previous time, there is no linkage from the previous repetitions ... So in a way you don't know if you are doing better today than you did yesterday ... The quality of how I'm doing them. [Acute 2]

I suppose it's nice to see it really, but she needs to undergo a great makeover ... Just a bit more human the graphics ... I mean even if it was more a cartoon figure or something it doesn't really matter. [Post-Acute 4]

Finally, a small number of participants talked about gamification ideas, yet there were mixed opinions on the relevance and the benefit of incorporating gamified features and customisation within the system:

If there was a games element to it you know you have unlocked the next level ... or a medal or something. [Acute 4]

I think that'd be a mistake because then you are going to end up turning it into playtime rather than exercise time. I think it'll lose the point of it. I don't think you should be able to manipulate too much unless it is information gathering or correcting the programme. For me this is a medical instruction for exercise to improve your health... you'd end up wasting time and not doing the exercise. [Acute 9]

In summary, the SUS and uMARS results, in combination with the interview data, suggest that the system had a high degree of usability and functionality, however there are programming issues causing inaccuracies in feedback that can be improved upon in future iterations to further enhance the user experience of the system. Participants in the acute group demonstrated a mean adherence rate of 79% (range 42%–100%) compared to the recommended number of exercise sessions in their rehabilitation programme. The results suggest that such a system may provide additional support and motivation in the rehabilitation process and improve adherence to the exercise programme, with patients highlighting features such as an extended exercise library and a joint angle measurement tool to further improve engagement and potential impact.

4. Discussions

This study investigated patient perceptions of using a custom-built interactive exercise biofeedback system with wearable technology during orthopaedic rehabilitation. Few studies have explored the opinions of the end-user in this population despite the increasing commercial prevalence of such systems [25], therefore this study adds to the current base of literature. Patients largely showed a positive reaction to the use of such a system, with numerous perceived benefits reported, a view that has been shared by clinicians [23]. The results offer fresh insights that can be used to inform the design of such systems, with suggestions to encourage user-engagement, improve usability and optimise impact.

The results indicate that using wearable sensors to offer biofeedback in support of the home-exercise programme prescribed following orthopaedic surgery improves the patient experience and has potential benefits to the clinical outcome. This perceived value may be measured in exercise adherence, patient satisfaction, and clinical effectiveness of the intervention, supporting similar previous suggestions in the literature [20,34], and advocating the ongoing development and evaluation of such systems.

Previous research has demonstrated clinician concern that usability would be a significant barrier to engagement with such systems [23]. However, the results from this study show that, provided the system is built with a user-centred focus, it may be possible to mitigate these concerns, including those of reduced digital literacy within the target demographic. The SUS results reinforce the interview data, as this system scored above the 95th percentile and is comparable to other systems developed for exercise biofeedback [5,25,30]. However few studies have evaluated the usability of a system with a mixed-methods approach over a period of several days as is recommended in the current literature [17].

While usability can be defined as the "effectiveness, efficiency and satisfaction with which specified users achieve specified goals in particular environments", it is also important to explore the user experience, that is "the users' perceptions and responses that result from the use of a system" [35]. Results suggest that this system can contribute to an increased sense of routine in the patient's rehabilitation regime and provide greater levels of enjoyment as they exercise. This in turn may reduce the perceived burden of, and barriers to, self-management [36], thus facilitating better engagement and adherence. However, it also shows how technical issues or wording of feedback can negatively impact user-experience. Particularly given the exercises may be challenging and often painful for patients, they may have a reduced tolerance for technological flaws in a system such as this than they would in other contexts.

It is notable that the uMARS score for the 'engagement' section demonstrated distinctly lower mean scores than the other sections. When analysing the individual questions, it is clear that the lack of customisation of sound, content and notifications (mean 1.9) along with the inability to set reminders and allow for interactivity (mean 3.2) had a negative impact on engagement. Arguably though the level of interactivity was misunderstood by participants, as the system will not function without user input from the sensor data. Additionally, an interesting finding from the uMARS was that the aesthetics of the prototype were not of concern, despite the clear graphical issues discussed in the interview data, further highlighting the benefits of the mixed-methods approach.

The usage data would suggest engagement was not as much of an issue as the uMARS would illustrate. The mean adherence rate to the specified number of exercise sessions was relatively high at 79%, with only one participant, who reported negatively on their overall experience in their interview data, demonstrating any kind of drop-off in engagement over time. This patient was one of only three to have received a UKR and was progressed on from these exercises within the study period. These adherence levels are similar to those reported in the recent evaluation of a camera-based biofeedback system for joint replacement rehabilitation [5], and are greater than the varying reports of 35–67% in the wider exercise adherence literature [37,38]. It is also widely documented that there is currently no valid and reliable measurement tool for exercise adherence [38,39]. The use of IMU based biofeedback solutions can therefore not only address factors that affect adherence by providing feedback, goal-setting and self-monitoring, but also offer a more reliable method of measurement of adherence rates [22].

The role of feedback was continuously mentioned throughout this study, with results suggesting it is crucial for habit formation and creating sustained engagement. In current clinical practice there is no ability to monitor or provide feedback to patients between clinic appointments, with a reliance on the patient's own self-management skills [23]. A system such as this therefore has the ability to offer feedback on exercise technique and clinical progress outside of the clinic setting. This in turn has the potential to provide added incentive to continue engaging with rehabilitation, increasing adherence, and maximising clinical outcomes [40]. Users requested additional features for further feedback such as a joint angle measure, and gamification ideas including unlocking levels of new and more challenging exercises in order to sustain engagement. This highlights the need for user-centred design approaches, as designers cannot assume what the user needs or sees as important [41]. Of particular interest was the role of monitoring and the perceived impact this had, as some patients were motivated by the ability to self-monitor, while others reported greater engagement and adherence as they were aware that their behaviours could be tracked by their clinician.

The lack of real-world validation of exercise biofeedback systems consisting of IMU based sensing platforms in the literature is of concern [10,18]. In this case, users were able to detect what they considered to be inaccurate feedback which has previously been reported as an important criterion for users [42]. These results reinforce the need for field evaluations to become a mainstream methodology, particularly for systems aimed at supporting treatment, where accuracy is key to ensure patient engagement and successful clinical decisions [10].

This study is not without its limitations however, particularly as the sample was selected from a single private hospital. This therefore may not be representative of the wider population, as the majority of patients were degree educated and from more affluent socio-economic backgrounds, which are determinants of better self-management and health outcomes [43,44]. While a sample size of 15 participants is standard for usability testing, this does not guarantee the opinions discussed are generalisable beyond this population. It is important to note that the impact discussed in this study is based solely on participant perceptions from analysis of interview data and uMARS results, and further objective investigation of impact is recommended. As the aim of this paper was to explore user perceptions on usability and perceived impact, there is no reference to the quantitative performance and accuracy of the system in measuring patient exercise technique in the 'real-world'. Therefore, until this validation is completed, the adherence rates stated could only be calculated by the number of exercise sessions, rather than the exact number of repetitions completed during each session.

Despite these limitations, patients believe exercise biofeedback systems consisting of IMUs and mobile technology can offer significant value to the rehabilitation experience, potentially maximising adherence, satisfaction, and therefore clinical outcome. Few other studies have been published that investigate these perceptions in similar systems, despite the importance of a user-centred focus in the design process. Further research is required to objectively assess whether these perceived benefits are demonstrated in clinical practice, and to rigorously validate the technical aspects of any such system. The development of patient recommended features can also be undertaken to improve the impact and user-experience in this biofeedback system, including a range of motion measurement, additional exercises for progression and gamification elements.

5. Conclusions

The emergence of ubiquitous mobile technologies and wearable sensors offer the opportunity to provide novel and effective methods of supporting patients in exercise rehabilitation. Patients perceive the use of wearable exercise biofeedback systems such as the prototype evaluated can offer additional motivation and feedback to enhance adherence, and positively impact patient experience and clinical outcome. However, there is a need for such systems to demonstrate real-world accuracy validation.

By involving patients in the development of such systems in a user-centred design manner, it is possible to maximise engagement and effectiveness, and highlight shortcomings or areas for further research early in the development cycle. The prototype system can be considered highly usable and the findings support the ongoing development and evaluation of such sensor-based biofeedback systems.

Ethical Approval: The research ethics committee of Beacon Hospital approved this study (REF: BEA0065).

Supplementary Materials: The following are available online at http://www.mdpi.com/1424-8220/19/2/432/s1, Supplementary File 1: Video of system usage, Supplementary File 2: Interview topic guide, Supplementary File 3: Additional quotations from interviews.

Author Contributions: R.A., P.S., A.D. and B.C. conceived and designed the study. R.A. conducted the recruitment and data collection with the assistance of P.S., A.D. and M.N. A.B. contributed to the development of the prototype biofeedback system. R.A. and P.S. conducted the data analyses and drafted and revised the manuscript. All authors read and approved the final manuscript.

Funding: This project forms part of the CHESS (Connected Health Early Stage Researcher Support System) Innovation Training Network and has received funding from the European Union's Horizon 2020 research and innovation programme under the Marie Sklodowska-Curie grant agreement No. 676201.

Conflicts of Interest: The authors declare no conflict of interest.

Abbreviations

IMU	inertial measurement unit
SUS	system usability
SD	standard deviation
TKR	total knee replacement
UKR	unicompartmental knee replacement
uMARS	user version of the Mobile Application Rating Scale

References

1. Caulfield, B.M.; Donnelly, S. What is Connected Health and why will it change your practice? *QJM* **2013**, *106*, 703–707. [CrossRef] [PubMed]
2. Brennan, D.M.; Mawson, S.; Brownsell, S. Telerehabilitation: Enabling the remote delivery of healthcare, rehabilitation, and self management. *Stud. Health Technol. Inform.* **2009**, *145*, 231–248. [PubMed]
3. Kairy, D.; Lehoux, P.; Vincent, C.; Visintin, M. A systematic review of clinical outcomes, clinical process, healthcare utilization and costs associated with telerehabilitation. *Disabil. Rehabil.* **2009**, *31*, 427–447. [CrossRef] [PubMed]
4. Giggins, O.M.; Persson, U.; Caulfield, B. Biofeedback in rehabilitation. *J. NeuroEng. Rehabil.* **2013**, *10*, 60. [CrossRef] [PubMed]
5. Chughtai, M.; Kelly, J.J.; Newman, J.M.; Sultan, A.A.; Khlopas, A.; Sodhi, N.; Bhave, A.; Kolczun, M.; Mont, M.A. The Role of Virtual Rehabilitation in Total and Unicompartmental Knee Arthroplasty. *J. Knee Surg.* **2019**, *32*, 105–110. [CrossRef] [PubMed]
6. Smittenaar, P.; Erhart-Hledik, J.C.; Kinsella, R.; Hunter, S.; Mecklenburg, G.; Perez, D. Translating Comprehensive Conservative Care for Chronic Knee Pain into a Digital Care Pathway: 12-Week and 6-Month Outcomes for the Hinge Health Program. *JMIR Rehabil. Assist. Technol.* **2017**, *4*, e4. [CrossRef] [PubMed]
7. Correia, F.D.; Nogueira, A.; Magalhães, I.; Guimarães, J.; Moreira, M.; Barradas, I.; Teixeira, L.; Tulha, J.; Seabra, R.; Lains, J.; et al. Home-based Rehabilitation with A Novel Digital Biofeedback System versus Conventional In-person Rehabilitation after Total Knee Replacement: A feasibility study. *Sci. Rep.* **2018**, *8*, 11299. [CrossRef] [PubMed]
8. Bergmann, J.H.M.; Anastasova-Ivanova, S.; Spulber, I.; Gulati, V.; Georgiou, P.; McGregor, A. An Attachable Clothing Sensor System for Measuring Knee Joint Angles. *IEEE Sens. J.* **2013**, *13*, 4090–4097. [CrossRef]
9. Burns, A.; Greene, B.R.; McGrath, M.J.; O'Shea, T.J.; Kuris, B.; Ayer, S.M.; Stroiescu, F.; Cionca, V. SHIMMERTM—A Wireless Sensor Platform for Noninvasive Biomedical Research. *IEEE Sens. J.* **2010**, *10*, 1527–1534. [CrossRef]

10. O'Reilly, M.; Caulfield, B.; Ward, T.; Johnston, W.; Doherty, C. Wearable Inertial Sensor Systems for Lower Limb Exercise Detection and Evaluation: A Systematic Review. *Sports Med.* **2018**, *48*, 1221–1246. [CrossRef]
11. Giggins, O.M.; Sweeney, K.T.; Caulfield, B. Rehabilitation exercise assessment using inertial sensors: A cross-sectional analytical study. *J. NeuroEng. Rehabil.* **2014**, *11*, 158. [CrossRef] [PubMed]
12. O'reilly, M.A.; Whelan, D.F.; Ward, T.E.; Delahunt, E.; Caulfield, B.M. Technology in Strength and Conditioning: Assessing Bodyweight Squat Technique with Wearable Sensors. *J. Strength Cond. Res.* **2017**, *31*, 2303–2312. [CrossRef] [PubMed]
13. O'Reilly, M.A.; Whelan, D.F.; Ward, T.E.; Delahunt, E.; Caulfield, B. Classification of lunge biomechanics with multiple and individual inertial measurement units. *Sports Biomech.* **2017**, *16*, 1–19. [CrossRef] [PubMed]
14. Bevilacqua, A.; Huang, B.; Argent, R.; Caulfield, B.; Kechadi, T. Automatic classification of knee rehabilitation exercises using a single inertial sensor: A case study. In Proceedings of the 2018 IEEE 15th International Conference on Wearable and Implantable Body Sensor Networks (BSN), Las Vegas, NV, USA, 4–7 March 2018; pp. 21–24.
15. Kurtz, S.; Ong, K.; Lau, E.; Mowat, F.; Halpern, M. Projections of Primary and Revision Hip and Knee Arthroplasty in the United States from 2005 to 2030. *J. Bone Joint Surg. Am. Vol.* **2007**, *89*, 780–785.
16. Perry, M.A.; Hudson, H.S.; Meys, S.; Norrie, O.; Ralph, T.; Warner, S. Older adults' experiences regarding discharge from hospital following orthopaedic intervention: A metasynthesis. *Disabil. Rehabil.* **2011**, *34*, 267–278. [CrossRef] [PubMed]
17. Zapata, B.C.; Fernández-Alemán, J.L.; Idri, A.; Toval, A. Empirical Studies on Usability of mHealth Apps: A Systematic Literature Review. *J. Med. Syst.* **2015**, *39*, 1–19. [CrossRef] [PubMed]
18. Peake, J.M.; Kerr, G.; Sullivan, J.P. A Critical Review of Consumer Wearables, Mobile Applications, and Equipment for Providing Biofeedback, Monitoring Stress, and Sleep in Physically Active Populations. *Front. Physiol.* **2018**, *9*, 743. [CrossRef] [PubMed]
19. Michie, S.; Yardley, L.; West, R.; Patrick, K.; Greaves, F. Developing and Evaluating Digital Interventions to Promote Behavior Change in Health and Health Care: Recommendations Resulting from an International Workshop. *J. Med. Internet Res.* **2017**, *19*, e232. [CrossRef] [PubMed]
20. Bergmann, J.H.M.; McGregor, A.H. Body-Worn Sensor Design: What Do Patients and Clinicians Want? *Ann. Biomed. Eng.* **2011**, *39*, 2299–2312. [CrossRef] [PubMed]
21. Nicolson, P.J.; Hinman, R.S.; French, S.D.; Lonsdale, C.; Bennell, K.L. Improving adherence to exercise: Do people with knee osteoarthritis and physical therapists agree on the behavioural approaches likely to succeed? *Arthr. Care Res. Hoboken* **2018**, *70*, 388–397. [CrossRef]
22. Argent, R.; Daly, A.; Caulfield, B. Patient Involvement with Home-Based Exercise Programs: Can Connected Health Interventions Influence Adherence? *JMIR mHealth uHealth* **2018**, *6*, e47. [CrossRef]
23. Argent, R.; Slevin, P.; Bevilacqua, A.; Neligan, M.; Daly, A.; Caulfield, B. Clinician perceptions of a prototype wearable exercise biofeedback system for orthopaedic rehabilitation: A qualitative exploration. *BMJ Open* **2018**, *8*, e026326. [CrossRef] [PubMed]
24. Dowsey, M.M.; Choong, P.F.M. The Utility of Outcome Measures in Total Knee Replacement Surgery. *Int. J. Rheumatol.* **2013**, *2013*, 1–8. [CrossRef] [PubMed]
25. O'Reilly, M.A.; Slevin, P.; Ward, T.; Caulfield, B. A Wearable Sensor-Based Exercise Biofeedback System: Mixed Methods Evaluation of Formulift. *JMIR mHealth uHealth* **2018**, *6*, e33. [CrossRef] [PubMed]
26. Gutmann, J. Qualitative research practice: A guide for social science students and researchers (2nd edition). *Int. J. Mark. Res.* **2014**, *56*, 407. [CrossRef]
27. Brooke, J. SUS: A 'quick and dirty' usability scale. In *Usability Evaluation in Industry*; Jordan, P., Thomas, B., McClelland, I., Weerdmeester, B., Eds.; Taylor and Francis: London, UK, 1996; pp. 189–194.
28. Stoyanov, S.R.; Hides, L.; Kavanagh, D.J.; Wilson, H. Development and Validation of the User Version of the Mobile Application Rating Scale (uMARS). *JMIR mHealth uHealth* **2016**, *4*, e72. [CrossRef]
29. Bangor, A.; Kortum, P.T.; Miller, J.T. An Empirical Evaluation of the System Usability Scale. *Int. J. Hum.-Comput. Interact.* **2008**, *24*, 574–594. [CrossRef]
30. Bangor, A.; Kortum, P.; Miller, J. Determining what individual SUS scores mean: Adding an adjective rating scale. *J. Usability Stud.* **2009**, *4*, 114–123.
31. Stoyanov, S.; Hides, L.; Kavanagh, D.J.; Zelenko, O.; Tjondronegoro, D.; Mani, M. Mobile App Rating Scale: A New Tool for Assessing the Quality of Health Mobile Apps. *JMIR mHealth uHealth* **2015**, *3*, 27. [CrossRef]

32. Fereday, J.; Muir-Cochrane, E. Demonstrating Rigor Using Thematic Analysis: A Hybrid Approach of Inductive and Deductive Coding and Theme Development. *Int. J. Qual. Methods* **2006**, *5*, 80–92. [CrossRef]
33. Boeije, H. A Purposeful Approach to the Constant Comparative Method in the Analysis of Qualitative Interviews. *Qual. Quant.* **2002**, *36*, 391–409. [CrossRef]
34. Papi, E.; Belsi, A.; McGregor, A.H. A knee monitoring device and the preferences of patients living with osteoarthritis: A qualitative study. *BMJ Open* **2015**, *5*, 007980. [CrossRef] [PubMed]
35. International Organization for Standardization. *ISO 9241-11 Ergonomics of Human-System Interaction-Part 11: Usability: Definitions and Concepts*; Ergonomics of Human-System Interaction: Geneva, Switzerland, 2018.
36. Jack, K.; McLean, S.M.; Moffett, J.K.; Gardiner, E. Barriers to treatment adherence in physiotherapy outpatient clinics: A systematic review. *Man. Ther.* **2010**, *15*, 220–228. [CrossRef] [PubMed]
37. Alexandre, N.M.C.; Nordin, M.; Hiebert, R.; Campello, M. Predictors of compliance with short-term treatment among patients with back pain. *Rev. Panam. Salud Publica* **2002**, *12*, 86–95. [CrossRef] [PubMed]
38. Peek, K.; Sanson-Fisher, R.; MacKenzie, L.; Carey, M.; Information, P.E.K.F.C. Interventions to aid patient adherence to physiotherapist prescribed self-management strategies: A systematic review. *Physiotherapy* **2016**, *102*, 127–135. [CrossRef] [PubMed]
39. Bollen, J.; Dean, S.G.; Siegert, R.J.; Howe, T.E.; Goodwin, V.A.; Nepogodiev, D.; Chapman, S.J.; Glasbey, J.C.D.; Kelly, M.; Khatri, C.; et al. A systematic review of measures of self-reported adherence to unsupervised home-based rehabilitation exercise programmes, and their psychometric properties. *BMJ Open* **2014**, *4*, 005044. [CrossRef] [PubMed]
40. Van Gool, C.H.; Penninx, B.W.J.H.; Kempen, G.I.J.M.; Rejeski, W.J.; Miller, G.D.; Van Eijk, J.T.M.; Pahor, M.; Messier, S.P. Effects of exercise adherence on physical function among overweight older adults with knee osteoarthritis. *Arthr. Rheum.* **2005**, *53*, 24–32. [CrossRef] [PubMed]
41. Beyer, H.R.; Laplante, P.A. *User-Centered Design*; Informa UK Limited: London, UK, 2010; pp. 1308–1317.
42. Steele, R.; Lo, A.; Secombe, C.; Wong, Y.K. Elderly persons' perception and acceptance of using wireless sensor networks to assist healthcare. *Int. J. Med. Inform.* **2009**, *78*, 788–801. [CrossRef]
43. Blyth, F.M.; March, L.M.; Nicholas, M.K.; Cousins, M.J. Self-management of chronic pain: A population-based study. *PAIN* **2005**, *113*, 285–292. [CrossRef]
44. Power, C.; Matthews, S. Origins of health inequalities in a national population sample. *Lancet* **1997**, *350*, 1584–1589. [CrossRef]

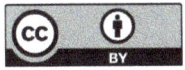 © 2019 by the authors. Licensee MDPI, Basel, Switzerland. This article is an open access article distributed under the terms and conditions of the Creative Commons Attribution (CC BY) license (http://creativecommons.org/licenses/by/4.0/).

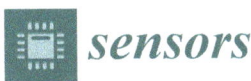

Article

Feature Extraction and Similarity of Movement Detection during Sleep, Based on Higher Order Spectra and Entropy of the Actigraphy Signal: Results of the Hispanic Community Health Study/Study of Latinos

Miguel Enrique Iglesias Martínez [1], Juan M. García-Gomez [2,*], Carlos Sáez [2], Pedro Fernández de Córdoba [3] and J. Alberto Conejero [3]

1. Departamento de Telecomunicaciones, Universidad de Pinar del Río, Pinar del Río, Cuba, Martí #270, CP: 20100; Instituto Universitario de Matemática Pura y Aplicada, Universitat Politècnica de València (UPV), Camino de Vera s/n, 46022 Valencia, España; migueliglesias2010@gmail.com
2. Biomedical Data Science Lab (BDSLab), Instituto Universitario de Tecnologías de la Información y Comunicaciones (ITACA), Universitat Politècnica de València (UPV), Camino de Vera s/n, 46022 Valencia, España; carsaesi@ibime.upv.es
3. Instituto Universitario de Matemática Pura y Aplicada, Universitat Politècnica de València (UPV), Camino de Vera s/n, 46022 Valencia, España; pfernand@mat.upv.es (P.F.d.C.); aconejero@upv.es (J.A.C.)
* Correspondence: juanmig@ibime.upv.es; Tel.: +34-963-877-000 (ext. 75278)

Received: 19 October 2018; Accepted: 30 November 2018; Published: 6 December 2018

Abstract: The aim of this work was to develop a new unsupervised exploratory method of characterizing feature extraction and detecting similarity of movement during sleep through actigraphy signals. We here propose some algorithms, based on signal bispectrum and bispectral entropy, to determine the unique features of independent actigraphy signals. Experiments were carried out on 20 randomly chosen actigraphy samples of the Hispanic Community Health Study/Study of Latinos (HCHS/SOL) database, with no information other than their aperiodicity. The Pearson correlation coefficient matrix and the histogram correlation matrix were computed to study the similarity of movements during sleep. The results obtained allowed us to explore the connections between certain sleep actigraphy patterns and certain pathologies.

Keywords: actigraphy; bispectrum; entropy; feature extraction

1. Introduction

Actigraphy is now being increasingly used to explore sleep patterns in sleep laboratories. Its main advantages include its easy setup, its low cost, and the fact that prolonged records can be obtained over time, permitting patient activity in ambulatory conditions without interfering with their daily routines. It is considered to be a valuable tool for controlling and monitoring circadian alterations and insomnia, as well as avoiding false positives in the assessment of daytime sleepiness tests, such as the multiple sleep latency test, and the wakefulness maintenance test [1–5].

Many recent studies have validated the practice of actigraphy, for example, in [6] several wrist-worn sleep assessments, actigraphy devices were compared. A relationship has been found between sleep disorders and their effects on certain conditions, such as hypertension and obesity [7], and it is now even possible to analyze sleep depth by actigraphy signals [8].

A review of the current state of higher-order statistics (HOS) and their use in biosignal analysis can be found in [9]. As most of the biomedical signals are non-linear, non-stationary, and non-Gaussian in nature, iHOS (Higher Order Statistics) analysis is preferable to second-order correlations and power spectra [9]. On this issue, several studies, such as [10] have been published on the screening of pediatric sleep apnea–hypopnea syndrome, and the automated classification of glaucoma stages in [11].

Concerning the detection of similarity of movements, in [12,13] although classification patterns were obtained from sleep/awake states according to the characteristics of the actigraphy signal, they were not based on higher order spectra. In fact, the common approach is to analyze individual actigraphy records over several days, so that the studies cited above were not focused on the analysis of the activity signal as a random process that is dependent on the movement of a certain part of the body.

The present work is based on the bispectral analysis of actigraphy signals and their relationship with bispectral entropy. The increase of movements as a form of feature extraction measurement, and the detection of similarities of movements during sleep are shown as features to be considered. The results obtained indicate the potential of this approach for the study of sleep disorders, and their connection with other conditions. The work is organized as follows: Materials and Methods are described in Section 2, the results are given in Section 3, the Discussion in Section 4, and the Conclusions and future work are outlined in Section 5.

2. Materials and Methods

2.1. Data Acquisition

The experiments were carried out on 20 samples of actigraphy signals obtained from the Hispanic Community Health Study/Study of Latinos (HCHS/SOL) Database [14–17] chosen at random, through the use of the "randi" Matlab function. The Sueño Ancillary Study recruited 2252 HCHS/SOL participants to wear wrist-worn actigraphy devices (Actiwatch Spectrum, Philips Respironics, Royal Philips, Netherlands,) between 2010 and 2013. The participants were instructed to wear the watch for a week. Records were scored by a trained technician of the Boston Sleep Reading Center [17].

2.2. Methods

Actigraphy signals have a random nature that can be visualized in terms of uniformity in the bispectrum. This uniformity depends on the non-impulsive characteristics of the signal, which are reflected in the spectrum as frequency peaks. Since the bispectrum is a function that presents unique characteristics for each signal in terms of frequency and phase it can easily be seen in a graph. This led us to explore an entire methodology based on calculating the bispectrum and the bispectral entropy, which would be able to detect similar characteristics in movement patterns during sleep. Twenty cases of actigraphy signals were analyzed to extract their characteristics, which were then used to determine similarities and differences among the signals.

The activity signals were first normalized to 1, and then segmented to determine the subjects' daily activity record. The bispectrum of the total sample of the activity signal recorded was seven days. The experiments were conducted on two age groups between 18 and 44 years old, and 45 and 64 years old.

2.3. Theoretical Foundations: Bispectrum

Let $\{x(n)\}_n$, $n = 0, \pm 1, \pm 2, \ldots$ be a stationary random vector, and let us also suppose that we can compute its higher order moments [18,19], where:

$$m_k^x(\tau_1, \tau_2, \ldots, \tau_{k-1}) = E(x(n) \cdot x(n + \tau_1) \ldots x(n + \tau_{k-1})) \tag{1}$$

represents the moment of order k of that vector. This moment only depends on the different time slots $\tau_1, \ldots, \tau_{k-1}$ where $\tau_i = 0, \pm 1, \ldots$ for all i. The cumulants are similar to the moments, but the difference is that the moments of a random process are derived from the characteristic function of the random variable, while the cumulant generating function is defined as the logarithm of the characteristic function of that random variable. The k-th order cumulant of a stationary random process $\{x(n)\}_n$ can be written as [20]:

$$c_k^x(\tau_1, \tau_2, \ldots, \tau_{k-1}) = m_k^x(\tau_1, \tau_2, \ldots, \tau_{k-1}) - m_k^G(\tau_1, \tau_2, \ldots, \tau_{k-1}), \quad (2)$$

where $m_k^G(\tau_1, \tau_2, \ldots, \tau_{k-1})$ is the k-th order moment of a process with an equivalent Gaussian distribution that presents the same mean value and autocorrelation function as the vector $\{x(n)\}_n$.

It is evident from (2) that a process following a Gaussian distribution has null cumulants for orders greater than 2, since $m_k^x(\tau_1, \tau_2, \ldots, \tau_{k-1}) = m_k^G(\tau_1, \tau_2, \ldots, \tau_{k-1})$, and so that $c_k^x(\tau_1, \tau_2, \ldots, \tau_{k-1}) = 0$ [20,21].

In practice, we estimate cumulants and polyspectra from a finite amount of data $\{x(n)\}_{n=0}^{N-1}$. These estimates are also random and are characterized by their bias and variance [22]. Let $\{x(n)\}_n$. denote a zero mean stationary process; we assume that all relevant statistics exist, and that they have finite values. The third order cumulant sample estimate is given by [21]:

$$C_3(\tau_1, \tau_2) = \frac{1}{N} \sum_{n=N_1}^{N_2} x(n) \cdot x(n+\tau_1) \cdot x(n+\tau_2) \quad (3)$$

where N_1 y and N_2 are chosen such that the sums only involve $x(n)$ for $n = 0, \ldots, N-1$, N being the number of samples in the cumulant region. Likewise, the bispectrum estimation is defined as the Fourier Transform of the third-order cumulant sequence [22]:

$$B_x^N(f_1, f_2) = \sum_{\tau_1=-N-1}^{N-1} \sum_{\tau_2=-N-1}^{N-1} C_3(\tau_1, \tau_2) \cdot e^{-2\pi f_1 \tau_1} \cdot e^{-2\pi f_2 \tau_2} = \frac{1}{N^2} X^*(f_1+f_2) \cdot X(f_1) \cdot X(f_2) \quad (4)$$

where f_1 and f_2 are the spectral frequency vectors of the sequence $\{x(n)\}_{n=0}^{N-1}$, and $X(f_i)$, $i = 1, 2$, is its Fourier Transform.

2.4. Bispectral Entropy Analysis

Entropy provides a measure for quantifying the information content of a random variable in terms of the minimum number of bits per symbol that are required to encode the variable. It is an indicator of the amount of randomness or uncertainty of a discrete random process [23]. Consider a random variable Z with M states $z_1, z_2, \ldots z_M$, and state probabilities $p_1, p_2, \ldots p_M$, that is, $P(Z = z_i) = p_i$, the entropy of Z is defined as:

$$H(Z) = -\sum_{i=1}^{M} p_i \log_2(p_i) \quad (5)$$

The entropy of a discrete-valued random variable attains a maximum value for a uniformly distributed variable. In order to extend this notion from the spatial to the frequency domain, we introduce bispectral entropy as a way of measuring the uniformity of the spectrum [21]. The bispectral entropy is defined as:

$$E_{bx}^N(f_1, f_2) = -\sum_{\tau_1=-N-1}^{N-1} \sum_{\tau_2=-N-1}^{N-1} P_x^N(f_1, f_2) \cdot \log_2 P_x^N(f_1, f_2) \quad (6)$$

where the energy probability is computed in terms of the bispectrum estimation:

$$P_x^N(f_1, f_2) = \frac{B_x^N(f_1, f_2)}{\sum_{\tau_1=-N-1}^{N-1} \sum_{\tau_2=-N-1}^{N-1} B_x^N(f_1, f_2)} \quad (7)$$

3. Results

The actigraphy signals that measured the movements of individuals while sleeping were analyzed. These movements have an intrinsically random nature, since they can occur with non-specific probabilities and durations. This can be checked by analyzing the frequency spectrum of the activity signal and comparing it with a noise pattern. The probabilistic distribution function of the spectral pattern depends on the nature and uniformity of the movements, which may follow a normal distribution or another, such as a uniform distribution, depending on the random nature of the process.

3.1. Application of the Bispectrum to the Actigraphy Signal

A spectral analysis based on the one-dimensional Fourier transform is not recommended for the detection of traits in a random signal, such as the actigraphy signal. For these, this analysis only provides information relative to the magnitude-frequency or phase-frequency distribution. In other words, what is visualized in the spectrum is noise, which in our case, is in fact the useful information from which certain characteristics and features have to be extracted. The frequency spectrum of two actigraphy signals is shown in Figure 1, where it can be seen that the one-dimensional Fourier Transform is not able to identify the discriminant features in this type of signal.

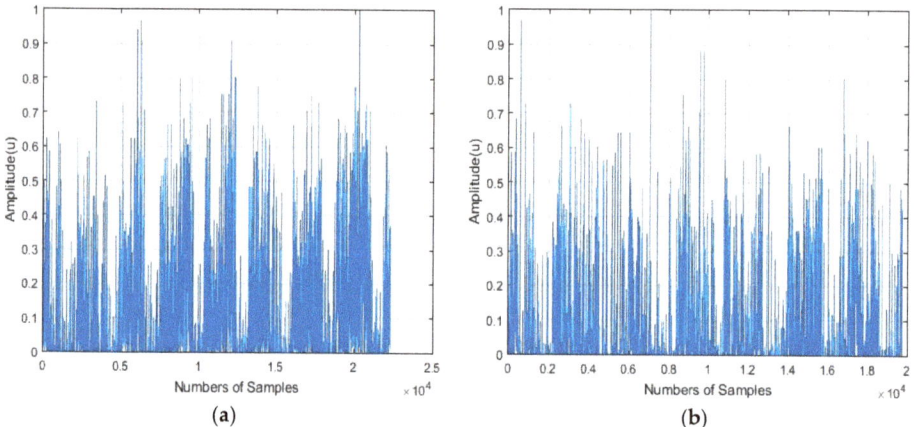

Figure 1. Ilustration of: (**a**,**b**) Examples of the frequency spectrum of two actigraphy signals obtained from their respective one-dimensional Fourier transforms.

Unlike the one-dimensional frequency spectrum, the bispectrum of an activity signal can provide information on the spatial distribution of the amplitude, and on the frequency components (see Equation (4)). This information can be represented in a matrix that can be used to obtain the particular identification features of each signal. The bispectrum of the actigraphy signal was simulated in MatLab, using the Higher Order Spectra Analysis toolbox. Figures 2 and 3 show the contours of the bispectrum surface of the actigraphy signal, where f1 and f2 are the normalized spectral frequency vectors generated from the calculation of the bidimensional Fourier Transform.

We found that the bispectrum can indicate variables that measure specific characteristics of the movement during sleep, based on the uniformity of the activity data and the disorder of the sample. Here, a greater frequency disorder at a bispectral level may imply an excess of movement during the analyzed period, which can even be an identifying feature of sleep, and be linked to patients. For the sake of completeness, we can see in Figures 2–5 that the bispectrum is a unique variable for each actigraphy signal.

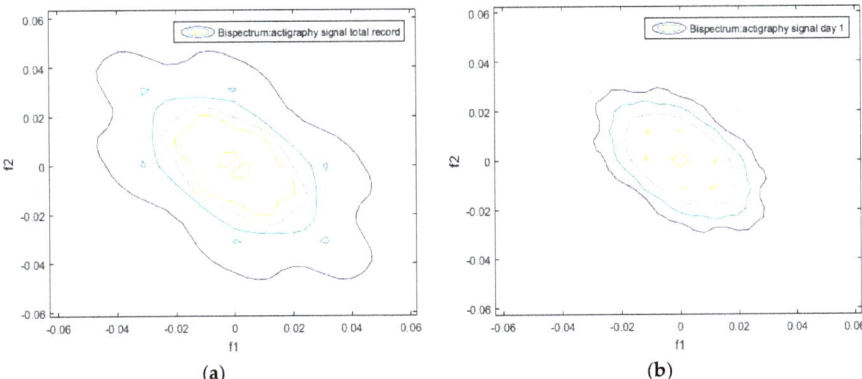

Figure 2. (a) Bispectrum of the activity record over seven days, and (b) bispectrum of the activity record on day 1 of the actigraphy data sample hchs-sol-sueno-00163225.

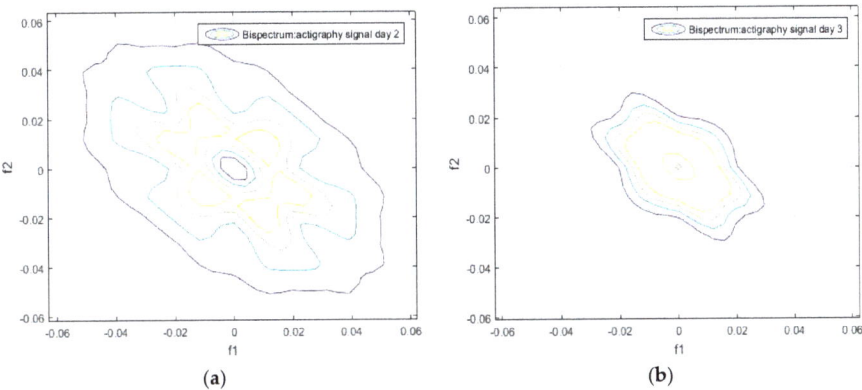

Figure 3. (a) Bispectrum of the activity record on day 2, and of (b) bispectrum of the activity record on day 3 of the actigraphy data sample hchs-sol-sueno-00163225.

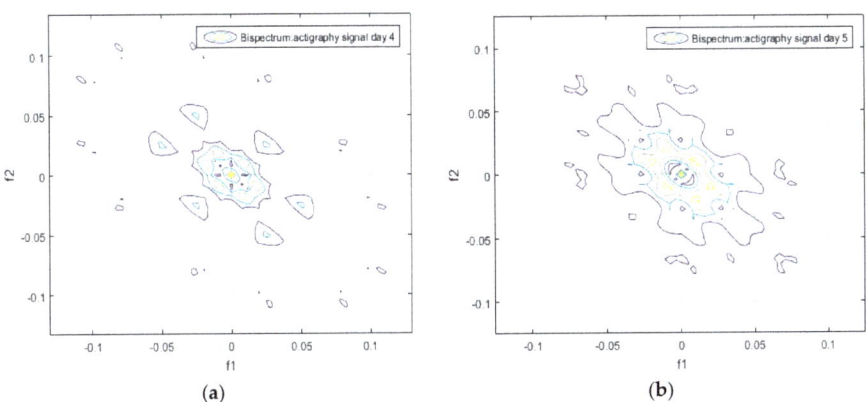

Figure 4. (a) Bispectrum of the activity record on day 4, and (b) bispectrum of the activity record on day 5 of the actigraphy data sample hchs-sol-sueno-00163225.

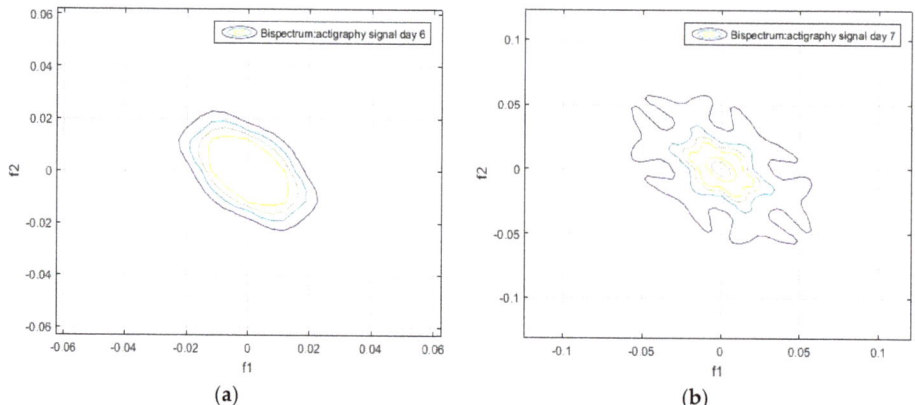

Figure 5. (a) Bispectrum of the activity record on day 6, and (b) bispectrum of the activity record on day 7 of the actigraphy data sample hchs-sol-sueno-00163225.

It can also be seen that the daily bispectrum registrations are all different from each other, showing that all these registers form an identification pattern, which we have named the bispectral pattern of the activity signal.

A bispectrum analysis was performed on 20 different activity signal records. We tried to identify each one with a specific spectral sleep pattern per day, and to find a possible relationship between an individual's movement patterns during sleep. The results obtained are shown in Figures 6–8, which give the bispectrum of the actigraphy signal for the first 10 of the 20 analyzed actigraphy signals from the HCHS/SOL database.

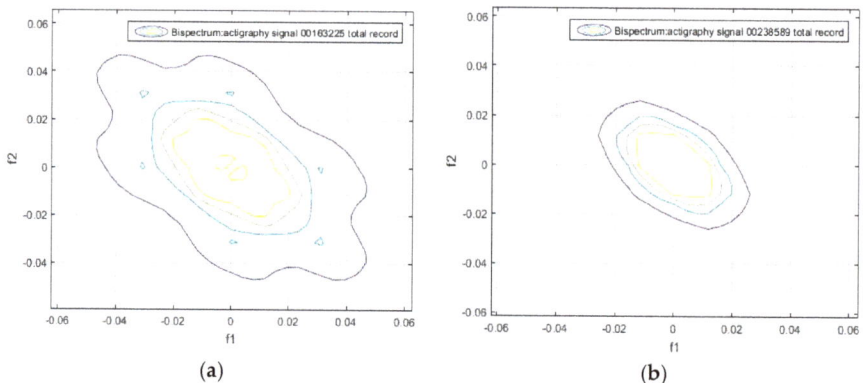

Figure 6. Bispectrum obtained from the 7-day activity record of the samples (a) hchs-sol-sueno-00163225 and (b) hchs-sol-sueno-00238589.

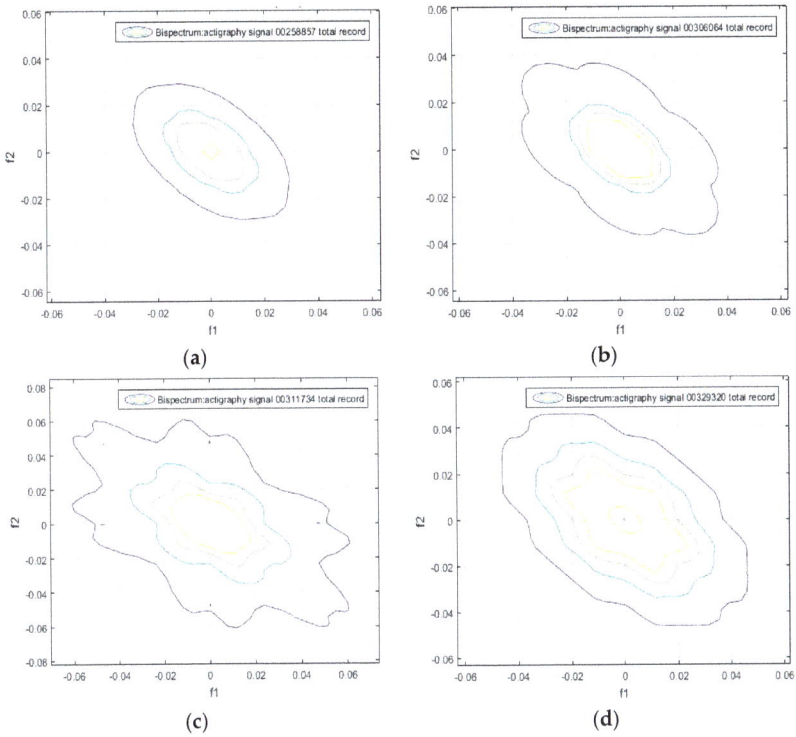

Figure 7. Bispectrum obtained from the 7-day activity record of the samples (**a**) hchs-sol-sueno-00258857, (**b**) hchs-sol-sueno-00306064, (**c**) hchs-sol-sueno-00311734, and (**d**) hchs-sol-sueno-00329320.

It can be seen that there are unique identifiable characteristic features that can be used to obtain patterns of movement during sleep. For instance, Figures 5–8 have similar contours. This means individuals can be divided into groups according to the similarity of their sleep patterns.

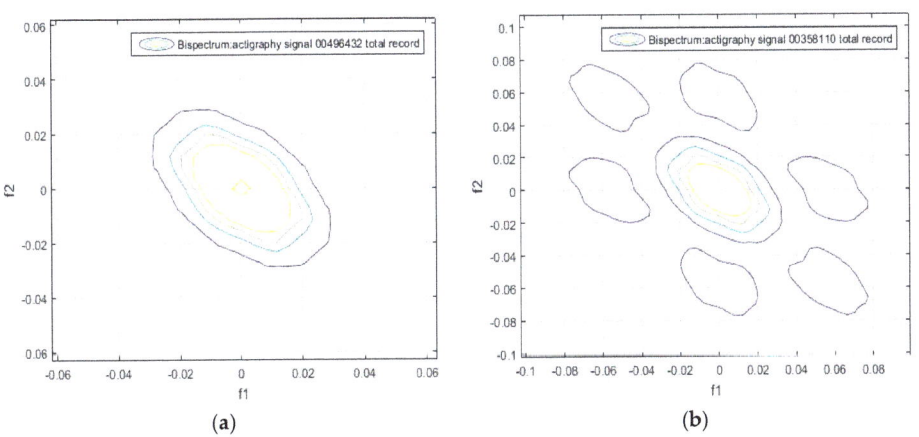

Figure 8. *Cont.*

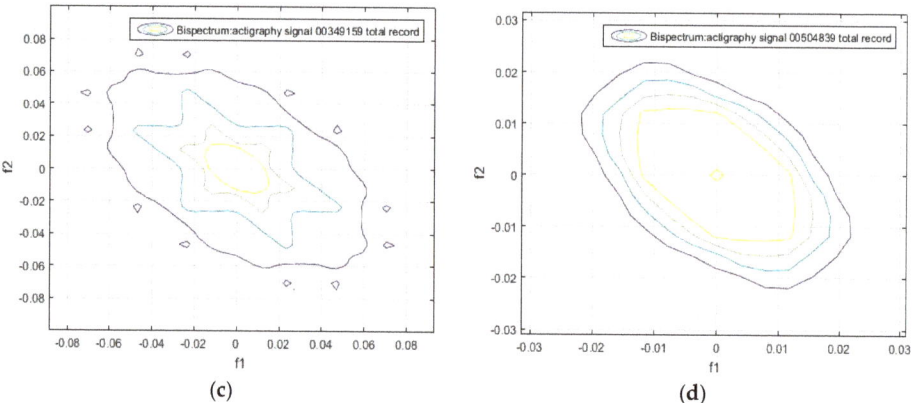

Figure 8. Bispectrum obtained from the 7-day activity record of the samples (**a**) hchs-sol-sueno-00349159 (**b**) hchs-sol-sueno-00358110 (**c**) hchs-sol-sueno-00496432 (**d**) hchs-sol-sueno-00504839.

To further illustrate these results, we correlated the bispectrum of the seven days of signals by computing the Pearson correlation coefficients for every pair of samples to find similarities between the two signals. The results are given in the correlation matrix R in Table 1. For example, R_{1-2} is the Pearson correlation coefficient between the bispectrum of samples 1 and 2 from hchs-sol-sueno-00163225 and hchs-sol-sueno-00238589.

In order to determine subgroups in the set of samples, and to identify the pairs of signals that give correlation values closest to 1, we selected the pairs with correlation values of greater than 0.97. This was done to satisfy the hypothesis of the similarity of the sleep movement patterns of two signals, since there must be as few differences as possible, and therefore, also minimal differences in their bispectral patterns. The results of similar pairs are shown in black in Figure 9, in which the values with the lowest correlation are indicated with red dashed lines to show different activity patterns. For this latter case, we considered values of below 0.8. Although these values are relatively high in comparison with other applications, we have considered its use for the search of dissimilar sleep patterns.

Table 1. Correlation matrix obtained from the analysis of the bispectrum comparison of the 7-day activity signal for the 20 Hispanic Community Health Study/Study of Latinos (HCHS/SOL) database samples analyzed.

0.898	0.944	0.934	0.965	0.957	0.899	0.899	0.947	0.825	0.966	0.976	0.971	0.950	0.979	0.911	0.972	0.970	0.973	0.945
0.961	0.935	0.875	0.881	0.767	0.860	0.957	0.981	0.823	0.935	0.953	0.949	0.869	0.991	0.884	0.876	0.923	0.919	-
0.965	0.944	0.914	0.837	0.911	0.961	0.909	0.892	0.970	0.976	0.970	0.917	0.970	0.937	0.925	0.959	0.933	-	-
0.931	0.886	0.860	0.899	0.949	0.887	0.886	0.949	0.954	0.950	0.895	0.945	0.920	0.916	0.936	0.885	-	-	-
0.938	0.914	0.926	0.927	0.809	0.962	0.969	0.951	0.945	0.949	0.890	0.973	0.965	0.967	0.913	-	-	-	-
0.847	0.832	0.899	0.817	0.948	0.951	0.936	0.915	0.971	0.896	0.974	0.926	0.945	0.972	-	-	-	-	-
0.849	0.844	0.688	0.889	0.892	0.854	0.864	0.870	0.773	0.889	0.888	0.863	0.799	-	-	-	-	-	-
0.908	0.799	0.887	0.929	0.911	0.904	0.862	0.867	0.881	0.921	0.920	0.849	-	-	-	-	-	-	-
0.913	0.891	0.957	0.976	0.956	0.913	0.965	0.912	0.921	0.955	0.926	-	-	-	-	-	-	-	-
0.739	0.871	0.898	0.905	0.791	0.966	0.819	0.810	0.861	0.860	-	-	-	-	-	-	-	-	-
0.946	0.924	0.892	0.964	0.841	0.960	0.960	0.941	0.922	-	-	-	-	-	-	-	-	-	-
0.977	0.964	0.958	0.942	0.964	0.963	0.976	0.953	-	-	-	-	-	-	-	-	-	-	-
0.975	0.953	0.966	0.957	0.954	0.981	0.949	-	-	-	-	-	-	-	-	-	-	-	-
0.921	0.954	0.952	0.944	0.970	0.906	-	-	-	-	-	-	-	-	-	-	-	-	-
0.888	0.970	0.961	0.960	0.957	-	-	-	-	-	-	-	-	-	-	-	-	-	-
0.899	0.886	0.937	0.931	-	-	-	-	-	-	-	-	-	-	-	-	-	-	-
0.962	0.971	0.937	-	-	-	-	-	-	-	-	-	-	-	-	-	-	-	-
0.967	0.912	-	-	-	-	-	-	-	-	-	-	-	-	-	-	-	-	-
0.938	-	-	-	-	-	-	-	-	-	-	-	-	-	-	-	-	-	-

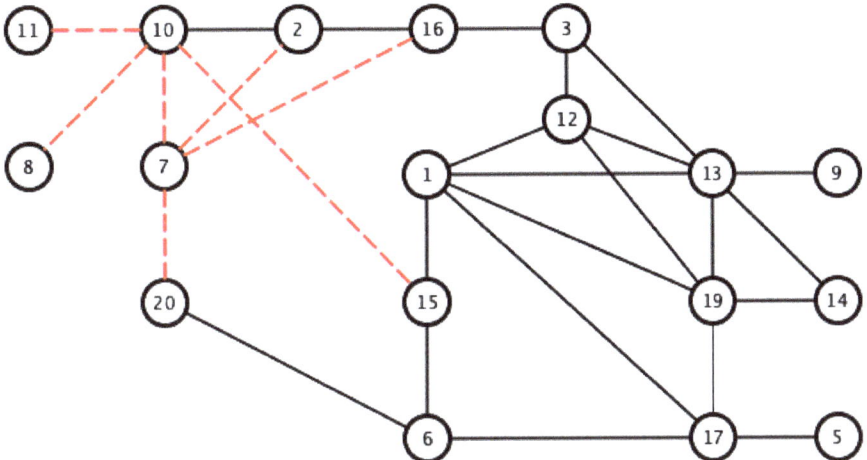

Figure 9. Visualization of pairs with Pearson correlation coefficients greater than 0.97 (black line) and lower than 0.8 (red dashed line).

The correlation values given in Table 1 and Figure 9 show that there may be a similarity in sleep movement patterns. In Table 1, the maximum distance value is 0.3122 and the minimum is 10^{-6}, the mean is 0.0538, and the statistical mode (the most frequent value in an array) is 0.001. Figure 10 gives a comparative measurement of the values in Table 1 by rearranging the columns of the matrix into a vector, and considering it as a time series, in which the x-coordinate is the position in the vector and the y-coordinate, the corresponding value of the coefficient. In this arrangement, the groups indicate almost repetitive terms that represent signals with similar characteristics.

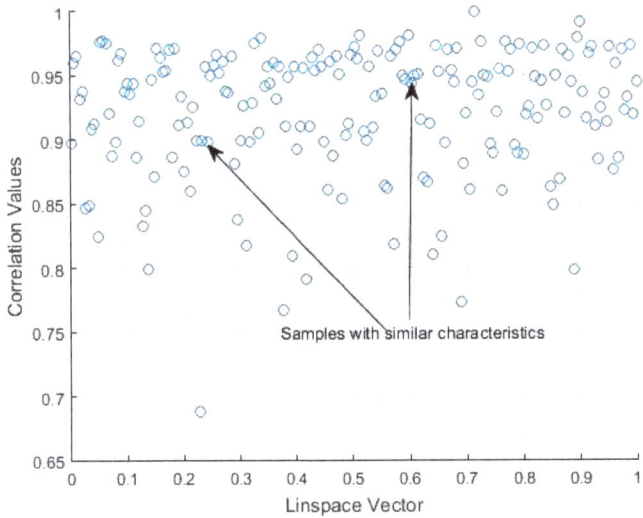

Figure 10. Scatter plot of the correlation matrix shown in Table 1.

In order to better distinguish the differences and similarities between the sleep signals, we performed another analysis using the bispectral entropy as the method of characterizing the disorder/uniformity of the processed signals.

3.2. Application of Bispectral Entropy as a Measure of Actigraphy Disorder

The experiment was based on a similarity analysis, analogous to that of the bispectrum. We calculated the bispectral entropy of each activity sample for the whole period of seven days, to obtain a measure of the degree of uniformity of the sleep movement pattern, taking the degree of randomness of the activity signal into account. We considered the maximum value of the bispectral entropy as a way of describing the degree of uniformity of a random process.

The bispectral entropy of the signals was computed in a minimum window of eight samples, to represent the temporal displacement index of the signals. The results obtained are shown in Figure 11, together with the mean value of the bispectral entropy of each actigraphy signal.

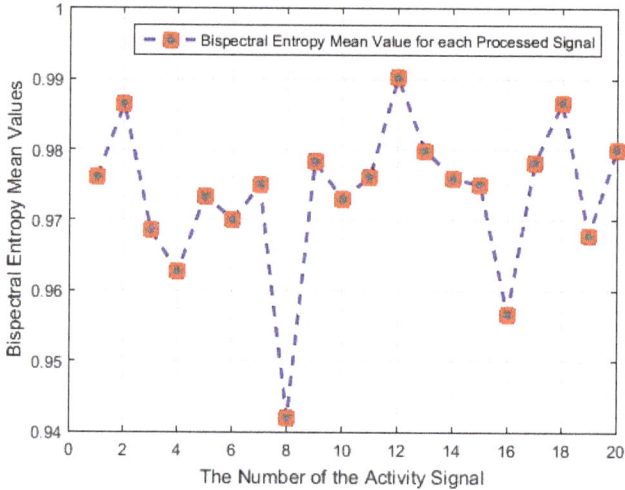

Figure 11. Mean bispectral entropy values of the 20 actigraphy signals considered.

It can be seen that signals 8 and 16 have the lowest bispectral entropy values, due to the non-uniformity of the bispectrum frequency distribution. This can also be identified in some of the previous graphs; for instance, in Figure 8b, the high-frequency components are characterized by the outer points (in blue), and the disconnected regions are the lowest frequency values.

In Figure 11 there are also samples with similar values of bispectral entropy of between 0.98 and 0.99, which indicates that they may be related to the hypothesis that activity samples with a similar correlation at the bispectral level may have the same level of uniformity of their value distributions. The opposite is also true with the minimum values of bispectral entropy, shown in Figure 11, as are those of samples 8, 10, 7, and 16, and other visible relationships, whose correlation values are under 0.8 in Table 2, and in Figure 11 are related to different uniformity patterns.

Given the analogy of the activity signal with the random process, the maximum entropy value would mean a greater uniformity of movement in the subject in the time interval studied, i.e., a high uniformity in the randomness of the movements. Conversely, occasional movements would be associated with impulsive noise, which has a non-uniform randomness, and thus, it would be associated with minimum entropy.

To also visualize the frequency of the maximum uniformity of sleep movements, histograms were made of the 7-day bispectral entropy of each activity signal. The frequencies of the entropy values for each processed sample are shown in Figures 12 and 13. These histograms provide information on the number of repetitions of the entropy values in each sample, i.e., the number of times the value in the data vector is repeated.

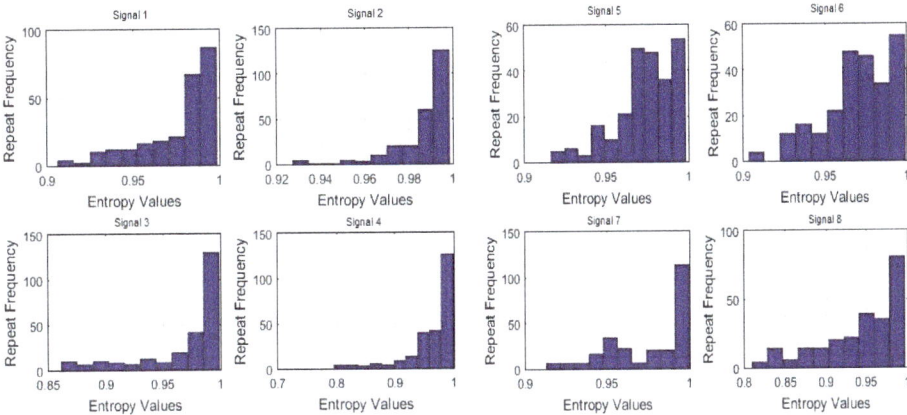

Figure 12. Histograms of the 7-day bispectral entropy of each activity signal (Signals 1 to 8, processed samples).

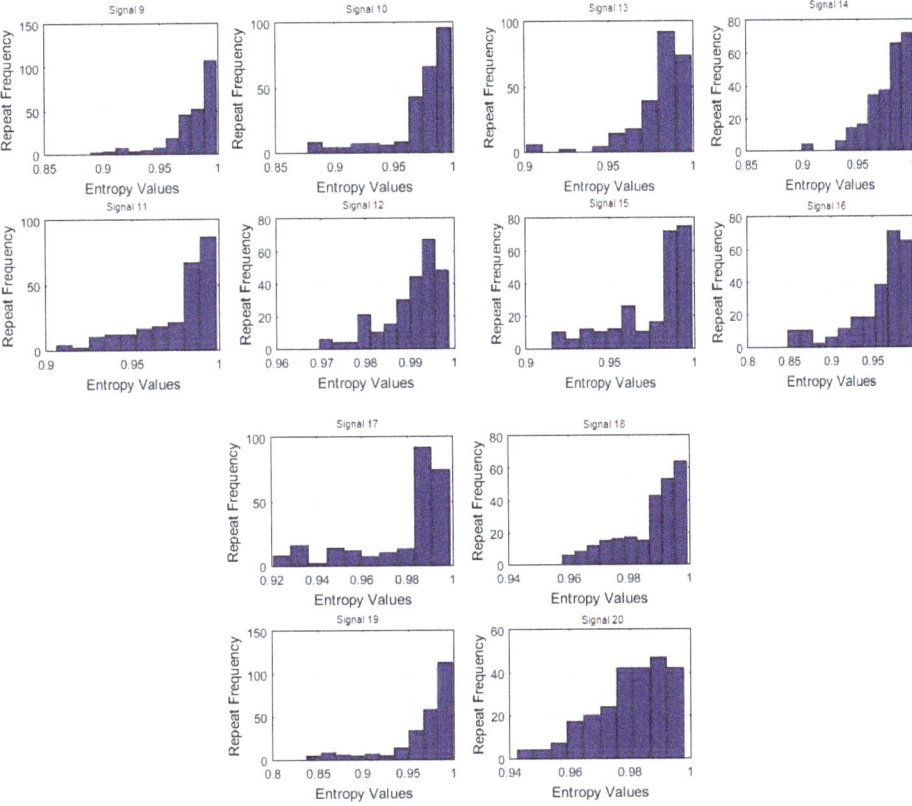

Figure 13. Histograms of the 7-day bispectral entropy of each activity signal (Signals 9 to 20, processed samples).

Although none of the histograms is repeated in Figures 12 and 13, some of them show certain similarities that could indicate similar sleep patterns. To verify this, the histograms were correlated to each other, with the criteria for the entropy values as well as for the data repetition frequency. The results are shown below in Table 2.

Table 2. Correlation matrix obtained from the analysis of the bispectral entropy histograms of the 20 analyzed samples from the HCHS/SOL database.

0.966	0.906	0.908	0.681	0.702	0.791	0.889	0.934	0.957	1.000	0.828	0.928	0.938	0.972	0.931	0.927	0.931	0.957	0.720	
0.976	0.973	0.699	0.714	0.880	0.944	0.967	0.948	0.966	0.725	0.842	0.893	0.906	0.865	0.841	0.889	0.985	0.650	-	
0.979	0.593	0.623	0.937	0.930	0.943	0.906	0.906	0.583	0.731	0.783	0.840	0.763	0.748	0.827	0.964	0.504	-	-	
0.715	0.732	0.913	0.979	0.985	0.945	0.908	0.677	0.780	0.845	0.824	0.818	0.740	0.894	0.983	0.621	-	-	-	
0.981	0.514	0.802	0.774	0.711	0.681	0.816	0.706	0.853	0.558	0.730	0.511	0.762	0.703	0.934	-	-	-	-	
0.553	0.805	0.790	0.715	0.702	0.793	0.697	0.848	0.575	0.708	0.490	0.773	0.713	0.926	-	-	-	-	-	
0.886	0.845	0.788	0.791	0.429	0.559	0.665	0.709	0.615	0.589	0.729	0.863	0.430	-	-	-	-	-	-	
0.975	0.929	0.889	0.731	0.786	0.874	0.798	0.834	0.717	0.913	0.958	0.720	-	-	-	-	-	-	-	
0.976	0.934	0.779	0.859	0.908	0.855	0.887	0.789	0.947	0.989	0.714	-	-	-	-	-	-	-	-	
0.957	0.840	0.927	0.925	0.912	0.947	0.878	0.975	0.980	0.708	-	-	-	-	-	-	-	-	-	
0.828	0.928	0.938	0.972	0.931	0.927	0.931	0.957	0.720	-	-	-	-	-	-	-	-	-	-	
0.937	0.932	0.796	0.928	0.825	0.898	0.756	0.910	-	-	-	-	-	-	-	-	-	-	-	
0.955	0.934	0.992	0.931	0.937	0.865	0.800	-	-	-	-	-	-	-	-	-	-	-	-	
0.889	0.962	0.863	0.939	0.897	0.899	-	-	-	-	-	-	-	-	-	-	-	-	-	
0.929	0.950	0.887	0.892	0.646	-	-	-	-	-	-	-	-	-	-	-	-	-	-	
0.924	0.954	0.892	0.802	-	-	-	-	-	-	-	-	-	-	-	-	-	-	-	
0.846	0.845	0.618	-	-	-	-	-	-	-	-	-	-	-	-	-	-	-	-	
0.932	0.801	-	-	-	-	-	-	-	-	-	-	-	-	-	-	-	-	-	
0.657	-	-	-	-	-	-	-	-	-	-	-	-	-	-	-	-	-	-	

Table 2 contains the results based on the histogram of the bispectral entropy of the activity signals to provide a criterion for the similarity of the data, based on the uniformity of the bispectrum. This table can be interpreted similarly to Table 1, which was based on the algorithm that describes the matrix correlation in Figure 9.

According to the previous analysis, the upper threshold was 0.97, and the lower threshold was a little lower than previously found. We considered 0.7 to distinguish between the similarities and clear differences among the signals (see Figure 14).

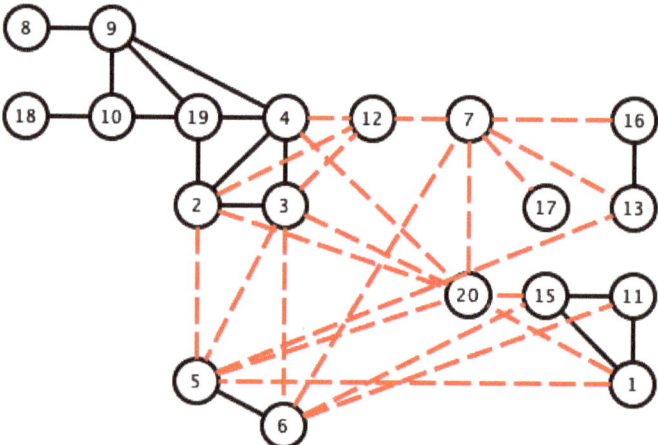

Figure 14. Visualization of pairs with Pearson correlation coefficients greater than 0.97 (black line) and lower than 0.7 (red dashed line).

It can thus be seen that several histograms are highly correlated, which indicates that this activity signal presents a high level of data uniformity, i.e., bispectral entropies with similar values, and also a high correlation value in terms of the bispectrum comparison. The dispersion graph of the correlation values obtained from Table 2 is shown in Figure 15. The data with similar values are seen to be grouped. The maximum value of the distance matrix is 0.6715, and the minimum is 10^{-5}. The mean value of the distance matrix was 0.1407, and the statistical mode was 10^{-5}, which indicates data groups with similar characteristics associated with the same type of movement, as can be seen in Figure 15.

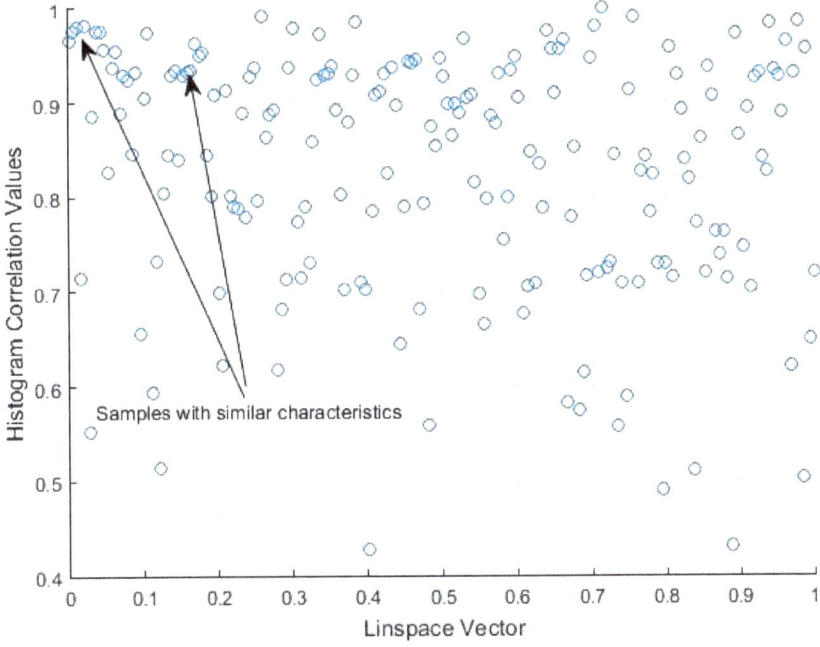

Figure 15. Scatter plot for the correlation matrix shown in Table 2.

4. Discussion

In order to associate the results with clinical diagnoses, several variables were taken from the HCHS/SOL database as the clinical characteristics of the 20 actigraphy samples. First, we considered the following variables:

CDCR_SUENO: self-report of cerebrovascular disease & carotid revascularization.
CHD_SELF_SUENO: combination of self-reports of coronary revascularization or heart attack.
DIABETES_SELF_SUENO: indicates a self-report of diabetes.
DIABETES _SUENO: indicates diabetes.
DM_AWARE_SUENO: describes the awareness of diabetes.
Hypertension_SUENO: indicates hypertension status.
STROKE_SUENO: checks for a self-report of stroke history.
STROKE_TIA_SUENO: checks for medical history of stroke, mini-stroke or TIA (transient ischemic attack).

These variables are of the 0/1 type, i.e., '0' for a negative response and '1' for a positive. Their values for the 20 individuals whose actigraphy signals were processed can be found in Table 3.

Table 3. Clinical characteristics of each individual analyzed for each actigraphy sample.

Samples	CDCR_SUENO	CHD_SELF_SUENO	DIABETES_SELF_SUENO	DIABETES_SUENO	DM_AWARE_SUENO	HYPERTENSION_SUENO	STROKE_SUENO	STROKE_TIA_SUENO
1	0	0	0	0	0	1	0	0
2	1	1	1	1	1	1	0	0
3	0	0	0	0	0	1	0	0
4	0	0	0	0	0	0	0	0
5	0	0	0	0	0	0	0	0
6	0	0	0	0	0	0	0	0
7	0	0	0	1	0	1	0	0
8	0	0	0	0	0	1	0	0
9	0	0	0	0	0	0	0	0
10	0	0	0	0	0	1	0	0
11	0	0	0	0	0	0	0	0
12	0	0	0	0	0	0	0	0
13	0	0	0	0	0	0	0	0
14	0	0	0	0	0	0	0	0
15	0	0	0	0	0	0	0	0
16	0	0	0	0	0	1	0	0
17	0	0	0	1	0	0	0	0
18	0	1	0	0	0	1	0	0
19	0	0	1	1	1	1	0	0
20	0	0	0	0	0	1	0	0

To relate the clinical characteristics of the patients with the obtained results, the correlation was first used, which is a measure of the similarity of data. We show these results, although the obtained correlations are weak, in part, for the limited number of signals used, and for the limitations of the information content embedded in the used signals database.

We opted to consider the HYPERTENSION_SUENO variable to study relationships within the actigraphy signals, since its value varies in several samples. First, we saw that 47.62% of the pairs whose bispectrum correlates with a value greater than 0.97 share the same clinical diagnosis. However, in Figure 9, it can be seen that the pairs with the same positive or negative diagnosis tend to cluster, which indicates a stronger hidden relationship that cannot be obtained by simply correlating the bispectrum of the signals (see Figure 16).

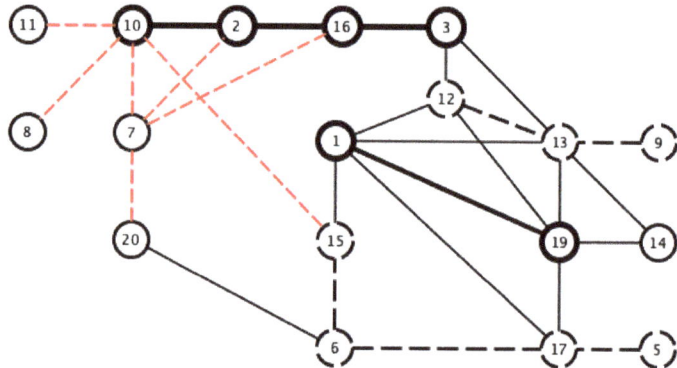

Figure 16. Pairs of bispectrum signals correlated with a coefficient that is greater than 0.97 (black lines) or lower than 0.7 (red dashed line). The thick black line indicates pairs that share a hypertension diagnosis, while the dashed black line indicates pairs in which neither has hypertension.

A similar effect was found in the comparison of the bispectral entropy histograms. Only 41.17% of the pairs correlated with a coefficient of 0.97 or higher present the same hypertension diagnoses. However, in the pairs with the same diagnosis in Figure 14 those sharing the hypertension diagnosis are seen to be connected (see Figure 17).

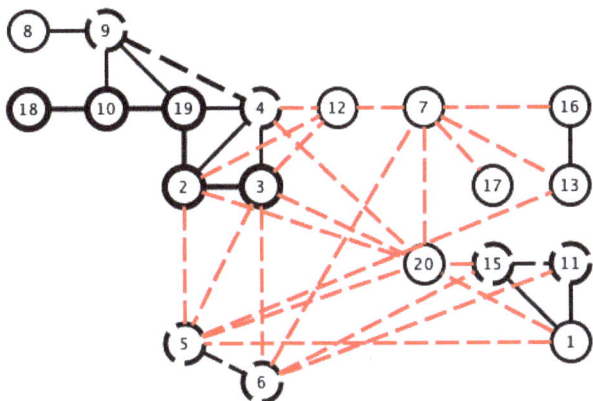

Figure 17. Pairs of bispectral entropy histograms correlated with a coefficient greater than 0.97 (black lines), and lower than 0.7 (red dashed line). The thick black line indicates pairs with a shared hypertension diagnosis, while the dashed black line indicates pairs in which neither has hypertension.

Although, the results shown in Figures 16 and 17 are not conclusive, they do suggest a further in-depth study of the characteristics of bispectrum signals that can contribute most to these similarities. It is also worth mentioning that the limited number of cases considered in this study advise a more systematic study of larger database samples.

5. Conclusions

This paper has shown that the application of higher-order statistical analysis to actigraphy signals can contribute to determining the traits and patterns of movement during sleep. These criteria can be based on part of the spatial information provided by the bispectrum and the bispectral entropy, both of which can help us to determine effective criteria for measuring the uniformity of data randomness.

The actigraphy signal experiments suggest the possible application of these criteria for the extraction and comparison of patterns of sleep movements. This would have a potential use in medicine, since similar pathologies may have similar associated movement patterns.

In future work we propose to use high-order statistical techniques, as for instance in [23]. We also want to experiment with data from chest actigraphy or other actigraphy signal measures, to corroborate the potential use of sleep actigraphy signals for purposes of diagnosis.

Our next step will be to increase the number of cases analyzed to cover the entire HCHS/SOL database, and also to experiment with other clinical characteristics in patients and pathologies associated with specific sleep disorders or brain-associated diseases.

Author Contributions: Conceptualization, M.E.I.M., J.M.G.-G., C.S., P.F.d.C., and J.A.C.; Methodology, M.E.I.M.; Software, M.E.I.M.; Validation, M.E.I.M., J.M.G.-G., C.S., P.F.d.C., and J.A.C.; Formal Analysis, M.E.I.M.; Investigation, M.E.I.M., J.M.G.-G., C.S., P.F.d.C., and J.A.C.; Resources, M.E.I.M., J.M.G.-G., C.S., P.F.d.C. and J.A.C.; Data Curation, M.E.I.M. and C.S.; Writing—Original Draft Preparation, M.E.I.M., J.M.G.-G., C.S., P.F.d.C., and J.A.C.; Writing—Review & Editing, M.E.I.M., J.M.G.-G., C.S., P.F.d.C., and J.A.C.; Visualization, M.E.I.M.; Supervision, C.S.S., J.A.C.; Project Administration, J.A.C.

Funding: Funding for this study was provided by the authors' departments. J.A.C. acknowledges support from the Ministerio de Economía, Industria y Competitividad, Grant MTM2016-75963-P. J.M.G.-G. y C.S. Ministerio de Ciencia Tecnología y Telecomunicaciones, Grant DPI2016-80054-R. J.A.C., J.M.G.-G. and C.S. acknowledge support from the European Commission, CrowdHealth project (H2020-SC1-2016-CNECT No. 727560).

Acknowledgments: Special thanks to the Hispanic Community Health Study/Study of Latinos (HCHS/SOL) Database. The HCHS/SOL dataset was used under the Data Access and Use Agreement approval from the National Sleep Research Resource.

Conflicts of Interest: The authors declare no conflict of interest. The founding sponsors had no role in the design of the study, in the collection, analyses or interpretation of data, in the writing of the manuscript, or in the decision to publish the results.

References

1. Kushida, C.A.; Chang, A.; Gadkary, C.; Guilleminault, C.; Carrillo, O.; Dement, W.C. Comparison of actigraphic, polysomnographic, and subjective assessment of sleep parameters in sleep-disordered patients. *Sleep Med.* **2001**, *2*, 389–396. [CrossRef]
2. Jean-Louis, G.; Kripke, D.F.; Mason, W.J.; Elliott, J.A.; Youngstedt, S.D. Sleep estimation from wrist movement quantified by different actigraphic modalities. *J. Neurosci. Methods* **2001**, *105*, 185–191. [CrossRef]
3. Ancoli-Israel, S.; Cole, R.; Alessi, C.; Chambers, M.; Moorcraft, W.; Pollak, C.P. The role of actigraphy in the study of sleep and circadian rhythms. *Sleep* **2003**, *26*, 342–392. [CrossRef] [PubMed]
4. de Souza, L.; Benedito, A.A.; Nogueira, M.L.; Poyares, D.; Tufik, S.; Calil, H.M. Further validation of actigraphy for sleep studies. *Sleep* **2003**, *26*, 1–5. [CrossRef]
5. Taraldsen, K.; Chastin, S.F.; Riphagen, I.I.; Vereijken, B.; Helbostad, J.L. Physical activity monitoring by use of accelerometer-based body-worn sensors in older adults: A systematic literature review of current knowledge and applications. *Maturitas* **2012**, *71*, 13–19. [CrossRef]
6. Martin, J.L.; Hakim, A.D. Wrist Actigraphy. *Chest* **2011**, *139*, 1514–1527. [CrossRef]
7. Ray, M.A.; Youngstedt, S.D.; Zhang, H.; Robb, S.W.; Harmon, B.E.; Jean Louis, G.; Bo, C.; Hurley, T.G.; Herbert, J.R.; Bogan, R.K.; et al. Examination of wrist and hip actigraphy using a novel sleep estimation procedure. *Sleep Sci.* **2014**, *7*, 74–81. [CrossRef]
8. Giménez, S.; Romero, S.; Alonso, J.F.; Mañanas, M.Á.; Pujol, A.; Baxarias, P.; Antonijoan, R.M. Monitoring sleep depth: Analysis of bispectral index (BIS) based on polysomnographic recordings and sleep deprivation. *J. Clin. Monit. Comput.* **2017**, *31*, 103–110. [CrossRef]
9. Chua, K.C.; Chandran, V.; Acharya, U.R.; Lim, C.M. Application of higher order statistics/spectra in biomedical signals: A review. *Med. Eng. Phys.* **2010**, *32*, 679–689. [CrossRef]
10. Vaquerizo-Villar, F.; Álvarez, D.; Kheirandish-Gozal, L.; Gutiérrez-Tobal, G.C.; Barroso-García, V.; Crespo, A.; Del Campo, F.; Gozal, D.; Hornero, R.G. Utility of bispectrum in the screening of pediatric sleep apnea-hypopnea syndrome using oximetry recordings. *Comput. Methods Programs Biomed.* **2018**, *156*, 141–149. [CrossRef]
11. Noronha, K.P.; Acharya, U.R.; Nayak, K.P.; Martis, R.J.; Bhandary, S.V. Automated classification of glaucoma stages using higher order cumulant features. *Biomed. Signal Process* **2014**, *10*, 174–183. [CrossRef]
12. Long, X.; Fonseca, P.; Foussier, J.; Haakma, R.; Aarts, R. Sleep and wake classification with actigraphy and respiratory effort using dynamic warping. *IEEE J. Biomed. Health* **2014**, *18*, 1272–1284. [CrossRef] [PubMed]
13. Matthews, K.A.; Patel, S.R.; Pantesco, E.J.; Buysse, D.J.; Kamarck, T.W.; Lee, L.; Hall, M.H. Similarities and differences in estimates of sleep duration by polysomnography, actigraphy, diary, and self-reported habitual sleep in a community sample. *Sleep Health* **2018**, *4*, 96–103. [CrossRef] [PubMed]
14. Dean, D.A., 2nd; Goldberger, A.L.; Mueller, R.; Kim, M.; Rueschman, M.; Mobley, D.; Sahoo, S.S.; Jayapandian, C.P.; Cui, L.; Morrical, M.G.; et al. Scaling up scientific discovery in sleep medicine: The National Sleep Research Resource. *Sleep* **2016**, *39*, 1151–1164. [CrossRef] [PubMed]
15. Zhang, G.Q.; Cui, L.; Mueller, R.; Tao, S.; Kim, M.; Rueschman, M.; Mariani, S.; Mobley, D.; Redline, S. The National Sleep Research Resource: Towards a sleep data commons. *J. Am. Med. Inform. Assoc.* **2018**, to appear. [CrossRef]

16. Redline, S.; Sotres-Alvarez, D.; Loredo, J.; Hall, M.; Patel, S.R.; Ramos, A.; Shah, N.; Ries, A.; Arens, R.; Barnhart, J.; et al. Sleep-disordered breathing in Hispanic/Latino individuals of diverse backgrounds. The Hispanic Community Health Study/Study of Latinos. *Am. J. Respir. Crit. Care Med.* **2014**, *189*, 335–344. [CrossRef]
17. Patel, S.R.; Weng, J.; Rueschman, M.; Dudley, K.A.; Loredo, J.S.; Mossavar-Rahmani, Y.; Ramirez, M.; Ramos, A.R.; Reid, K.; Seiger, A.N.; et al. Reproducibility of a standardized actigraphy scoring algorithm for sleep in a US Hispanic/Latino Population. *Sleep* **2015**, *38*, 1497–1503. [CrossRef]
18. Mendel, J.M. Tutorial on higher-order statistics (spectra) in signal processing and system theory: Theoretical results and some applications. *IEEE Proc.* **1991**, *79*, 278–305. [CrossRef]
19. Nikia, C.L.; Mendel, J.M. Signal Processsing with higher-order spectra. *IEEE Signal Process. Mag.* **1993**, *10*, 10–37. [CrossRef]
20. Swami, A.; Mendel, J.M.; Nikias, C.L. *Higher-Order Spectral Analysis Toolbox User's Guide, Version 2*; United Signals & Systems, Inc.: Ranco Palos Verde, CA, USA, 2001.
21. Vaseghi, S.V. *Advanced Digital Signal Processing and Noise Reduction*, 4th ed.; John Wiley & Sons: Hoboken, NJ, USA, 2008.
22. Bao, M.; Zheng, C.; Li, X.; Yang, J.; Tian, J. Acoustical vehicle detection based on bispectral entropy. *IEEE Signal Process. Lett.* **2009**, *16*, 378–381. [CrossRef]
23. Murua, A.; Sanz-Serna, J.M. Vibrational resonance: A study with high-order word-series averaging. *Appl. Math. Nonlinear Sci.* **2016**, *1*, 239–246. [CrossRef]

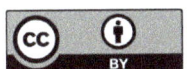

© 2018 by the authors. Licensee MDPI, Basel, Switzerland. This article is an open access article distributed under the terms and conditions of the Creative Commons Attribution (CC BY) license (http://creativecommons.org/licenses/by/4.0/).

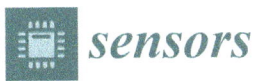

Article

Data Analytics of a Wearable Device for Heat Stroke Detection

Shih-Sung Lin *, Chien-Wu Lan, Hao-Yen Hsu and Sheng-Tao Chen

Department of Electrical and Electronic Engineering, Chung Cheng Institute of Technology, National Defense University No. 75, Shiyuan Rd., Daxi District, Taoyuan City 33551, Taiwan; chienwulan@gmail.com (C.-W.L.); shihaoyen@gmail.com (H.-Y.H.); iiccanffly@gmail.com (S.-T.C.)
* Correspondence: shihsunglin@gmail.com; Tel.: +886-910-608-121

Received: 31 October 2018; Accepted: 6 December 2018; Published: 9 December 2018

Abstract: When exercising in a high-temperature environment, heat stroke can cause great harm to the human body. However, runners may ignore important physiological warnings and are not usually aware that a heat stroke is occurring. To solve this problem, this study evaluates a runner's risk of heat stroke injury by using a wearable heat stroke detection device (WHDD), which we developed previously. Furthermore, some filtering algorithms are designed to correct the physiological parameters acquired by the WHDD. To verify the effectiveness of the WHDD and investigate the features of these physiological parameters, several people were chosen to wear the WHDD while conducting the exercise experiment. The experimental results show that the WHDD can identify high-risk trends for heat stroke successfully from runner feedback of the uncomfortable statute and can effectively predict the occurrence of a heat stroke, thus ensuring safety.

Keywords: heat stroke; filtering algorithm; physiological parameters; exercise experiment

1. Introduction

According to the 2017 global climate report published by the National Oceanic and Atmospheric Administration of the United States [1], the global temperature in 2017 reached the third highest recorded in history. Moreover, the global temperature was also found to increase 0.07 °C every ten years. These findings indicate an evident trend of global warming occurring in recent decades. This trend has had a significant impact on Taiwan as well. The main island of Taiwan is located on the Tropic of Cancer. The northern part of Taiwan falls within the subtropical zone whereas the southern part is within the tropical climate zone. Nevertheless, both parts of Taiwan are surrounded by a hot and humid climate. Affected by global warming, heat waves are now becoming increasingly frequent and intense in Taiwan, which has led to an increasing number of heat-related illnesses, including heat cramps, heat exhaustion, and heat stroke. Among these illnesses, heat stroke is the most severe, which often occurs in a high temperature and calm weather.

As sports are becoming a more popular component of daily life, many wearable devices capable of detecting physiological information, automatically recording physical data, and tracking the user's location have been developed to offer convenience and improve safety in sport activities. The improvement in safety is particularly important because the detection of physiological information enabled by these wearable devices can monitor the physical condition and predict potential safety risks for the user, thereby effectively reducing the possibility of getting injured in sports. Table 1 summarizes the pathological features and the corresponding physiological risk factors of heat stroke, obtained from relevant literature studies [2,3]. These findings can be used to increase the chance of early detection of heat stroke.

Table 1. Pathological features and the corresponding physiological risk factors of heat stroke.

Pathological Feature	Physiological Risk Factor	Use of Sensors
Body temperature is always greater than 40.6 °C, heat cannot be dissipated normally from the body	Body temperature	Yes
High-temperature and high-humidity environment	Environmental temperature and humidity	Yes
Lack of sweating or the opposite behavior for heat stroke during sport activity	Skin conductance	Yes
Individuals performing intense exercise	Running	Experimental scenario
Rapid heartbeat or low systolic blood pressure	Heart rate	Yes
Individuals with abnormal BMI, obese individuals, and seniors	Height, weight, and age	Prior investigation

In their heat stroke prevention studies, Naoya Mizota et al. [4] proposed the concept of showing a heat stroke alert on users' smartphones based on the environmental temperature—humidity index. Other studies have also suggested that the change in body temperature for individuals of different ages is also an indicator of potential heat stroke [5–7]. Many other wearable devices equipped with physiological information sensors can monitor changes in a patient's condition using physiological information signals, such as electrocardiogram, electromyography, and electroencephalogram signals [8,9]. However, a simple device for assessing heat stroke risk based on pathological features and their physiological information that can be carried easily by individuals is still lacking. Such a device can advise the users to take appropriate precautions in case of potential heat stroke risk, and therefore, prevent heat injury.

Wearable devices have been used widely in everyday life with substantial impact on the way that we live. By integrating physiological sensors in wearable devices, the physiological information of an individual exercising (e.g., running) can now be monitored automatically and instantaneously. This information can be combined with recorded environmental conditions to predict the risk of heat stroke and further advise the user to take proper precautions. Because ordinary wearable devices have limited computational power, the physiological information collected by the sensors is usually first sent back to a paired smartphone through Bluetooth wireless communication and then processed by the smartphone [10]. Bluetooth wireless communication embedded in smart handheld devices has the advantage of low power consumption and easy connection [11]. While the operating range of Bluetooth communication is officially claimed to be 100 m, experiments have shown that the practical communication range is between 5 and 10 m [12]. Although such a distance can satisfy the requirements in most conditions [13–18], the ultimate distance between the sensor and the smart handheld device is still limited by the maximum available wireless communication distance if one wishes to monitor the physiological information of an outdoor runner instantaneously. For individuals performing outdoor sports activities, increasing the wireless communication distance of the wearable device can offer more convenience. A summary of the technical specifications of different wireless communication systems [19] is provided in Table 2. As shown in the table, LoRa is a promising wireless technology that can resolve the aforementioned issue owing to its advantageous transmission distance, transmission power consumption, and standby current. Specifically, it has a longer range of wireless signal transmission, a lower sensitivity, and a lower power consumption [12] than other wireless communication technologies. Therefore, it is an ideal candidate for use as a communication module in wearable devices.

In addition, fuzzy logic is different from the traditional binary logic, in which the state can be only described by 0 or 1. In fuzzy logic, a membership function with output values changing continuously between 0 and 1 is used to describe the state of a phenomenon [20]. Using binary logic to describe heat stroke can result in potential danger because heat injury has already occurred when a heat stroke is detected. Using fuzzy logic to describe the heat stroke can prevent potential heat injury based on the level of heat stroke derived by the fuzzy rule. Thus, fuzzy logic is suitable for use in heat stroke prevention.

Table 2. Comparison of the technical specifications of different low-power wireless communication systems.

Type of Technology	Low-Power WiFi	Bluetooth	LoRa	NB-IoT
Frequency	2.4 GHz / 5 GHz	2.4 GHz	868 MHz / 915 MHZ	7–900 MHz
Transmission speed	16 Mbps	1 Mbps	12.5 kbps	200 kbps
Transmission power	±17 dBm	±10 dBm	±18 dBm	±23 dBm
Sensitivity	−92 dBm	−89 dBm	−136 dBm	−141 dBm
Transmission range	100 m	30 m	3–15 km	2–20 km
Current consumption (during transmission)	350 mA	22 mA	120 mA	120–300 mA
Standby current	58 μA	1.3 μA	1 μA	5 μA
Topology	Star shape	Star shape	Star shape	Star shape
Node capacity	<30	<30	>10,000	>20,000

In our previous work [21], we developed a wearable heat stroke detection device (WHDD) and demonstrated its heat stroke prediction capability for running. It should be noted that the usage of WHDDs is not limited to running alone. The WHDDs can be used to monitor body temperature and prevent the occurrence of heat stroke in any activity or exercise that carries the risk of heat stroke. In this study, we perform a more detailed analysis and experimental investigation from the perspective of information analysis and experimental subjects. Our results further demonstrate the superior applicability of the WHDD.

2. Materials and Methods

2.1. System Description

As shown in Figure 1, the architecture of the WHDD comprises three main parts: a wearable device, a wireless transmission module, and a back-end monitoring system. The complete WHDD is shown in Figure 2. Detailed descriptions of the different components of the device can be found in our previous work [21].

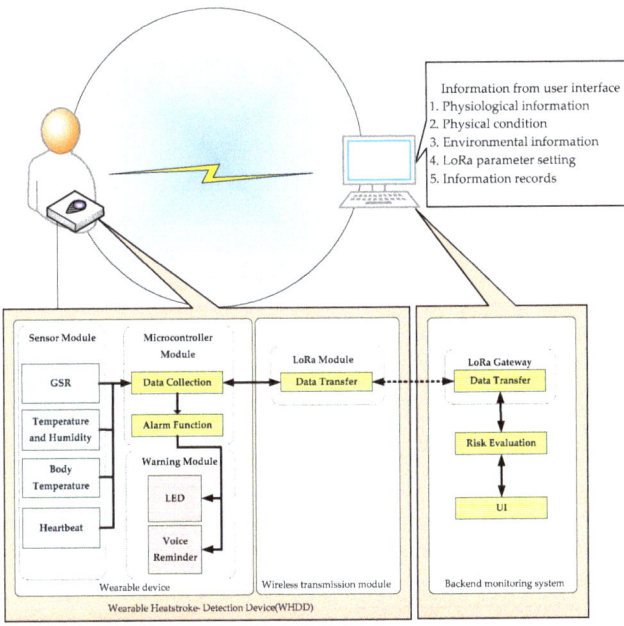

Figure 1. Architecture of the system.

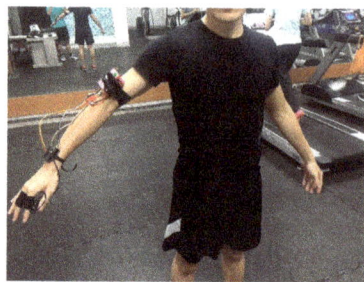

Figure 2. Photograph of the wearable heat stroke detection device (WHDD) on a human body.

2.1.1. Wearable Device

The wearable device is further composed of three parts: the microcontroller, the sensor module, and the alert module. The microcontroller, based on an Arduino Nano board, is responsible for performing basic processing of the front-end data collected by the sensors, data filtering, and signal filtering. Subsequently, the microcontroller packs the data and passes them to the LoRa wireless transmission module, from where they are transmitted to the back-end monitoring system. The sensor module comprises four individual sensors that measure heart rate (World Famous Electronic), body temperature (MLX90614), environmental temperature and humidity (SHT75), and skin resistance (Grove-GSR) separately. The sensor module captures the main physiological information from the user's body. This information is then transmitted to the back-end monitoring system by the wireless transmission module. Once the back-end system evaluates the risk of heatstroke from the received data, based on the risk level, the control buzzer warns the runner as follows: no alert means Safe situation, the LED turns on without the buzzer in Attention mode, the LED blinks and the buzzer beeps smoothly in Warning status, and the LED blinks and the buzzer beeps rapidly in Interdiction mode. The system suggests to the runner to ensure that appropriate measures are immediately taken in a dangerous situation to avoid heat stroke. The details of these procedures can be found in our previous work [21].

2.1.2. Wireless Transmission Module

To achieve a large-distance, low-power, and low-cost design target, the LoRa module developed by iFrogLab is used in the wireless transmission module of our device. The LoRa transmission module enables transmission of the information collected by the sensors from the wearable device to a terminal device. The wireless transmission module employs universal asynchronous receiver/transmitter (UART) for signal communication. Control of the data transmission is achieved using the attention (AT) command system. These approaches facilitate the integration of different components to construct the device.

2.1.3. Back-End Monitoring System

After collecting and transmitting the physiological information using the sensors and LoRa, respectively, this information is received by the back-end monitoring system, where the heat stroke risk is analyzed. The primary functions of the back-end monitoring system include recording the user's physiological information, physical status, and environmental information, as well as setting the parameters for LoRa.

2.2. Planning and Design of Heat Stroke Detection Workflow

After introducing the system architecture of the WHDD, we define the desired operation of the device as well as the associated techniques and hardware required. In this section, we discuss the design of the workflow for heat stroke detection and for the specific functions associated with each of the three architectures (the wearable device, the wireless transmission module, and the back-end monitoring system). Figure 3 shows the workflow of the entire system.

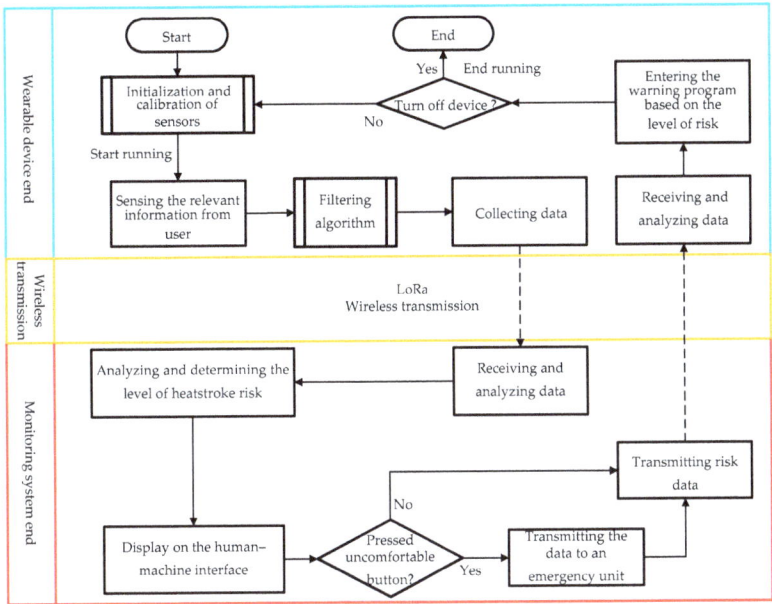

Figure 3. Workflow of the WHDD.

2.2.1. Wearable Device

This section describes the workflow for the target function of the WHDD. The overall workflow can be divided into two stages, namely, the stage before running and during running. The workflow for each section is described in detail below.

During the first stage (before running), the physiological information of the user is recorded. This information will be compared with the physiological information of the user during running. The change in the physiological information before and during running is an important factor for predicting heat stroke risk. Two physiological features, the heart rate and the skin resistance, of the user are recorded by the sensors during this stage. The overall workflow is shown in Figure 4.

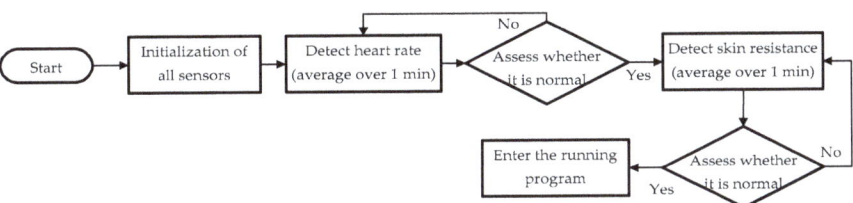

Figure 4. Workflow for collecting physiological information before running.

This workflow comprises the following steps:

1. Initialization of all the sensors.
2. The heart rate sensor monitors the user's heart rate for 1 min with a sampling frequency of 2 Hz (one sample every 0.5 s). After 1 min, a total of 120 measurement points are obtained, whose average value is considered as the user's heart rate before running.

3. Determine whether the heart rate is normal. The heart rate of a normal adult ranges from 50 to 90 bpm [22]. If the heart rate cannot be detected by the sensor, equals zero, or falls within the range associated with an adult in a non-resting condition, then an abnormal phenomenon is identified, and the heart rate is measured again.
4. The user's skin resistance is measured through the galvanic skin response for 1 min with a sampling frequency of 2 Hz (one sample every 0.5 s). A total of 120 measurement points are obtained and the average value is used as the user's skin resistance before running.
5. Determine whether the user's skin resistance falls within the normal range. The skin resistance of an adult under resting conditions is approximately 10–50 µS [23]. If the skin resistance cannot be measured, equals zero, or falls within the range associated with an adult in non-resting conditions, then an abnormal phenomenon is identified and the skin resistance is measured again.

In the second stage (during running), the wearable device mainly captures information about the surrounding environment and the user's physiological condition. Subsequently, this information is packaged and transmitted to the monitoring end by the LoRa wireless transmission module. The main workflow is shown in Figure 5.

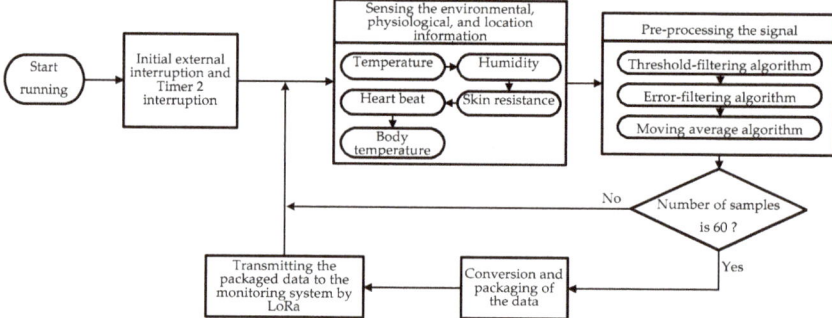

Figure 5. Workflow for extracting information on the surrounding environment and the user's physiological condition (main program).

This workflow comprises the following steps:

1. Initial timer interruption program and external interruption program. The timer interruption program allows the wearable device to receive the heat stroke risk level from the monitoring system on a regular basis. The external interruption program enables the user to ask for help by pressing a button on the device. In this case, the device immediately sends the physiological and environmental information back to the monitoring end.
2. Determine whether the device must be turned off, namely, by removing the battery from the device and shutting down the program.
3. Collection of the user's physiological and environmental information by the sensors (e.g., temperature and humidity sensor). The information is collected in the following order: environmental temperature and humidity, skin resistance, heart rate, and body temperature. This information is collected at intervals of 3 ms. Therefore, 15 ms are required to complete an entire cycle of information collection.
4. The heart rate and body temperature signals are preprocessed, first by a threshold-filtering algorithm, then by an error-filtering algorithm, and finally by a moving-average algorithm. When the number of samples reaches 60, all the filtered information is packaged and transmitted to the monitoring system by LoRa. The interval between each data transmission is approximately 15 ms × 60 = 900 ms (approximately 1 s)

5. When the number of samples is less than 60 or the data transmission is finished, the device continues executing the workflow from step 2.

The detailed signal processing workflows for the two most important indices for evaluating the heat stroke risk, i.e., the heart rate and body temperature, are discussed below.

Because the heart rate sensor is designed to be positioned on the user's wrist, the movement of the arms while running can potentially induce errors in the heart rate measurements. To resolve this issue, a threshold-filtering, error-filtering, and moving-average strategy is adopted to preprocess the heart rate signal and mitigate measurement errors. The code of the program is shown in Algorithm 1.

Algorithm 1 Heart rate filtering

1:   Global Variables:
2:       $TrueHR$ △$TrueHR$ is the final filtered value of user's heart rate
3:       $count = 0$, $mincount = 0$, $maxcount = 0$
4:       Let $HR[60]$ to be a new array
5:       $HR[0] = RelaxHR$ △$RelaxHR$ is the user's relax heart rate
6:       **function** $HRThresholdFilter(Value)$ △$Value$ comes from HR sensor
7:           $count++$
8:           **if** $50 \leq value \leq 190$ **then**
9:               $HR[count] = Value$
10:          **else**
11:               $HR[count] = HR[count - 1]$
12:          **end if**
13:          Call function $HRErrorFilter(HR[count])$
14:          **if** $count = 59$ **then**
15:               Call function $HRMovingAverage()$
16:          **end if**
17:   **end function**
18:       **function** $HRErrorFilter(Value)$
19:           $Error = Value - HR[count - 1]$
20:           **if** $Error < -10$ **then**
21:               $mincount++$
22:               **if** $mincount \leq 6$ **then**
23:                   $HR[count] = Value - Round(Error * 1.05)$
24:               **else**
25:                   $HR[count] = HR[count - 1]$
26:                   $mincount = 0$
27:               **end if**
28:           **else if** $Error > 25$ **then**
29:               $maxcount++$
30:               **if** (then$maxcount \leq 2$)
31:                   $HR[count] = Value - Round(Error \times 0.6)$
32:               **else**
33:                   $HR[count] = HR[count - 1]$
34:                   $maxcount = 0$
35:               **end if**
36:           **else**
37:               Keep $HR[count]$
38:           **end if**
39:       **end function**

In the heart rate threshold-filtering program, heart rate signals falling outside the range of 50 to 190 bpm are filtered out. This is because the heart rate of an adult at rest ranges between 50 and 90 bpm [22]. Therefore, 50 bpm is selected as the lower limit of the heart rate. The upper limit is selected based on the study by Tanaka et al. [24], who proposed in 2001 that the maximum heart rate (HR_{Max}) of an individual during exercise should be calculated based on the age instead of the gender. Roy et al. [25] in 2015 reviewed all the existing equations for calculating the maximum heart rate during exercise. They found that the equation proposed by Tanaka is rather accurate. This equation is given by

$$HR_{Max} = 208 - 0.7 \times age \tag{1}$$

Here, we assume the age to be 26 and derive the maximum heart rate to be approximately 190. Therefore, the upper limit of the heart rate is selected to be 190.

In the heart rate error-filtering program, each measured heart rate (HR_t) is compared with the heart rate recorded in the previous cycle. The error between neighboring measurements is given by

$$Error = HR_t - HR_{t-1} \tag{2}$$

This difference is used to revise the heart rate measurement based on a comparison between the performance of the heart rate sensor used in this study and that of a commercial heart rate belt. A fixed equation is derived to convert the measured heart rate to the actual value based on the difference between neighboring heart rate measurements. The revised heart rate is given by the following equation

$$\begin{cases} HR_{fix} = HR_t - Error \times 1.05, & Error < -10 \\ HR_{fix} = HR_t - Error \times 0.6, & Error > 25 \end{cases} \tag{3}$$

Finally, when the number of heart rate measurements reaches 60, a heart rate moving-average program is executed to obtain the average value of the heart rate measurements obtained over 60 cycles. The final value is used as the anticipated heart rate (HR_{True}), which is given by

$$HR_{True} = \frac{\sum_0^t HR_t}{60}, \quad t = 1 \ldots 60 \tag{4}$$

The sensor used for measuring body temperature in this study is a non-intrusive sensor. First, it measures the human skin temperature using an infrared sensor and then it converts that to the adult body temperature using a conversion equation. This temperature sensor is placed on the inner side of the user's wrist. Owing to the low thickness of the skin, this location is the most suitable place for measuring body temperature. According to a study by John Gammel [26], the following equation, together with the parameters (α) listed in Table 3, are used to convert skin temperature to core temperature.

$$T_{Core} = T_{Skin} + \alpha \times (T_{Skin} - T_{Ambient}) \tag{5}$$

Table 3. Parameter α for different body parts.

Body Part	α
Rectal	0.0699
Head	0.3094
Torso	0.5067
Hand	0.7665
Foot	2.1807

However, we found that the sweat generated during exercise reduces the surface temperature of the skin, and therefore, results in a lower body temperature. This impact also varies significantly with different levels of sweating for different people. Specifically, the measured skin temperature is increasingly smaller than the actual skin temperature for those generating a larger amount of sweat during exercise and vice versa. Therefore, the error of the core temperature obtained using the conversion equation is greater with increasing exercise time. To reduce the error induced by this physical phenomenon, the temperature data are filtered and processed using the program code shown in Algorithm 2.

Algorithm 2 Body Temperature filtering

1:    Global Variables:
2:    *BodyTemp* △*BodyTemp* is the final filtered value of user's body temperature
3:    *TempDiff* = 0
4:    Let *Temp*[60] to be a new array
5:    **function** *TempThresholdFilter(Value)* △*Value* comes from MLX90614 sensor
6:        **if** 28 <= *Value* <= 35 **then**
7:            *Temp* = 35 − *Value*
8:            **if** *Temp* != *TempDiff* **then**
9:                *TempDiff* = *Temp*
10:               *Temp*[count] = *Value* + *TempDiff* × 1.5
11:           **else**
12:               *Temp*[count] = *Temp*[count − 1]
13:           **end if**
14:        **else if** 35 < *Value* < 40 **then**
15:            *Temp*[count] = *Value*
16:        **else**
17:            *Temp*[count] = 36
18:        **end if**
19:        **if** *count* = 59 **then**
20:            Call function *TempMovingAverage()*
21:        **end if**
22:    **end function**

After converting the skin temperature to the core temperature (T_{Core}), the core temperature is processed by a temperature-threshold filter to yield a reasonable body temperature. This revision is based on a comparison between the body temperature measured using the system developed in this study and the value measured using an ear thermometer. A compensation equation is derived from this comparison to revise the core temperature measured by our device. The equation and the applicable temperature ranges are given by

$$\begin{cases} T_{Fix} = T_{Core} + (35 - T_{Core}) \times 1.5, & 31 \leq T_{Core} \leq 35 \\ T_{Fix} = T_{Core}, & 35 < T_{Core} < 40 \\ T_{Fix} = 36, & \text{else abnormal condition} \end{cases} \qquad (6)$$

When the measured core temperature (T_{Core}) is in the range 31–35 °C, the real body temperature is obtained by compensating the difference between the core temperature and 35 °C proportionally. When the measured core temperature is 35–40 °C, no further revision is required. If the measured core temperature is outside the above ranges, it is assigned with a constant value of 36.0 °C, as explained below. According to Reference [27], humans are warm-blooded animals, and the normal body temperature (no disease) of an adult human range between 35.0 and 37.0 °C based on forehead temperature measured by an infrared temperature gun. Therefore, all abnormal body temperatures were converted to the average human body temperature of 36.0 °C in this study.

Finally, similar to the process used for the heart rate and skin resistance signals, the body temperature data are also processed by a moving-average program that calculates the average value of 60 temperature measurements. Equations (3) and (4) are used to yield the final body temperature of the user (T_{Body}).

2.2.2. Monitoring System End

After the user's information is transmitted from the wearable device to the monitoring system, it is imported by the monitoring system to the fuzzy controller designed in this study. The physiological information measured by the sensors and collected by the microcontroller, such as skin resistance, safety factor, human body temperature, and heart rates, is used as input variables for performing fuzzy inference based on a fuzzy rule database, after these input variables are fuzzified. The final results are defuzzified to yield the instantaneous risk level of the user automatically. The details of this process can be found in our previous work [21]. Additionally, a human–machine user interface (UI) was developed by combining the back-end monitoring system with a C# program. This UI is used to display the physiological information of the user.

2.3. Experiment

This section discusses the experimental process and compares data measured in static conditions (before exercising) and dynamic conditions (during exercise) to confirm the applicability of the WHDD.

2.3.1. Static Experiment

Heart rate and body temperature are the two most important indices for detecting heat stroke [28,29]. To validate the accuracy of these two indices, as measured using the proposed device, we performed a 90-s static experiment. The original heart rate and body temperature measured by the sensors were compared with the results obtained after applying the numerical-filtering algorithm and the conversion formula proposed in this paper. Such a comparison allows us to evaluate the stability of the sensor and the performance of the filtering algorithm. Additionally, the values recorded by the heart rate and body temperature sensors every 10 s were also compared with measurements obtained with existing commercial products to verify the accuracy of our device. Specifically, the CK-102S [30] instrument, purchased from CHANG KUN, was used to measure the heart rate with a ±5% accuracy. The UE-0042 [31] instrument, purchased from nac nac, was used to measure the ear temperature with a ±0.2% accuracy. The deviation between the raw values detected by each sensor and those obtained from the commercial instruments were explored by experiments.

2.3.2. Dynamic Experiment

Four adults between the ages of 25–37 participated in the dynamic experiment, as shown in Table 4. The participants were required to wear the WHDDs and run on a treadmill for 15 min in an indoor environment with a temperature of 28.9 °C and a humidity of 68.2%. The participants performed the exercise at different intensities. The entire test comprised three stages, including warm-up (running at 8 km/h for 10 min), accelerating (running at 10 km/h for 2 min), and intense exercise (running at 12 km/h for 3 min). Increases in running intensities will increase the discomfort of the runners, but the amount of discomfort felt by each individual will be different because they have different levels of fitness. Therefore, the users could press the button on the device to send feedback when they felt uncomfortable while running. This feedback was used for experimental data analysis and validation.

Additionally, when the user was running, the movement of the arm caused the wearable device to loosen, which resulted in errors in the sensor measurements. Although such a scenario was inevitable, the filtering algorithm could detect and remove these abnormal signals. Particularly, because the heart rate and body temperature were measured by non-intrusive methods, their values suffered from the greatest errors. Furthermore, because the heart rate and temperature sensors were only fixed on the skin surface, they could be affected substantially by the user's motion. Therefore, the commercial product HRM-Ru [32] was used to obtain the heart rate under exercise conditions, as shown in Figure 6. A FLIR ONE [33] thermal camera was used together with a smartphone application to obtain the instantaneous body temperature, as shown in Figure 7. These measurements were compared with those obtained by the WHDD.

Table 4. Physiological differences between users.

User	User 1	User 2	User 3	User 4
Age	25	37	23	23
BMI	22.9 (normal)	27.3 (mildly obese)	23.2 (upper limit of normal weight)	25 (overweight)
Exercising habits	Twice per week	Three times per week	Irregular	Irregular
Remark	No exercise before test	Exercise before test	Warm-up before test	Warm-up before test

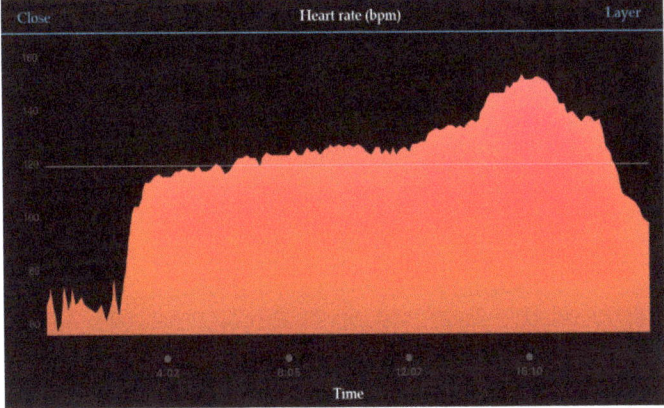

Figure 6. Heart rate data measured with the commercial heart rate belt.

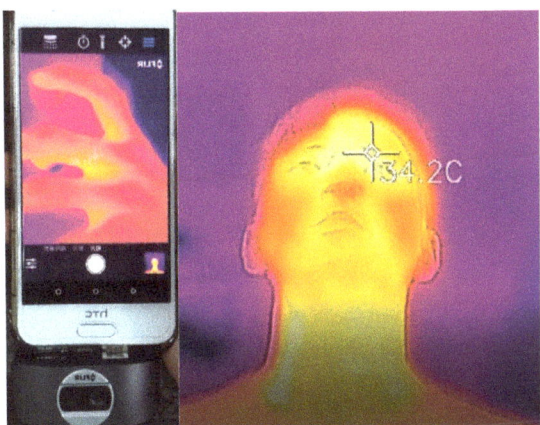

Figure 7. Thermal camera and measured dynamic body temperature map.

To probe the effectiveness of the WHDD in outdoor exercises, an outdoor running test was conducted with five adults in the evening. The test environment was a standard 400 m track, and the ambient temperature and humidity were 23.5 °C and 80%, respectively, which is equivalent to an environmental danger coefficient of 31.5. The test was carried out by having the test subjects run five continuous laps (2 km) around this track within their individual limits. The physiological differences between the test subjects are shown in Table 5.

Table 5. Physiological differences between users for outdoor experiment.

User	User 1	User 2	User 3	User 4	User 5
Age	37	36	24	24	24
BMI	27.3 (mildly obese)	22.8 (normal)	24.0 (upper limit of normal weight)	31 (mildly obese)	23.2 (normal)
Exercising habits	Four times per week	Twice per week	Irregular	Irregular	Irregular

3. Results

3.1. Static Experiment

3.1.1. Heart Rate

As shown in Figure 8, all the original heart rate values fall within the normal range (50–90 bpm) [22] when the user is at rest. The data obtained after filtering by the microcontroller were found to overlap with the original data. This finding suggests that the sensor can measure the heart rate accurately when the user is at rest. Additionally, no significant measurement fluctuation was observed during the test and there was almost no difference between the original data and the filtered data.

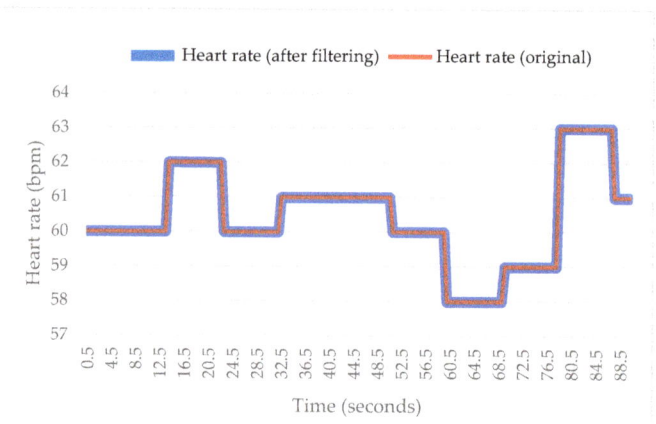

Figure 8. Comparison between original and filtered heart rate when the user was at rest.

Additionally, the average heart rate measured using the commercial wrist sphygmomanometer was approximately 56 bpm. The differences between the data measured using the commercial instrument and the data measured using the WHDD after filtering are summarized in Table 6. These results show that the average difference between the measurement obtained using the commercially available sphygmomanometer and the device developed in this study is approximately 0.1. Therefore, the sensor integrated in the WHDD can be used to measure the heart rate.

3.1.2. Body Temperature

As shown in Figure 9, no significant difference was observed between the original data measured by the sensor and the filtered data when the user was at rest. This is primarily because all of the body temperatures obtained after conversion are within a reasonable range (between 35 °C and 40 °C), with an average value of approximately 36.5 °C. Additionally, we see in the figure that the sensor measurement is rather stable when the user is at rest. The maximum error was less than 1 °C, which confirms that the sensor integrated in our device can be used to measure body temperature.

Table 6. Errors of the heart rates measured in this experiment with respect to data measured using a commercially available sphygmomanometer.

Experimental Runs	Heart Rate (After Filtering)	Average Heart Rate (Commercial Instrument)	Error
1	74	81	−7
2	80	78	2
3	75	80	−5
4	77	75	2
5	73	80	−7
6	91	88	3
7	93	91	2
8	85	78	7
9	84	81	3
10	81	80	1
Average			0.1

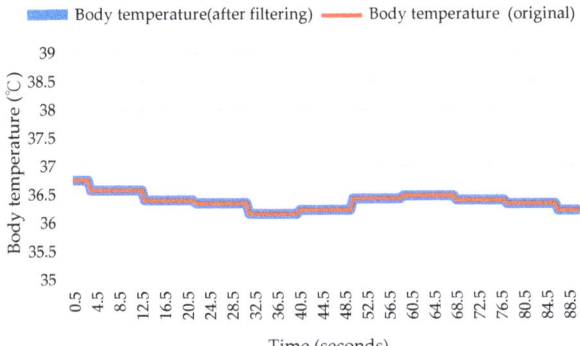

Figure 9. Comparison between the original and filtered body temperature when the user was at rest.

Next, a commercial infrared ear thermometer was used to measure the body temperature when the user was at rest. The average body temperature measured by the commercial instrument varied by 0.14 °C from the temperature measured by the proposed device. The error comparison is shown in Table 7.

Table 7. Difference between the body temperature measured in this experiment and that measured using a commercially available infrared temperature gun.

Experimental Runs	Body Temperature (°C) (After Filtering)	Body Temperature (°C) (Commercial Instrument)	Error (°C)
1	36.89	36.3	0.59
2	36.75	36.4	0.35
3	36.33	36.4	−0.07
4	36.85	36.4	0.45
5	36.19	36.5	−0.31
6	36.41	37	−0.59
7	36.59	36.4	0.19
8	36.61	36.5	0.11
9	36.71	36.4	0.31
10	36.81	36.4	0.41
Average			0.14

3.2. Dynamic Experiment

3.2.1. Heart Rate and Body Temperature

The heart rate and body temperature exhibited the greatest errors among all the physiological information indices by the sensors. Therefore, the dynamic experiment was focused on investigating these two indices. The heart rates measured by the WHDD during running were compared with those measured using a commercially available commercial heart rate belt and the associated smartphone application. This comparison is shown in Table 8.

Table 8. Comparison between heart rates measured with the WHDD and with a commercially available heart rate belt during running.

Heart Rate [bpm]	Test Time (min)					
	2	4	6	12	15	Average
WHDD (after filtering)	78	106	140	157	157	131
commercial product	81	125	125	140	155	125
Error	−3	−19	+15	+17	+2	+6

Next, the dynamic temperature data obtained during running were compared with the instantaneous body temperature measured using a commercial thermal camera in combination with a smartphone application, as shown in Table 9.

Table 9. Comparison between body temperatures measured with WHDD and with a commercially available infrared temperature gun during running.

Body Temperature (°C)	Test Time (min)					
	2	4	6	12	15	Average
WHDD (after filtering)	36.5	36.3	32.4	30.1	30.3	32.3
commercial product	33.8	33.8	32.8	32.5	31.9	32.9
Error	+2.7	+2.5	−0.4	−2.4	−1.6	−0.6

3.2.2. Heat Stroke Risk Indicator

Figure 10 shows a comparison between the physiological data and the feedback signals of the four users during running. Here, user 5 and user 1 are the same participant. Because the change in environmental temperature and humidity were negligible and all of the users exercised under suitable temperature and humidity conditions, the relationship between the environmental temperature/humidity and heat stroke risk are not discussed in this paper.

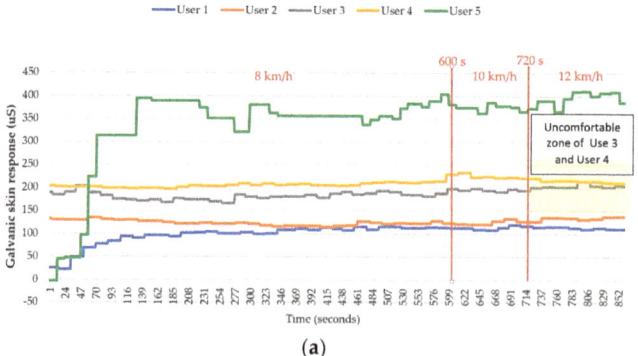

(a)

Figure 10. Cont.

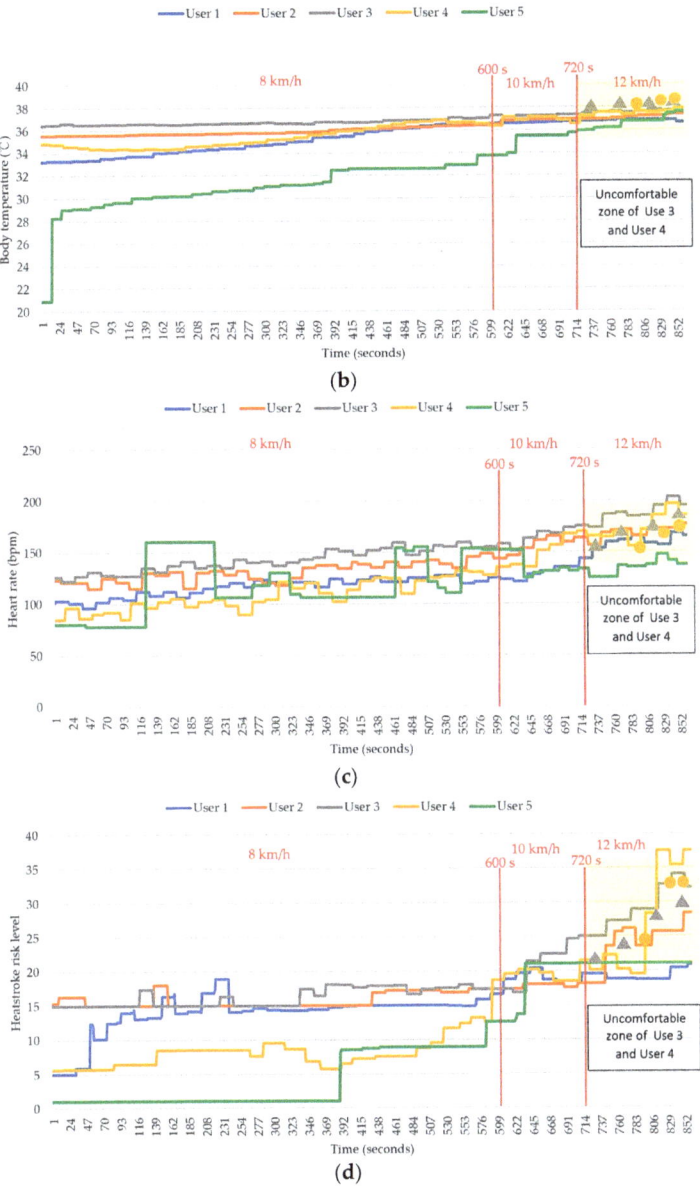

Figure 10. Comparison between the physiological data and the feedback signals of the four users during running. (**a**) Galvanic skin response (GSR); (**b**) body temperature; (**c**) heartbeat; and (**d**) heatstroke risk level.

First, we found that the data associated with user 5 was very different from those associated with the other four users because they did not undergo the filtering process developed in this study. Instead, these data were extracted directly from the raw measurements to predict the heat stroke risk level. Particularly, the body temperature and heart rate of user 5 varied more significantly from those of the other four users. Although the data still exhibited a reasonable trend, in accordance with the model of an individual performing exercise, the large data fluctuations in a continuous time period resulted in large fluctuations in the heat stroke risk indicator. Therefore, very different heat stroke risk predictions are provided by the device in a short time. Such a high instability issue could cause the user and the system to make wrong assessments. In contrast, the data associated with the other four users were very stable. Therefore, the heat stroke risk levels were also found to be stable for these users.

Next, a detailed analysis was performed on the conditions of the remaining four users. As shown in Figures 11 and 12, both user 3 and user 4 provided "uncomfortable" feedback to the system, while user 1 and user 2 did not provide any uncomfortable feedback during the exercise. The results were divided into two groups based on the feature of "uncomfortable" and analyzed by comparing the numerical values. With respect to the change in skin inductance (skin resistance), both data groups showed a stable condition in the measurements. This finding indicates that all four users experienced continuous sweating while running. Therefore, the skin resistance changed accordingly during the process. However, the skin inductance of individual was determined by the reference value of the static skin resistance. In other words, the skin resistance is always different for different individuals. Therefore, we infer that the occurrence of uncomfortable conditions in this group was apparently not caused by the lack of sweating but by other physiological factors.

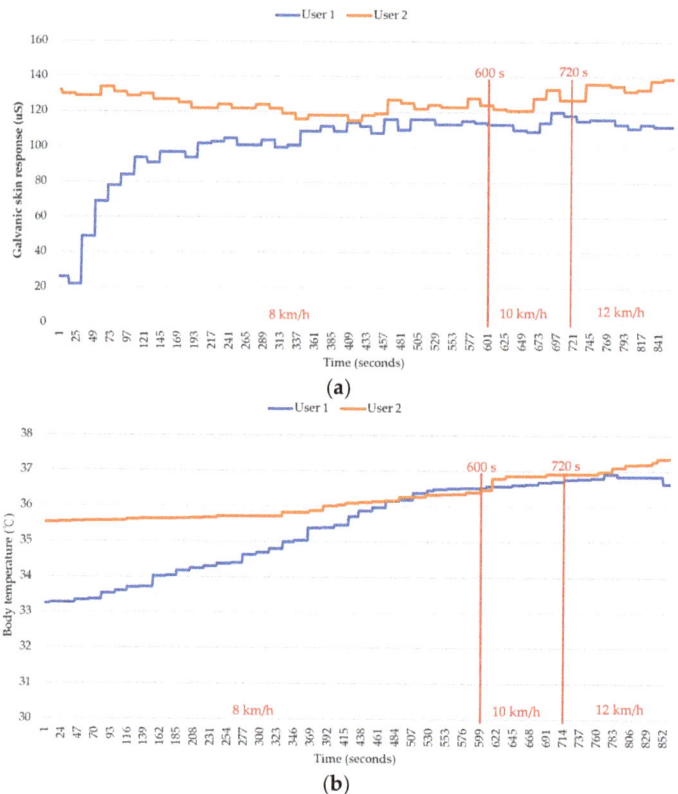

Figure 11. Cont.

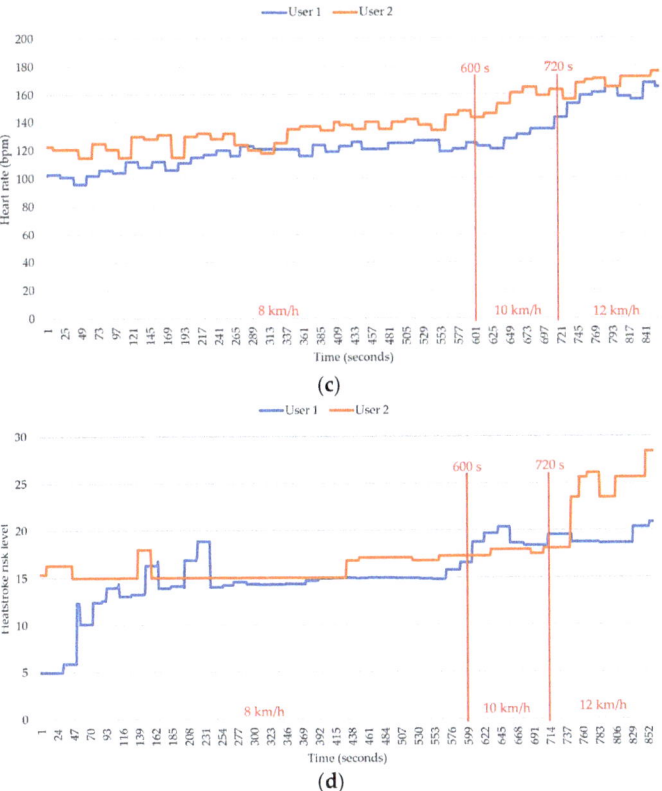

Figure 11. Comparison of skin inductance values in the testing group that did not report uncomfortable conditions (user 1 and 2). (**a**) Galvanic skin response (GSR); (**b**) body temperature; (**c**) heartbeat; and (**d**) heatstroke risk level.

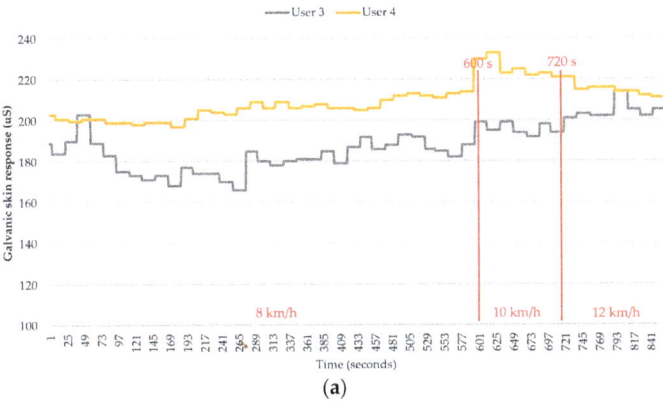

Figure 12. *Cont.*

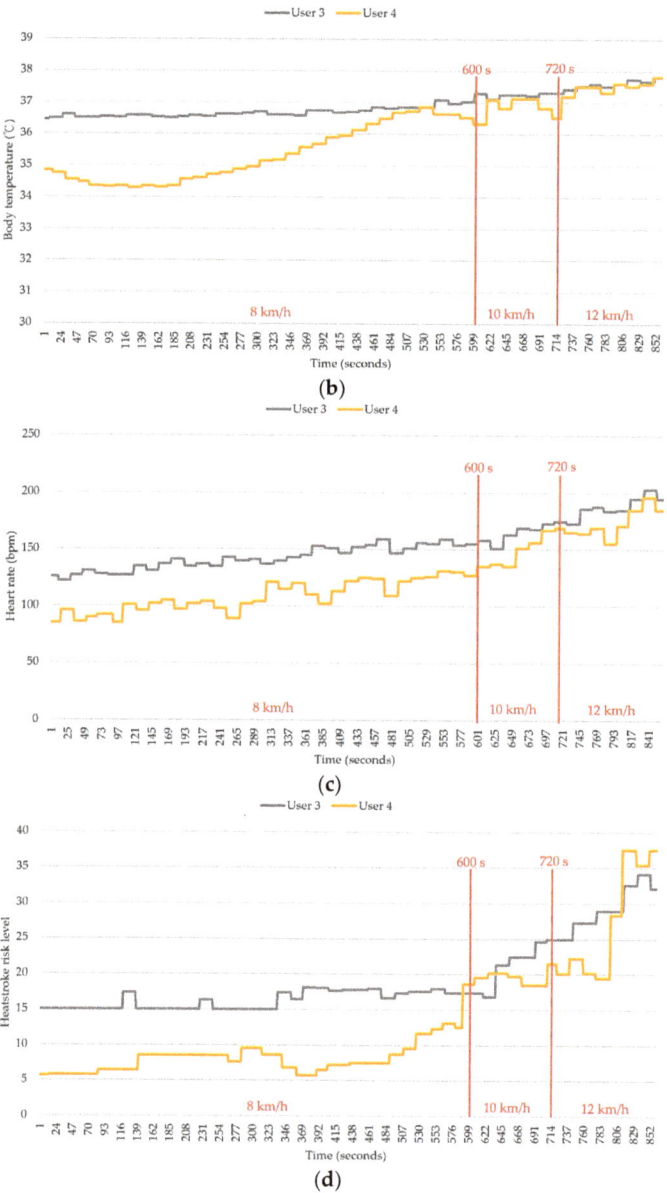

Figure 12. Comparison of skin inductance values in the testing group that reported uncomfortable conditions (user 3 and 4). (**a**) Galvanic skin response (GSR); (**b**) body temperature; (**c**) heartbeat; and (**d**) heatstroke risk level.

Figure 13 shows the results of the outdoor WHDD experiment. Because the physical condition of each test subject was different, the durations in which they completed the 2-km run were all different. User 1, who exercises regularly, completed the 2-km run in the shortest amount of time, whereas User 5, who had the worst physical condition, required the longest duration of time to complete the run. Furthermore, because the environmental danger coefficient of this experiment was lower than that of the indoor experiment (31.5 versus 35.72), it was observed that the risk of heat stroke in this low-risk environment, as evaluated by the WHDD system, was generally lower than that of the indoor experiment.

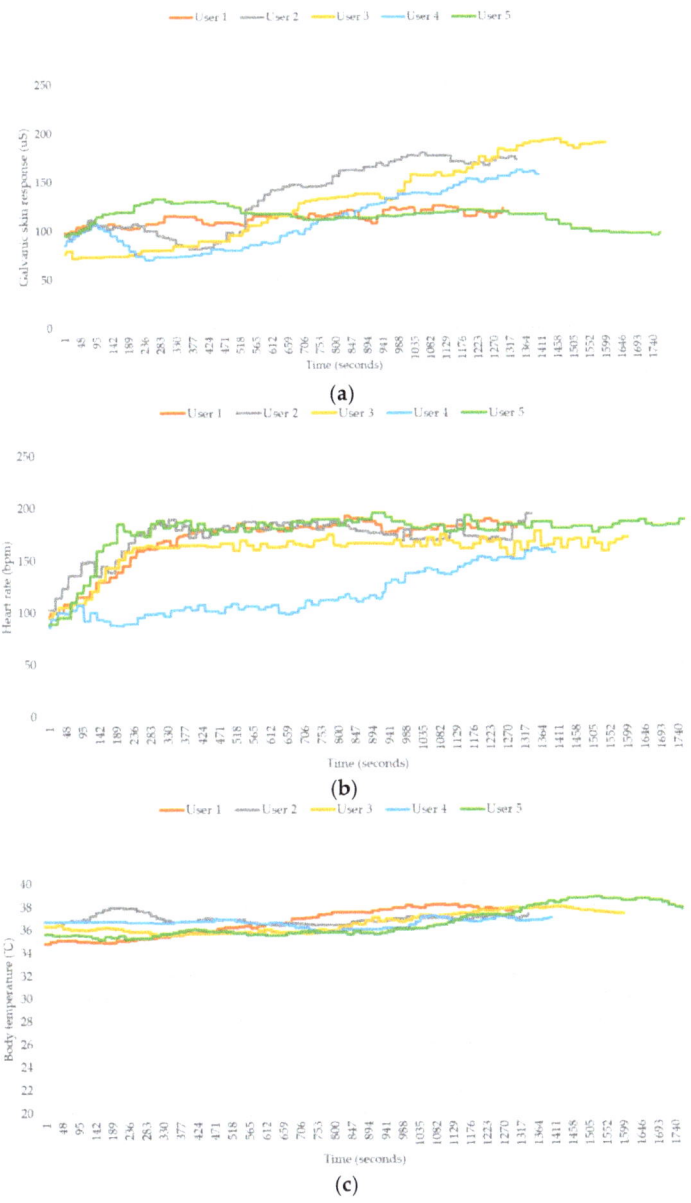

Figure 13. Cont.

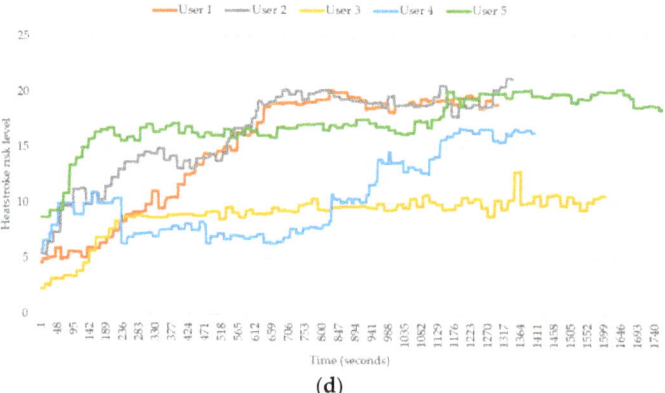

(d)

Figure 13. Comparison between the physiological data and the feedback signals of the five users during running outdoors. (**a**) Galvanic skin response (GSR); (**b**) body temperature; (**c**) heartbeat; and (**d**) heatstroke risk level.

4. Discussion

The rise of body temperature is a common phenomenon for humans when running. Additionally, the highest temperature of all four users never reached a dangerous level (40 °C). This finding suggests that the central control of the human body functions properly to maintain a normal body temperature. However, close examination reveals that the body temperatures of the users in the first group were higher than those in the second group. Although their body temperatures were still within a normal range, a high body temperature can still significantly increase the risk of heat stroke in the calculation. Nevertheless, no substantial difference in body temperature was observed between different users. Therefore, the body temperature is unlikely to be the factor causing an uncomfortable feeling. However, a reasonable guess is that if all four users keep running continuously, there is a high possibility that the body temperature of some users will eventually exceed 40 °C. This could result in a significant increase in heat stroke risk and to a dangerous situation.

The last physiological factor, the "individual heart beat," is presumed to be the main factor causing an uncomfortable feeling. It can be seen in the Figure 10 that the conditions of all four users are rather normal during the initial stage—particularly, in the first 10 min, when the users were jogging at 8 km/h. When the users started running at 10 km/h, a significant increase in heart rate was observed for users 2, 3, and 4. This phenomenon is consistent with the physiological changes that occur in the human body when performing exercise. No uncomfortable condition was observed during this stage, which indicates that the heart rate of each user was within a reasonable range associated with exercise. When the users started running at 12 km/h, the heart rate of user 3 was found to increase greatly and to be considerably higher than that of the other three users. Next, an uncomfortable signal was sent from user 4 when the total exercise time approached 800 s. Afterwards, the heart rate of user 4 increased suddenly as well. Although the increased heart rate of user 4 was still lower than that of user 3, it was still much higher than those of the other two users. Although the heart rate of user 2 was also rather high, it only increased slightly and remained mostly stable during the stage in which the users were running at 12 km/h. This indicates that the high heart rate associated with the exercise load was still acceptable for the user.

By combining the physiological information and the feedback signals of each user, three conclusions can be drawn from the study:

First, from the perspective of individual data, it can be seen that the heat stroke risk indicator of the users who gave uncomfortable feedback falls within the alert (21–30) and dangerous (31–40) zone. For the users that did not give uncomfortable feedback, however, the highest heat stroke risk indicator falls only within the alert zone (21–30). Therefore, we conclude that the heat stroke risk indicator obtained by the fuzzy controller can be used as a reference for predicting the danger of heat stroke. However, the actual body condition of an individual with a heat stroke risk indicator in a fuzzy area (e.g., the alert zone) can only be known by questioning the person. Only by doing so can we determine the possibility of heat stroke for this individual.

Second, from the perspective of individual data, the physiological factor and the actual physiological reaction of each individual are found to be in good agreement. We can infer with confidence that the heart rate is the major reason causing the uncomfortable feeling to the user. A second factor is the body temperature, which incurs a reaction slightly later than the reaction induced by the heart rate. This is because the rise of body temperature is a normal phenomenon for humans performing exercise. A body temperature reaching 39 °C can still be considered as normal. However, if the individual keeps running with a high heart rate (high load), the body temperature will inevitably rise to a dangerous level. The last factor related to heat stroke is the skin resistance. The reaction induced by skin resistance occurs even later than that induced by body temperature. This is because the human body must dissipate excessive heat by sweating to maintain a constant temperature. The skin resistance starts changing significantly (decrease from large to small, accompanied by a reduction in sweat) only when the body temperature becomes too high. This scenario indicates a shift from normal sweating to a no-sweating condition. Therefore, the heat cannot be dissipated effectively from the human body. At this stage, the user is most likely already affected by heat stroke. Therefore, it is necessary to use the WHDD to predict the possibility of heat stroke and the associated uncomfortable symptoms for a particular user. In this case, an appropriate reminder can be provided to the user to avoid suffering a heat stroke.

A systematic assessment of the relationship between the heart rate, body temperature, and heat stroke risk value was performed. The heat stroke risk value was calculated by the fuzzy controller. Fuzzy theory is mainly based on expert systems—i.e., the experience of the user—whereas the fuzzy rules are obtained from the literature, users' feedback, and repetitive tests. In the previous section, an analysis of the numerical values obtained from the actual experiments was performed based on Figure 10. From this analysis, we can obtain the order of reaction to each physiological factor associated with heat stroke, which is: heart rate > body temperature > skin resistance. Therefore, a similar result is expected when analyzing the relationship between heart rate and temperature with heat stroke risk using the heat stroke fuzzy controller designed in this study. Figure 14 shows the relationship between these three factors, obtained by analyzing the results in MATLAB, as the figure clearly shows that the slope associated with the relationship between heart rate and heat stroke is much larger than that associated with the relationship between body temperature and heat stroke risk. This finding also confirms that the device developed in this study can truly reflect the possibility of suffering heat stroke during exercise for an individual with certain physiological characteristics.

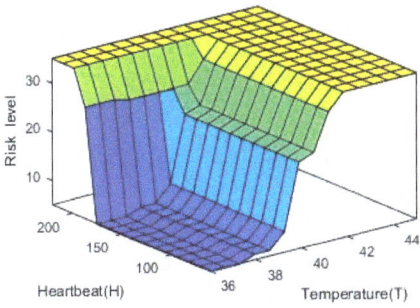

Figure 14. Three-dimensional relationship map between heart rate, temperature, and heat stroke risk level.

Subsequently, the feedback of the users who reported an uncomfortable feeling was compared and validated against the predictions of our system. The analysis of the comparison shown in Figure 15 yields the results shown in Tables 10 and 11. Based on the data of user 3, the system indicates a "dangerous" condition after 816 s. This prediction is 84 s (1 min 24 s) later than the first feedback provided from the user (732 s). For user 4, however, the system indicates a "dangerous" condition starting at 814 s. This prediction is only 2 s earlier than the first feedback provided by user 4 (816 s). Based on the analysis results on these two individuals, we can first conclude that the heat stroke detection function of our system can be affected by the physiological differences between different individuals and their distinct exercising habits. However, the system developed in this study is capable of detecting potential heat strokes. If the time factor is excluded, our system can effectively reflect the physiological condition of a user, predict the possibility of suffering heat stroke, and assist in cases of danger. To resolve the issue of the differences between different individuals, we can modify the parameters of the fuzzy controller according to the characteristics of the individual. Thus, the system can be revised to better match the condition of a particular individual. In the future, we expect to introduce the concept of machine learning to our system, which can automatically correct the associated parameters and therefore resolve this issue.

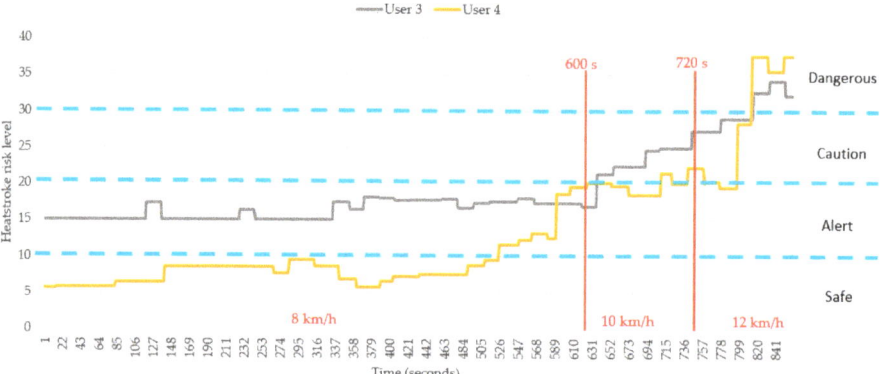

Figure 15. Comparison of heat stroke risk indicators for users feeling uncomfortable during the experimental tests (users 3 and 4).

Table 10. Comparison between feedback data and system prediction results for user 3.

Testing Time (s)	732		766		804		841	
User	Reported	System	Reported	System	Reported	System	Reported	System
3	Yes	Caution	Yes	Caution	Yes	Caution	Yes	Caution

Table 11. Comparison between feedback data and system prediction results for user 4.

Testing Time (s)	816		830		848		851	
User	Reported	System	Reported	System	Reported	System	Reported	System
4	Yes	Dangerous	Yes	Dangerous	Yes	Dangerous	Yes	Dangerous

5. Conclusions

Based on our previous work of a designed and implemented WHDD, this study performs further static and dynamic experiments to verify the availability and effectiveness of WHDD. In the static experiment, the heart rate and body temperature parameters are corrected by applying the proposed filtering algorithm. In addition, various intensity running experiments are conducted on several runners who wore the WHDD. The experimental results show that the WHDD can successfully identify the high-risk trends of heat stroke when the runners respond to discomfort information, so the device can effectively predict the occurrence of heat stroke and ensure the safety of runners.

Author Contributions: All the authors work at the design and realization of the work. S.-S.L. developed the idea of the proposed plan and directed the experiments. C.-W.L. supervised both the technical and experimental activities. H.-Y.H. integrated the electronic measurement devices with the wearable sensors and performed the experiments. S.-T.C. wrote the paper and made all revisions.

Funding: This research was funded by Ministry of Science and Technology of Taiwan, R.O.C. with Grant number MOST-107-2221-E-606-012.

Acknowledgments: The authors thank the financial support from Ministry of Science and Technology of Taiwan, R.O.C. with Grant number. MOST-107-2221-E-606-012.

Conflicts of Interest: The authors declare no conflict of interest.

References

1. Global Climate Report—Annual 2017. Available online: https://www.ncdc.noaa.gov/sotc/global/201713 (accessed on 14 October 2018).
2. Guidelines for the Identification of Professional Diseases Caused by Heat Hazards. Available online: https://www.osha.gov.tw/1106/1176/1185/1190/1194/ (accessed on 30 October 2018).
3. Gerrett, N.; Redortier, B.; Voelcker, T.; Havenith, G. A comparison of galvanic skin conductance and skin wettedness as indicators of thermal discomfort during moderate and high metabolic rates. *J. Therm. Boil.* **2013**, *38*, 530–538. [CrossRef]
4. Mizota, N.; Lu, H.; Nakashima, S.; Zhang, L.; Serikawa, S.; Kitazono, Y. Proposal of alert system for prevention of heat stroke. In Proceedings of the 2012 IEEE/SICE International Symposium on System Integration (SII), Fukuoka, Japan, 16–18 December 2012; pp. 111–116. [CrossRef]
5. Casper, R.; Schlosser, K.; Pascucci, R.; Feldman, J. Is it exertional heatstroke or something more? A case report. *J. Emerg. Med.* **2016**, *51*, e1–e5.
6. Zeller, L.; Novack, V.; Barski, L.; Almog, Y. Exertional heatstroke: Clinical characteristics, diagnostic and therapeutic considerations. *Eur. J. Int. Med.* **2013**, *22*, 296–299. [CrossRef] [PubMed]
7. Veltmeijer, M.T.; Eijsvogels, T.M.; Barteling, W.; Verbeek-Knobbe, K.; Heerde, W.L.; Hopman, M.T. The impact of exercise-induced core body temperature elevations on coagulation responses. *J. Sci. Med. Sport* **2017**, *20*, 202–207. [CrossRef] [PubMed]
8. Fujinami, K.; Kouchi, S.; Xue, Y. Design and Implementation of an On-body Placement-aware Smartphone. In Proceedings of the 32nd International Conference on Distributed Computing Systems Workshops, Macau, China, 18–21 June 2012; pp. 69–74.
9. Tomasini, M.; Benatti, S.; Milosevic, B.; Farella, E.; Benini, L. Power Line Interference Removal for High-Quality Continuous Biosignal Monitoring With Low-Power Wearable Devices. *IEEE Sens. J* **2016**, *16*, 3887–3895. [CrossRef]
10. Suzuki, Y.; Toyozumi, N.; Takahashi, L.; Guillaume, L.; Hosaka, H.; Itao, K. Wearable Individual Adapting Cooling System Using Smartphone and Heart Beat Sensor. In Proceedings of the SICE Annual Conference, Tsukuba, Japan, 20–23 September 2016; pp. 531–536.
11. Wang, J.M.; Yang, M.T.; Chen, P.L. Design and Implementation of an Intelligent Windowsill System Using Smart Handheld Device and Fuzzy Microcontroller. *Sensors* **2017**, *17*, 830. [CrossRef] [PubMed]
12. Augustin, A.; Yi, J.; Clausen, T.; Townsley, W. A Study of LoRa: Long Range & Low Power Networks for the Internet of Things. *Sensors* **2016**, *16*, 1466.
13. Chou, C.H. Design and Implementation for Wearable Sensor System Based on Bluetooth 4.0. Master's Thesis, National Taipei University of Technology, Taipei, Taiwan, 2014.
14. Liu, L.W. The Use of Low-Power Bluetooth Wireless Transmission—A Case Study in Mountaineering. Master's Thesis, National Cheng Kung University, Tainan, Taiwan, 2015.
15. Yang, H.C. Classifying Head Gestures by Wearable Devices through Machine Learning. Master's Thesis, National Chiao Tung University, Hsinchu, Taiwan, 2016.
16. Hsu, J.Y. Using Wearable Devices for Detection and Tracking Falls of Elders. Master's Thesis, Tamkang University, Taipei, Taiwan, 2017.

17. Choi, M.; Koo, G.; Seo, M.; Kim, S.W. Wearable Device-Based System to Monitor a Driver's Stress, Fatigue, and Drowsiness. *IEEE Trans. Instrum. Meas.* **2018**, *67*, 634–645. [CrossRef]
18. Cheng, S.H.; Huang, J.C. An Intelligent Sleep Quality Detection System Based On Wearable Device. In Proceedings of the 2017 International Conference on Machine Learning and Cybernetics (ICMLC), Ningbo, China, 9–12 July 2017; pp. 493–498.
19. Wireless Networking Technology to Promote the Use of Internet of Things Gateways. Available online: http://www.2cm.com.tw/2cm/zh-tw/magazine/-CoverStory/C9636801F9DF433FB70909B87B8BDAF4 (accessed on 14 October 2018).
20. Zadeh, L.A. Fuzzy sets. *Inf. Control.* **1965**, *8*, 338–353. [CrossRef]
21. Chen, S.T.; Lin, S.S.; Lan, C.W.; Hsu, H.Y. Design and Development of a Wearable Device for Heat Stroke Detection. *Sensors* **2017**, *18*, 17. [CrossRef] [PubMed]
22. Exercise and Heart Beat. Available online: http://www.epsport.idv.tw/sportscience/scwangshow.asp?repno=4&page=1 (accessed on 14 October 2018).
23. Design of Wearable Skin Electric Response Measuring Device. Available online: https://www.edntaiwan.com/news/article/20160530TA01-GSR (accessed on 14 October 2018).
24. Tanaka, H.; Monahan, K.D.; Seals, D.R. Age-Predicted Maximal Heart Rate Revisited. *J. Am. Coll. Cardiol.* **2001**, *37*, 153–156. [CrossRef]
25. Roy, S.; Mccrory, J. Validation of Maximal Heart Rate Prediction Equations Based on Sex and Physical Activity Status. *Int. J. Exerc. Sci.* **2015**, *8*, 318–330. [PubMed]
26. High-Precision Temperature Sensing for Core Temperature Monitoring in Wearable Electronics. Available online: https://www.ecnmag.com/article/2016/11/high-precision-temperature-sensing-core-temperature-monitoring-wearable-electronics (accessed on 30 October 2018).
27. Is There a Fever? Different Measurement Tools Have Different Standards. Available online: http://www.ilong-termcare.com/Article/Detail/262 (accessed on 30 October 2018).
28. Hamatani, T.; Uchiyama, A.; Higashino, T. HeatWatch: Preventing Heatstroke Using a Smart Watch. In Proceedings of the 2017 IEEE International Conference on Pervasive Computing and Communications Workshops (PerCom Workshops), Kona, HI, USA, 13–17 March 2017; pp. 661–666.
29. Antonio, P.O.; Rocio, C.M.; Vicente, R.; Carolina, B.; Boris, B. Heat stroke detection system based in IoT. In Proceedings of the 2017 IEEE Second Ecuador Technical Chapters Meeting (ETCM), Salinas, Ecuador, 16–20 October 2017; pp. 420–425.
30. CK-102S Blood Pressure Monitor. Available online: http://www.spicgz.com/en/Products/52.html (accessed on 7 December 2018).
31. Nac Nac Infrared Ear Thermometer (UE-0042). Available online: https://www.fda.gov.tw/MLMS/H0001D3.aspx?LicId=05003964 (accessed on 14 October 2018).
32. HRM-Run. Available online: https://buy.garmin.com/en-US/US/p/530376#specs (accessed on 14 October 2018).
33. FLIR ONE Infrared Camera. Available online: http://www.donho.com.tw/products_3.php?gid=7 (accessed on 14 October 2018).

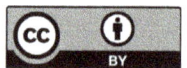

© 2018 by the authors. Licensee MDPI, Basel, Switzerland. This article is an open access article distributed under the terms and conditions of the Creative Commons Attribution (CC BY) license (http://creativecommons.org/licenses/by/4.0/).

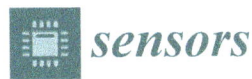

Article

Wearable Fall Detector Using Recurrent Neural Networks

Francisco Luna-Perejón *, Manuel Jesús Domínguez-Morales and Antón Civit-Balcells

Architecture and Computer Technology Department (Universidad de Sevilla), E.T.S Ingeniería Informática, Reina Mercedes Avenue, 41012 Seville, Spain; mdominguez@atc.us.es (M.J.D.-M.); civit.anton@gmail.com (A.C.-B.)
* Correspondence: fralunper@atc.us.es or flunaperejon@gmail.com

Received: 14 October 2019; Accepted: 4 November 2019; Published: 8 November 2019

Abstract: Falls have become a relevant public health issue due to their high prevalence and negative effects in elderly people. Wearable fall detector devices allow the implementation of continuous and ubiquitous monitoring systems. The effectiveness for analyzing temporal signals with low energy consumption is one of the most relevant characteristics of these devices. Recurrent neural networks (RNNs) have demonstrated a great accuracy in some problems that require analyzing sequential inputs. However, getting appropriate response times in low power microcontrollers remains a difficult task due to their limited hardware resources. This work shows a feasibility study about using RNN-based deep learning models to detect both falls and falls' risks in real time using accelerometer signals. The effectiveness of four different architectures was analyzed using the SisFall dataset at different frequencies. The resulting models were integrated into two different embedded systems to analyze the execution times and changes in the model effectiveness. Finally, a study of power consumption was carried out. A sensitivity of 88.2% and a specificity of 96.4% was obtained. The simplest models reached inference times lower than 34 ms, which implies the capability to detect fall events in real-time with high energy efficiency. This suggests that RNN models provide an effective method that can be implemented in low power microcontrollers for the creation of autonomous wearable fall detection systems in real-time.

Keywords: accelerometer; deep learning; embedded system; fall detection; wearable; recurrent neural networks

1. Introduction

Falls are major public health problems worldwide for elderly people. Reports from the World Health Organization (W.H.O.) indicate that approximately 28%–35% of seniors over 65 years old suffer at least one fall per year [1]. The reports also show that this rate increases when considering people over 70 years old. The analysis of the records of emergency departments reported in [2] identified that fall victims suffered at least one new fall every six months. A major factor that influences this fact is that many elderly people lose confidence and adopt a more sedentary life, losing mobility, quality of life and, thus, increasing the probability of falling because of their poor shape [3,4]. Direct consequences of falls can be injuries to muscles or ligaments, bone fractures and head trauma with consequent brain damage, among others. Major injuries pose significant risk for post-fall morbidity and mortality. In addition to that, it has strong economic impacts on family and public health. For instance, it was estimated that the United States spent $19 billion as a consequence of fall related hospitalizations in 2006 [5]. This topic is gaining importance due to the progressive increase in the elderly population [6,7].

Fall detection systems (FDS) are devices that monitor user activity and ideally alert when a fall has occurred. Their main goal can be summarized as distinguishing between two states: Activity of daily living (ADL) and fall events (alerting when this one happens) [8]. These devices allow sending an accident notification immediately to medical entities, caregivers and family members for quick assistance.

The detection of falls through technological systems is a very active field of study, given the importance of the subject. The literature review in [8] distinguishes between context-aware and wearable systems. The first one uses sensors such as cameras, pressure sensors or microphones, deployed in the environment. Their main advantages are that it is not necessary to wear any special device, and that acquisition sensors can be more complex for an increased effectiveness as they do not have significant computational or energy supply limitations. However, these kinds of solutions are limited to their deployment area, which usually implies having to perform an installation of sensors in the different rooms where the user lives or is monitored. These facts mean that these systems are not suitable in some situations, for instance if the user lives in sparsely populated areas such as small towns and leaves home often. In addition, these systems are generally expensive because of the installation they require and the sensors they use, which could make them economically unfeasible for some population niches. Another important aspect is that its installation in public health systems could be difficult because these systems would not only collect information from the target patients, but from other people, undermining their privacy.

On the other hand, wearable devices allow continuous monitoring without any dependence from environment-based sensors. That makes them ubiquitous systems that only acquire user-related data, which favors its use in hospitals and many other scenarios. In addition, they usually use simple sensors, commonly accelerometers and gyroscopes, that require low-power consumption. Several review studies have been done about this topic and one of them is presented in this work [9]. This fact allows to reduce the size of the devices and to increase their battery life. This also usually implies lower economical costs compared to context-aware systems. As disadvantages, these devices need to be worn by the user and must be charged periodically. In order to make these systems autonomous, they must combine efficiency and effectiveness: Fall detection techniques require a continuous sensor monitoring process (several times per second) that may demand a high power consumption if the data is processed externally (in order to obtain better results); but, if the detection is done inside the embedded system itself (to reduce power consumption), the detection algorithm may reduce the fall detection accuracy and the system could have high response times if the algorithm implemented is computationally expensive.

Among the different algorithms that exist for wearable devices, we can find two main types: Threshold based and machine learning based algorithms. While threshold based algorithms show very high performance [10] in terms of detection effectiveness and low computational complexity, they present many difficulties when trying to adapt them to new types of falls and user characteristics [11]. Machine learning methods are considered more sophisticated approaches to solving this problem, but they require a high number of samples to achieve high effectiveness rates, and nowadays there is a scarcity of datasets for study these events [12]. Other functionalities that can be investigated for this type of system is the prevention of falls or the possibility of damage mitigation [13].

Recurrent neural networks (RNN) such as long short-term memory units (LSTM) and gated recurrent units (GRU) are deep learning networks specifically designed to process sequences. Recent studies shed some light on the potential of RNNs for dynamic signals classifications [14] and more precisely for accelerometer data [15,16]. However, these algorithms have a high computational cost due to the large number of algebraic operations they perform. Running these models on low power microcontrollers with limited features, suitable for wearable devices, can lead to long response times and high power consumption, even for simple tasks [17]. This fact makes difficult to create real-time wearable fall detectors based on RNN.

The research described in this paper aims to assess the feasibility of implementing a wearable system for the detection of both falls and fall hazards using RNN architectures which has a good performance in terms of computational complexity and real-time effectiveness.

The article is organized as follows: the current Section 1 continues with the description of the most recent works in the literature that use machine learning algorithms for fall detection, implemented on wearable devices, as well as the basis of the two types of RNN used, that is, Long Short Term Memory (LSTM) and Gated Recurrent Units (GRU); Section 2 describes the proposed materials and methodology used for the assessment of the RNN-based wearable fall detector systems; Section 3 presents the results and discussion regarding the effectiveness of the trained deep learning models, the performance obtained after their integration into an embedded system, as well as an analysis of energy consumption; and Section 4 includes the conclusions and points out possible future works.

1.1. Previous Works

Fall detection systems are a very active research area. In this section we consider several of the most recent studies that are based on the use of wearable devices to detect falls. Table 1 summarizes these works highlighting information about the methodology and results.

Table 1. Summary of most recent studies about wearable fall detector systems using machine learning.

Ref.	Detector System	Dataset	Type of Sensor	N Users	N Records	N Classes	Body Sensor Localization	Algorithms	Accuracy (%)	Sensitivity (%)	Specificity (%)
[18]	Simulation on PC	1. [19] 2. [20]	Accelerometer	30 30	4500 NS	7	Waist	K-NN ANN QSVM EBT	85.8 91.8 96.1 97.7	NS	NS
[21]	Android application	Acquired in the study	Accelerometer	20	346 381	2	1. Waist 2. Thigh	TBM + (MLK-SPV)	97.8 91.7	99.5 95.8	95.2 88.0
[22]	Simulation on PC	SisFall [23]	Accelerometer	38		2	Waist	SVM	99.9	99.5	99.44
[11]	Embedded system	Acquired in the study	Accelerometer, Gyroscope and Magnetometer	22	NS	2	Wrist	K-NN LDA LR DT SVM	99.0 96.4 97.4 95.8 97.4	100 99.0 97.9 97.9 97.9	97.9 93.8 96.9 93.8 96.9
[24]	Embedded system	SisFall [23]	Accelerometer	38	3820	4	Waist	DT	91.7	91.7	97.2
[13]	External gateway	Acquired in the study	Surface electromyography	15	423	2	Lower leg	LDA	88.0	91.3	89.5
[25]	Embedded system + Android Application	Acquired in the study	Accelerometer	20	660	2	Waist (front-pocket)	TBM + K-NN	90.0	83.0	97.0
[26]	Embedded system	SisFall [23]	Accelerometer	38	4510	3	Waist	RNN (LSTM)	95.51	92.7	94.1

In [18] four different machine learning algorithms were analyzed using two combined datasets: k-nearest neighbors (K-NN), artificial neural network (ANN), quadratic support vector machine (QSVM) and ensembled bagged tree (EBT). The main contribution to this research area is the proposal of a set of new features obtained from accelerometer information, so these can be used as output from the machine learning algorithms. The best accuracy obtained (97.7%) was obtained with the ensembled bagged tree algorithm, a type of decision tree algorithm. The study shown in [22] also proposed new features, based on the first and second order moments, extracting 12 new features that were used with a Support Vector Machine algorithm. The results are very good, with an accuracy of 99.9% when using the features.

The work in [21] combines threshold based metrics (TBM) with multiple kernel learning support vector machine (MKL-SVM). The system was implemented in an Android app, and was trained to identify falls with the mobile phone located near both the waist and the thigh. The first TBM stages allow to discard false positives resulting from performing a daily activity that has sharp acceleration moments, such as lying on a bed. The best results were obtained when the mobile was located in the waist, with an accuracy of 97.8%.

The study in [11] also considers the effectiveness of different algorithms, that is, k-NN, linear discriminant analysis (LDA), logistic regression (LR) and classic decision tree (DT). In this case, the fall detector system consist of an ATMega32 Arduino microcontroller located in the user wrist. Thus, the features considered as output of these algorithms have to identify arm movement key values. In this work, k-NN algorithm had the best results with a 99.0% of accuracy, a 100% sensitivity and 97.9% specificity. In this case, three sensors were used: An accelerometer, a gyroscope and a magnetometer.

The work in [24] showed a fall detection system architecture design that combines big data techniques used for a continuous improvement of a decision tree algorithm. Initially, the algorithm was trained with a subset of activities from the SisFall dataset [23] to classify three different classes of falls, and ADL. It was tested with data obtained from empirical experiments, with good results. While the wearable device only acts as an accelerometer signal acquisition tool, it would be possible to create a version that dumps the updated decision tree in the embedded system periodically to get improved alert times.

A more unusual detection system is described in [13], where the used signals consist of muscle impulses measured by a surface electromyography sensor. The study analyzes the capacity of a LDA algorithm to identify the initial phases of a fall and prevent damage with an actuator system. The results obtained showed that these signals can also be used to detect falls and can complement the most common acquisition systems to reduce the number of false positives.

The study in [25] also combined TBM with Machine Learning. The TBM stage detected potential falls and was implemented in an embedded system with accelerometer located in the user front-pocket. The potential falls were finally classified using a k-NN algorithm implemented in an Android app. The system was empirically tested with 20 users who simulated falls and activities of daily living. With this approach short execution times were achieved, which allow real-time classification and good accuracy.

Finally, the proposal in [26] is unique, to the best of our knowledge, as it assesses the use of a RNN-based algorithm to detect falls. The used approach, which we address in this work as well, is the detection of both falls and fall hazards. The obtained effectiveness was exceptionally good, considering that it is possibly the first study that uses this technology for fall detection using accelerometers, that the architecture used comes from other studies and no modifications were made to adapt it to this problem, and that the algorithm inputs are raw sensor samples without preprocessing or calculating any feature. However, the main problem lies in its computational cost, which ruled out its use in real time when executed on a microcontroller. One of the reasons that made real-time execution non viable were the high sampling rates and the complexity of the used RNN architecture. The term architecture refers to the number and type of layers that configure a specific neural network based algorithm.

In this work we assess architectures where execution times are improved without losing effectiveness. We also perform tests with different sampling frequencies.

1.2. Gated RNNs

Gated recurrent neural networks are RNN architectures that provides an effective solution to the vanishing gradient problem [27] and the exploding gradient problem [28] that affected backpropagation through time [29] in previous RNN versions. The central idea behind these architectures is a memory cell with nonlinear gating units. The memory cells hold information separated, maintaining its state over time. The information is managed through a set of activation functions, named gates. During the training process, each cell adjusts the activation weights, that is, learns to close or open its gates, according to the relevance of the information obtained from the sequence and the information currently stored. This information is used in the learning process of the classical RNN part. Since the information contained in the cells is isolated from the flow of the conventional RNN, they are not affected by the vanishing and exploding problems.

long short-term memory units [30] were the first proposed Gated RNN. They contain three gates, two of which, called input and forget gates, are responsible for evaluating the addition of new information into memory and the deletion of part of the stored information, respectively. A third one, called output gate, controls what information is provided to the next step of the neural network in the training process. The set of vector formulas that rule a LSTM layer can be expressed mathematically as

$$\mathbf{h}_t = \mathbf{o}^t \circ \tanh(\mathbf{c}^t) \tag{1}$$

$$\mathbf{o}^t = \sigma(\mathbf{W}_{xo}\mathbf{x}^t + \mathbf{W}_{ho}\mathbf{h}^{t-1} + \mathbf{w}_{co} \circ \mathbf{c}^t + \mathbf{b}_o) \tag{2}$$

$$\mathbf{c}^t = \mathbf{f}^t \circ \mathbf{c}^{t-1} + \mathbf{i}_t \circ \tilde{\mathbf{c}}^t \tag{3}$$

$$\tilde{\mathbf{c}}^t = \tanh(\mathbf{W}_{xc}\mathbf{x}^t + \mathbf{W}_{hc}\mathbf{h}^{t-1} + \mathbf{b}_c) \tag{4}$$

$$\mathbf{f}^t = \sigma(\mathbf{W}_{xf}\mathbf{x}^t + \mathbf{W}_{hf}\mathbf{h}^{t-1} + \mathbf{w}_{cf} \circ \mathbf{c}^{t-1} + \mathbf{b}_f) \tag{5}$$

$$\mathbf{i}_t = \sigma(\mathbf{W}_{xi}\mathbf{x}^t + \mathbf{W}_{hi}\mathbf{h}^{t-1} + \mathbf{w}_{ci} \circ \mathbf{c}^{t-1} + \mathbf{b}_i) \tag{6}$$

where $\mathbf{h}^t$ is the unit state. $\mathbf{c}^t$ represents the cell memory, while $\tilde{\mathbf{c}}^t$ is the new information coming from the recurrent neural network. $\mathbf{o}^t$, $\mathbf{f}^t$, $\mathbf{i}^t$ are the results of the output gate, forget gate and input gates, respectively. σ and tanh represent the sigmoid and hyperbolic tangent activation functions, respectively. Vectorial pointwise multiplication is denoted by $\circ$. We get the following weights:

- Input weights: $\mathbf{W}_{xo}, \mathbf{W}_{xc}, \mathbf{W}_{xf}, \mathbf{W}_{xi} \in \mathbb{R}^{N \times M}$
- Recurrent weights: $\mathbf{W}_{ho}, \mathbf{W}_{hc}, \mathbf{W}_{hf}, \mathbf{W}_{hi} \in \mathbb{R}^{N \times N}$
- Cell weights: $\mathbf{w}_{co}, \mathbf{w}_{hc}, \mathbf{w}_{cf}, \mathbf{w}_{ci} \in \mathbb{R}^{N}$
- Bias weights: $\mathbf{b}_o, \mathbf{b}_c, \mathbf{b}_f, \mathbf{b}_i \in \mathbb{R}^{N}$

where N is the number of LSTM units, and M the number of inputs.

On the other hand, gated recurrent units (GRU) [31] are more recent cells similar to LSTM. They are distinguished mainly by the lack of the output gate and, thus, what is stored in the memory by the cell is dumped into the neural network completely during the entire training process. The remaining gates are named update and reset, which add new input information and clear data stored from previous iterations, respectively. The equations are quite different from those modeling the LSTM, mainly as a result of the absence of output gate:

$$\mathbf{h}^t = (1 - \mathbf{z}^t) \circ \mathbf{h}^{t-1} + \mathbf{z}^t \circ \tilde{\mathbf{h}}^t \tag{7}$$

$$\mathbf{z}^t = \sigma(\mathbf{W}_{xz}\mathbf{x}^t + \mathbf{W}_{hz}\mathbf{h}^{t-1} + \mathbf{b}_z) \tag{8}$$

$$\tilde{\mathbf{h}}^t = tanh(\mathbf{W}_{xc}\mathbf{x}^t + \mathbf{W}_{hc}(\mathbf{r}^t \circ \mathbf{h}^{t-1})) \tag{9}$$

$$\mathbf{r}^t = \sigma(\mathbf{W}_{xr}\mathbf{x}^t + \mathbf{W}_{hr}\mathbf{h}^{t-1} + \mathbf{b}_r) \tag{10}$$

where $\mathbf{z}^t$, $\mathbf{r}^t$ are the result of the update gate, and reset gates, respectively. For this architecture, there are fewer weights involved:

- Input weights: $\mathbf{W}_{xz}, \mathbf{W}_{xc}, \mathbf{W}_{xr} \in \mathbb{R}^{N \times M}$
- Recurrent weights: $\mathbf{W}_{hz}, \mathbf{W}_{hc}, \mathbf{W}_{hr} \in \mathbb{R}^{N \times N}$
- Bias weights: $\mathbf{b}_z, \mathbf{b}_r \in \mathbb{R}^N$

Both RNN layer alternatives have shown to be similarly effective [32], but GRUs have a slightly lower computational cost because of the absence of the output gate.

2. Materials and Methods

2.1. Dataset

The research protocol and results presented in this work were performed using the SisFall dataset [23]. It is composed of several simulated activities mainly classified in falls and ADL. The participants in the data collection were 38, among which there are 23 adults and 15 elderly people. Each sample contains accelerometer and gyroscope measurements obtained from a device fixed to the user's waist and acquired at 200 Hz. This dataset was complemented in [16] with a labeling proposal. Each temporary sample was classified according to whether it belonged to a fall event, a fall hazard or an activity of daily life. To our best knowledge this is the only public fall dataset that contemplates fall hazard events, consisting of moments before a fall, or during a dangerous situation where the user was able to avoid a fall.

As mentioned in previous sections, the inputs of recurrent neural networks consist of a sequence of values with a fixed length. That length is named width. Each value in the sequence has a fixed dimension. In the context of this problem, the values consist of a tuple with three elements corresponding to the three axes of the accelerometer. From now on, throughout the manuscript we will refer to each tuple with the term sample. In the same way, each sequence of samples with fixed width will be referred as block. To train a RNN model, each block must have an associated label, corresponding to the event class that contemplates. We used the proposal established in [16], in which each block is classified according to the percentage of appearance of the most relevant class. The classes in order of relevance refer to a fall event (FALL), a risk of falling (ALERT) and others, labeled as background (BKG). Background or BKG class considers the rest of time intervals, that mainly includes activities of daily life, other activities not related to a fall, such as jumping, and also the time that the user remains lying after a fall. The classification criteria are schematized in Figure 1 (left). This rule was applied to each activity record from the dataset, establishing a block width of 256 samples, equivalent to 1.28 seconds. A 50% stride was applied.

Lastly, three additional versions from the resulting dataset were created, reducing the number of samples per block, that is, the width. It is intended to evaluate the performance of the models when they are trained with less information, simulating a lower sampling rate. The process of reduction of samples consisted in eliminating the samples in even position of each block (see Figure 1, right). It was performed three times with each resulting dataset, obtaining blocks with a width of 128, 64 and 32 samples, which correspond to 100 Hz, 50 Hz and 25 Hz sampling frequency, respectively.

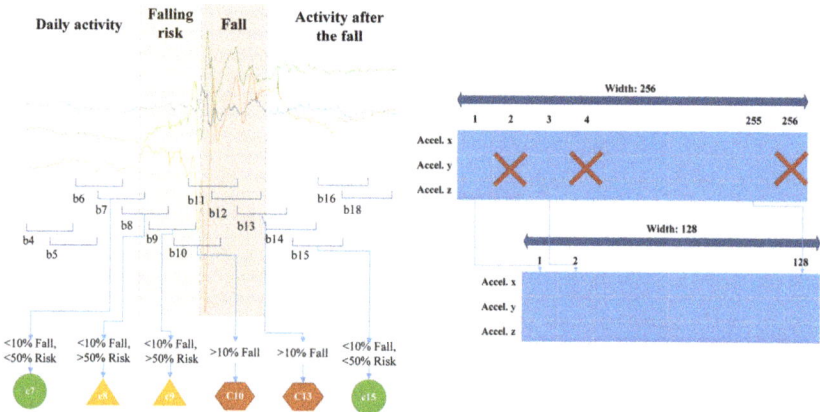

Figure 1. On the left: Recording segmentation and labeling process. Green circles, yellow triangles and red hexagons indicate the block is classified as a background (BKG), a risk of falling (ALERT) or a fall event (FALL), respectively. On the right: Block width reduction process. In the case illustrated, a 256-width block, corresponding to a frequency sampling of 200 Hz, is reduced to 128 samples to obtain a frequency sampling of 100 Hz. The same process was performed with 128-width and 64-width blocks to obtain 64-width (50 Hz) and 32-width (25 Hz) datasets, respectively.

2.2. RNN Architectures

Results obtained in [33] showed that the regularization of sample values substantially improves the effectiveness. To achieve this, a batch normalization layer is included at the beginning of the architecture. A recent study [34] revealed that this smooths the objective function to improve the performance. A 10-fold cross validation study [35] determined that this was not effective for obtaining non-sequential characteristics. Based on these results, in this work we deepened our study and analyzed the feasibility of integration for four different architectures. These architectures are those with higher performance determined in previous studies.

The two simplest architectures consist of batch normalization, a RNN layer and a fully-connected output layer (see Figure 2). Softmax is used to determine the event class. The difference between one and the other is the use of LSTM or GRU as the recurrent layer. The other two architectures contain a second RNN layer of the same type as the previous one. While the computational cost in the most complex versions is higher, their effectiveness is also slightly higher.

In order to optimize the results, we adjusted batch size and learning rate hyperparameters by grid search. Dropout [36] technique was also applied to the inputs of the fully-connected layer.

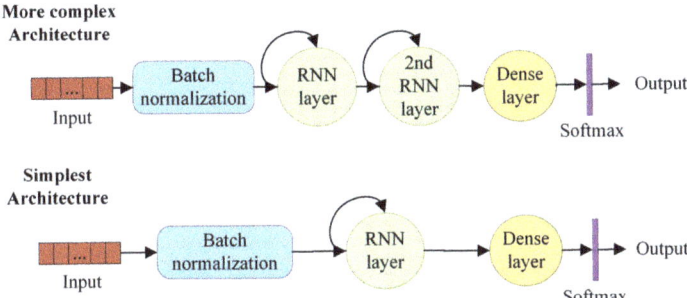

Figure 2. Diagram of the four recurrent neural network (RNN) architectures analyzed in this study.

2.3. Embedded System Features

We chose two STM32 32-bit microcontrollers (MCUs) for the integration and performance analysis of the trained models. Both are based on the high-performance ARM Cortex-M4 processors, with features that allow real-time capabilities, digital signal processing and low-power operation.

The first device selected is a STM32L476RG, part of the ultra-low-power catalog with the specified ARM processor MCU. It operates at a frequency up to 80MHz, contents 1 Mbyte of flash memory and 128 Kbyte of SRAM. The second device is a STM32F411RE, that offers a higher processing performance. It operates at a frequency up to 80 MHz, 512 Kbytes of flash memory and 128 Kbyte of SRAM. Both feature a floating point unit for a better precision in data-processing.

2.4. Protocol

The feasibility analysis consisted in a set of tests, divided into three stages. The first aims to study the algorithm effectiveness before the training, optimizing the hyperparameters. Secondly, the performance of the modes were assessed once they are integrated in the microcontroller. Lastly, a power consumption analysis was performed.

2.4.1. Effectiveness Analysis

The architectures were trained using the data from 30 users, (near of 80% of the dataset), while the rest, corresponding to 8 users, were used for the final evaluation. The users for each subset were randomly chosen, but maintaining an equitable distribution between adults and elderly. The training subset were the used in [35] applying 10-fold cross validation and estimate the goodness of the models with a correct reliability. In a first stage, five training processes for each architecture with different sampling frequencies were performed, in order to determine those with the best performance. In a second stage, we used smart grid search for optimizing the architectures with better results in the first stage.

Due to the dataset being highly unbalanced, the overall classification accuracy is not an appropriate way to measure the effectiveness of the system. We compared the effectiveness employing the macro F1-score [37], that measures the relations between data's positive labels and those given by a classifier through a harmonic mean of macro-precision ($precision_m$) and macro-recall ($recall_m$).

$$F1 - score_m = 2 * \frac{precision_m * recall_m}{precision_m + recall_m} \tag{11}$$

$$Precision_m = \sum_c \frac{TP_c}{TP_c + FP_c}, c \in classes \qquad (12)$$

$$Recall_m = \sum_c \frac{TP_c}{TP_c + FN_c}, c \in classes \qquad (13)$$

where m index refers to macro metric and $classes = \{BKG, ALERT, FALL\}$. TP_c, FP_c and FN_c denotes the number of true positives, false positives and false negatives of each class $c \in classes$, respectively.

While the F1-score is an appropriate metric for a multi-class problem, it is not usual to assess the performance of a FDS. In this context, sensitivity and specificity metrics are more commonly used. Sensitivity is another term to refer to recall. The formula for specificity is

$$Specificity = \sum_c \frac{TN_c}{TN_c + FP_c}, c \in classes \qquad (14)$$

where TN_c denotes the number of true negatives of each class $c \in classes$. These metrics are also considered in this work.

2.4.2. Performance on Embedded Systems

Two main aspects were analyzed for the embedded devices with each proposed model. First, the time spent processing a block, that is, the execution time of the integrated model. This parameter seeks to locate those architectures that can work in real time, that is, that are capable of providing a response in the time that elapses until a new sample of the accelerometer is read. Secondly, we assessed the differences on the inference outputs of the models optimized for their execution on the embedded systems. This is obtained by calculating the relative L2 error:

$$e = \frac{\|F_{generated} - F_{original}\|}{\|F_{generated}\|} \qquad (15)$$

where $F_generated$ refers to the flatten array of the generated model last output layer and $F_original$ refers to the flatten of the original model.

2.4.3. Power Usage Analysis

We assessed if the implementation of these kinds of models in an embedded system provides some advantage in terms of energy consumption. For this, two fall detector system designs were considered (see Figure 3). The alternative version consisted in using the embedded system as only an acquisition and transmission tool, so that its tasks are reading of the accelerometer measures and transmitting each new sample to an external device with greater computational capacity and no energy related constraints. We considered Bluetooth as the communication technology. This first scenario was compared with the target version, consisting of an embedded system which integrates the RNN model and executes it in real-time. This version has as main tasks the accelerometer reading, the execution of the implemented model and an alert transmission to an external device, only in case of an alert or a fall event. The power consumption for each task was calculated based on the technique specifications for the embedded systems and the auxiliary modules: The bluetooth module and the triaxial accelerometer. The execution time for each task was also estimated based on the hardware features and the RNN execution time.

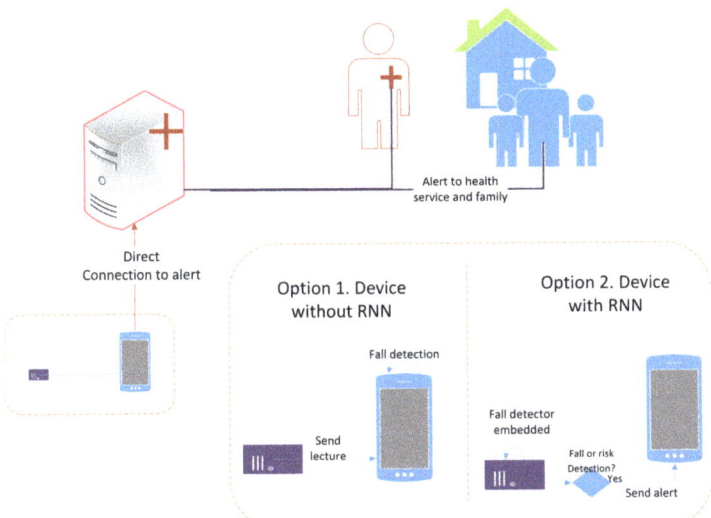

Figure 3. Fall detector system versions. In option 1, the microcontroller sends the accelerometer readings, and a master device executes the RNN algorithm. In option 2, the RNN model is implemented in the microcontroller, and only sends a notification when a fall or a fall hazard event happens.

3. Results and Discussion

3.1. Models Analysis

The number of blocks per each subset from the dataset is shown in Table 2. As mentioned in the methods section, the number of blocks from classes ALERT and FALL are much lower than BKG. This is due to the short duration of risk and fall events. For the training process, we used a graphic processor unit NVIDIA GTX 1080 Ti and the CuDNN versions of this RNN layer provided, implemented in the Keras framework. The use of CuDNN RNN layers improves the training speed substantially, 8 to 10 times faster.

Table 2. Dataset distribution for each subset.

Subset	Users		Blocks			
	Adults	Elderly	Total	BKG	Alert	Fall
Training	19	11	94,667	90,173	1172	3322
Test	4	4	22,321	21,425	201	695

The results of F1-score with cross-validation using the training set (Figure 4, left) indicate that the reduction of the number of samples per block does not affect the results negatively. The standard deviation (around ±0.25 and ±0.35) reveals a slight dependence on training and validation subsets. Each architecture was trained five times with initial random weights. Figure 4 (right) shows the macro F1-score average results using the subset reserved for test. Both architectures presented similar effectiveness. The architecture with two GRU layers shows a sightly better F1-score. However, we did not consider the differences between the models substantial enough to discard any model in terms of effectiveness. On the other hand, since the computational efficiency of these models was greatly influenced by the reduction in the number of samples processed, the rest of the study was conducted with blocks of 32 samples (25 Hz).

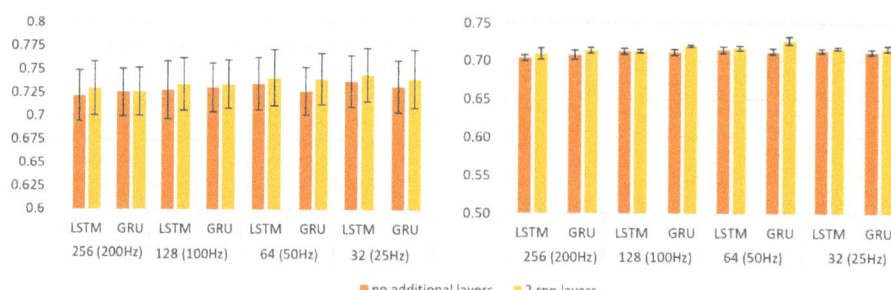

Figure 4. Macro F1-score results for each architecture and different input width (frequency sampling). On the left: The results applying 10-fold cross validation with the training subset. On the right: Results with the training subset and evaluated with the test subset (average results from training five times each model).

Table 3 covers the values considered for the hyperparameters and the dropout for grid search. The best results obtained for each model and the associated hyperparameters are shown in Table 4. The accuracy is greater than the most recent works which consider a multi-class problem. However, the sensitivity is quite lower. We have assessed the architectures using 10-fold cross-validation to ensure the results are independent from the test subset used. The effectiveness deviation depending on the test subset that reveals Figure 4 (left) can explain the differences in the results with [16], where a typical 80%/20% dataset split was used.

Table 3. Grid search values for exhaustive parameters optimization.

Parameter	Value 1	Value 2	Value 3
Learning rate	0.001	0.0005	0.0001
Batch size	32	48	64
Dropout	0	0.2	0.35

Table 4. Best results obtained after grid search optimization.

RNN Architecture	Learn. Rate	Batch Size	RNN Drop.	Accuracy	Precision	F1-Score	Specificity	Sensitivity
One LSTM layer	0.0005	32	0	0.963	0.695	0.726	0.964	0.882
Two LSTM layers	0.001	48	0.2	0.961	0.683	0.724	0.971	0.902
One GRU layer	0.001	32	0.35	0.964	0.682	0.725	0.963	0.882
Two GRU layers	0.0005	32	0	0.967	0.681	0.730	0.968	0.875

Macro F1-score results are mainly affected by the low macro precision metric value which, in turn, is low due to the low precision value in the ALERT class. This is due to the scarcity of data for this class. A small percentage of BKG events are wrongly predicted as ALERT, but comparing with the amount of blocks of the ALERT class this is a very significant percentage. This fact reveals the difficulty in training machine learning algorithms with unbalanced data. A larger quantity of datasets is necessary, something difficult for this problem, since falls can only be obtained from simulations and they imply putting at risk the health of the participants, especially if the participants are elderly, which is unfortunately the target population.

The receiver operating characteristic (ROC) curves (see Figure 5) per each model and class reveal a good reliability in the inference of event classes. These curves were obtained from the results for each node of the output layer by modifying the confident threshold. The areas under the curve (AUCs) are higher than 96%. The confusion matrix for each model (see Figure 6) shows high accuracy values, but in addition, it reveals the previously mentioned problem about the scarcity of ALERT events and the percentage of BKG predicted as ALERT.

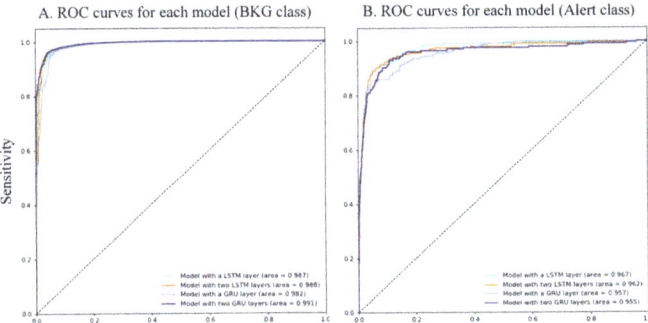

Figure 5. *Cont.*

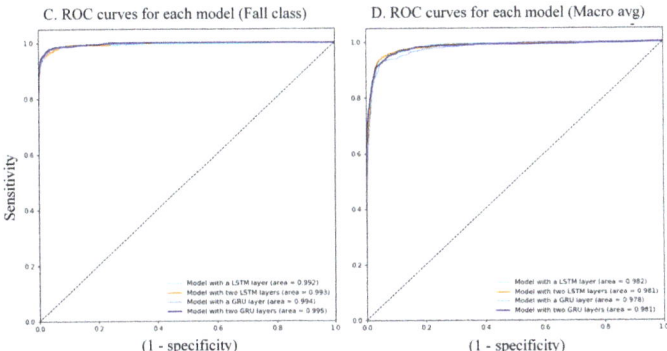

Figure 5. Receiver operating characteristic (ROC) curves of the best models for each architecture considered (at 25 Hz).

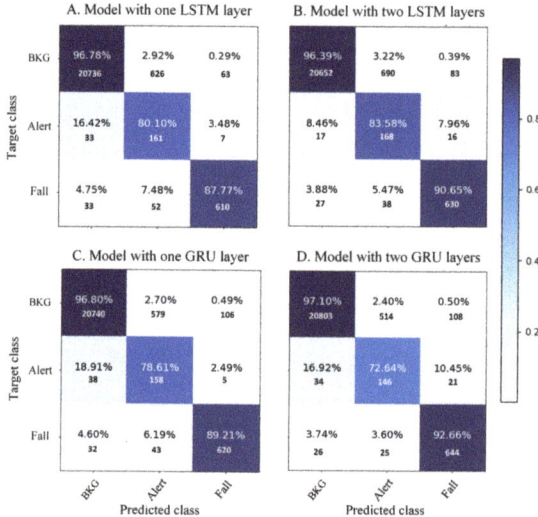

Figure 6. Confusion matrix of the best models for each architecture considered (at 25 Hz).

3.2. Integrated Model Performance

The different RNN models were integrated in the ST-Nucleo boards using the X-CUBE-AI STM32CubeMX expansion pack. It allows the conversion of pre-trained models optimized for their execution on SMT32 devices. Furthermore, it provides tools for measuring the execution times of the model more accurately, as well as for the comparison between the original algorithm version and the C-model running on the microcontroller. It is important to mention that, due to the models being trained using CuDNN versions for the RNN layers, it was needed to transmit and adapt the weights to non-CuDNN equivalent layers, before their conversion to optimized c-models. The framework allows this. To verify that the change did not affect to the model effectiveness, it was checked that the classification of the test subset matched to the results shown in the previous section. There were no differences in the classification.

To evaluate the variation in the effectiveness of the models after their conversion to optimized versions for ST32 devices, we compared the values of the outputs of the last layer for both cases. The outputs per block inference consists of three values, one for each class considered, with ranges between 0 and 1, in floating point. The L2 error for LSTM model (see Table 5) was less than 10^{-6}, which indicates very little variation in the generated models. However, the L2 error obtained is much lower in LSTM models than GRU ones. This fact can be due to differences in Keras and X-CUBE-AI libraries that affect the GRU layer implementation.

Table 5. L2 error per each model (trained model vs. generated c-model).

RNN Architecture	200 Hz	100 Hz	50 Hz	25 Hz
One LSTM layer	8.85×10^{-7}	6.47×10^{-7}	5.14×10^{-7}	2.35×10^{-7}
Two LSTM layers	5.08×10^{-7}	3.78×10^{-8}	3.78×10^{-8}	9.30×10^{-7}
One GRU layer	3.80×10^{-3}	1.92×10^{-1}	1.38×10^{-1}	3.75×10^{-1}
Two GRU layers	$2.23E \times 10^{-1}$	1.83×10^{-1}	2.26×10^{-1}	9.82×10^{-2}

Figure 7 shows the time required for each inference, that is, the classification of a unique block. It is calculated as the average execution time for 10 executions per model and block size. The lines in the chart indicate the accelerometer sampling rate, which implies approximately the available deadline of each model to run in real time. In case of the F411RE device, only the simplest models complied with the required running time, with a sampling frequency of 25 Hz, equivalent to 32 samples per block. For the L476RG, only the simplest GRU model satisfied the time requirements, but it was very close to the sampling rate (35.8 ms per classification). Due to the fact that the microcontroller also has to perform other operations such as the accelerometer reading, the L476RG device had to be discarded.

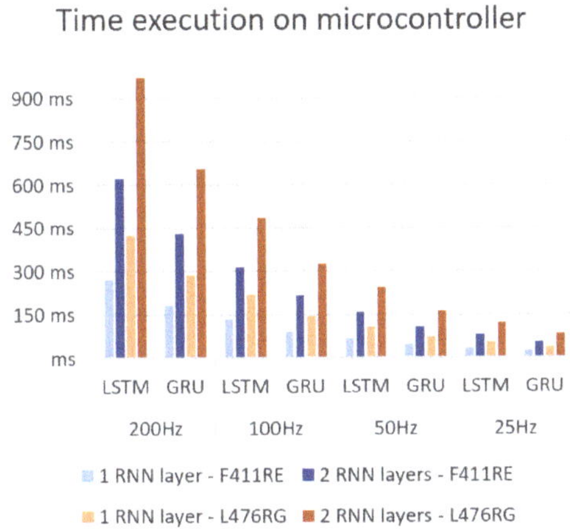

Figure 7. RNN model execution times.

Since the system can operate in real time, at a frequency of 25 Hz, this implies that the system is capable of sending an alert notification in less than 40 ms. Based on the criteria used to classify the dataset blocks, a fall would be detected in less than 180 ms since it starts. Additionally, an alert event could be detected in less than 680 ms since it begins. This implies that these types of systems can be a preventive tool, connected to some element such as a portable airbag.

3.3. Power Consumption Estimations

The components that conform the systems are a ADXL345 accelerometer and a Bluetooth HC-06 module connected to a F411RE microcontroller, and a general-purpose device as receptor. During the tests, this receptor was a personal computer, but in a real environment it would be ideally a portable device with a continuous connection to a health emergency center. The transmission protocol used for the accelerometer was I2C.

According to the technical features of the F411RE microcontroller, the current consumption when executing from Flash memory should be as low as 100 µA/MHz. In stop mode the power consumption is lower than 10 µA, which can be considered negligible. Using an I2C protocol for the accelerometer register values from the ADXL345 sensor the current estimated during the reading process is 5 mA. In case of the device without an integrated RNN, the battery is mainly used in the transmission of data, that is determined by the sampling frequency. The current for stage, consisting in transform the values to be sent, was estimated in 5 mA, and the sample sending via Bluetooth was 43 mA considering the power consumption in the specifications. At 25 Hz, the device battery life would be approximately 9.9 h if it is powered with a 150 mAh battery.

Regarding to the device with the simplest LSTM model implemented, the energy consumption comes mainly from the accelerometer values reading and the execution of the algorithm. The current estimated during the RNN execution is 5 mA, although the time spent running it is considerably longer than the transformation of values performed in the previous case (82.5% running for the simplest LSTM model and 57.5% for the simplest GRU model). The remaining power consumption depends on the number of transmissions made to alert on a fall or a risk event detection. According to [1,38], the number of falls of an elderly person is near to once a year. However, we consider in this analysis unfavorable cases, such as the case of people with poor balance or motor difficulties. Figure 8 shows the battery life considering different number of events. Considering a large number of events, up to 100 K, the device's battery life is over 35 h when implementing the LSTM model, and over 56 h if it is running the GRU model.

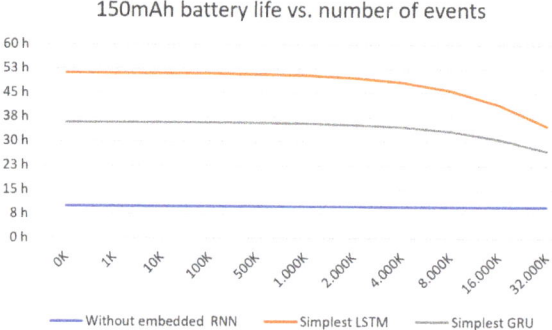

Figure 8. Battery life with the power consumption estimation for each device and feasible real-time RNN model.

Results obtained improve the battery life reported by other works with machine learning solutions [22,26]. Due to this, it can be possible to add new characteristics, such as a wifi module or connection to mobile networks, instead of bluetooth, to directly transmit information without the need for an auxiliary device.

Given the scarcity of datasets that currently exists from falls, that is the biggest problem currently for the improvement of deep learning algorithms, the system should be improved with an infrastructure based on big data analysis, as proposed in [24]. In order not to affect the battery consumption while in use, these wearable devices could integrate a data storage module that saves the data registered during the day, to be synchronized in the cloud when charging the device. This would allow this anonymized data to be used to improve the algorithm.

4. Conclusions

This work provides a study of the feasibility for the creation of wearable fall detector systems in real time using RNN architectures. The obtained results reveal that the architectures with 1 RNN layer at 25 Hz sampling frequency can be executed into a low power microcontroller in real time. The assessment of the trained models reveals that the reduction in the sampling frequency only affects the effectiveness very slightly. The estimated consumption indicates that it is possible to use small batteries. It allows to design a miniaturized device that is easy and comfortable to wear by the users.

The results in accuracy and specificity are greater or similar to other multi-class fall detector classifiers using accelerometer signals. However, sensitivity is slightly lower. The lack of data on the optimal values used and absence of F1-score metric in these studies did not allow us to make a more exhaustive comparison of effectiveness. In this study, 10-fold cross-validation has been used for greater result reliability, independently of the training subset. This reveals an F1-score deviation depending of the subset used and can explain the differences in sensitivity with other studies with evaluation methods that may be influenced by the dataset split used. In any case, this work focuses mainly on the integration of this type of model in low performance embedded systems. The execution times obtained with the proposed models are much higher than those obtained in [26], allowing real-time prediction using low power microcontrollers and higher battery life.

Due to the fact that these systems can be executed in real time, we consider that this work shows that deep learning RNN architectures are a new approach to the creation of more effective wearable fall detection systems. Therefore, we encourage research on these models, for instance by applying techniques that are already used in traditional machine learning models such as the introduction of features as input data, or reducing the complexity of the proposed models.

In future works a complete fall detection system based on this model will be thoroughly tested with new participants in order to verify the effectiveness in real scenarios.

Author Contributions: Conceptualization: F.L.-P. and A.C.-B.; Formal analysis: F.L.-P., M.J.D.-M. and A.C.-B.; Funding acquisition, A.C.-B.; Investigation: F.L.-P. and M.J.D.-M.; Methodology: F.L.-P. and M.J.D.-M.; Software: F.L.-P.; Supervision: M.J.D.-M. and A.C.-B.; Validation: M.J.D.-M.; Writing—original draft: F.L.-P.; Writing—review & editing: M.J.D.-M. and A.C.-B.

Funding: This work has been partially supported by the Telefonica Chair "Intelligence in Networks" of the Universidad de Sevilla, Spain.

Conflicts of Interest: The authors declare no conflict of interest.

Abbreviations

The following abbreviations are used in this manuscript:

RNN	Recurrent Neural Network
FDS	Fall detection system
ADL	Activity of Daily Living
LSTM	long short-term memory
GRU	Gated Recurrent Unit
K-NN	k-Nearest Neighbors
ANN	Artificial Neural Network
QSVM	Quadratic Support Vector Machine
EBT	ensembled bagged tree
TBM	Threshold based Metrics
MKL-SVM	Multiple Kernel Learning Support Vector Machine
LDA	linear discriminant analysis
LR	logistic regression
DT	decision tree
MCU	Microcontroller Unit
ROC	Receiver Operating Characteristic
AUC	Area Under the Curve

References

1. Organization, W.H.; Course, A.L.; Halth, F.C. *WHO Global Report on Falls Prevention in Older Age*; World Health Organization: Geneva, Switzerland, 2008.
2. Sri-On, J.; Tirrell, G.P.; Bean, J.F.; Lipsitz, L.A.; Liu, S.W. Revisit, subsequent hospitalization, recurrent fall, and death within 6 months after a fall among elderly emergency department patients. *Ann. Emerg. Med.* **2017**, *70*, 516–521. [CrossRef] [PubMed]
3. Rubenstein, L.Z. Falls in older people: Epidemiology, risk factors and strategies for prevention. *Age Ageing* **2006**, *35*, ii37–ii41. [CrossRef] [PubMed]
4. Aschkenasy, M.T.; Rothenhaus, T.C. Trauma and falls in the elderly. *Emerg. Med. Clin.* **2006**, *24*, 413–432. [CrossRef] [PubMed]
5. Stevens, J.A.; Corso, P.S.; Finkelstein, E.A.; Miller, T.R. The costs of fatal and non-fatal falls among older adults. *Inj. Prev.* **2006**, *12*, 290–295. [CrossRef] [PubMed]
6. Carone, G.; Costello, D. Can Europe afford to grow old. *Financ. Dev.* **2006**, *43*, 1–9.
7. Werner, C.A. *The Older Population: 2010. 2010 Census Briefs, 2011*; US Census Bureau: Washington, DC, USA, 2011.
8. Igual, R.; Medrano, C.; Plaza, I. Challenges, issues and trends in fall detection systems. *Biomed. Eng. Online* **2013**, *12*, 66. [CrossRef] [PubMed]
9. Rucco, R.; Sorriso, A.; Liparoti, M.; Ferraioli, G.; Sorrentino, P.; Ambrosanio, M.; Baselice, F. Type and location of wearable sensors for monitoring falls during static and dynamic tasks in healthy elderly: A review. *Sensors* **2018**, *18*, 1613. [CrossRef] [PubMed]
10. Pannurat, N.; Thiemjarus, S.; Nantajeewarawat, E. Automatic fall monitoring: A review. *Sensors* **2014**, *14*, 12900–12936. [CrossRef] [PubMed]
11. de Quadros, T.; Lazzaretti, A.E.; Schneider, F.K. A movement decomposition and machine learning-based fall detection system using wrist wearable device. *IEEE Sens. J.* **2018**, *18*, 5082–5089. [CrossRef]
12. Khan, S.S.; Hoey, J. Review of fall detection techniques: A data availability perspective. *Med. Eng. Phys.* **2017**, *39*, 12–22. [CrossRef] [PubMed]
13. Rescio, G.; Leone, A.; Siciliano, P. Supervised machine learning scheme for electromyography-based pre-fall detection system. *Expert Syst. Appl.* **2018**, *100*, 95–105. [CrossRef]
14. Gao, C.; Neil, D.; Ceolini, E.; Liu, S.C.; Delbruck, T. DeltaRNN: A power-efficient recurrent neural network accelerator. In Proceedings of the 2018 ACM/SIGDA International Symposium on Field-Programmable Gate Arrays, Monterey, CA, USA, 25–27 February 2018; ACM: New York, NY, USA, 2018; pp. 21–30.
15. Yu, S. Residual Learning and LSTM Networks for Wearable Human Activity Recognition Problem. In Proceedings of the 2018 37th IEEE Chinese Control Conference (CCC), Wuhan, China, 25–27 July 2018; pp. 9440–9447.
16. Musci, M.; De Martini, D.; Blago, N.; Facchinetti, T.; Piastra, M. Online fall detection using recurrent neural networks. *arXiv* **2018**, arXiv:1804.04976.
17. Canziani, A.; Paszke, A.; Culurciello, E. An analysis of deep neural network models for practical applications. *arXiv* **2016**, arXiv:1605.07678.
18. Chelli, A.; Pätzold, M. A Machine Learning Approach for Fall Detection and Daily Living Activity Recognition. *IEEE Access* **2019**, *7*, 38670–38687. [CrossRef]
19. Anguita, D.; Ghio, A.; Oneto, L.; Parra, X.; Reyes-Ortiz, J.L. A public domain dataset for human activity recognition using smartphones. In Proceedings of the ESANN European Symposium on Artificial Neural Networks, Computational Intelligence and Machine Learning, Bruges, Belgium, 24–26 April 2013.
20. Ojetola, O.; Gaura, E.; Brusey, J. Data set for fall events and daily activities from inertial sensors. In Proceedings of the 6th ACM Multimedia Systems Conference, Portland, OR, USA, 18–20 March 2015; ACM: New York, NY, USA, 2015; pp. 243–248.
21. Shahzad, A.; Kim, K. FallDroid: An automated smart-phone-based fall detection system using multiple kernel learning. *IEEE Trans. Ind. Inform.* **2018**, *15*, 35–44. [CrossRef]

22. Saleh, M.; Jeannès, R.L.B. Elderly fall detection using wearable sensors: A low cost highly accurate algorithm. *IEEE Sens. J.* **2019**, *19*, 3156–3164. [CrossRef]
23. Sucerquia, A.; López, J.; Vargas-Bonilla, J. SisFall: A fall and movement dataset. *Sensors* **2017**, *17*, 198. [CrossRef] [PubMed]
24. Yacchirema, D.; de Puga, J.S.; Palau, C.; Esteve, M. Fall detection system for elderly people using IoT and big data. *Procedia Comput. Sci.* **2018**, *130*, 603–610. [CrossRef]
25. Fortino, G.; Gravina, R. Fall-MobileGuard: A smart real-time fall detection system. In Proceedings of the 10th EAI International Conference on Body Area Networks, Sydney, Australia, 28–30 September 2015; ICST (Institute for Computer Sciences, Social-Informatics and Telecommunications Engineering): Brussels, Belgium, 2015; pp. 44–50.
26. Torti, E.; Fontanella, A.; Musci, M.; Blago, N.; Pau, D.; Leporati, F.; Piastra, M. Embedded real-time fall detection with deep learning on wearable devices. In Proceedings of the 2018 2first IEEE Euromicro Conference on Digital System Design (DSD), Prague, Czech Republic, 29–31 August 2018; pp. 405–412.
27. Hochreiter, S. The vanishing gradient problem during learning recurrent neural nets and problem solutions. *Int. J. Uncertainty Fuzziness Knowl.-Based Syst.* **1998**, *6*, 107–116. [CrossRef]
28. Bengio, Y.; Simard, P.; Frasconi, P. Learning long-term dependencies with gradient descent is difficult. *IEEE Trans. Neural Netw.* **1994**, *5*, 157–166. [CrossRef] [PubMed]
29. Williams, R.J.; Zipser, D. Gradient-based learning algorithms for recurrent. In *Backpropagation: Theory, Architectures, and Applications*; Psychology Press: London, UK, 1995; Volume 433.
30. Hochreiter, S.; Schmidhuber, J. Long short-term memory. *Neural Comput.* **1997**, *9*, 1735–1780. [CrossRef] [PubMed]
31. Cho, K.; Van Merriënboer, B.; Bahdanau, D.; Bengio, Y. On the properties of neural machine translation: Encoder-decoder approaches. *arXiv* **2014**, arXiv:1409.1259.
32. Chung, J.; Gulcehre, C.; Cho, K.; Bengio, Y. Empirical evaluation of gated recurrent neural networks on sequence modeling. *arXiv* **2014**, arXiv:1412.3555.
33. Luna-Perejon, F.; Civit-Masot, J.; Amaya-Rodriguez, I.; Duran-Lopez, L.; Dominguez-Morales, J.P.; Civit-Balcells, A.; Linares-Barranco, A. An Automated Fall Detection System Using recurrent neural networks. In Proceedings of the Conference on Artificial Intelligence in Medicine in Europe, Poznan, Poland, 26–29 June 2019; Springer: New York, NY, USA, 2019; pp. 36–41.
34. Santurkar, S.; Tsipras, D.; Ilyas, A.; Madry, A. How does batch normalization help optimization? In *Advances in Neural Information Processing Systems*; MIT Press: Cambridge, MA, USA, 2018; pp. 2483–2493.
35. Luna-Perejón, F.; Civit-Masot, J.; Muñoz-Saavedra, L.; Durán-López, L.; Amaya-Rodríguez, I.; Domínguez-Morales, J.P.; Vicente-Díaz, S.; Linares-Barranco, A.; Civit-Balcells, A.; Domínguez-Morales, M. Sampling Frequency Evaluation on recurrent neural networks Architectures for IoT Real-time Fall Detection Devices. In Proceedings of the International Joint Conference on Computational Intelligence (INSTICC), Vienna, Austria, 17–19 September 2019; pp. 536–541.
36. Srivastava, N.; Hinton, G.; Krizhevsky, A.; Sutskever, I.; Salakhutdinov, R. Dropout: A simple way to prevent neural networks from overfitting. *J. Mach. Learn. Res.* **2014**, *15*, 1929–1958.
37. Sokolova, M.; Lapalme, G. A systematic analysis of performance measures for classification tasks. *Inf. Process. Manag.* **2009**, *45*, 427–437. [CrossRef]
38. Petronila Gómez, L.; Aragón Chicharro, S.; Calvo Morcuende, B. Caídas en ancianos institucionalizados: Valoración del riesgo, factores relacionados y descripción. *Gerokomos* **2017**, *28*, 2–8.

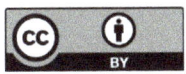

© 2019 by the authors. Licensee MDPI, Basel, Switzerland. This article is an open access article distributed under the terms and conditions of the Creative Commons Attribution (CC BY) license (http://creativecommons.org/licenses/by/4.0/).

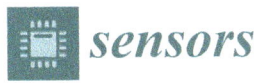

Article

Analyzing Spinal Shape Changes During Posture Training Using a Wearable Device

Katharina Stollenwerk [1,*], Jonas Müller [2], André Hinkenjann [1] and Björn Krüger [2]

1   Hochschule Bonn-Rhein Sieg, Institute of Visual Computing, 53757 Sankt Augustin, Germany
2   Gokhale Method Institute, Stanford, CA 94305, USA
*   Correspondence: katharina.stollenwerk@h-brs.de; Tel.: +49-2241-865-773

Received: 31 July 2019; Accepted: 16 August 2019; Published: 20 August 2019

Abstract: Lower back pain is one of the most prevalent diseases in Western societies. A large percentage of European and American populations suffer from back pain at some point in their lives. One successful approach to address lower back pain is postural training, which can be supported by wearable devices, providing real-time feedback about the user's posture. In this work, we analyze the changes in posture induced by postural training. To this end, we compare snapshots before and after training, as measured by the Gokhale *SpineTracker*™. Considering pairs of before and after snapshots in different positions (standing, sitting, and bending), we introduce a feature space, that allows for unsupervised clustering. We show that resulting clusters represent certain groups of postural changes, which are meaningful to professional posture trainers.

Keywords: posture analysis; spinal posture; accelerometer; wearable sensor

1. Introduction

Back pain is experienced by a large percentage of the world's population. Approximately 70% of the world's population experience lower back pain, contributing to the worldwide burden of disease. Levels of intensity and disability vary [1]:

- Grade I: low-intensity, low disability symptoms are experienced by 49%.
- Grade II: high-intensity, low disability symptoms are experienced by 12%.
- Grade III/IV: high-intensity, high disability symptoms are experienced by 11%.

In the U.S., 28% of the American workforce experiences lower back pain of various intensities at any given time, and during any given year 8% of the working population will be disabled due to low back pain [2,3]. According to Rubin and Devon [4], a majority of the population will suffer from a back problem at some point in their lives. This makes back pain the largest factor in the decline in productivity of workers, resulting in estimated economic costs ranging from $200 billion to $600 billion per year in the United States [5].

There is a wide range of treatments for back pain in use. This includes invasive methods, medication, exercise, supportive clothing, and postural change. The crowd-sourcing platform healthoutcome.org collects patients' ratings about all available treatments. In total more then 160,000 patient ratings have been collected for back pain, so far. Peleg et al. [6] report that results from this platform correspond to findings of randomized control trials. According to the crowd-sourcing platform itself, postural modifications are the highest-ranked interventions in terms of positive success. Posture training can be supported by wearable devices [7,8] to provide both, the user and the trainer, with real-time feedback about the student's posture.

In their review of works in the field of wearable technology for spine movement assessment [9], Papi et al. point out that the majority of articles in that field reported on the validity of their system with relatively few works making use of real-world data. They additionally state that the systems used were usually rather cumbersome. While their systematic review focussed on dynamic task performance only including papers themed in this direction, they excluded only three papers from their original compilation of 1610 qualifying papers (1566 of these were excluded based on their title or abstract) because the paper did not focus on *dynamic* task performance. This leads us to the valid assumption that real-world data is generally not widely used in dynamic or non-dynamic movement assessment of the spine.

Methods for analyzing changes in spine shape or posture [10–14] usually need a predefined 'normal' state to compare to or prevalently use statistical test to attempt differentiation between two defined groups. Section 2 on related work goes into detail on the aforementioned works.

We aim to address these gaps by systematically analyzing geometric changes in posture as a result of postural training by a Gokhale Method teacher and captured by the *SpineTracker*™ wearable (http://spinetracker.com, accessed 31 July 2019). To this end, we compare snapshots of the measured spine curve before training and the most recent target set by the teacher during or at the end of posture training. Our analysis does not rely on the definition of a global 'normal' spine shape.

The main contributions of this paper are:

1. The analysis of postural change in a large real-world data base of posture data, recorded using the SpineTracker wearable, by

    - devising a medium dimensional feature set from the spine curve data, well suited for further analysis and
    - showing how these data can be embedded into a two-dimensional feature space using a combination of standard dimensionality reduction techniques.

2. The demonstration that simple unsupervised clustering in the defined feature space results in a data separation which is geometrically and semantically meaningful.

The novelty of our approach lies in the fact that (a) works making use of real-world data to assess spinal movement, especially with wearables, are very rare, and that (b) we do not rely on any predefined 'normal' state to compare to.

Throughout this document we make use of the following terms: we use position to describe a passive, static state, e.g., standing, sitting. The realization of such a state by a person is called posture, emphasizing its execution as a multi-factor dynamic (active) process of both, skeletal alignment and muscle activation. When looking at a temporal sequence of motion data (here posture data), snapshot refers to a single element in that sequence.

The remainder of this work is organized as follows: We give an overview of related works in Section 2. A detailed description of the used materials and methods is given in Section 3. We present the results of our approach in Section 4 and discuss our findings in Section 5. Finally, the paper is concluded in Section 6.

2. Related Work

Human motion capturing refers to the recording of human movement and transforming them into a digital 3D representation. Full-body motion capture systems include optical and non-optical systems. Optical systems generally rely on imaging sensors and computer vision algorithms to capture a person with or without a set of passive or active markers attached to their body. Non-optical systems include motion capturing based on e.g., exoskeletons and inertial measurement unit (IMU) based systems. Optical systems generally suffer from being restricted to a capturing volume. Using inertial systems is one way to lift such restrictions.

2.1. IMU-Based Full-Body Motion Capture and Reconstruction

Roetenberg et al. [15] describe the Xsens (https://www.xsens.com, accessed 31 July 2019) IMU-based full-body human motion capturing relying on biomechanical models and sensor fusion algorithms. The system uses a set of 17 sensors. Earlier, Tautges et al. [16] enabled full-body animation through four 3D accelerometers attached to wrists and ankles in combination with a large database of motion clips recorded with a marker-based optical motion capture system. Extending on the aforementioned work, Riaz et al. [17] use accelerometer data of wrists and the lower trunk together with ground contact information (computed from trunk sensor) for data-driven motion reconstruction.

2.2. Capturing of Body Parts, Specifically the Shape of the Spine

Sometimes it is desirable to only capture data from specific body parts in order to capture these in finer detail. Examples include capturing of the face [18,19], arms [20], legs [21], hands [22,23], and spine [7,10,12,24–30].

There have been different technologies for measuring the curvature of the spine reaching from image-based surface reconstruction methods (e.g., static and dynamic rasterstereography [24,25], CT scans [10], laser-triangulation [26]) over a ribbon of (eight) fibre-optic sensors, e.g., Williams et al. [27], strips of (twelve) strain-gauge elements, e.g., Consmüller et al. [28], and accelerometers, e.g., Stollenwerk et al. [7], to inertial sensors, e.g., Wong and Wong [12], Cajamarca et al. [29], and Voinea et al. [30].

Wong and Wong [12] developed a smart garment with three inertial sensors (3D accelerometer, three 1D gyroscopes) for posture training. Sensors were mounted between T1 and T2, between T11 and L1, and on S1 (The human spine [31] is divided into four segments (from top to bottom): cervical spine (neck region), thoracic spine (mid-back), lumbar spine (lower back), and sacrum (base of the spine). Each of these regions consists of several vertebrae (here listed from top to bottom). The cervical spine consists of seven vertebrae, abbreviated C1 through C7. The following twelve vertebrae belong to the thoracic spine and are abbreviated T1 through T12. Beneath the thoracic spine are the five lumbar vertebrae, L1–L5. The sacrum is a triangular-shaped bone located below L5. It consists of five fused sacral vertebrae S1–S5). The authors estimated inclination angles in the sagittal and coronal plane of thoracic and lumbar spine and measured posture change as a change in inclination between pairs of neighboring sensors. They also included a small study on the garment's posture feedback system concluding that it helped participants to avoid poor postures.

Cajamarca et al. [29] built StraightenUp+, a low-cost wearable device for monitoring posture explicitly designed for older persons. StraightenUp+ is a backpack-shaped waist-adjustable harness vest in which three inertial sensors (3D gyroscopes and 3D accelerometers), along with other necessary hardware, are attached to the vertical rear strap. Sensors are distributed equidistantly along the vertical strap covering approximately the full length of the back. They use the sensor data to identify a fixed set of eight physical activities.

Voinea et al. [30] and Stollenwerk et al. [7] describe a 2D reconstruction model for the shape of the human spine based on inertial sensors and plain accelerometers. Although Voinea et al.'s sensors are capable of outputting 3D orientations, they only use a single angle for spine shape reconstruction. In their setup, the five sensors are distributed equidistantly between C7 and L4 vertebrae. While from a reconstruction image their model looks a lot like the one used in [7], Voinea et al.'s models are designed to explicitly represent a C-shaped spine (kyphosis) and an S-shaped spine (normal), the authors of [7] do not make that assumption. Another difference is that [7] puts the first sensor on the L4 vertebra but distributes the following sensors equidistantly over a fixed-length segment independent of the person's spine length.

An overview of commonly used technologies for spine movement assessment along with respective spine outcomes is reported in the Papi et al. review of works in the field of wearable technology for spine movement assessment [9]. As explained in detail in the introduction (Section 1), this work gave rise to our assumption that in general, real-world data is rarely used in the movement assessment of the spine, neither in dynamic nor in non-dynamic settings.

2.3. Methods for Data Analysis

Hay et al. [10] compare spine curves extracted from CT images to a model spine curve computed from multiple individuals without spinal disorders and a history of back pain. Aiming at the detection and quantification of pathologies, the comparison is based on the amount of curve deviation from the model, the deviation of the curvature as well as the torsion along the curve.

In their paper, Brink et al. [11] evaluate the amount of postural change in adolescent computer users after a period of twelve months in order to understand associations between postural change and upper quadrant musculoskeletal pain. For this purpose, different sitting postural angles were recorded and individually analyzed with respect to magnitude and orientational change using univariate and multivariate linear regression models. Sitting postural angles considered were head flexion, neck flexion, craniocervical angle, and trunk flexion. These angles mainly target the upper spinal region. In a small three-day posture feedback study (first day without feedback, second and third day with feedback) Wong and Wong [12] compare average trunk angles between days with and without feedback as well as between days with feedback.

Franklin and Conner-Kerr [13] investigated the relationship of postural changes during pregnancy and back pain. They measured and compared means and standard deviations as well as state analysis of variance (ANOVA) results for a total of nine postural variables (seven postural angles and head and shoulder displacements) of women in the first and third trimesters of pregnancy. Gonzáles-Sanchez et al. [14] compare thoracolumbar curvature angles between two groups (normal weighted and obese persons) using Student's t-test (parametric test for independent data) and Wilcoxon's test (non-parametric tests) in order to find out if there are statistically significant differences between the two groups.

As stated before (Section 1), methods summarized here either rely on a predefined 'normal' state to compare to or use statistical tests to compare two defined groups. In contrast to this, we aim at an analysis of changes in spinal shape essentially comparing two arbitrary spine curves of one person at two points in time, one before (unguided) and one after posture training (guided). To the best of our knowledge, there is no method for the geometric analysis of that change.

3. Materials and Methods

In this section we describe the system used for data recording in Section 3.1, the data we worked with (Section 3.2) as well as the derived feature space (Section 3.3) and dimensionality reduction techniques in Sections 3.4 and 3.5. The following Section 3.6 contains information on minimum spanning trees and how they can be used for clustering. We detail our processing pipeline in Section 3.7 and conclude with an explanation of visualization methods used to present results (Section 3.8).

3.1. Wearable

The system used for capturing the spinal shape is the *SpineTracker* developed by Gokhale Method Enterprises, Stanford, CA, USA. It consists of five individual accelerometer-based sensors (Figure 1a) which are attached to the lower back of the user as shown in Figure 1b,c. In contrast to single-device posture wearables, the five-sensor approach enables the capture of more detailed spinal curvature information also covering a larger portion of the spine.

All five sensor units were technically identical. The sensors connected and streamed data wirelessly to one host via bluetooth; currently this may be an iOS device or a computer. The sensors support sample rates of up to 50 Hz, thus allowing for a variety of applications, ranging from slow-motion measurements, e.g., sitting, to faster movements such as brisk walking.

More detailed technical information on the wearable as well as the model used for reconstruction of a spine shape from the accelerometer readings and the systematic evaluation of the system's accuracy (sensors and reconstruction method) can be found in [7].

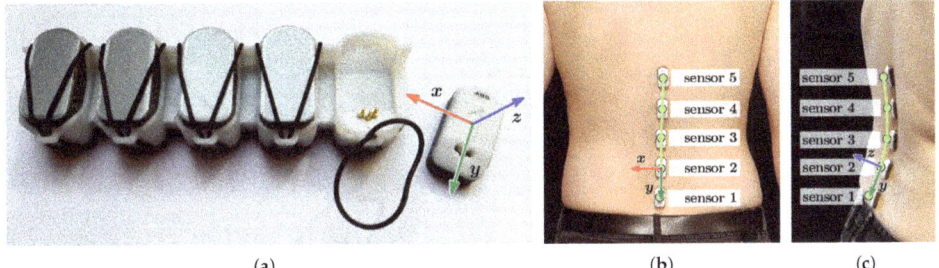

Figure 1. Photos of the *SpineTracker* sensor system. (**a**) Four of the five sensors are sitting in the charger. The sensor outside the charger is shown with its local coordinate system. A single sensor has the dimensions 33 mm × 16 mm × 10 mm. Each sensor is attached to a person's lumbar spine with double sided tape. (**b**,**c**) Back and side view of sensor positioning on the lumbar spine including directions of the sensor coordinate system. Sensors are overlayed with a reconstructed spine curve (green dots and line).

3.2. Data

The data representing the shape of the spine is usually either a set of angles or a set of 2D positions: when streaming data from the sensors, spine shape information is stored as a sequence of forward tilts $\tau_{acc,i}, i = 1, \ldots, 5$ of the five *SpineTracker* sensors ordered by sensor ID. Using the spine curve model described in [7], these five angles are transformed into a 2D spine curve consisting of six 2D points P_j (a base point P_0 and five sensor positions $P_i, i = 1, \ldots, 5$) and arc segments connecting these points. For consistent visualization, the spine curve is positioned in space in a way that the first sensor lies in the origin, $P_1 = (0, 0)$.

The *SpineTracker* sensor system can also capture single frames ("snapshots") from the data stream that will represent the shape of the spine at that point in time. We used a database of such snapshots of three distinct positions: standing, sitting, and (hip) hinging. Snapshots can be unguided or guided. In an unguided snapshot, a person assumed one of the positions on their own and without a trainer's intervention or support. A guided snapshot was taken when the position was assumed under the guidance of a posture trainer. Each single snapshot in this database was labelled either "guided" or "unguided".

From this database, we considered per-user snapshot pairs. These pairs consist of one unguided posture and one teacher-guided posture in which the highest amount of change is to be expected. i.e., for the unguided postures, we extracted the respective initial posture snapshot of a position (t_0 snapshot). For the guided postures, we used the latest guided snapshot (t_1 snapshot) available. The t_0 *snapshots* hence represent the most unlearned realizations of the position and the t_1 *snapshots* contain the current best imitation of the position the user aims for at the moment of capture. As a consequence, we use exactly one pair per user and position even if more snapshots of that user are available for a specific position. For ethical reasons all data was anonymized. Table 1 gives details on the size of the database used, split by position, as well as overall. It additionally shows statistics on the time passed between unguided and guided snapshots.

In order to show that there was a significant difference in angles between the t_0 and t_1 snapshot pairs in one or more sensors, indicating plausibility of further analysis, we considered each sensor individually and conducted a paired samples Wilcoxon test (also called the Wilcoxon signed-rank test) [32].

Table 1. General statistics of the data basis used for our analysis. The column labelled # samples contains information on the number of snapshot pairs per position. The # users states how many different users recorded such pairs. The last four columns state the minimum, average, median, and maximum time passed between the snapshots in each pair. Time is displayed as a tuple of days (d), hours (hh), minutes (mm), and seconds (ss).

	# Samples	# Users	\multicolumn{4}{c}{Time Difference, Format: "d hh:mm:ss"}			
			Minimum	Mean	Median	Maximum
standing	393	393	0 00:30:07	30 01:34:18	2 00:39:43	443 03:38:05
sitting	386	386	0 00:30:13	23 23:03:02	2 01:16:43	399 00:23:05
hip hinging	362	362	0 00:37:44	24 11:23:42	2 00:54:51	385 21:39:54
full	1141	425	0 00:30:07	26 05:26:02	2 01:08:07	443 03:38:05

The database of (t_0, t_1) posture pairs used in this work is publicly available at https://skylab.vc.h-brs.de/kstoll2m/PosturePairsDB19/ (Supplementary Materials).

3.3. Feature Extraction

For each pair of snapshots in the database of position-posture-pairs we compute a feature vector F. F is composed of the normalized difference d_j of the sensor positions in the t_0 and t_1 snapshots and the length l_j of the difference

$$l_j = \left\| P_{j|t_1} - P_{j|t_0} \right\|_2 \tag{1}$$

$$d_j = \frac{P_{j|t_1} - P_{j|t_0}}{l_j}, \tag{2}$$

where $P_{j|t_0}$ ($P_{j|t_1}$) is the j-th 2D spine curve point in snapshot t_0 (t_1). This way, spinal shape change is expressed by the 2D directional change between the two snapshots and the 1D amount of change. This results in a 15 dimensional feature vector, five 2D directions d_j and five 1D lengths l_j, $j \in \{0, 2, 3, 4, 5\}$, for each snapshot pair. We only considered five of the six spine curve points leaving out the sensor positioned in zero (P_1). For general statistics we continue to use the sensor angle data $\tau_{acc,i|t}$, $i = 1, \ldots, 5, t \in \{t_0, t_1\}$.

3.4. Principal Component Analysis

Principal component analysis (PCA) [33] is one of the oldest and most widely used linear dimensionality reduction techniques. It is based on the eigendecomposition of the data's covariance matrix. Its eigenvectors are sorted by their respective eigenvalue forming the new orthogonal coordinate axes (principal component) of the underlying data set. The directions of the new coordinate axes coincide with the directions of maximum variation of the original data points. Geometrically spoken, PCA rotates the Cartesian coordinate system of a high dimensional point set in a way that maximizes the variance of the data along each axis. After the transform, axes are sorted by descending variance. Dimensionality reduction is achieved by retaining only the first n principal components.

3.5. T-Stochastic Neighbor Embedding

T-stochastic neighbor embedding (t-SNE) [34] is a more recent non-linear dimensionality reduction technique for mapping high-dimensional data to a low-dimensional space (often called a map). It is based on the following:

- A fix data similarity matrix of conditional distances between pairs of data points in the original high-dimensional space. Conditional distances are computed based on a combination of the pairwise Euclidean distances and a point-specific Gaussian distribution.

- A similar point-wise neighborhood estimation in the low-dimensional target space (map similarity matrix), exchanging the Gaussian distribution with a one degree-of-freedom Student's t-distribution.

The goal is to iteratively adapt the map similarity matrix to best fit the data similarity matrix. This is achieved by minimization of the Kullback–Leibler divergence [35] of the two probability distributions underlying the two similarity matrices.

3.6. Minimum Spanning Tree and Clustering

A minimum spanning tree (MST) is a graph theory concept fulfilling the following criteria: given an undirected graph $G = (V, E)$ of vertices V and weighted edges E, an MST is a tree $(V, E' \subseteq E)$ including all vertices of G using a minimum number of edges E' such that the total weight of the edges is minimal. The MST is unique if all edge weights are distinct, which is a reasonable assumption for real-world scenarios.

MSTs can be used for clustering. Let $G = (V, E)$ be a fully connected graph of the data points (V) of a data set. Let the weight of each edge $e = \{v, w\} \in E$ be defined as e.g., the Euclidean distance between the data points v and w it connects. This graph is used to construct an MST which is then used for clustering: Subsequent cutting of edges with highest weight increases the number of connected components in this graph. Connected components represent clusters.

3.7. Processing Pipeline

An overview of our processing pipeline is given in Figure 2. For each pair of snapshots in our database, we compute each posture's 2D spine curve and extract one feature vector per snapshot pair as described above (Section 3.3). We perform PCA to the set of extracted features to reduce the dimensionality of the data while retaining over 95% of the feature data's variance. We additionally use t-SNE to further reduce the dimensionality to two dimensions. PCA, as well as other linear dimensionality reduction techniques, preserves the global structure of the data. This preservation of global structure results from maintaining a high variability in the data which in turn translates in a separation of dissimilar data points. The non-linear dimensionality reduction t-SNE tries both, keep similar data points close together and dissimilar data points far apart. This is particularly interesting for finding clusters of data points in higher dimensional space.

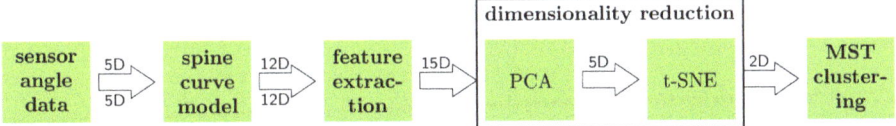

Figure 2. Overview of the processing pipeline used. Individual steps are marked by boxes, arrows indicate the direction of the pipeline. Each arrow is annotated with dimensionality of the data output by the preceding step. Two dimension labels indicate that the data from the two postures in each posture pair is not yet combined.

Clustering generally groups data points sharing a set of properties. Even though postural training is a highly individual process, we assume that the recorded data will exhibit certain differences and commonalities. This in turn will allow us to combine posture pairs into distinct clusters. We apply MST-clustering to the two-dimensional t-SNE map of the chosen feature space, as there is no prior knowledge on the general structure of clusters in the 2D t-SNE map. We compute the Euclidean distance between all pairs of t-SNE map points, which results in a similarity matrix of the map. The MST is constructed on this similarity matrix. Using MST-clustering is a reasonable choice due to the following properties:

1. The t-SNE map equalizes the density of neighboring data points in the higher dimensionality evening out distances between neighboring points in the map. As a consequence condensed clusters are spread and spread clusters are contracted.
2. In MST-clustering, data points are grouped together by proximity and need neither be separable by a regular geometric curve nor grouped around a centroid.

3.8. Visualization of Results

We visualize clustering results using the 2D t-SNE map of the data coloring each point by its cluster ID. We compute the angle difference between the t_1 and t_0 snapshots, $\tau_{acc,i|t_1} - \tau_{acc,i|t_0}$, $i = 1, \ldots, 5$. This set of difference angles was used to reconstruct an *offset spine shape*. The resulting offset base position $P_{offset,0}$ and offset sensor positions $P_{offset,i}$, $i = 1, \ldots, 5$, ordered by increasing y-coordinate, represent the computed differences as offset from a vertical line. Figure 3b shows an example of such an *offset spine shape*. The underlying two reconstructed spine shapes are illustrated in Figure 3a.

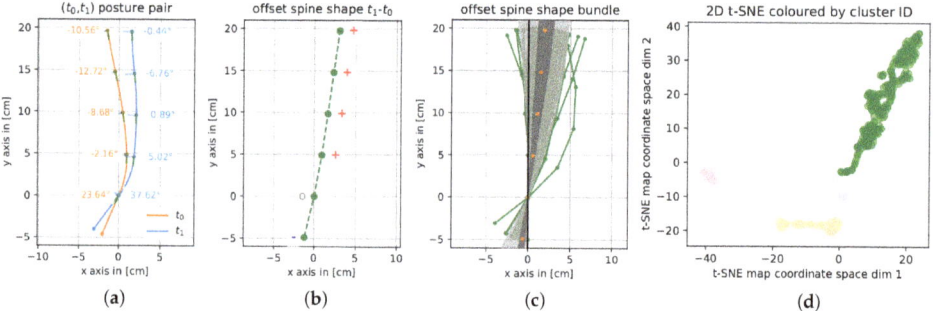

Figure 3. (**a**) Two spine shapes reconstructed from the t_0 and t_1 input angles and (**b**) resulting *offset spine shape*. (**c**) Offset spine shape bundle representing a data cluster in the feature set's T-stochastic neighbor embedding (t-SNE) map (**d**), colored by cluster ID.

Spine shapes are annotated with the sensor angle data they were constructed from and an indication to which side the person is looking: the line in each sensor position points away from the person's back.

Offset spine shapes are annotated with the sign of each offset position's x-coordinate. A red '+' stands for positive, a grey 'o' for zero, and a blue '-' for a negative horizontal offset from a vertical line positioned in zero.

As each data point in a cluster represents the difference of two spine shapes, we also visualize clusters by overlaying all offset spine shapes of each cluster as displayed in Figure 3c. The light grey area in this visualization represents the region between the 1st-percentile and 99th-percentile of the horizontal distribution of the data. Covering the central 50% of the horizontal extent of the offset spine shapes (at each point level), the dark grey area shows the region between the 25th-percentile and the 75th-percentile. Orange dots mark the median of the horizontal extent of the data. This overlay serves as visualization of the main orientation of the offset spine shapes in a specific cluster.

4. Results

In the following, we first list the results of the angle data analysis (Section 4.1) and motivate why this analysis is relevant. We then describe the behavior of the clustering under variation of the t-SNE parameter perplexity in Section 4.2. For this section, too, we state reasons for analyzing results from this variation. The last Section 4.3 presents and analyzes the results of the clustering of the posture data divided by position based on their geometry.

4.1. Analysis of the Angle Data

As normality test (Shapiro-Wilk [36], Anderson-Darling [37], Q-Q Plot [38]) indicated that the data is not normally distributed, we use the non-parametric paired samples Wilcoxon test (also called the Wilcoxon signed-rank test) [39] to check whether there was a difference in posture for the unguided and guided snapshots already on a single sensor level. We could confirm that for all positions, there was at least one sensor in which the median change in angle between the unguided t_0 snapshots and the guided t_1 snapshot pairs was significantly different from zero.

For standing, there was a significant difference in angle between the t_0 and t_1 snapshot pairs for all sensors ($p < \varepsilon = 10^{-6}$). For sitting the difference between the two snapshots is significant for only the first sensor ($p < \varepsilon$). Finally, the angle difference between t_0 and t_1 snapshot pairs is below the standard significance threshold $\alpha = 0.05$ for all but one sensor for hip hinging ($p < \varepsilon$ for four out of five sensors).

Descriptive statistics of both snapshots for all positions and sensors are listed in Table 2. The last column of the table marks the previously reported sensors for which $p < \alpha$. Figure 4 provides additional information on the distribution of the five sensors' angle data for each position.

Table 2. Mean, standard deviation (sd), minimum (min), maximum (max), and median (med) values as well as the interquartile range (IQR) of all five sensor's angle data for t_0 and t_1 snapshots. A star in the last column stands for a rejected null hypothesis of the Wilcoxon signed-rank test ($p < 0.05$).

	t_0 Snapshots					t_1 Snapshots					
	Mean (SD)	Min	Max	Med	IQR	Mean (SD)	Min	Max	Med	IQR	
standing											
sensor 1	19.6 (10.3)	−24.6	57.8	19.4	11.8	22.5 (8.0)	−4.5	48.2	22.7	10.2	*
sensor 2	10.1 (10.7)	−19.8	54.1	10.0	13.0	13.8 (9.2)	−14.4	51.4	13.3	12.4	*
sensor 3	−4.1 (10.3)	−40.4	53.8	−4.5	11.1	−0.1 (9.0)	−27.9	54.1	−0.9	10.4	*
sensor 4	−12.3 (8.9)	−29.6	82.0	−13.1	8.5	−8.2 (6.6)	−30.1	45.3	−8.3	7.0	*
sensor 5	−12.0 (9.5)	−28.2	115.7	−12.8	8.3	−7.6 (7.3)	−24.9	77.2	−7.7	7.5	*
sitting											
sensor 1	12.0 (10.0)	−34.1	45.2	11.8	13.4	16.7 (10.2)	−22.3	56.1	16.2	11.4	*
sensor 2	6.0 (9.4)	−21.6	35.1	5.6	12.3	6.3 (8.5)	−16.0	43.2	5.9	9.8	
sensor 3	−0.6 (8.7)	−26.9	37.1	−0.7	10.6	−1.0 (7.1)	−25.1	35.3	−0.9	7.8	
sensor 4	−6.8 (7.4)	−32.5	32.0	−6.7	9.9	−6.9 (6.9)	−30.3	40.6	−6.6	8.2	
sensor 5	−6.9 (8.2)	−84.7	36.8	−7.3	9.1	−6.7 (5.9)	−20.5	22.0	−6.8	7.7	
hip hinging											
sensor 1	75.5 (18.1)	2.7	114.8	77.7	22.7	81.8 (14.5)	21.9	116.9	83.7	19.1	*
sensor 2	77.4 (18.8)	−9.7	121.0	80.1	22.8	79.9 (14.5)	33.1	116.3	81.0	19.8	
sensor 3	79.1 (20.1)	−16.9	128.1	81.7	23.6	75.1 (15.1)	27.7	111.4	75.7	20.4	*
sensor 4	82.1 (21.6)	−22.2	128.5	85.2	24.9	69.3 (15.1)	20.2	109.1	71.2	19.5	*
sensor 5	87.8 (22.6)	−26.3	142.0	90.7	25.3	69.1 (14.6)	9.4	111.8	70.5	17.8	*

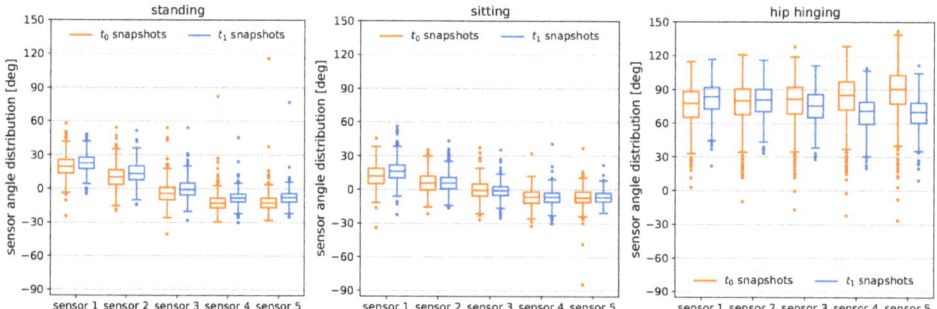

Figure 4. Boxplots of the angle distribution of the t_0 and t_1 snapshots grouped by sensor. The box frames the lower (Q_1) to upper (Q_3) quartile values of the data. The horizontal line inside each box marks the data's median. Whiskers include data between $Q_1 - 1.5$ IQR and $Q_3 + 1.5$ IQR, where IQR $= Q_3 - Q_1$ abbreviates the interquartile range. Outliers outside the whisker range are marked with dots.

4.2. Clustering under Varying t-SNE Perplexity

The t-SNE parameter *perplexity* reflects the number of neighbors expected in its distance optimization process. In their paper [34] van der Maaten and Hinton state that variation of perplexity has little influence on the performance of t-SNE. In order to assert clustering of our data is prevalently consistent under variation of perplexity, we show the results of clustering the 2D t-SNE map into four (six for hip hinging) clusters for perplexity values ranging from 25 to 40 in steps of five in Figure 5.

As Figure 5 shows, most of the time the general size of the clusters were approximately identical under variation of perplexity. This was also true for the data represented by these clusters. The only noteworthy exception is observed in *sitting* when using a perplexity value of 40, also see Figure 6a,b in comparison to Figure 6c, which is drawn using a perplexity value of 25 but is the same for 30 and 35. While the general shape of the t-SNE map superficially appears unchanged, distances between groups of data points slightly shift. The three segments of cluster 1 were pulled apart and partially moved closer to cluster 0, thus changing the split position of clusters 0 and 1 and associating about 25 data points more (less) to cluster ID 0 (1) than for lower perplexity values.

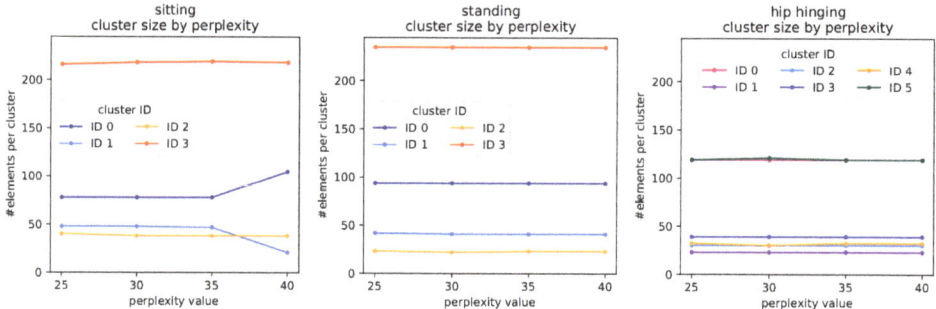

Figure 5. The number of elements per cluster under variation of the perplexity value, plotted by cluster ID.

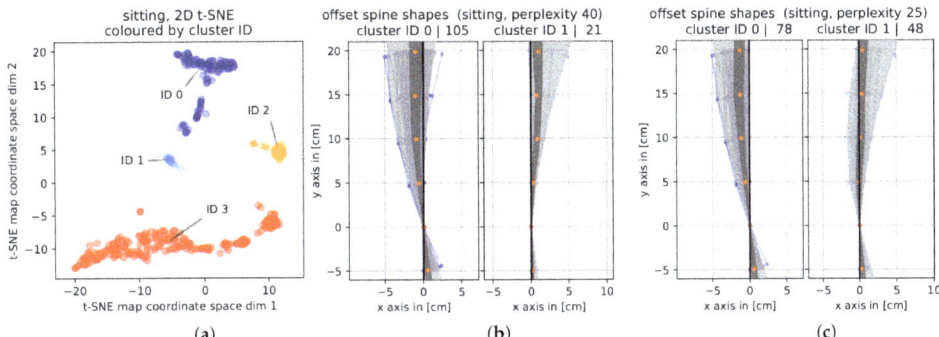

Figure 6. Visual comparison of changes in clustering when varying perplexity. (**a**) A 2D t-SNE map and (**b**) offset spine shape bundles per cluster for a perplexity value of 40. (**c**) offset spine shape bundles per cluster for a perplexity value of 25. The offset spine shape bundles displayed represent the only two clusters that changed for a perplexity value of 40. All axis titles of the offset spine shape bundles contain information of the cluster ID and the number of elements in that cluster.

Inspecting the data (offset spine shape bundles) more closely, we see that with a perplexity value of 40, almost all offset spine shapes in cluster ID 1 havd a positive x-coordinate, while this was not the case for lower perplexity values. For lower values, these two clusters are predominantly split based on the horizontal offset from zero in the base position P_0 and the topmost position P_5. The data in the other clusters remain identical throughout parameter variation.

Choice of Parameters for Cluster Analysis

Throughout the results presented in this paper we used the following parameters. The number of PCA components was chosen such that the resulting lower dimensional space still captures over 95% of the feature data variance. For the computation of the 2D t-SNE map, we fixed the cost parameter perplexity to 30, which is approximately the centre of achieving repeatedly stable results for clustering (see Figure 5). Optimization parameters of t-SNE are left to the implementation defaults [40] as these in general only affect the rate of convergence [41]. Upon initial inspection of the data, and after confirming that clusters would be stable when varying parameters in repeated computations, we set the number of clusters to four for standing and sitting and to six for hip hinging.

4.3. Analysis of Clusters per Position

The following three sections analyze results from clustering from a geometric point of view, assigning a geometric meaning to each cluster. The analysis is separated into the three positions: standing Section 4.3.1, sitting Section 4.3.2, and hip hinging Section 4.3.3.

4.3.1. Standing

Figure 7 illustrates the results of clustering the data from posture pairs of *standing* into four components in form of their 2D t-SNE map and in form of offset spine shape bundles. For the visualization of cluster representatives (t_0 and t_1 posture pairs and $t_1 - t_0$ offset spine shapes), please see Figure A2 in the Appendix A.

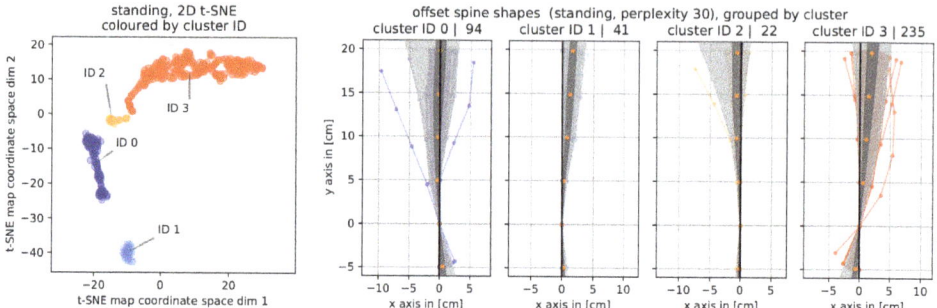

Figure 7. Results for clustering posture pairs of *standing*. (**left**) The T-SNE map labelled with and colored by cluster ID. (**right**) Corresponding cluster bundles of *offset spine shapes* including information about the cluster ID and the number of elements in that cluster in each axis title.

Geometrically, the four clusters were separated mainly based on the position of the offset spine shapes' base points and further by the orientation of the upper part. For the first and second cluster (IDs 0 and 1), the offset spine shapes all had positive base point x-coordinates while these were negative for the third and fourth cluster (IDs 2 and 3). The first and second cluster differ in the position representing the second sensor ($P_{\text{offset},2}$), for ID 0 its x-coordinate is always negative while it was always positive for ID 1). The upper part of the offset spine shape bundle of cluster ID 0 shared no particular orientation, this part is clearly leaning in positive x direction. This pattern was repeated for the third and fourth cluster (IDs 2 and 3), in which the third cluster tends to negative values and the fourth cluster leans to positive values. Again a clear geometric separation can only be seen for the offsets in $P_{\text{offset},2}$.

4.3.2. Sitting

Figure 8 shows the results of clustering the data from sitting posture pairs into four components using the 2D t-SNE map and the offset spine shape bundles per cluster. Again, we show representative spine curve shapes and offset spine curve shapes for each cluster in the Appendix A, Figure A4.

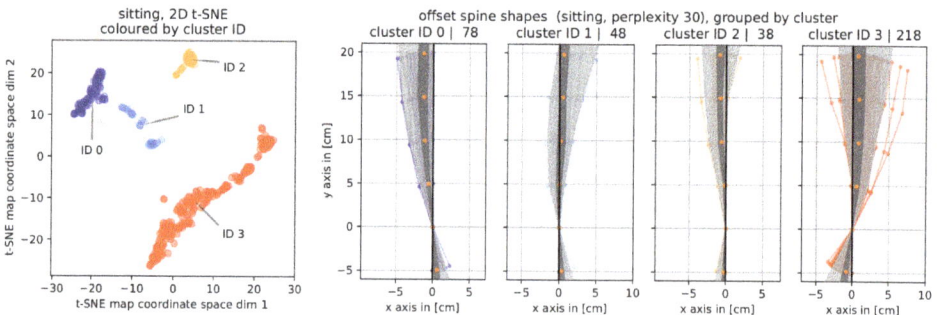

Figure 8. Results for clustering posture pairs of *sitting*. (**left**) The t-SNE map labelled and colored by cluster ID. (**right**) Corresponding cluster bundles of *offset spine shapes* including information about the cluster ID and the number of elements in that cluster.

The geometric pattern observed in *standing* repeats for *sitting*: the four clusters are separated mainly based on the position of the offset spine shapes' base points and further by the orientation of the upper part: For the first and second cluster (IDs 0 and 1), the offset spine shapes all have positive base point x-coordinates while these are negative for the third and fourth cluster (IDs 2 and 3). The two groups can each be further separated into positive slanted clusters (IDs 1 and 3) and negative slanted clusters (IDs 0 and 2). While only sensor 1 shows a significant difference between the angular data of the unguided and guided snapshot pairs on a per sensor level (see Section 4.1 and Table 2), the combined information on all five sensors allows for a class separation into four clusters.

4.3.3. Hip Hinging

The results of clustering t_0 and t_1 posture pairs of the position hinging into six clusters are presented in Figure 9. As before, we show the 2D t-SNE map colored by cluster ID along with the corresponding offset spine shape bundles. For representative spine curves for each cluster, please refer to the Appendix A, Figure A6.

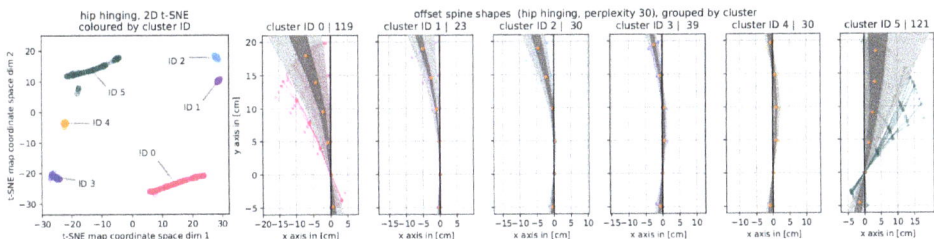

Figure 9. Results for clustering posture pairs of *hip hinging*. (**left**) The t-SNE map labelled with and colored by cluster ID. (**right**) Corresponding cluster bundles of *offset spine shapes*.

Here, the geometry of the offset spine shapes reveals a clear pattern. Again, an initial distinction between the clusters can be made based on the position of the base points. One cluster (ID 0) had only positive *x*-valued base points while this is purely negative for four of the five others (IDs 1–4) and almost purely negative (except for seven samples) for the last cluster (ID 5). In the upper part, all samples in the first cluster (ID 0) more or less strongly slanted to the left, all upper offset spine shape points having a negative *x*-coordinate. This was also the case for the upper part of the second cluster (ID 1). For the subsequent clusters (IDs 2–5) the position at which the offset spine shapes of that cluster cross the thought vertical line passing through $x = 0$ moved stepwise up. For cluster ID 1 there was no crossing. In cluster ID 1, the offset spine shapes cross that line between $P_{\text{offset},2}$ and $P_{\text{offset},3}$, i.e., the *x*-coordinate of all $P_{\text{offset},2}$ is > 0 and it is < 0 for all $P_{\text{offset},k}, k \in \{3,4,5\}$. For the next cluster (ID 2), the crossing is between $P_{\text{offset},3}$ and $P_{\text{offset},4}$. This progression continues up to the last cluster (ID 5) in which there is no crossing in the observed area, meaning that all offset spine curves slant in positive direction ($x > 0$ for $P_{\text{offset},k}, k \in \{2,3,4,5\}$). These properties defines the separation of clusters with IDs 1–5.

5. Discussion

This section shortly summarizes results (Sections 5.1 and 5.2), puts this work in context with existing research (Section 5.3), and lists limitations in Section 5.4.

5.1. Summary of Results

For all three positions, sitting, standing, hip hinging, we found a significant change in posture between the sets of guided and unguided snapshot pairs. We used a Wilcoxon signed-rank test on the sensor angle data representation of the posture pairs. This results indicated that is is plausible to further analyze posture pairs in our data base with respect to postural change.

We confirmed that our clusters remain stable under variation of the t-SNE parameter perplexity.

In the geometric analysis of the clusters for each position, it turned out that clusters formed based on the position of offset spine shapes, the base points, and the direction of the upper part. This underlines the necessity of a multi-sensor system to achieve a meaningful separation into different clusters. The separation of the upper part was more fine-grained as there are six clusters for hip hinging.

Showing several samples per cluster to a professional posture trainer, the samples and clusters, that are based on our geometric feature, had a meaning for her. Her assessments are summarized in the following section.

5.2. Sample-Based Evaluation per Cluster by a Professional Posture Trainer

Several samples of unguided and guided posture pairs per cluster were shown to a professional posture teacher. She has experience in comparing such posture pairs and is able to understand how the change in posture within such a posture pair affects the shape of the spine as well as posture in general. This information is important to give semantic meaning to our clusters which formed based on geometric features.

A professional posture trainer interprets clusters for *standing* (see Figure 7) the following way: Cluster ID 0 represents a loss of pelvic anteversion and often (but not always) a reduction in sway. The second cluster (ID 1) stands for a group of users who have sacrificed a little in pelvic anteversion and very much straightened out a sway. The most notable property of the third cluster (ID 2) was a high reduction of sway. The second property which this cluster shares with the last cluster but to a smaller degree is an increased pelvic anteversion. The last cluster cluster could not be attributed with a definitive property describing the changes in the upper part.

From the perspective of a professional posture trainer, in *sitting* (see Figure 8), cluster ID 0 represents cases that have less curvature in the upper lumbar area and (possibly due to having reduced that curvature) reduced pelvic anteversion. The second cluster (ID 1) stands for sacrificing (a little) pelvic anteversion and straightening out a sway. Both remaining clusters (IDs 2 and 3) exhibit an increase in pelvic anteversion. Only cluster ID 2 could clearly be associated with a reduced sway while for the fourth cluster (ID 3) there was no clear attribution to a consistent change in posture valid throughout the cluster.

The posture trainer's assessments of the clustering for *hip hinging* (see Figure 9) was this: Cluster ID 0 in the guided t_1 snapshots did not go as far with the pelvis as in the unguided t_0 snapshot and learned to stop rounding the upper part of the back in order to reach deeper. People in cluster ID 1 go further down in t_1 than in t_0 or as deep as in t_0 in the lowest part of the pelvis and also stopped rounding the upper back. The next cluster (ID 2) represents students who stopped rounding in the upper lumbar area and who have increased their pelvic anteversion. Cluster four (ID 3) is a group with more anteversion in the pelvis and a straighter upper back. This general pattern repeats for cluster ID 4: rounding in t_0, not rounded any more in the t_1 snapshot and slightly more pelvic anteversion. In the last cluster (ID 5) the posture trainer sees students who use a sway to overcome their inability to tip their pelvis (alone), thus their pelvic tip increases but so does their sway.

5.3. Relation to Existing Research

Previous work on spine shape analysis has for a long time been majorly interesting in medicine. There, analysis is mainly driven by pathology quantification, by relation investigation, or by evaluation of a new technology. Pathology quantification (e.g., Hay et al. [10], 24 participants) is often tightly tied to a definition of a 'normal' spine shape, determining and assessing a given spine shape by its deviation from the 'normal' one. Relation driven investigations give answer to questions like *is there a relation between weight groups (normal, obese) and differences in spinal curvatures?* ([14], 39 participants), or *is there a relation of back pain and changes in spine curvature during pregnancy?* ([13], twelve participants), or *is upper back pain related to the amount of postural change in young computer users?* ([11], 153 participants). Relation driven questions are tested for significance and hypothesis confirmation using statistical tests, e.g., ANOVA, Student's t-test, or Wilcoxon's test.

Wearables have become an increasingly promising tool for posture monitoring and analysis. Posture change comparisons here are also often based on a 'neutral' or 'normal ' position: In an evaluation study, Wong and Wong [42] (three participants, three repetitions of each position) use accelerometers to measure postural change in terms of curvature variation from a *neutral sitting* position for three pre-defined modifications: sitting with left (right) lateral bending, and sitting while flexing forward. They computed curvature variation with respect to *neutral sitting*.

Without the notion of a 'normal' state for spine shape or posture and without pre-defined groups to put into relation to one another, we invert the process described above: Based on a database of spine shapes of unguided and guided posture pairs, we cluster changes in spinal shape. Clusters form based on the geometry of the change and represent a semantically meaningful separation of the data according to the assessment of a professional posture trainer.

5.4. Limitations

Our database did not have information on gender, age, height, or weight of the users. Therefore, we could not separate our analysis based on such criteria. However, these factors can have a considerable impact on the shape of the spine: Nachemson et al. [43] reported a minor tendency for the influence of age on increased stiffness of intervertebral discs. The authors also found that in bending, female motion segments are more flexible than male. According to Hay et al. [10], the BMI, which is based on weight and height, is related to thoracic sagittal kyphosis. Youdas et al. [44] found an association between BMI and pelvic inclination.

Another limitation of our presented work is the choice of the number of clusters. These were mainly based on observations in the 2D t-SNE map. Especially in light of the posture trainer's evaluation of the clusters, it is easily seen that the number of clusters suggested by the geometry does not necessarily reflect the number of clusters found by the posture trainer. Therefore it would be highly beneficial to include several posture trainer's knowledge on patterns in change into the clustering approach and maybe even into feature design.

We showed several samples per cluster to only one professional posture trainer for postural change evaluation. As this work aimed at describing a general methodology for analysis of changes in spine shape, we did not do a blind-test cross-validation with several posture trainers, removing any information relating a sample to a cluster and have several posture trainers assess the samples. However, this would make the evaluation of the postural change in the clusters independent and improve the reliability of the clusters that formed based on geometric features and the trainers' assessments.

6. Conclusions and Future Work

This work aimed at analyzing the change of the spinal shape under posture training in three different positions: sitting, standing, and hip hinging. In particular, it compared snapshots of an unguided-guided posture pair based on features computed from the 2D spine curve geometry. Clustering was used to group posture changes with common geometric characteristics. The results from clustering our spine-shape-geometry inspired features could be identified with specific changes in posture by a professional posture trainer. Our large data base consists of real-world spine curves of over 350 single-user posture pairs and is pathology-unrelated. Our analysis is independent from a definition of a global *normal* spine shape. Instead, it is a highly individual process based on each individual's spine shape before and after posture training. This makes the successful separation of change in spinal shape into geometrically and semantically meaningful clusters (second contribution stated in the introduction, see Section 1) both interesting and important. We believe that this is the first work in the field of wearable-sensor-based evaluation of spine curves that analyzes this many distinct data points based on geometric features without relying on the definition of a *normal* spine shape.

Future work includes blind-test cross-validation of multiple sample posture pairs per clusters by several posture trainers as well as a more detailed grouping of our data based on additional information about e.g., age and gender. Further research could also include comparison against pain ratings using standard questionnaires, e.g., the low back pain specific Roland Morris questionnaire, or targeting general health status measurement SF12 and SF36, and eventually associate pain levels or changes therein with certain groups of posture change.

Furthermore it will be interesting to integrate feedback based on common features in spinal shape change, represented by clusters, into posture training. This could e.g., be implemented by also categorising posture training exercises based on a student's progress and suggest exercises tailored to their group of shape change. Moving partially away from clustering postural change towards analysis of spinal shape change of an individual user could provide them with helpful instant feedback on which region they need improvement on and how to get there. This also could be realized using e.g., an exercise specifically designed to improve the identified region. It would need a previously taken guided snapshot to compare the current user snapshot to.

Supplementary Materials: The following are available online at https://skylab.vc.h-brs.de/kstoll2m/PosturePairsDB19/: Database of (t_0, t_1) posture pairs used in this work.

Author Contributions: conceptualization, B.K., K.S., J.M., A.H.; methodology, K.S., B.K.; software, K.S.; validation, K.S., B.K., J.M., A.H.; formal analysis, K.S.; resources, A.H., B.K., J.M.; data curation, K.S., B.K.; writing—original draft preparation, K.S., B.K.; writing—review and editing, J.M., K.S., B.K., A.H.; visualization, K.S.; supervision, B.K.; all authors critically revised the manuscript and approved the content of the submission.

Funding: This research received no external funding.

Acknowledgments: We would like to extend our sincere thanks to Esther Gokhale who has gone through and assessed all posture samples we showed to her.

Conflicts of Interest: Jonas Müller and Björn Krüger work for Gokhale Method Enterprise Inc. and developed the Gokhale *SpineTracker* wearable. They had no role in the decision to publish the results.

Appendix A. Sample Spine Curve of Posture Pairs per Cluster

On the following pages, we will show representative spine curve posture pairs for each cluster. For better overview and localization of presented sample (cluster representative), we re-plot the t-SNE map and corresponding cluster bundles from the results. Each cluster in the t-SNE maps is additionally annotated with the location of the cluster representatives. Figures A1 and A2 draw the results of clustering and sample posture pairs for *standing*. Clusters and representatives for the position *sitting* are displayed in Figures A3 and A4. Finally, Figures A5 and A6 depict clusters and cluster representatives for *hip hinging*.

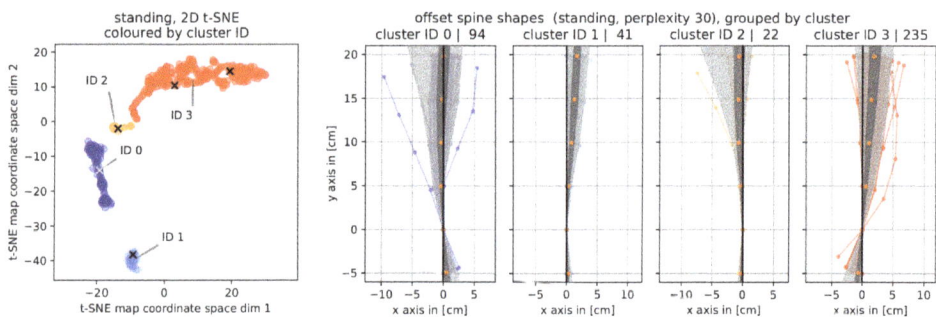

Figure A1. Results for clustering posture pairs of *standing*. (**left**) The t-SNE map labelled with and colored by cluster ID. An 'x' marks the position of a cluster representative. (**right**) Corresponding cluster bundles of *offset spine shapes*.

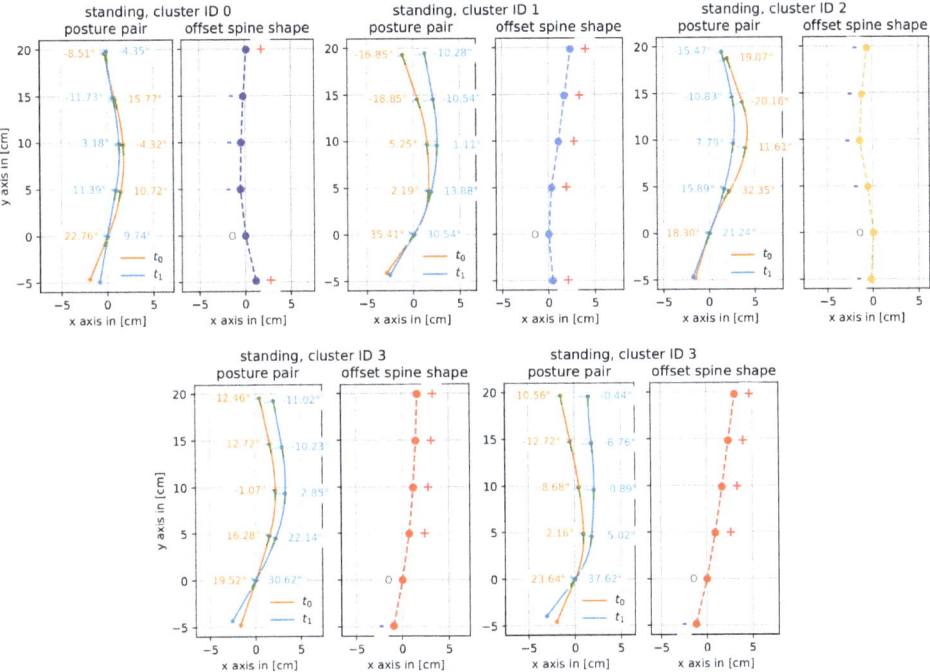

Figure A2. Results for clustering posture pairs of *sitting*: Cluster representative sample posture pairs and offset spine shapes for each cluster. Each sample's position within its cluster is marked by an 'x' in the colored t-SNE map.

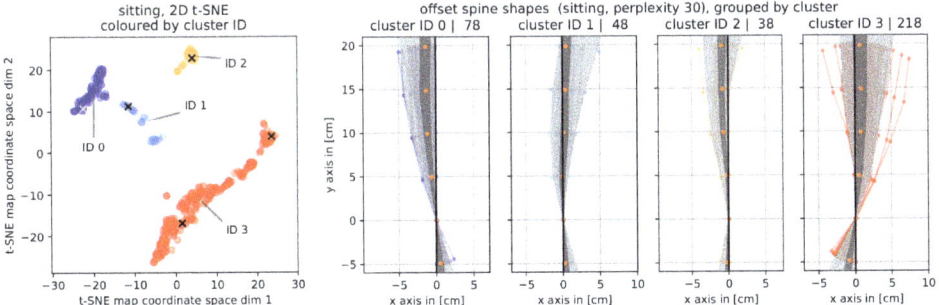

Figure A3. Results for clustering posture pairs of *sitting*. (**left**) The t-SNE map colored by cluster ID. An 'x' marks the position of a cluster representative. (**right**) Corresponding cluster bundles of *offset spine shapes*.

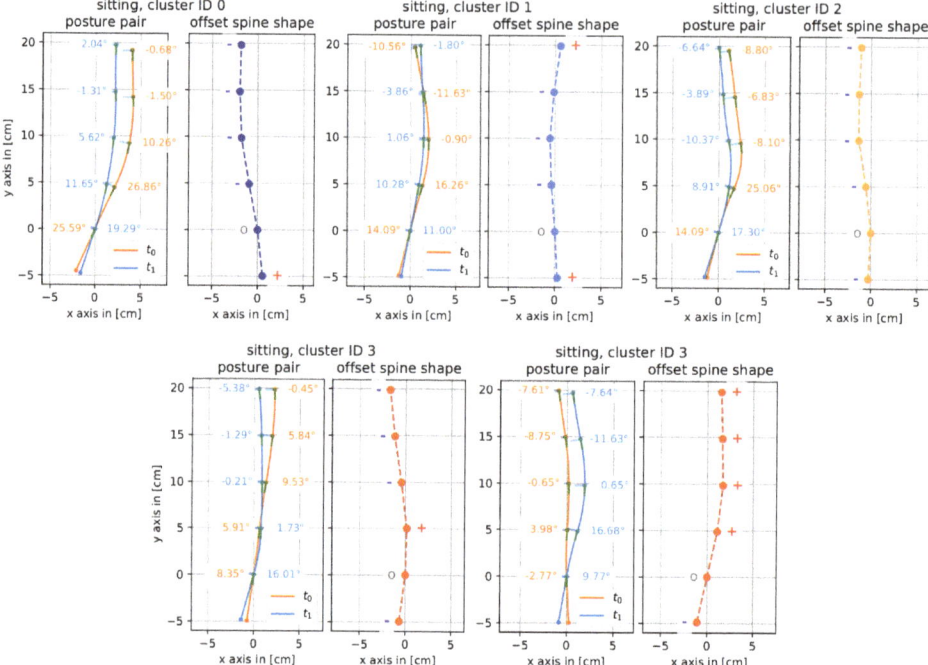

Figure A4. Results for clustering posture pairs of *sitting*: Cluster representative sample posture pairs and offset spine shapes for each cluster. Each sample's position within its cluster is marked by an 'x' in the colored t-SNE map.

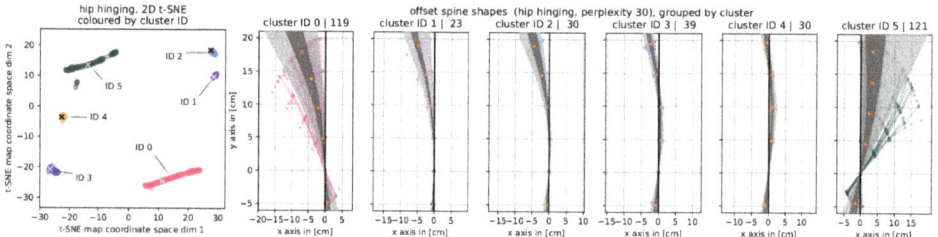

Figure A5. Results for clustering posture pairs of *hip hinging*. (**left**) The t-SNE map colored by cluster ID. An 'x' marks the position of a cluster representative. (**right**) Corresponding cluster bundles of *offset spine shapes*.

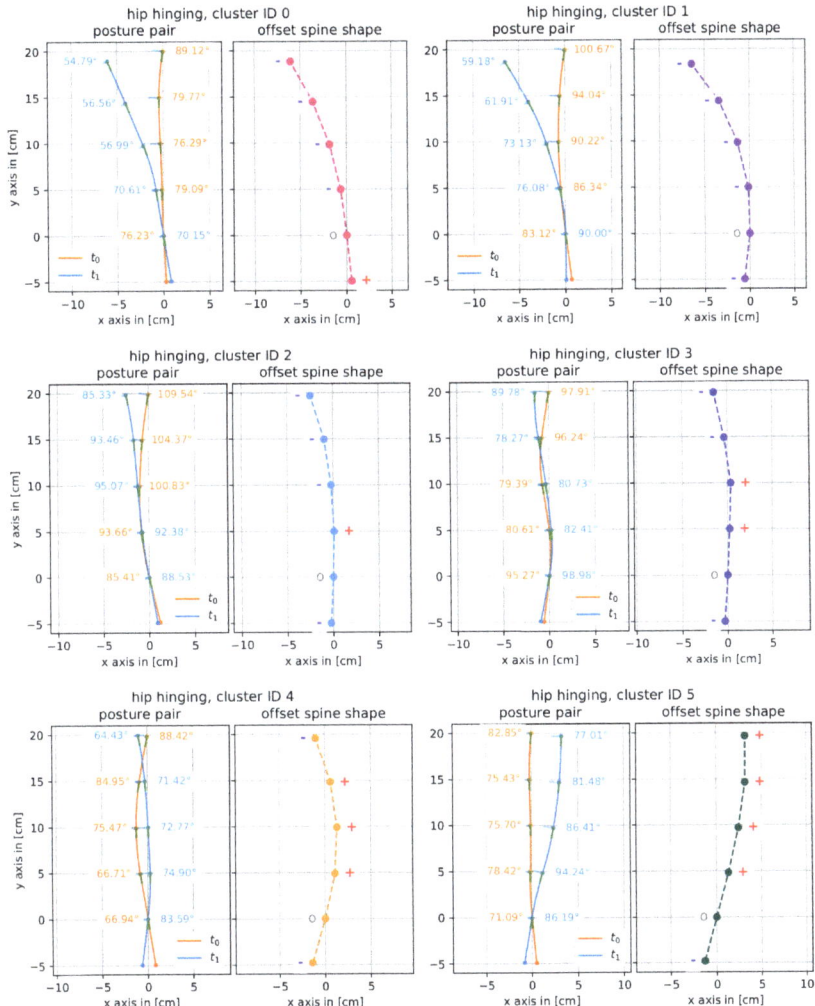

Figure A6. Results for clustering posture pairs of *hip hinging*. Cluster representative sample posture pairs and offset spine shapes for each cluster. Each sample's position within its cluster is marked by an 'x' in the colored t-SNE map. The two posture snapshots are additionally rotated about the origin such that the topmost sensor of the unguided t_0 snapshot lies on the y-axis.

References

1. Manchikanti, L.; Singh, V.; Falco, F.J.E.; Benyamin, R.M.; Hirsch, J.A. Epidemiology of Low Back Pain in Adults. *Neuromodul. Technol. Neural Interface* **2014**, *17*, 3–10. [CrossRef] [PubMed]
2. Hoy, D.; March, L.; Brooks, P.; Blyth, F.; Woolf, A.; Bain, C.; Williams, G.; Smith, E.; Vos, T.; Barendregt, J.; et al. The Global Burden of Low Back Pain: Estimates From the Global Burden of Disease 2010 Study. *Ann. Rheum. Dis.* **2014**, *73*, 968–974. [CrossRef] [PubMed]
3. Nelson, R.J. The Rape of the Spine. *Spine J.* **2015**, *15*, S11–S12. [CrossRef] [PubMed]
4. Rubin, D.I. Epidemiology and Risk Factors for Spine Pain. *Neurol. Clin.* **2007**, *25*, 353–371. [CrossRef] [PubMed]
5. Gaskin, D.J.; Richard, P. The Economic Costs of Pain in the United States. *J. Pain* **2012**, *13*, 715–724. [CrossRef] [PubMed]

6. Peleg, M.; Leung, T.I.; Desai, M.; Dumontier, M. Is Crowdsourcing Patient-reported Outcomes The Future of Evidence-based Medicine? A Case Study of Back Pain. In Proceedings of the Conference on Artificial Intelligence in Medicine in Europe, Vienna, Austria, 21–24 June 2017; Springer: Berlin/Heidelberg, Germany, pp. 245–255.
7. Stollenwerk, K.; Müllers, J.; Müller, J.; Hinkenjann, A.; Krüger, B. Evaluating an Accelerometer-based System for Spine Shape Monitoring. In Proceedings of the Computational Science and Its Applications—ICCSA 2018, Melbourne, VIC, Australia, 2–5 July 2018.
8. Peper, E.; Krüger, B.; Gokhale, E.; Harvey, R. Comparing Muscle Activity and Spine Shape in Various Sitting Styles. In *Biofeedback*; Allen Press: Lawrence, KS, USA, in press.
9. Papi, E.; Koh, W.S.; McGregor, A.H. Wearable Technology for Spine Movement Assessment: A Systematic Review. *J. Biomech.* **2017**, *64*, 186–197. [CrossRef] [PubMed]
10. Hay, O.; Hershkovitz, I.; Rivlin, E. Spine Curve Modeling for Quantitative Analysis of Spinal Curvature. In Proceedings of the 2009 Annual International Conference of the IEEE Engineering in Medicine and Biology Society, Minneapolis, MN, USA, 3–6 September 2009; pp. 6356–6359. [CrossRef]
11. Brink, Y.; Louw, Q.; Grimmer, K. The Amount of Postural Change Experienced by Adolescent Computer Users Developing Seated-related Upper Quadrant Musculoskeletal Pain. *J. Bodyw. Mov. Ther.* **2018**, *22*, 608–617. [CrossRef]
12. Wong, W.Y.; Wong, M.S. Trunk Posture Monitoring with Inertial Sensors. *Eur. Spine J.* **2008**, *17*, 743–753. [CrossRef]
13. Franklin, M.E.; Conner-Kerr, T. An Analysis of Posture and Back Pain in the First and Third Trimesters of Pregnancy. *J. Orthop. Sport. Phys. Ther.* **1998**, *28*, 133–138. [CrossRef]
14. González-Sánchez, M.; Luo, J.; Lee, R.; Cuesta-Vargas, A.I. Spine Curvature Analysis between Participants with Obesity and Normal Weight Participants: A Biplanar Electromagnetic Device Measurement. *Biomed. Res. Int.* **2014**, *2014*, 935151. [CrossRef]
15. Roetenberg, D.; Luinge, H.; Slycke, P. *Xsens MVN: Full 6DOF Human Motion Tracking Using Miniature Inertial Sensors*; Technical Report 1; Xsens Motion Technologies B.V.: Enschede, The Netherlands, 2013.
16. Tautges, J.; Zinke, A.; Krüger, B.; Baumann, J.; Weber, A.; Helten, T.; Müller, M.; Seidel, H.P.; Eberhardt, B. Motion Reconstruction using Sparse Accelerometer Data. *ACM Trans. Graph.* **2011**, *30*, 18:1–18:12. [CrossRef]
17. Riaz, Q.; Guanhong, T.; Krüger, B.; Weber, A. Motion Reconstruction Using Very Few Accelerometers and Ground Contacts. *Graph. Model.* **2015**. [CrossRef]
18. Weise, T.; Bouaziz, S.; Li, H.; Pauly, M. Realtime Performance-based Facial Animation. *ACM Trans. Graph.* **2011**, *30*, 77:1–77:10. [CrossRef]
19. Cao, C.; Hou, Q.; Zhou, K. Displaced Dynamic Expression Regression for Real-time Facial Tracking and Animation. *ACM Trans. Graph.* **2014**, *33*, 43:1–43:10. [CrossRef]
20. Hoffmann, J.; Brüggemann, B.; Krüger, B. Automatic Calibration of a Motion Capture System based on Inertial Sensors for Tele-Manipulation. In Proceedings of the 7th International Conference on Informatics in Control, Automation and Robotics (ICINCO), Funchal, Portugal, 15–18 June 2010.
21. Ma, C.Z.H.; Ling, Y.T.; Shea, Q.T.K.; Wang, L.K.; Wang, X.Y.; Zheng, Y.P. Towards Wearable Comprehensive Capture and Analysis of Skeletal Muscle Activity during Human Locomotion. *Sensors* **2019**, *19*, 195. [CrossRef]
22. Zhao, W.; Chai, J.; Xu, Y.Q. Combining Marker-based Mocap and RGB-D Camera for Acquiring High-fidelity Hand Motion Data. In Proceedings of the ACM SIGGRAPH/Eurographics Symposium on Computer Animation, Lausanne, Switzerland, 29–31 July 2012; pp. 33–42.
23. Stollenwerk, K.; Vögele, A.; Krüger, B.; Hinkenjann, A.; Klein, R. Automatic Temporal Segmentation of Articulated Hand Motion. In Proceedings of the Computational Science and Its Applications—ICCSA 2016: 16th International Conference, Beijing, China, 4–7 July 2016; Part II; Springer International Publishing: Berlin/Heidelberg, Germany, 2016; pp. 433–449. [CrossRef]
24. Drerup, B.; Hierholzer, E. Automatic Localization of Anatomical Landmarks on the Back Surface and Construction of a Body-fixed coordinate System. *J. Biomech.* **1987**, *20*, 961–970. [CrossRef]
25. Betsch, M.; Wild, M.; Johnstone, B.; Jungbluth, P.; Hakimi, M.; Kühlmann, B.; Rapp, W. Evaluation of a Novel Spine and Surface Topography System for Dynamic Spinal Curvature Analysis during Gait. *PLoS ONE* **2013**, *8*, e70581. [CrossRef]

26. Poredoš, P.; Čelan, D.; Možina, J.; Jezeršek, M. Determination of the Human Spine Curve Based on Laser Triangulation. *BMC Med. Imaging* **2015**, *15*, 2. [CrossRef]
27. Williams, J.M.; Haq, I.; Lee, R.Y. Dynamic Measurement of Lumbar Curvature Using Fibre-optic Sensors. *Med. Eng. Phys.* **2010**, *32*, 1043–1049. [CrossRef]
28. Consmüller, T.; Rohlmann, A.; Weinland, D.; Druschel, C.; Duda, G.N.; Taylor, W.R. Comparative Evaluation of a Novel Measurement Tool to Assess Lumbar Spine Posture and Range of Motion. *Eur. Spine J.* **2012**, *21*, 2170–2180. [CrossRef]
29. Cajamarca, G.; Rodríguez, I.; Herskovic, V.; Campos, M.; Riofrío, J.C. StraightenUp+: Monitoring of Posture during Daily Activities for Older Persons Using Wearable Sensors. *Sensors* **2018**, *18*, 3409. [CrossRef] [PubMed]
30. Voinea, G.D.; Butnariu, S.; Mogan, G. Measurement and Geometric Modelling of Human Spine Posture for Medical Rehabilitation Purposes Using a Wearable Monitoring System Based on Inertial Sensors. *Sensors* **2017**, *17*, 3. [CrossRef] [PubMed]
31. Gray, H.; Williams, P.L.; Bannister, L.H. Chapter 6: Skeletal System–Vertebral Column, Ribs, Thorax, Skull. In *Gray's Anatomy*, 38th ed.; Churchill Livingstone: New York, NY, USA, 1995.
32. Wilcoxon, F. Individual Comparisons of Grouped Data by Ranking Methods. *J. Econ. Entomol.* **1946**, *39*, 269–270. [CrossRef] [PubMed]
33. Hotelling, H. Analysis of a Complex of Statistical Variables into Principal Components. *J. Educ. Psychol.* **1933**, *24*, 417–441. [CrossRef]
34. Van der Maaten, L.; Hinton, G. Visualizing Data Using t-SNE. *J. Mach. Learn. Res.* **2008**, *9*, 2579–2605.
35. Kullback, S.; Leibler, R.A. On Information and Sufficiency. *Ann. Math. Stat.* **1951**, *22*, 79–86. [CrossRef]
36. Shapiro, S.S.; Wilk, M.B. An Analysis of Variance Test for Normality (Complete Samples). *Biometrika* **1965**, *52*, 591–611. [CrossRef]
37. Stephens, M.A. EDF Statistics for Goodness of Fit and Some Comparisons. *J. Am. Stat. Assoc.* **1974**, *69*, 730–737. [CrossRef]
38. Wilk, M.B.; Gnanadesikan, R. Probability Plotting Methods for the Analysis of Data. *Biometrika* **1968**, *55*, 1–17. [CrossRef]
39. Wilcoxon, F. Individual Comparisons by Ranking Methods. *Biom. Bull.* **1945**, *1*, 80–83. [CrossRef]
40. Pedregosa, F.; Varoquaux, G.; Gramfort, A.; Michel, V.; Thirion, B.; Grisel, O.; Blondel, M.; Prettenhofer, P.; Weiss, R.; Dubourg, V.; et al. Scikit-learn: Machine Learning in Python. *J. Mach. Learn. Res.* **2011**, *12*, 2825–2830.
41. Van der Maaten, L.; Hinton, G. Visualizing Non-metric Similarities in Multiple Maps. *Mach. Learn.* **2012**, *87*, 33–55. [CrossRef]
42. Wong, W.Y.; Wong, M.S. Detecting Spinal Posture Change in Sitting Positions with Tri-axial Accelerometers. *Gait Posture* **2008**, *27*, 168–171. [CrossRef]
43. Nachemson, A.L.; Schultz, A.B.; Berkson, M.H. Mechanical Properties of Human Lumbar Spine Motion Segments: Influences of Age, Sex, Disc Level, and Degeneration. *Spine* **1979**, *4*, 1–8. [CrossRef]
44. Youdas, J.W.; Garrett, T.R.; EganMayo, K.S.; Therneau, T.M. Lumbar Lordosis and Pelvic Inclination in Adults with Chronic Low Back Pain. *Phys. Ther.* **2000**. [CrossRef]

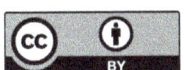

© 2019 by the authors. Licensee MDPI, Basel, Switzerland. This article is an open access article distributed under the terms and conditions of the Creative Commons Attribution (CC BY) license (http://creativecommons.org/licenses/by/4.0/).

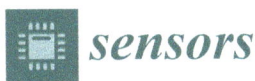

Article

P-Ergonomics Platform: Toward Precise, Pervasive, and Personalized Ergonomics using Wearable Sensors and Edge Computing

Mario Vega-Barbas [1,*], Jose A. Diaz-Olivares [2], Ke Lu [1], Mikael Forsman [1,2], Fernando Seoane [3,4,5] and Farhad Abtahi [1,2,*]

1. Institute of Environmental Medicine, Karolinska Institutet, Solnavägen 1, 17177 Solna, Sweden; ke.lu@ki.se (K.L.); mikael.forsman@ki.se (M.F.)
2. School of Engineering Sciences in Chemistry, Biotechnology and Health, KTH Royal Institute of Technology, Hälsovägen 11C, 14157 Huddinge, Sweden; jadiaz@kth.se
3. Department of Clinical Science, Intervention and Technology, Karolinska Institutet, Hälsovägen 7, 14157 Huddinge, Sweden; fernando.seoane@ki.se
4. Swedish School of Textiles, University of Borås, Allégatan 1, 50190 Borås, Sweden
5. Departm and t of Biomedical Engineering, Karolinska University Hospital, 1, 17176 Solna, Sweden
* Correspondence: mario.vega.barbas@ki.se (M.V.-B.); farhad.abtahi@ki.se (F.A.)

Received: 14 February 2019; Accepted: 6 March 2019; Published: 11 March 2019

Abstract: Preventive healthcare has attracted much attention recently. Improving people's lifestyles and promoting a healthy diet and wellbeing are important, but the importance of work-related diseases should not be undermined. Musculoskeletal disorders (MSDs) are among the most common work-related health problems. Ergonomists already assess MSD risk factors and suggest changes in workplaces. However, existing methods are mainly based on visual observations, which have a relatively low reliability and cover only part of the workday. These suggestions concern the overall workplace and the organization of work, but rarely includes individuals' work techniques. In this work, we propose a precise and pervasive ergonomic platform for continuous risk assessment. The system collects data from wearable sensors, which are synchronized and processed by a mobile computing layer, from which exposure statistics and risk assessments may be drawn, and finally, are stored at the server layer for further analyses at both individual and group levels. The platform also enables continuous feedback to the worker to support behavioral changes. The deployed cloud platform in Amazon Web Services instances showed sufficient system flexibility to affordably fulfill requirements of small to medium enterprises, while it is expandable for larger corporations. The system usability scale of 76.6 indicates an acceptable grade of usability.

Keywords: disease prevention; occupational healthcare; P-Ergonomics; precision ergonomics; musculoskeletal disorders; smart textiles; wearable sensors; wellbeing at work

1. Introduction

Musculoskeletal disorders (MSDs) are still common in the working population, causing individual suffering and an economic burden for companies and societies [1,2]. Further, the challenge of an aging population—an increased percentage of elderly individuals in the overall population—has occurred for more than two decades and its consequences, e.g., increasing costs, a lack of healthcare personnel, and more complex combinations of chronic diseases [3], have emerged. For economic reasons, a longer life expectancy requires an increase in the retirement age. These increases have already occurred in some countries and are planned in others [4,5].

To facilitate a prolonged work life for the general population, a balance between work demands and human capabilities must be found, especially for blue-collar workers [5]. This is in line with suggested approaches for chronic disease management to reduce the healthcare burden [6].

Interventions aiming to reduce MSD risk factors at work are not new. Ergonomists and work psychologists have tried to identify risk factors at specific workplaces to design and suggest physical, organizational, and when relevant, behavioral changes to reduce the risks. Work psychologists may use self-reports, and ergonomists often use observation-based assessment tools to identify these risks [7,8]. Observation methods are easy to use, inexpensive, and widely accessible, but the inter- and intra-observer reliability of such methods are relatively poor [7,9,10]. There are also substantial inter-method differences in risk assessments [11]. Another source of variance in risk assessments is the short observation time; the ergonomist often observes a minor part of the workday, which is then supposed to represent the full day. There are also differences in anthropometrics and work techniques between different workers, so risk assessments should include several workers to increase reliability.

Popular ergonomic risk assessment methods are mostly based on evaluation of the workplace and the workers by ergonomists and experts who coach the workers or suggest the redesign of workplaces. This approach faces at least two challenges; the first is due to differences in workers' individualities, e.g., height and body size. The solution to a risk factor, e.g., unforced demanding posture, may be to coach the workers towards a less demanding and less risk-inducing work technique. However, it is often difficult to change a habitual pattern of movement. In large organizations with manufacturing and assembly lines, regular inspection and coaching by ergonomists is often used to customize the workplace to the workers, e.g., providing the possibility for shorter persons to work in an assembly line. In cases where there is a need to modify a worker's technique, changing is trickier. A few coaching sessions might appear to be sufficient to train the workers toward more ergonomic work behavior. However, people tend to go back to their old working habits, reducing the effect of these training efforts [12].

Direct measurement techniques provided by accelerometers, gyroscopes, magnetometers, electromyogram (EMG), and heart rate recorders have been used in ergonomics research since the nineties [13–15]. However, these systems are relatively expensive, complicated to use in the data collection and analysis phases, and have not been widely used by ergonomists and occupational healthcare providers. Electronic sensors, e.g., inertial measurement units (IMUs), have advanced dramatically during the past two decades, making them widely accessible, more affordable, and more compact in form. Additionally, wearable sensors, such as sensorized garments, smart watches, and wristbands, are changing the traditional interaction with users in welfare and healthcare. Wearable solutions may be a natural way to improve the usability of measurement systems by avoiding the use of cables and sticky electrodes and ensuring correct electrode placement by novice users [16].

The use of wearable sensing technologies enables continuous and long-term monitoring (i.e., full work days) for as many work days as needed, successively or at repeated time intervals (e.g., once a month) for a reliable assessment or successful work technique intervention. Long-term usage allows for a personalized coaching approach with continuous feedback and risk trend analysis. Informing people about their behavior and risks could be a first step toward behavioral changes, which can be supported with strategies such as gamification. Gamification is the use of gaming elements, e.g., points, badges, trophies, and awards, in a collaborative or competitive environment to support behavioral changes [17].

In this work, we present a platform that enables precise risk assessments and personalized automatized coaching. Because it is precise, pervasive, and personalized, we call it the P-Ergonomic platform. The platform is designed for producing a generic assessment and coaching by using in-house developed garments and a mobile application, as well as third party solutions. The platform has a generic base and may be used for other applications, e.g., in sports and medical kinetic training; the current application is focused on MSD prevention and changing sedentary work behavior.

In the following sections, the specification of the system and proposed architecture are described in detail, followed by the methods for technical validation. The results of the technical evaluation are presented in Section 5, followed by the discussion and conclusion.

2. System Specification

The main objective of the p-Ergonomics platform is to provide a reliable and flexible foundation for data collection, storage, analysis, and feedback to the end users, i.e., workers, employers, coaches, and occupational healthcare providers. The business cases for p-Ergonomics include small- to medium-sized businesses, as well as large enterprises. Since these businesses have different budgets and policies, the system architecture should consider the flexibility of deploying the platform at local or cloud servers using a cost-effective approach, which is scalable for big enterprises and affordable for small businesses, e.g., self-employed hairdressers or ergonomic coaches.

Security aspects are important features to ensure the privacy of workers. Authentication and authorization should be implemented to ensure accredited access to specific actions according to the user's role and granted permissions. Action logs should provide the possibility of auditing the activities. The confidentiality and integrity of the data should be ensured with different measures, e.g., encryption. The security features should provide the possibility for compliance with restrictive data and information regulations, e.g., the General Data Protection Regulation (GDPR) [18].

The system should be flexible, which means a layered architecture to allow for changing different modules, e.g., sensors, third party integration, and analytics, without modifying the entire system. Considering the performance, a minimum required performance of 500 concurrent users for each deployed instance of the system should be tested for a target availability of 24/7.

The system should handle internationalization (i18n), providing support for i18n in the presentation layer and other layers, e.g., the analytic layer. Usability is another important requirement; the system should be easy to deploy, learn, and use by different stakeholders, such as occupational healthcare providers, administrators, and end users, i.e., workers.

3. Proposed Architecture

The system collects data generated by wearable sensors, processes it for the purposes of risk assessment, intervention, and evaluation, and delivers the data to different stakeholders, including the worker, coach, and manager. The proposed system architecture is illustrated in Figure 1. The system consists of three layers: a wearable sensing layer, a mobile computing layer, and a server layer. The wearable sensing layer provides various physiological and biomechanical measurements and preprocesses the raw signals. At the mobile computing layer, data from each sensor node is collected, synchronized, and processed into variables reflecting exposure. The risk levels are then assessed according to defined ergonomic criteria and real-time feedback can be sent to the individual for intervention. Data from each individual is collected and stored at the server layer, where further analyses at both individual and group levels occurs. The server layer also employs user management for data logging and information access.

3.1. Wearable Sensing System

The wearable sensor system consists of a t-shirt or vest, reported in other studies [19–25], which includes four textile electrodes made of conductive fabric. A pair of electrodes is used for the current injection and the other pair senses the electric potential. An ECGZ2 device (Z-Health Technologies AB, Borås, Sweden) was used as the recorder for electrocardiography (ECG) and electrical bioimpedance and was placed in a pocket on the shoulder strap of the vest or front of the t-shirt, as shown in Figure 2. ECG and thoracic impedance signals were recorded with sampling rates of 250 Hz and 100 Hz, respectively. One and two LPMS-B2 inertial measurement units (IMUs) (LP Research, Tokyo, Japan) were placed in the pocket on the back of the t-shirt or vest and t-shirt sleeves, respectively.

The Polar A370 wristband smart watch (Polar Electro, Kempele, Finland) was included to monitor the daily activity and nightly sleep outside of working hours.

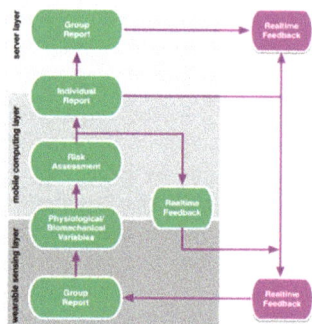

Figure 1. The proposed system architecture, hardware layers, and information flow.

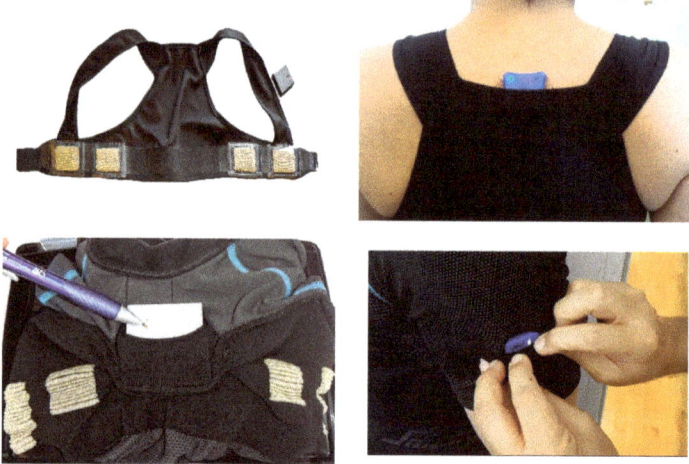

Figure 2. Vest (**top**) and t-shirt (**bottom**), including textrodes and ECGZ2 and IMUs.

3.2. Personal Analytics and Coaching App

Analysis of the data from the different wearable sensors and the provision of feedback to the user is done through different software layers. The software runs on an edge-computing node in the form of a smartphone device with an Android operation system. Figure 3 illustrates the different layers of the system. This approach facilitates independence between layers, allowing for the update or substitution of any of them without hindering the system's performance.

3.2.1. Data Acquisition Layer

Data are acquired from the different wearable sensors, which make use of the Bluetooth communication standard to connect to the smartphone device, emulating a body area network operation. The user can select from a list of sensing devices based on the needs of different ergonomics variables of the assessment. The options are inertial measurement units (IMUs), and electrocardiogram (ECG) and thoracic bioimpedance recording devices. The smartphone connects to the sensors, initially configuring them based on preset specifications, emphasizing the frequency control of data acquisition and communication, filtering implementation, and data formatting.

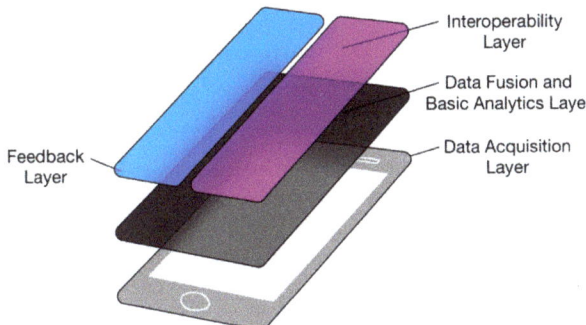

Figure 3. Distribution of the four layers that comprise the Edge node.

This layer also controls and applies calibration algorithms, which require a direct interaction with the configuration functions of the sensing devices' firmware, enabling treatment of the raw data from the sensors to calibrate the referential systems for inertial measurement units and other referential-type sensors.

This layer formats the acquired raw data to a standard format to be used by the subsequent layers. Synchronization of recordings from different sensors is done by adding timestamps to the data.

3.2.2. Data Fusion and Basic Analytics Layer

This layer provides the system with the capability to transform the raw information extracted from the sensors into added-value information that can be analyzed to perform real-time multimodal risk assessments.

Firstly, preprocessing of the standardized raw data is performed. Data from the sensors is transformed from their original units, i.e., quaternions from IMUs or voltage from electrocardiographic recording devices, into units or information that are interpretable by the risk evaluation algorithms, i.e., transforming quaternions into Euler angles or voltage from electrocardiographic measurements into heart rate frequency. This process also includes data fusion from different sensors to produce additional useful information for the assessment, i.e., relative angles and angular velocity between two IMUs located in the body area network.

Processing and sensor fusion results in dramatic reduction of data sent to the cloud data warehouse. As an example, data from IMUs includes 3-axis gyroscope, a 3-axis accelerometer, and a 3-axis magnetometer sampled at sampling rates around 20−100 Hz depends on application. However, processed data from sensor fusion might just include the limb angles at a rate of 1 Hz sent to the cloud data warehouse. In some working scenarios, such as production lines, it might be interesting to look at workload at specific working or break cycles. To cover this scenarios, an extra processing of data can be done by allowing categorization of data based on sensor data, e.g., location data showing a station or even manual time stamps.

Finally, action policies are applied to enable the production of risk assessments based on the requirements established by the users and existing risk assessment algorithms, such as Risk Assessment and Management tool for manual handling Proactively (RAMP) screening [26].

3.2.3. Feedback Layer

Given the possibility of estimating the risks, the real-time analysis of the measured parameters allows for the production of feedback in real time, based on the triggering of different events abiding to the different action policies chosen by the users. The feedback for this system prioritizes user-friendly notifications, descriptions, and instructions that are easily understood by different users.

Different types of feedback can be used to adapt to different scenarios. Visual feedback, such as the display of information through the graphical display of the smartphone, can provide different levels of information based on the user's profile and display different parameters continuously, e.g., heart rate and activity recognition. Visual feedback could be a detailed report of the session or simply color-coded icons representing the different levels of risk, as well as a description of what caused that problem, enabling the users to minimize it.

The system is not limited to visual feedback. In most common working scenarios, the workers might not be able to interact with the screen, so an audio feedback system is preferred. A series of predefined coaching messages are given to the worker if an activity has been recognized as exceeding a risk threshold. The audio feedback is given at time intervals defined by the user. Haptic feedback using the actuators integrated in the wearables has also been tested and showed promising preliminary results.

3.2.4. Interoperability Layer

This layer provides the body area network with the possibility of connecting to a remote server solution to send the information processed by the data analytics and fusion layer. By formatting the time-stamped processed data into a JavaScript Object Notation (JSON) message, it is possible to use the Hypertext Transfer Protocol (HTTP) Representational State Transfer (REST) service to upload the data to a cloud platform or to a local server, depending on the restrictions of the deployment environment. In this sense, this layer offer to users the possibility to specify the server that has implemented similar REST APIs, described in Tables 1–3.

By default, the accumulated data of the previous five minutes is uploaded, but the user can change this uploading speed to as fast as every second, allowing for the use of the information of the body area network for remote monitoring in a close-to-real-time manner. At the end of a work-day, the total work exposure is saved on the server, and a statistical summary may be generated, with variables that may be compared the recommended action levels, and to the levels of other occupations [27,28]. Especially when a group of workers have been using the system at the same workplace, this is a very time efficient way of objectively obtaining precise work exposure, and risk analyses, at a work group level.

3.3. Data Warehousing and Business Logic

The server was developed following a RESTful software architecture approach. This means all resources or services offered by the system on the server side are offered through HTTP methods. The data is stored in an open source relational database, PostgreSQL version 9.6.8, with a management layer by TimeScaleDB (Timescale Inc, NYC, US) added for the treatment of time-series records.

The Node.js 10.13.0 programming language was used for implementation of the server. Due to its nature, Node.js is oriented to the development of web applications, facilitating the encapsulation of all functions and procedures of the server into small RESTful services. Through a RESTful API, these services are offered to the other components of the system as simple web resources, identified by a textual representation. Figure 4 shows an overview of the relationships between the server side solutions and the other elements through the RESTful API.

The internal design of the architecture is based on modules. Each module brings together the functions and resources related to a specific objective: identity and security management, log management, data management, communication with third-party applications, and management of action policies. Figure 5 shows an overview of the architecture and the interaction between modules. These interactions can be generated by the direct action of the user (solid arrow) or as a consequence of an internal process (dashed arrow). The following sections define each of the modules.

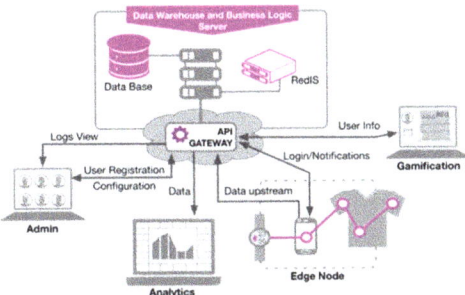

Figure 4. Data Warehouse and Business Logic Server overview and its interoperation with the other elements of the system.

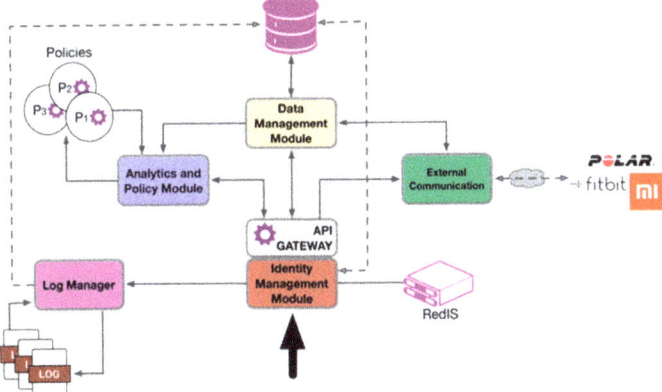

Figure 5. Distribution of the modules that comprise the analytical server and the interactive processes between them.

3.3.1. Identity Management Module

The security management of the server is based on a simple access and identity management system. Secure communication is implemented through HTTPS channels between the clients and the server and the use of REDIS and PassportJS as a solution for the management of certificates, sessions, and cookies.

This module enables control of access to the resources offered by the server and management of the users. This module allows for the management of permissions to the resources to generate different user profiles. Thus, the system can discern and adapt the interactions according to whether it is an administrator user that is more focused on the management of the system, end users, whether they are information consumers (analysts and experts) or workers, and other profiles necessary for the correct deployment of the solution. The resources offered by this module are detailed in Table 1.

Table 1. Resources provided by the Identity Manager Module.

Resource	Method	Description
/auth/login	POST	Performs the login in the system. As a response, the system sends an authentication token.
/auth/register	POST	Registers new simple users in the system.
/auth/logout	GET	Log out from the system.
/auth/status	GET	Obtain the current status of the user and it informs users if they are logged or not.
/auth/regdevice	PUT	Register a new mobile device in the system. This mobile is syndicated to the user (authenticated previously) that uses this resource. See Section 3.3.3.

3.3.2. Log Manager

All actions in the system must be logged to ensure the integrity of users. Therefore, the Log Manager registers all activities carried out in the server to process. The recorded logs are stored following the Common Log Format [29]. Through collaboration with the Data Management module, this module allows for exporting logs to a CSV format file that can be analyzed by experts. This functionality is encapsulated in a service managed by the Data Management module (see Table 4).

3.3.3. Data Management Module

In general, the P-Ergonomics solution uses two types of data—those generated by wearable sensors, and those obtained from the evaluations of the user's state, e.g., questionnaires or expert comments. In addition, sensors might be placed on different body parts or different types of questionnaires and subjective assessments can be used. Therefore, the data management module offers the resources required to support different data structures. The data of the sensors correspond to the structure described in Table 2. The information collected from the questionnaires is managed following the data structure detailed in Table 3. The resources offered by the RESTful API of the system related to the information management module are defined in Table 4.

Table 2. Data Structure of a Sensory Measurement.

Data Field	Description	Value Example
tstamp	Time stamp when the data is stored into the system.	2018-07-23 12:37:37.206017+00
type	Short description or type of the measurement, i.e., calories, sleep time, etc.	Angle (Degrees)
position	Location of the sensor, if relevant, such as left arm, right wrist, back, etc.	Back/Trunk
sensor	Sensor type, i.e., IMUs, Polar watch, etc.	LPMS-B2 IMU
value	Final value stored in the system and its interpretation, conditioned by the type of data (type field).	−3.63287
id_user	User from whom the measure is taken.	6

Table 3. Data Structure of a Questionnaire Response.

Data Field	Description	Value Example
id_response	Unique identification of the stored response.	123
id_user	User who completed the form.	14
response_tstamp	Time stamp when the response is stored into the system.	2018-07-23 12:37:37.206017+00
response	Response structure, e.g., 5#4#5#2#2#3#1.	4#4#5#2#1#-#3#3#-#1#2#1
q_type	Type of form, indicating the policy to be applied for its analysis.	Stress-Energy

Table 4. Resources provided by the Data Management Module.

Resource	Method	Description
/api/v1/data/logs	GET	Obtain the logs of the system in CSV format.
/api/v1/data/msr	GET	Obtain all measures of all users. Only administrators can perform this action.
/api/v1/data/msr	POST	Store measurements in the database. This resource admits a set of several measurements or a single one.
/api/v1/data/msr/{id}	GET	Obtain all responses stored in the system. Only administrators can perform this action.
/api/v1/data/qtn	GET	Obtain the current status of the user, i.e., this resource informs users if they are logged or not.
/api/v1/data/qtn	POST	Store responses of a questionnaire in the database. This resource admits a set of several measurements or a single one.

3.3.4. External Communication Module

The interactions between the system and external agents are managed through the external communication module. In the presented version, interaction with wearable solutions from Polar Electro, Kempele, Finland, through the Polar AccessLink is implemented to retrieve the relevant user information, e.g., sleep time, daily activity, consumed calories, and resting heart rate. This integration is done through an Open Authorization (OAuth) protocol by asking users to share their Polar information with this platform. The access token and user identifier in the third-party system, e.g., Polar, are kept for the future operations, e.g., obtaining data from AccessLink (https://www.polar.com/accesslink-api/#authorization-endpoint). The resources associated with this module are detailed in Table 5.

Table 5. Resources provided by the External Communication Module.

Resource	Method	Description
/external/polar/auth	GET	Connect with Polar AccessLink API and start the authentication process.
/external/polar/callback	GET	Stores authentication credential (access token and user identification) of the user from the Polar AccessLink API.
/external/polar/register/{id}	GET	Registers a worker in the Polar AccessLink system. This action is mandatory to allow users to access their data.
/external/polar/delete	GET	Revokes the authorized access token provided by Polar.
/external/polar/listOf/{performance}	GET	Access and process the user's daily activity data from the Polar AccessLink and store them in the system database.

3.3.5. Analysis and Action Policy Module

The server offers the possibility to manage action policies based on the data collected by the sensors and questionnaires. These actions are based on previously designed analysis libraries that are included in the system before execution. The analysis results of the user data are managed following the guidelines established in the action policies, i.e., store or send to the user or to the coach.

In addition to internal feedback and notifications, this module allows for sending messages to third party applications. In the current version, it interacts with Pocket mHealth (ATOS, S.A., Madrid, Spain) [30]. The management of notifications in this third-party application is beyond the scope of the article. The resources offered by this module are described in Table 6.

Table 6. Resources provided by the Analysis and Action Policy Module.

Resource	Method	Description
/api/v1/notification/pmh/{msg}	GET	Send notifications and messages (msg) to external services. The system uses an external notification API based on Firebase [30].
/api/v1/notification/pmh	GET	Perform analysis related to the health at work policy associate. The policy is defined as a main function in a library.

The process followed by this module to manage the action policies defined in the system and the interactions involved are shown in Figure 6.

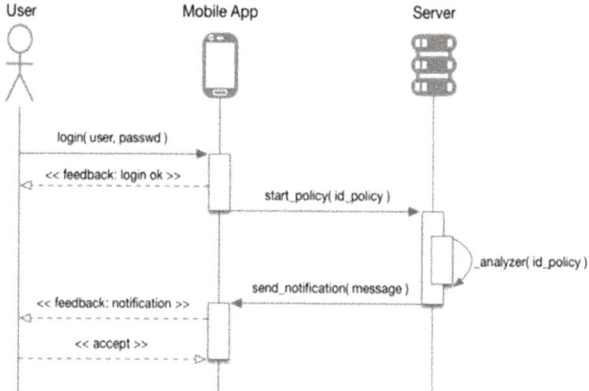

Figure 6. Sequence diagram of the action policy execution and interactions involved.

4. System Validation

The proposed architecture and its implementation were validated through a realistic testing scenario. The objective of this validation was to evaluate the functionality, performance, and efficiency of the system for real deployment environments. Therefore, two types of tests were defined: a performance evaluation and a usability assessment.

4.1. Usability Assessment

The first stage of validation is to measure the usability of the system. A quantitative usability test, the System Usability Scale (SUS), was used [31]. The SUS questionnaire is a simple tool based on ten items to give a global view of subjective assessments of usability; that is, the effectiveness, the efficiency, and the user satisfaction related with the use of the system in order to perform a specific task. This test was carried out with N = 20 users in 4 groups of 5 users. As Nielsen noted in previous studies [32,33], this set of users is sufficient to tackle most usability problems and provides an overall view of the usability of the system. These users were selected from two different work types—office work and hospital work—to represent white- and pink-collar workers. The tests were carried out over 4–5 h for at least a working day in Spain and Sweden. In addition, all issues that occurred during the execution of the work activities were logged by an expert, such as interruption of the workflow due to system malfunctions. All participants were fully informed about the study and provided written consent. Ethical permission for the tests and data collection were obtained from the Regional Ethical Review Board in Stockholm (Dnr 2017/1586-31) and the local ethical board at Atos S.A.

4.2. Performance Evaluation

Another important aspect is to test the functional viability of the system using a performance test. The design of this test is based on the common behavior of a user while interacting with the system, i.e., skipping the connection setup of the wearable sensors. This behavior model is shown as a state diagram defined in Figure 7.

Figure 7 shows the user interaction with the Edge App focuses on two main activities, the initialization or identification and the data collection. These two activities must be considered in the design of the performance test. Two processes comprise the information gathering, one related to the filling of questionnaires, and the other to the use of body sensors to measure movements and record physiological signals produced by the user. In both cases, the operation is similar: collect information, package it, and send it to the server to be stored and processed. However, the task of processing the data generated by the sensors is more complex due to the preprocessing performed in the Edge node.

Therefore, the information gathering activity is modeled focusing only on the user's interaction with the questionnaires, as it considerably simplifies the implementation of the test.

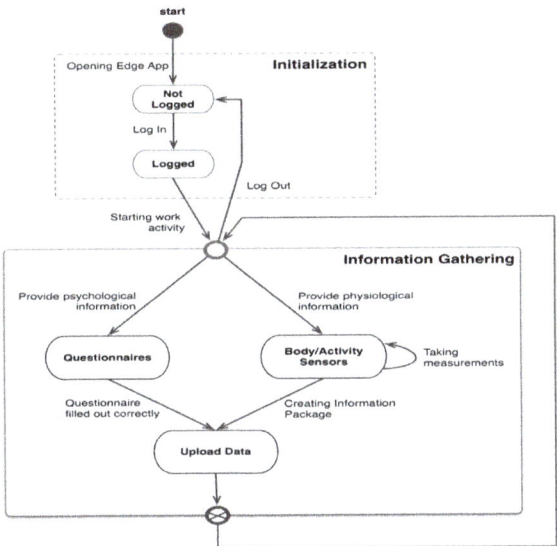

Figure 7. State diagram of common user activity with the Edge App.

A Node.js library, Artillery.js, was used to implement the test using a human-readable data serialization file (YAML). This file defines two functional scenarios, where a virtual user should sign in and send the information related to a questionnaire to the server, with a similar workload to sending sensor data. Considering the probability of each scenario in real life, a weight was assigned to each, 1–4% to log in and log out, and 96–99% to upload information to the server.

As noted in previous research [34], a common scenario for a normal large company (logistics, manufacturing, etc.) is to have 120 workers for the same work line. However, a set of 50 simultaneous users could represent small-medium enterprises (SMEs) and 200 to 500 is more suitable for large corporations with more than 120 simultaneous users to be analyzed, if applicable. Thus, the test was performed by simulating 50, 120, 200, 300, and 500 users.

In terms of hardware, an Amazon Elastic Compute Cloud (Amazon EC2) (Amazon, Seattle, WA, USA) instance running the Ubuntu Server 16.04 was used to deploy the server, starting with the most restrictive set of resources, Amazon EC2 instance t2.nano. The test increased the resources, i.e., the Amazon EC2 instance type, when a use case demanded more CPU or memory. The client for data generation was simulated in an Amazon EC2 instance type t2.medium with Ubuntu Server 16.04, with similar hardware features to those offered by the real edge nodes used by the system. A description of the Amazon EC2 instances is presented in the Table A1.

5. Results and Discussion

The platform was tested in two different real work scenarios—one corresponding to white-collar workers at the ATOS offices in Madrid, Spain, and the other corresponding to pink-collar workers at the sterilization unit of the New Karolinska University Hospital in Stockholm, Sweden. Twenty users were enrolled and the system was tested for 4–5 h during a workday. These trials generated 2,601,016 measurements, an average of 130,050.8 per user. These measurements were used and analyzed to determine new activity detection algorithms, define new ergonomic suitability comparisons between jobs, or evaluate new occupational risks. Figure 8 shows the classification of the stored measurements and how each sensor contributed to the total. The IMU sensors (3 in each T-shirt) generated 73.53% of the measurements stored, with the angle between them being the most common type of measurement (48.61%). The least information came from third-party devices (Polar) at 8% of the total, because the raw data is stored in the Polar Access link server and only the essential information for the ergonomic analysis is retrieved, processed, and filtered according to the needs of the final application, i.e., calories, activity levels, and active steps.

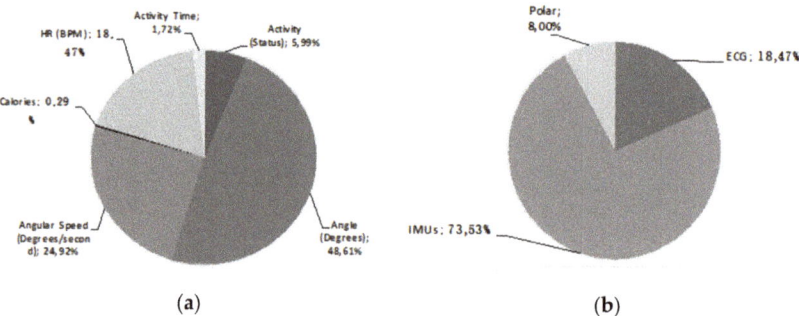

Figure 8. Distribution of the measures according to the type (**a**) and sensor that generated it (**b**).

The analysis of the answers obtained from the usability tests (N = 20) yields an SUS score of 75,625 out of 100. According to most interpretations [35], this score indicates that the system has an acceptable usability level, i.e., a C grade. However, as shown in Figure 9, there is room for improvement.

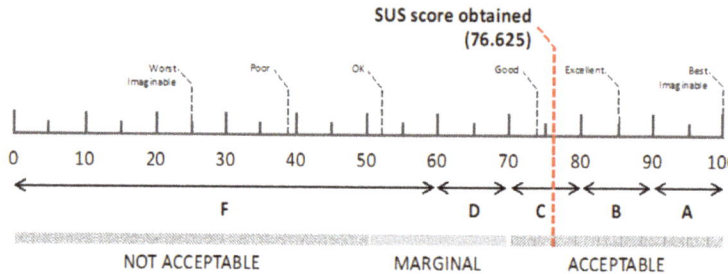

Figure 9. The SUS score of the system (dashed red line), with a visual explanation of adjective ratings, acceptability scores, and school grade scales in relation to the average SUS score [35].

This margin of improvement is visualized in the representation of the answers given to each question of the questionnaire outlined in Figure 10.

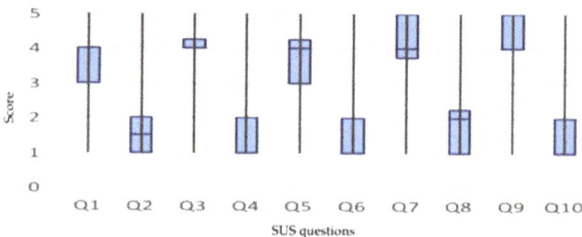

Figure 10. Graphic representation of the scores given by the users to each question of the SUS questionnaire. The questions are detailed in the Table A2.

Note that the even questions refer to positive aspects of the usability of the system and the odd questions refer to negative aspects. It has observed that the system must improve around questions

1, 5, and 8. Question 1 refers to the user's desire to use the system at all times. In this sense, the use of wearable elements and smart clothes appears to condition the final acceptance due to comfort aspects and doubts related to cleaning. Question 5 refers to the level of integration of the elements that comprise the system, that is, the functional coherence between the sensorized elements, such as the smart shirt, watch, and app. Question 8 refers to the comfort of the system, i.e., the wearable elements, which must be revised to increase the overall comfort of the system. The questions are detailed in the Table A2.

The performance test results are shown in Table 7. Depending on the number of users, it is possible to select a more restrictive Amazon EC2 instance type. The cost of each option is estimated by the amount of CPU credits used by the instance in 24 h (see Table A1 for the amount of credits offered for each instance type). The minimum amount of CPU credits necessary for a workday were estimated for each test. It is worth mentioning that performance numbers reported in Table 7 are heavily dependent on software implementation and cannot be generalized.

The performance scenario is designed as a worst case scenario, with simulation of request to the server at every second. However, in our actual scenario, one-second interval warehousing and cloud analysis of data is not required. Each limb data, from IMUs, was 150 bytes, and hence size of each packet corresponds to Header Bytes + (number of seconds * (number of sensors * 150)). In our pilots, we have used 300 s for synchronizing with the data warehouse, while the performance simulations are done in one second. Perhaps it might be desired to change to a binary communication in future to increase the efficacy.

Table 7. Summary of the performance test results.

Amazon EC2 Instance	User/sec	CPU Usage	Amazon EC2 Credits Used	Average Latency (ms)
T2.nano	50	37%	1.6	3.5 (p95 = 174.6)
T2.micro	120	72%	3.6	93.7 (p95 = 548.5)
T2.small	200	72%	3.5	61.3 (p95 = 420.7)
T2.medium	300	42%	3.5	75.2 (p95 = 468.8)
T2.medium	500	52%	3.6	154.7 (p95 = 658.8)
T2.large	500	59%	4.2	591.8 (p95 = 2485.7)
T2.nano	50	37%	1.6	3.5 (p95 = 174.6)

Figure 11 shows the difference between the minimum credits needed and those offered by each type of Amazon EC2 instance on dedicated Linux servers. Although the most affordable instances (t2.nano, t2.micro, and t2.small) offer adequate performance for few users, the final price can be altered due to the number of CPU credits used. In contrast, an instance of type t2.medium offers the best performance/credits-used ratio. With an annual advanced payment of $312, it is possible to handle up to 500 concurrent users with a CPU usage of 52%.

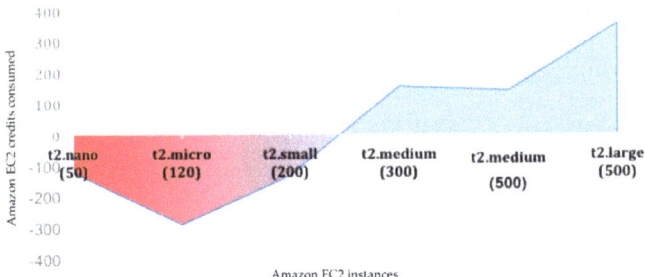

Figure 11. Graphical representation of difference between Amazon EC2 CPU credits offered by upfront payment for reserved Linux instances (type t2).

Another requirement of the system specification is the possibility to deploy the system on a local server. This is suitable for enterprises with highly restrictive policies about storing data on the cloud. The analytical part of the system, although it is implemented following a cloud service, can be deployed on private local servers. To achieve optimal performance similar to that offered by an Amazon EC2 t2.medium instance, the server specification is at least a dual-core processor and 4 GB of memory. Servers with such a specification are very affordable.

The development of the P-Ergonomics platform is in line with projects by our research group at the Royal Institute of Technology (KTH) and Karolinska Institutet, Sweden, and by our research partners. It is a part of the European Institute of Innovation and Technology (EIT) Health funded project [23], We@Work (http://weatwork.eu/). In a previous study [24], we demonstrated a wearable system integrating textrodes, motion sensors, and real-time data processing through a mobile application. Heart rate, respiration, and motion measurements obtained from a wearable system were fused to enhance the energy expenditure estimation [36,37]. Preliminary results of changing workers' behavior after giving feedback is also reported [38]. The aim is to develop a comprehensive solution to promote and support a healthy and safe working life. To the authors knowledge, this approach is novel and has not been reported elsewhere.

6. Conclusions and Future Work

The developed platform shows promising results in collecting data from the edge node (Android application). For its part, the functional analysis has been done with a specific platform (Amazon EC2) and different results could be achieved with other platforms, such as Google Cloud or Microsoft Azure. In addition, the performance and capacity could be expanded by software or operating system optimization, addition of hardware resources, or the detailed study of communication and data exchange between the node and the server, i.e., data compression algorithms. However, the results show that as a whole, the capacity and affordability of the implemented system meets the required specification.

Inclusion of protocols that make use of universal sensors is another possible expansion of the system that can increase its versatility. The usability tests show acceptable results, although the use of specific smart clothes seems to condition the final acceptance. This has caused the redesign of a new integration of the ECGZ2 device in the wearable garment by its integration into the t-shirt directly, avoiding the use of the vest. Thus, more detailed tests, including long-term usage of the new wearable systems, are planned for future work. A detailed test of the system for changing users' behavior by giving relevant feedback is ongoing. The use of gamification for engagement of workers is already planned and will be implemented. The use of pervasive and wearable technology in ergonomics could be a vital factor in enabling cost-effective ergonomic risk assessments and solutions in the near future.

Author Contributions: Conceptualization, M.V.-B., F.A., K.L., and J.A.D.-O.; funding acquisition, F.S., F.A., and M.F.; investigation, M.V.-B. and F.A.; methodology, M.V.-B., K.L., and F.A.; software, M.V.-B. and J.A.D.-O.; supervision, M.V.-B., F.A., F.S., and M.F.; validation, M.V.-B. and F.A.; writing—original draft, M.V.-B., F.A., J.A.D.-O., and K.L.; writing—review and editing, M.V.-B., F.A., F.S., and M.F.

Funding: This work was supported by EIT Health under project no. 18454 "Wellbeing, Health, and Safety @ Work".

Acknowledgments: Authors want to thanks Sterilization Unit at Karolinska Hospital and ATOS S.A. for their participation in the pilots.

Conflicts of Interest: Fernando Seoane is a co-founder and partial owner of Z-Health Technologies AB, Borås, Sweden. The other authors declare no conflicts of interest.

Appendix A

The Table A1 presents a summary of the features offered by Amazon for using Amazon EC2 Virtual Machines. This summary is only focused on the T2 Amazon EC2 instance, the most affordable modality, which is ideal for a variety of general purpose applications. In addition, the description of the T2 instances has been limited only to those used in the test, i.e., nano, micro, small, medium, and large.

Table A1. Characteristics of the Amazon EC2 instances.

Amazon EC2 instance	CPUs	Credits/hour	Memory (GiB)	Upfront Price ($)
T2.nano	1	3	0.5	39.00
T2.micro	1	6	1	77.00
T2.small	1	12	2	156.00
T2.medium	2	24	4	312.00
T2.large	2	36	8	625.00

Appendix B

The usability analysis has been carried out through the use of the System Usability Scale (SUS). For this, the tested and accepted questionnaire that provides this method has been used. Table A2 specifies the 10 questions that make up this questionnaire.

Table A2. SUS questionnaire.

Item	Question
Q1	I think that I would like to use this system frequently.
Q2	I found the system unnecessarily complex.
Q3	I thought the system was easy to use.
Q4	I think that I would need the support of a technical person to be able to use this system.
Q5	I found the various functions in this system were well integrated.
Q6	I thought there was too much inconsistency in this system.
Q7	I would imagine that most people would learn to use this system very quickly.
Q8	I found the system very cumbersome to use.
Q9	I felt very confident using the system.
Q10	I needed to learn a lot of things before I could get going with this system.

References

1. Hoy, D.; March, L.; Brooks, P.; Blyth, F.; Woolf, A.; Bain, C.; Williams, G.; Smith, E.; Vos, T.; Barendregt, J. The global burden of low back pain: Estimates from the Global Burden of Disease 2010 study. *Ann. Rheum. Dis.* **2014**, *73*, 968–974. [CrossRef] [PubMed]
2. U.S. Bureau of Labor Statistics. Nonfatal occupational injuries and illnesses requiring days away from work, 2015. Available online: https://www.bls.gov/news.release/osh2.nr0.htm (accessed on 24 November 2018).
3. Zweifel, P.; Felder, S.; Meiers, M. Ageing of population and health care expenditure: A red herring? *Health Econ.* **1999**, *8*, 485–496. [CrossRef]
4. Bloom, D.E.; Boersch-Supan, A.; McGee, P.; Seike, A. Population aging: Facts, challenges, and responses. *Benefits Compens. Int.* **2011**, *41*, 22.
5. Kadefors, R.; Nilsson, K.; Östergren, P.-O.; Rylander, L.; Albin, M. Social inequality in working life expectancy in Sweden. *Z. Gerontol. Geriatr.* **2019**, *52*, 52–61. [CrossRef] [PubMed]
6. Gavrilov, L.A.; Heuveline, P. Aging of Population. The Encyclopedia of Population. Available online: https://www.encyclopedia.com/social-sciences/encyclopedias-almanacs-transcripts-and-maps/aging-population (accessed on 20 November 2018).
7. Forsman, M. The search for practical and reliable observational or technical risk assessment methods to be used in prevention of musculoskeletal disorders. *Agron. Res.* **2017**, *15*, 680–686.
8. Lind, C. Assessment and Design of Industrial Manual Handling to Reduce Physical Ergonomics Hazards:–Use and Development of Assessment Tools. Ph.D. Thesis, KTH-Royal Institute of Technology, Stockholm, Sweden, 2017.
9. Eliasson, K.; Palm, P.; Nyman, T.; Forsman, M. Inter-and intra-observer reliability of risk assessment of repetitive work without an explicit method. *Appl. Ergon.* **2017**, *62*, 1–8. [CrossRef] [PubMed]
10. Takala, E.-P.; Pehkonen, I.; Forsman, M.; Hansson, G.-Å.; Mathiassen, S.E.; Neumann, W.P.; Sjøgaard, G.; Veiersted, K.B.; Westgaard, R.H.; Winkel, J. Systematic evaluation of observational methods assessing biomechanical exposures at work. *Scand. J. Work. Environ. Health* **2010**, *36*, 3–24. [CrossRef] [PubMed]

11. Chiasson, M.-È.; Imbeau, D.; Aubry, K.; Delisle, A. Comparing the results of eight methods used to evaluate risk factors associated with musculoskeletal disorders. *Int. J. Ind. Ergon.* **2012**, *42*, 478–488. [CrossRef]
12. De Korte, E.; Wiezer, N.; Roozeboom, M.B.; Vink, P.; Kraaij, W. Behavior Change Techniques in mHealth Apps for the Mental and Physical Health of Employees: Systematic Assessment. *JMIR mHealth uHealth* **2018**, *6*, e167. [CrossRef] [PubMed]
13. Dahlqvist, C.; Hansson, G.-Å.; Forsman, M. Validity of a small low-cost triaxial accelerometer with integrated logger for uncomplicated measurements of postures and movements of head, upper back and upper arms. *Appl. Ergon.* **2016**, *55*, 108–116. [CrossRef] [PubMed]
14. Veiersted, K.B.; Westgaard, R.H.; Andersen, P. Electromyographic evaluation of muscular work pattern as a predictor of trapezius myalgia. *Scand. J. Work Environ. Health* **1993**, *19*, 284–290. [CrossRef] [PubMed]
15. Hansson, G.Å.; Björn, F.; Carlsson, P. A new triaxial accelerometer and its application as an advanced inclinometer. In Proceedings of the 9th International Congress of ISEK, Florence, Italy, 29 June–2 July 1992.
16. Abtahi, F. Towards Heart Rate Variability Tools in P-Health: Pervasive, Preventive, Predictive and Personalized. Ph.D. Thesis, KTH-Royal Institute of Technology, Stockholm, Sweden, 2016.
17. Deterding, S.; Dixon, D.; Khaled, R.; Nacke, L. From game design elements to gamefulness: Defining gamification. In Proceedings of the 15th International Academic MindTrek Conference: Envisioning Future Media Environments, Tampere, Finland, 28–30 September 2011; pp. 9–15.
18. Regulation, G.D.P. Regulation (EU) 2016/679 of the European Parliament and of the Council of 27 April 2016 on the protection of natural persons with regard to the processing of personal data and on the free movement of such data, and repealing Directive 95/46. *Off. J. Eur. Union* **2016**, *59*, 294.
19. Seoane, F.; Ferreira, J.; Alvarez, L.; Buendia, R.; Ayllón, D.; Llerena, C.; Gil-Pita, R. Sensorized garments and textrode-enabled measurement instrumentation for ambulatory assessment of the autonomic nervous system response in the atrec project. *Sensors* **2013**, *13*, 8997–9015. [CrossRef] [PubMed]
20. De Rossi, D.; Carpi, F.; Lorussi, F.; Mazzoldi, A.; Paradiso, R.; Scilingo, E.P.; Tognetti, A. Electroactive fabrics and wearable biomonitoring devices. *AUTEX Res. J.* **2003**, *3*, 180–185.
21. Lanatà, A.; Scilingo, E.P.; Nardini, E.; Loriga, G.; Paradiso, R.; De-Rossi, D. Comparative evaluation of susceptibility to motion artifact in different wearable systems for monitoring respiratory rate. *IEEE Trans. Inf. Technol. Biomed.* **2010**, *14*, 378–386. [CrossRef] [PubMed]
22. Młyńczak, M.C.; Niewiadomski, W.; Żyliński, M.; Cybulski, G.P. Ambulatory impedance pneumography device for quantitative monitoring of volumetric parameters in respiratory and cardiac applications. In Proceedings of the Computing in Cardiology Conference (CinC), Cambridge, MA, USA, 7–10 September 2014; pp. 965–968.
23. Abtahi, F.; Yang, L.; Lindecrantz, K.; Seoane, F.; Diaz-Olivazrez, J.A.; Ke, L.; Eklund, J.; Teriö, H.; Mediavilla Martinez, C.; Tiemann, C. Big Data & Wearable Sensors Ensuring Safety and Health@ Work. In Proceedings of the Global Health 2017, The Sixth International Conference on Global Health Challenges, Barcelona, Spain, 12–16 September 2017.
24. Yang, L.; Lu, K.; Diaz-Olivares, J.A.; Seoane, F.; Lindecrantz, K.; Forsman, M.; Abtahi, F.; Eklund, J.A.E. Towards Smart Work Clothing for Automatic Risk Assessment of Physical Workload. *IEEE Access* **2018**, *6*, 40059–40072. [CrossRef]
25. Mohino-Herranz, I.; Gil-Pita, R.; Ferreira, J.; Rosa-Zurera, M.; Seoane, F. Assessment of mental, emotional and physical stress through analysis of physiological signals using smartphones. *Sensors* **2015**, *15*, 25607–25627. [CrossRef] [PubMed]
26. Lind, C.M.; Forsman, M.; Rose, L.M. Development and evaluation of RAMP I—A practitioner's tool for screening of musculoskeletal disorder risk factors in manual handling. *Int. J. Occup. Saf. Ergon.* **2017**, *25*, 165–180. [CrossRef] [PubMed]
27. Partnership for European Research in Occupational Safety and Health (PEROSH). Assessing Arm Elevation at Work with Technical Systems. Available online: http://www.perosh.eu/wp-content/uploads/2018/12/Report-Arm-Elevation.pdf (accessed on 10 October 2018).
28. Nordander, C.; Hansson, G.-Å.; Ohlsson, K.; Arvidsson, I.; Balogh, I.; Strömberg, U.; Rittner, R.; Skerfving, S. Exposure–response relationships for work-related neck and shoulder musculoskeletal disorders—Analyses of pooled uniform data sets. *Appl. Ergon.* **2016**, *55*, 70–84. [CrossRef] [PubMed]
29. Luotonen, A. The common log file format 1995. Available online: https://httpd.apache.org/docs/1.3/logs.html#common (accessed on 21 November 2018).

30. Rodríguez, J.M.; Aso, S.; Cavero, C.; Quintero, A.M.; Pérez, M.; Mediavilla, C.; Rodríguez, B. Towards Digital and Personalized Healthcare and Well-Being Solutions for the Workplace. In *Intelligent Environments 2018*; IOS Press: Amsterdam, The Netherlands, 2018; pp. 377–383.
31. Brooke, J. SUS-A quick and dirty usability scale. *Usability Eval. Ind.* **1996**, *189*, 4–7.
32. Nielsen, J. Quantitative studies: How many users to test. *Alertbox* **2006**, *26*, 2006.
33. Nielsen, J. Why you only need to test with 5 users 2000. Available online: https://www.nngroup.com/articles/why-you-only-need-to-test-with-5-users (accessed on 10 September 2018).
34. Wang, Q.; Owen, G.W.; Mileham, A.R. Determining numbers of workstations and operators for a linear walking-worker assembly line. *Int. J. Comput. Integr. Manuf.* **2007**, *20*, 1–10. [CrossRef]
35. Bangor, A.; Kortum, P.; Miller, J. Determining what individual SUS scores mean: Adding an adjective rating scale. *J. Susabil. Stud.* **2009**, *4*, 114–123.
36. Lu, K.; Yang, L.; Seoane, F.; Abtahi, F.; Forsman, M.; Lindecrantz, K. Fusion of Heart Rate, Respiration and Motion Measurements from a Wearable Sensor System to Enhance Energy Expenditure Estimation. *Sensors* **2018**, *18*, 3092. [CrossRef] [PubMed]
37. Lu, K.; Yang, L.; Abtahi, F.; Lindecrantz, K.; Rödby, K.; Seoane, F. Wearable Cardiorespiratory Monitoring System for Unobtrusive Free-Living Energy Expenditure Tracking. In *Proceedings of the World Congress on Medical Physics and Biomedical Engineering 2018*; Springer: Berlin/Heidelberg, Germany, 2019; pp. 433–437.
38. Mahdavian, N.; Lind, C.M.; Diaz Olivares, J.A.; Iriondo Pascual, A.; Högberg, D.; Brolin, E.; Yang, L.; Forsman, M.; Hanson, L. Effect of giving feedback on postural working techniques. In Proceedings of the Advances in Manufacturing Technology XXXII: Proceedings of the 16th International Conference on Manufacturing Research, incorporating the 33rd National Conference on Manufacturing Research, University of Skövde, Skövde, Sweden, 11–13 September 2018; Volume 8, p. 247.

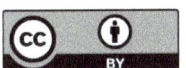

© 2019 by the authors. Licensee MDPI, Basel, Switzerland. This article is an open access article distributed under the terms and conditions of the Creative Commons Attribution (CC BY) license (http://creativecommons.org/licenses/by/4.0/).

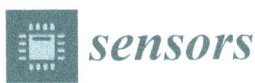

Article

Realization and Technology Acceptance Test of a Wearable Cardiac Health Monitoring and Early Warning System with Multi-Channel MCGs and ECG

Wen-Yen Lin [1,2], Hong-Lin Ke [1], Wen-Cheng Chou [1], Po-Cheng Chang [2], Tsai-Hsuan Tsai [2,3] and Ming-Yih Lee [2,4,*]

1. Department of Electrical Engineering, Center for Biomedical Engineering, Chang Gung University, Tao-Yuan 33302, Taiwan; wylin@mail.cgu.edu.tw (W.-Y.L.); k22060987@yahoo.com.tw (H.-L.K.); sito.19@gmail.com (W.-C.C.)
2. Division of Cardiology, Department of Internal Medicine, Chang Gung Memorial Hospital, Linkou, Tao-Yuan 33305, Taiwan; pccbrian@gmail.com (P.-C.C.); ttsai@mail.cgu.edu.tw (T.-H.T.)
3. Department of Industrial Design, Chang Gung University, Tao-Yuan 33302, Taiwan
4. Graduate Institute of Medical Mechatronics, Center for Biomedical Engineering, Chang Gung University, Tao-Yuan 33302, Taiwan
* Correspondence: leemiy@mail.cgu.edu.tw; Tel.: +886-3-211-8800 (ext. 5340)

Received: 9 September 2018; Accepted: 17 October 2018; Published: 19 October 2018

Abstract: In this work, a wearable smart clothing system for cardiac health monitoring with a multi-channel mechanocardiogram (MCG) has been developed to predict the myo-cardiac left ventricular ejection fraction (LVEF) function and to provide early risk warnings to the subjects. In this paper, the realization of the core of this system, i.e., the Cardiac Health Assessment and Monitoring Platform (CHAMP), with respect to its hardware, firmware, and wireless design features, is presented. The feature values from the CHAMP system have been correlated with myo-cardiac functions obtained from actual heart failure (HF) patients. The usability of this MCG-based cardiac health monitoring smart clothing system has also been evaluated with technology acceptance model (TAM) analysis and the results indicate that the subject shows a positive attitude toward using this wearable MCG-based cardiac health monitoring and early warning system.

Keywords: mechanocardiogram (MCG); smart clothes; heart failure (HF); left ventricular ejection fraction (LVEF); technology acceptance model (TAM)

1. Introduction

Mechanocardiogram (MCG) [1] or so-called Seismocardiogram (SCG) [2,3] was proposed in early 1990 using an inertial motion sensing device, i.e., an accelerometer, for cardiac activity monitoring. This technology is capable of identifying feature points of the cardiac activity events, such as the opening and closing of heart valves [4], as well as some heart systolic and diastolic characteristics, such as isovolumic movement (IM), isotonic contraction (IC), peak of rapid diastolic filling (RF), and peak of atrial systolic (AS) [5]. It has also turned into an emerging method for cardiac health monitoring as mature MEMS-based technology and the development of integrated circuit (IC) process [6].

Most of the related works employing MCG/SCG technologies used a single accelerometer placed on the sternum of the chest to record the mechanical composite vibration signal incurred from the complex heart beat activities within a cardiac cycle around the heart area on the surface of the chest. In this way, time delays and signal attenuations occur in only one detected signal, which is a combination of motion signals from different vibration sources in the heart, such as the four heart valves. Hence, Zanetti et al. [7] suggested using multiple accelerometers to reduce the influence of time delay and signal attenuation for the better detection of cardiac diseases. In the meantime, Lin et al. [8] identified six new feature points of cardiac activities, i.e., left ventricular lateral wall contraction peak velocity (LCV), septal wall contraction peak velocity (SCV), trans-aortic peak flow (AF), trans-pulmonary peak flow (PF), trans-mitral ventricular relaxation flow (MF_E), and atrial contraction flow (MF_A), which were not reported in any previous related works, with a novel multi-channel MCGs (or SCGs) system. With this system, more accurate timings of events have been identified among the previously found feature points. Some very important and meaningful cardia time intervals (CTIs) have then been calculated, such as the pre-ejection period (PEP), from ECG-Q to MCG-AO, and the left ventricular ejection time (LVET), from MCG-AO to MCG-AC. Reant et al. [9] proposed that the ratio of PEP to LVET, i.e., PEP/LVET, could also be an important index, known as the Contractility Coefficient (CC), for myo-cardiac functions. The key index used to justify the myo-cardiac functions, i.e., the left ventricular ejection fraction (LVEF), was also found to be strongly inversely correlated to the CC values in the study. Indeed, LVEF is an important clinical index for evaluating a human's cardiac functions, especially for heart failure (HF) patients with a reduced ejection fraction (HFrEF).

Unlike the popular diagnosis instruments which are widely used clinically for cardiac health monitoring and examination, such as magnetic resonance imaging (MRI), computerized tomography scan (CT scan), and echocardiography (Echo), this technology, by combining ECG and MCG signals, can support long-term continuous cardiac health monitoring of patients [10]. To benefit from this technology ubiquitously in daily life for long-term and continuous monitoring of cardiac health monitoring, efforts towards implementing these technologies as wearable devices are desired. In the past years, several efforts have been made to study wearable devices or the body-sensing-network (BSN) for cardiac health monitoring [11–14], but all of them employed ECG-based technologies for the monitoring of cardiac health. The only two portable products based on MCG/SCG technology for cardiac health monitoring are the "Cardio Pro" from Heart Force Medical Inc., Vancouver, BC, Canada [15], and the one by M. Di Rienzo et al. [16]. However, both of them use a single channel MCG/SCG signal and still incorporate the drawbacks of the single-channel MCG/SCG technology.

Ballistocardiography (BCG) is another similar technology with SCG for cardiac activity monitoring [17]. The difference between the SCG and BCG signals is not simply a matter of nomenclature. Because the BCG measures whole body vibrations, the BCG signal is less influenced by local anatomical and sensor placement factors, and thus provides a better indication of hemodynamic information (e.g., CO) [18–20]. However, BCG signals cannot be measured as readily as SCG signals with wearable devices, but rather with weighing scales, tables, beds, or chairs—devices that can capture whole body movements. Moreover, a few works [21,22] proposed novel methods of measuring BCG signals using cameras or optical imagine and gained high-quality signals, but these restrict the measurement to fixed sites and hence are not able to benefit from the technologies anytime, anywhere, as the wearable system can provide. Recently, serval groups have demonstrated that BCG signals can also be measured using wearable accelerometers [23,24] and extensive data processing works have been implemented for data analysis [25]. Nevertheless, the waveform of the data was more distorted when more data processing techniques were used and this would make the analysis of event identification less accurate.

Furthermore, with the increased attention in research on wearable devices and smart clothing technologies, studies have also focused on trying to understand users' perception of these smart technologies. Recent studies have used the technology acceptance model (TAM) [26], which is one of the most extensively used models to study an individual's acceptance of information and communication technologies, to explain a user's perception of wearable technology and smart clothes. For example, past studies [27–29] utilized the TAM to explain why users are more willing to adopt wearable technologies, such as smartwatches and wearable fitness products. Besides the original variables in the TAM, these studies also included other external constructs that were part of their research interests, such as visibility [27], affective quality, and mobility [28], as well as perceived health benefits [29].

However, even in recent studies that have sought to understand users' perceptions of smart clothes, the participants were mostly generally healthier rather than patients with cardiovascular disease (CVD). Therefore, in this study, we have proposed an extension of the original TAM by adding external variables with the goal to explore the effects of external factors on attitudes, behavioral intentions, and the decision to use smart clothing technology among patients with CVD.

The goals of this work can be summarized as follows:

(1) CHAMP: Design of the Cardiac Health Assessment and Monitoring Platform (CHAMP) with multi-channel MCGs/ECG data acquisition, processing, and the wireless communication framework for mobile cardiac health monitoring.
(2) Smart Clothes: Implementing the framework as a wearable smart clothing for cardiac health monitoring.
(3) Methods & Assessment of Cardiac health monitoring: Development of an efficient mechanism for cardiac health assessment and prediction of the left ventricular ejection fraction (LVEF) for HF patients with detected multi-channel MCGs and ECG data.
(4) Usability study: Analysis of the extended technology acceptance model in understanding users' behavioral intention to use a wearable cardiac health monitoring smart clothing system.

In this paper, the design and implementation of the wearable cardiac health monitoring and early warning system with multi-channel MCGs and ECG is described in Section 2, including: CHAMP; integration of CHAMP with textile-based technologies into smart clothing; methods of cardiac health assessment, especially for HF patients; and finally, the extended TAM model, the hypothesis proposition, and the details of data collection for this technology acceptance study. Section 3 presents the functional verification of the CHAMP, validations of the developed smart clothes, the analysis of output data from the system, and data correlation with myo-cardiac functions, as well as linkage to certain heart diseases, such as HFs, and the TAM results are also discussed. Finally, in Section 4, we conclude the entire paper. Some discussions and conclusions about the future direction of the work are drawn.

2. Materials and Methods

In this section, Section 2.1 describes the structure of CHAMP and its implementation for the synchronous multi-channel MCGs/ECG data acquisition, processing, and wireless data communication. The integration of the platform with textile-based technologies into wearable smart clothes is presented in Section 2.2. Section 2.3 introduces the CTIs that could be calculated from the system and how these can be used for the cardiac health assessment, such as how the LVEF can be derived from those CTIs and used for the cardiac health assessment of heart HF patients. Section 2.4 describes the extended TAM model, the hypothesis proposition, and the details of data collection for the usability and technology acceptance study.

2.1. CHAMP: Cardiac Health Assessment and Monitoring Platform

In order to simultaneously acquire data from multi-channel MCG units and a single channel ECG unit of the monitoring system, it is necessary to be able to read data from multiple accelerometers and digitized ECG data within a sampling period sequentially. To facilitate these requirements and considering mobility for support as wearable devices, a cardiac health assessment and monitoring platform, CHAMP, was designed and implemented. The block diagram of CHAMP is shown in Figure 1. The core architecture of CHAMP is a microcontroller to access four accelerometers through a four-channel I^{2}C bus switch and digitized ECG signal from ECG front-end circuitry sequentially within one sampling period. Then, data can be calculated and filtered by the firmware in the microcontroller and the processed data are transmitted using UART protocol through the BlueTooth module. Detailed functions and selection of the components are discussed below.

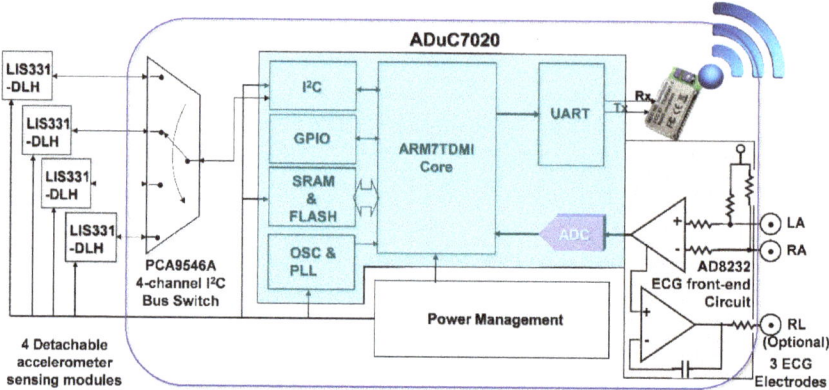

Figure 1. Block diagram of CHAMP (Cardiac Health Assessment and Monitoring Platform).

2.1.1. The Hardware Design of CHAMP

The main circuit of CHAMP is an embedded system with the microcontroller ADuC7020 from Analog Devices, Inc. (Norwood, MA, USA) as the core controller of this platform. The microcontroller has an internal crystal oscillator and can operate up to the core clock of 41.78 MHz, and the core is an ARM7TDMI core in 16-bit/32-bit RISC architecture with a 62 kB flash memory for program storage and 8 kB of SRAM for program execution. It includes multiple analog-to-digital converters (ADCs) providing a 12-bit resolution with a sampling rate up to 1 mega sampling per second (MSPS) on each channel. It also has built-in UART, I²C, and SPI on-chip peripherals and four general purpose timers. In the CHAMP design, an I²C interface is used to access multiple accelerometers, a UART peripheral is used to communicate with a Bluetooth module for wireless data transmission, an ADC is used to digitize the analog ECG signal so that it can be synchronized with multi-channel MCG data from accelerometers, and a timer is also set in the firmware to control the timing of event handling (data acquisition, processing, and transmission) for real-time data streaming to the receiver device.

Accelerometers used in this platform are LIS331DLH, from STMicroelectronics, Geneva, Switzerland. With the sampling rate of 400 Hz, these accelerometers are set at the sensing range of ± 2 g at a 12-bit resolution, so that a 1 mg sensitivity (1 mg = 2^{-10} g, i.e., 1/1024 g, where g is the gravity force) can be achieved. Raw data acquired from each accelerometer are the acceleration along the X-, Y-, and Z-axis, but only the Z-axis acceleration data (in the direction perpendicular to the chest surface area) were processed and transmitted wirelessly. In this multi-channel MCGs/ECG system design, the four accelerometers used are the same components from the manufacture, and hence these all have the same I²C address. The use of a single channel of the I²C interface built in the microcontroller, ADuC7020, is not enough to identify these accelerometers separately. To be able to access these four accelerometers separately, a four-channel I²C bus switch, PCA9546A, from Texas Instruments (Dallas, TX, USA), is used and the specific bits in its control register are set to define which channel of the I²C interface to use. Therefore, a specific accelerometer can be accessed through that selected slave I²C interface.

In this design, an ECG measurement front-end circuit, AD8232, a fully integrated single-lead ECG front end chip which is capable of providing high signal gain (G = 100) with dc blocking capabilities, from Analog Devices, Inc., with surrounded discrete components (resistors and capacitors), is integrated. The ECG signal can be extremely noisy, and the AD8232 circuit can work as an op amp to obtain a clear ECG analog signal. A Lead I limb ECG measurement circuit is implemented. With a positive reference electrode attached to the left arm (LA) and negative reference electrode attached to the right arm (RA), it can obtain an optimal ECG waveform, configured with a 0.5 Hz high-pass filter followed by a 40 Hz low-pass filter. The RLD circuit that drives the third electrode, which is usually attached to the right leg (RL), is used to cancel the common-mode interference. However, it is optional and in our smart clothes integration, this input is not connected. Since CHAMP is integrated into smart clothes, the electrodes for the LA and RA can only be located on the upper trunk.

To provide the capability of wireless data transmission, a Class 1, Bluetooth (BT) 2.1+EDR module, RN-41 from Microchip Technology Inc. (Chandler, AZ, USA), is integrated into CHAMP. This BT module is operated in a serial port profile (SPP) and configured with a 115,200 buad-rate and none parity bit, 8 data bits, and 1 stop bit (N-8-1) standard. The UART interface is used for the data communication between the microcontroller and BT module. As a result, the platform can stream the data either through a RS-232 cable or BT module under the same firmware control.

After finishing the schematic design of CHAMP, the PCB layout was completed with two metal layers with a size of 50 mm × 70 mm, as shown in Figure 2a. No special efforts were made to shrink the size of the PCB layout and hence there is still space to further reduce the size of the CHAMP PCB in future versions. Then, the PCB was fabricated with the FR4 panel and Figure 2b shows a photo of the actual system after all the components were soldered and the function of the board was tested. The total hardware cost of this platform, including the cost of PCB and all the components, is only around US$130. With larger quantities of hardware platforms made, a lower cost can be achieved.

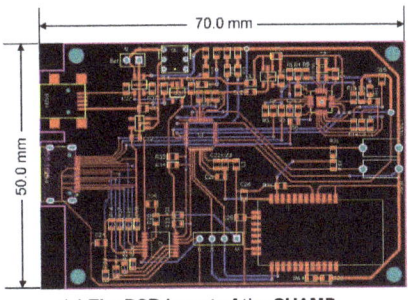
(a) The PCB layout of the CHAMP

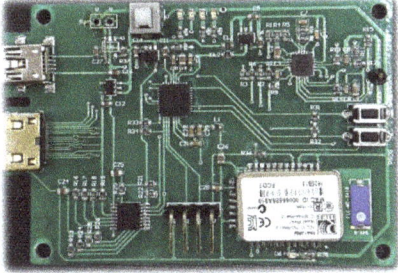
(b) The photo of soldered system

Figure 2. (a) The PCB layout of CHAMP; (b) the photo of the soldered system.

2.1.2. The Firmware Design of CHAMP

The firmware acts as the soul of CHAMP. Without proper implementation of the firmware, the functions of CHAMP would not perform as expected. Figure 3 shows the flowchart of the firmware, a simple interrupt driven program. Once the system is powered up, the firmware starts from its main program. In the main program, the system is initialized with proper configuration of the accelerometers (400 Hz sampling and output data rate, 0.5 Hz high-pass filter enabled), setting of the timer (every 2.5 ms), ADC configuration (400 SPS, 12-bit resolution), general purpose input-output (GPIO) configuration, UART initialization (115,200 bps, N-8-1 standard), and interrupt confirmation and enabling, etc. After the system has been initialized, the main program enters into an infinite loop waiting for the timer interrupt to occur. It is worth mentioning that the on-chip ADC is used to digitize the analog ECG signal from the ECG measurement front-end circuit. To save the power consumption of the microcontroller and to match the sampling rate with MCG signals, the sampling frequency of the ADC is set to use the timer signal.

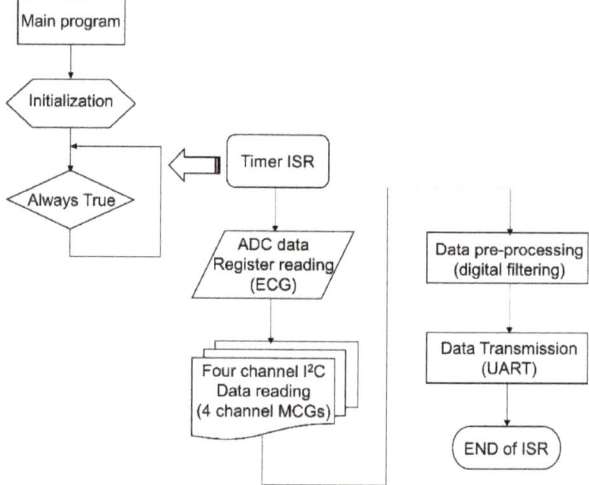

Figure 3. The flowchart of the firmware for CHAMP.

The timer interrupt is set to generate interrupt signals to the microcontroller for every 2.5 ms, i.e., 400 Hz frequency. Once the microcontroller receives the timer interrupt, the timer interrupt service routine (ISR) is executed. In the timer ISR, it disables any further interrupt from occurring, and then reads the ADC output data register. After reading ECG data from ADC, it uses the I^{2}C interface to go through the PCA9546A 4-channel I^{2}C bus switch and to read each of the digital outputs of the four accelerometers one by one. After the ECG and four-channel MCG data are retrieved, the signal pre-processing task follows. In the signal pre-processing, digital filtering of a 50 Hz low-pass filter through the single ECG and four-channel MCG data is performed. Then, the output data after filtering are transmitted out of the system through the UART peripheral via the BT module. Before exiting the timer ISR, all interrupts are enabled again and wait for the occurrence of the next interrupt event.

Because the timing is critical for this kind of high data rate (400 Hz) real-time system, only Z-axis data from each accelerometer for the MCG signals are processed and transmitted. In this platform, 13 byte of data are transmitted from the system with UART protocol at 115,200 bps. The output data packet is shown in Figure 4a. The data packet contains the header byte, 0xAA, 2 byte of data for ECG, and the four accelerometers' data (2 byte each), followed by an 8-bit counter value for the checking of continuity, and ends with a tail byte, 0xBB. The timing breakup of the firmware execution for the three major functional blocks, i.e., data retrieving, digital filtering, and UART transmission, is shown in Figure 4b, in a logic analyzer. With the microcontroller retrieving the ECG and 4 MCG data through I^{2}C, it takes 0.71 ms for data preprocessing of digital filtering for a single ECG; for 4 ECG data, it takes 0.551 ms; and finally, sending out the filtered data through UART takes 1.137 ms. Therefore, the total execution time of the timer ISR is 2.398 ms, which is still less than the timer interrupt period of 2.5 ms (i.e., 400 Hz). From the measurement, it can be concluded that the system is actually performing real-time data acquisition, processing, and streaming wirelessly.

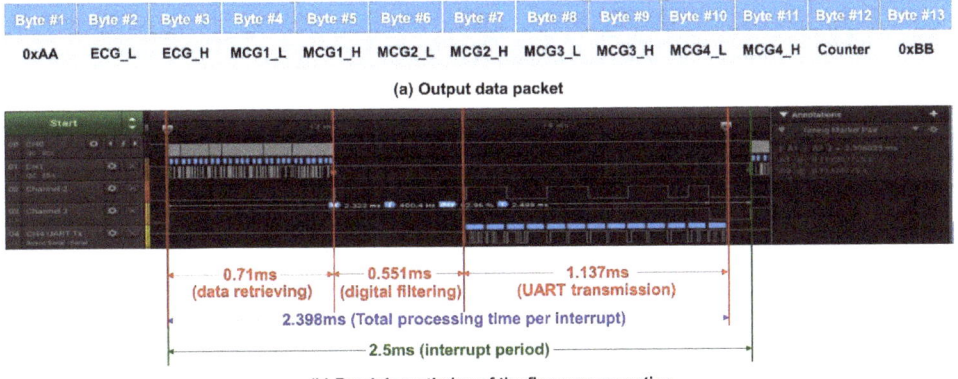

(a) Output data packet

(b) Breakdown timing of the firmware execution

Figure 4. (a) The output data packet of the system; (b) the timing breakdown of the firmware execution.

The raw data measured with accelerometers around the heart area on the chest surface can be extremely noisy. The signals have to be filtered for cleaner information and passed through the following processes. The ECG front-end circuit is already implemented with hardware high-pass and low-pass filters, so the major concerns are the MCG signals. The accelerometer used in the system is equipped with a built-in high-pass filter with certain cut-off frequency configurations. In the system, the accelerometer output data rate is set at 400 Hz and the built-in high-pass filter with a 1 Hz cut-off frequency is configured to block-out the dc value of acceleration due to the gravity and orientation of the accelerometer in use. To filter out the high frequency noise, the digital filtering process is desired for the raw MCG data. A low-pass FIR filter with a 50 Hz cut-off frequency and 60 dB signal drop-off at 60 Hz under a 400 Hz sampling frequency is designed with the FDATool in MATLAB®. With this FIR low-pass filtering design specification, a FIR digital filter with 79 taps is generated. With generated fixed-point coefficients and a filtering program implemented in C, the firmware incorporated with FIR digital filtering using fixed-point operations and a circular buffer mechanism is achieved within 0.551 ms of execution time for one ECG signal channel and four MCG signal channels.

2.2. The Multi-Channel MCGs/ECG Monitoring Smart Clothes

To avail benefits from this technology anytime, anywhere, and for any movement in daily life for long-term and continuous monitoring of cardiac health monitoring, CHAMP has been integrated into a wearable system, i.e., multi-channel MCGs/ECG monitoring smart clothes. With our previous experience [30] and understanding of the advanced textile-based conductive techniques, we teamed up with AiQ, a Smart Clothing company, to integrate CHAMP and sensors into proper locations of smart clothes and had it fabricated as the prototype of the multi-channel MCGs/ECG monitoring smart clothes, as shown in Figure 5.

Figure 5a shows the integration of the previously discussed hardware platform and sensors, i.e., CHAMP, into smart clothes. The smart clothes were fabricated as a stretchable vest, so that it is skin-tight enough to collect steady and reliable MCG and ECG signals. Four accelerometer sensors were placed at proper locations, as in a previously reported study in [8], as the green dots marked in Figure 5a,b. The ECG electrodes were made with fabric electrodes, which can deliver more than 37 dB of SNR, for the collection of ECG signals, and the quality of ECG signals measured with these electrodes was also verified and is described in Section 3.1.1. The main circuit board of CHAMP is embedded at the location near the neck area, as shown in Figure 5a. It is connected to the accelerometer sensors and ECG electrodes with electro-conductive fiber for the data collection. A battery was also placed at the back of the main board to provide the working power. As a matter of fact, the only rigid parts of this smart clothing are the CHAMP board, battery, and four accelerometer sensor modules

(10 mm × 7 mm each), and they weighed 70 g in total. The weight of the clothes is 245 g, including the rigid parts. Even so, from our usability study, patients still show a positive attitude towards using this system. Figure 5b shows the smart clothes worn by a human subject.

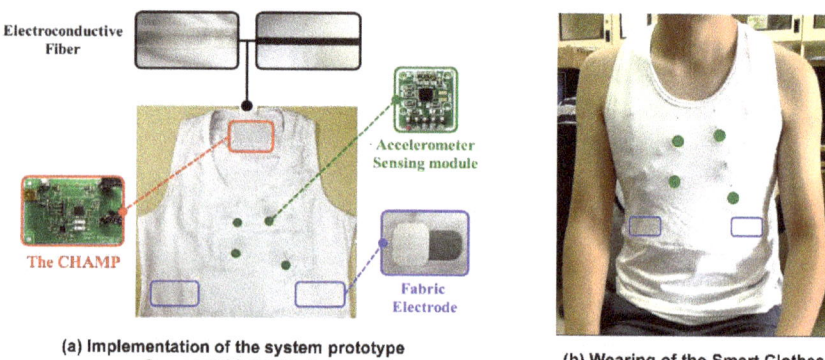

Figure 5. The prototype of multi-channel MCGs/ECG monitoring Smart Clothes.

2.3. Cardiac Health Assessment for Heart Failures

With the six newly identified feature points in the multi-channel MCG spectrum reported in Ref. [8] and the other feature points (FPs) which were identified and reported previously in Ref. [5], the time sequencing of these 15 feature points identified in the multi-channel MCGs/ECG data, along with the Q, R, and S points in the ECG signal, are plotted in Figure 6a. By calculating the time differences between certain FPs, some meaningful cardia time intervals (CTIs) can be obtained. For example, there are six CTIs related to the function of heart contraction, e.g., electro-mechanical delay (EMD) from the time point of ECG-Q to MCG-MC, iso-volumeric contraction time (IVCT) from MCG-MC to MCG-AO, pre-ejection period (PEP) from ECG-Q to MCG-AO, rapid ejection time (RET) from MCG-AO to MCG-AF (or RE), left ventricular ejection time (LVET) from MCG-AO to MCG-AC, and systole (SYS) from MCG-MC to MCG-AC. The time sequence of these feature points and the obtained CTIs are marked in Figure 6b.

Clinically, the left ventricular ejection fraction (LVEF) is the key index to justify the myo-cardiac functions, especially for HF patients with a reduced ejection fraction (HFrEF). A higher LVEF value indicates healthier myo-cardiac functions. Among these CTIs, Buell [9] proposed that the ratio of PEP to LVET, i.e., PEP/LVET, could also be an important index for myo-cardiac functions, i.e., the Contractility Coefficient (CC), as in Equation (1), and LVEF was also found to be inversely correlated to the CC values in the study.

$$CC = PEP/LVET, \qquad (1)$$

Hence, with the related feature points identified from the multi-channel MCGs and ECG signal, and with those CTIs calculated accordingly, the CC value can be derived and thereafter, the correlated LVEF can be obtained as the assessment index for myo-cardiac functions, which is especially helpful for the cardiac health monitoring of HF patients.

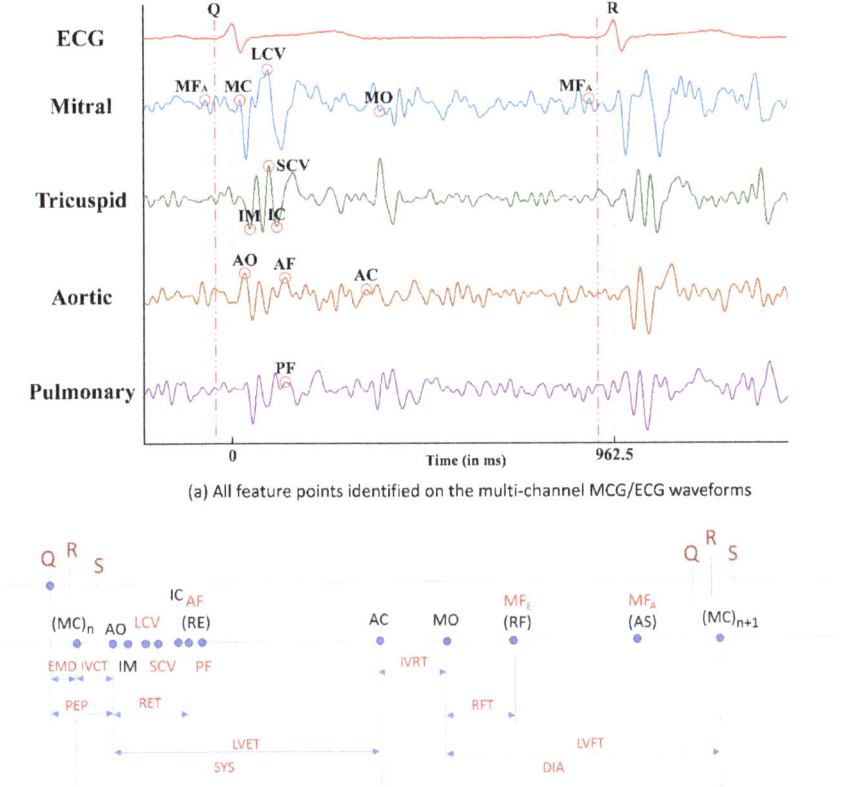

Figure 6. (a) All feature points identified on the multi-channel MCGs/ECG waveforms; (b) the time sequence of all feature points and related cardiac time intervals.

2.4. Extended TAM Verification–Models, Hypothesis, and Data Collection

The TAM has been shown to successfully explain users' perceptions of wearable technologies. In the TAM, perceived ease of use (PEOU) and perceived usefulness (PU) are two key psychological constructs that determine users' attitudes toward the use of a technology or service. That is, if a technology is perceived as easy and useful for accomplishing a task, then users will have a more positive attitude toward the technology. Furthermore, a user's attitude will later affect his/her intention to actually use the technology. Due to the explanatory ability of the TAM framework, the TAM has been consistently revised and validated in various fields of study. In this study, we extend the TAM to understand how other constructs, such as technology anxiety, perceived ubiquity, resistance to change, and benefit, would affect CVD patients' perceptions of wearable smart clothing technology. As a result, we postulated the following hypotheses:

Hypothesis 1. *Technology anxiety will be negatively associated with the perceived usefulness of a wearable cardiac health monitoring system among patients with cardiovascular disease.*

Hypothesis 2. *Perceived ubiquity will be positively associated with the perceived usefulness of a wearable cardiac health monitoring system among patients with cardiovascular disease.*

Hypothesis 3. *Perceived ubiquity will be positively associated with the perceived ease of use of a wearable cardiac health monitoring system among patients with cardiovascular disease.*

Hypothesis 4. *Perceived ubiquity will be negatively associated with resistance to change with respect to using a wearable cardiac health monitoring system among patients with cardiovascular disease.*

Hypothesis 5. *Perceived ubiquity will be positively associated with attitudes toward the use of a wearable cardiac health monitoring system among patients with cardiovascular disease.*

Hypothesis 6. *Resistance to change will be negatively associated with the behavioral intention to use a wearable cardiac health monitoring system among patients with cardiovascular disease.*

Hypothesis 7. *Benefit will be positively associated with the behavioral intention to use a wearable cardiac health monitoring system among patients with cardiovascular disease.*

Hypothesis 8. *Perceived usefulness will be positively associated with attitudes toward the use of a wearable cardiac health monitoring system among patients with cardiovascular disease.*

Hypothesis 9. *Perceived ease of use will be positively associated with the behavioral intention to use a wearable cardiac health monitoring system among patients with cardiovascular disease.*

Hypothesis 10. *Attitude will be positively associated with the behavioral intention to use a wearable cardiac health monitoring system among patients with cardiovascular disease.*

In total, 48 participants who were older than 20 years and were either diagnosed as having HF with a left ventricular ejection fraction <40% or severe valvular heart disease agreed to participate in the study. Ethical approval was obtained from the Institutional Review Board (IRB) of Chang Gung Hospital, Taoyuan, Taiwan (104-8175B). Among total subjects, 77% of the participants were male and 23% were female. In terms of age, 8% were between 20 and 29 years; 8% were between 30 and 39 years; 19% were between 40 and 49 years; 25% were between 50 and 59 years; 23% were between 60 and 69 years; 8% were between 70 and 79 years; 6% were between 80 and 89 years; and 2% were older than 90 years. Regarding education, 10% had graduated from a graduate school; 35% had graduated from a university; 21% had completed high school as their highest level of education; 8% had completed junior high school as their highest level of education; and 25% had completed elementary school as their highest level of education.

When a participant arrived in the clinical room for this research survey, the researchers first explained the purpose and the procedure of the study explicitly. Then, the participants signed the consent form. During the experimental stage, the participants' demographic data were collected. Subsequently, the researchers presented the developed wearable MCG-based cardiac health monitoring system to the participants so that they could actually feel the product and have a better sense of the texture and the functions of the wearable cardiac sensing technology. After completing the scenario presentation, the participant would then answer a technology acceptance questionnaire. The whole survey took approximately 30 min.

The technology acceptance questionnaire consisted of eight major sections that assessed technology anxiety, perceived ubiquity, resistance to change, benefit, perceived usefulness, perceived ease of use, attitude, and behavioral intention. All constructs were measured using five-point Likert-type scales, with 1 indicating strongly disagree and 5 indicating strongly agree. Each construct's corresponding questionnaire was derived and modified from a variety of sources to reflect the characteristics of smart clothes. The measures for technology anxiety and resistance to change were adapted from Guo et al. [31]. The measure for perceived ubiquity was adapted from Hsiao and Tan [32]. The measure for benefit was adapted from Demiris et al. [33]. The measures for perceived usefulness and perceived ease of use were derived from Davis [26]. The measure of attitude originated from Fishbein and Ajzen [34] and Ajzen [35], and the measure of behavioral intention originated from Venkatesh et al. [36]. The data analysis included two stages: the measurement model and the path analysis. The measurement model was used to test the reliability and the validity of the constructs by conducting a confirmatory factor analysis. The path analysis was used to test the proposed research hypotheses. SPSS 22 and LISREL 8.7 were used to respectively perform the analyses of the measurement model and the path analysis.

3. Results and Discussions

3.1. Functional Verifications of CHAMP

The major functions of CHAMP are presented in this section. It verifies the ECG signal measurement from the in-system AD8232 ECG acquisition circuit and performs signal verification of digital filtering for both ECG and MCG signals.

3.1.1. Verification of ECG Signal Measurement

The integration of the ECG monitoring circuit into CHAMP is a very important feature of the system. Therefore, the ECG signal measured from the on-board AD8232 ECG monitoring circuit is compared with the ECG signal measured from Bio Amplifier using commercially available electrodes simultaneously, as in the previous study [8], to confirm the correctness of the ECG measured signal from the on-board AD8232 circuit. As shown in Figure 7b, the timing of ECG signal feature points, i.e., P, Q, R, S, and T, measured from the on-board AD8232 circuit, is in-line with the one measured from Bio Amp and data acquired by PowerLab. In this comparison study, as shown in Figure 7a, not only the ECG signals are compared, and the positions of electrodes for AD8232 ECG measurement are attached on the upper trunk of the body instead of the hands and leg, which are the locations of electrodes attached in the conventional limb ECG measurement, such as the ECG measurement via Bio Amp in previous study. The comparison results concluded that the function and performance of the on-board AD8232 ECG monitoring circuit are reliable and the quality of ECG signals measured from fabric electrodes is about the same when compared with the commercial available electrodes.

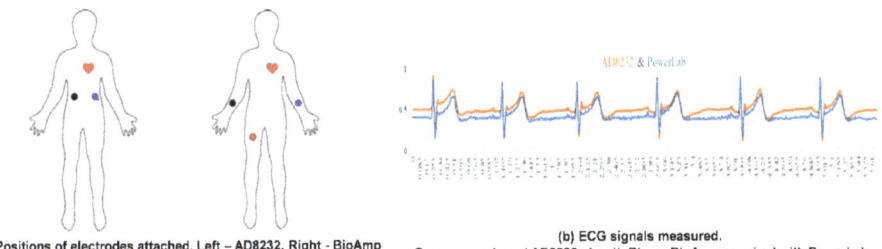

(a) Positions of electrodes attached. Left – AD8232, Right – BioAmp
(b) ECG signals measured.
Orange – on-board AD8232 circuit, Blue – BioAmp acquired with PowerLab

Figure 7. The verification of the on-board AD8232 ECG monitored signal. (**a**) Comparison of electrode positions; (**b**) ECG signal comparison.

3.1.2. Verification for Digital Filtering Implementation

To validate the digital filter implementation, and to verify if the output of the filtered signals meets the filter design specification, the frequency spectrum comparison of a single MCG channel signal before and after the digital filtering is shown in Figure 8. Figure 8a shows the original frequency spectrum of an MCG signal before digital filtering is applied and Figure 8b depicts the frequency spectrum of that MCG signal after applying the digital filtering. From Figure 8b, it can be observed that the signal starts to drop-off from 50 Hz and the magnitude almost drops to 0 after 60 Hz compared with the original spectrum shown in Figure 8a.

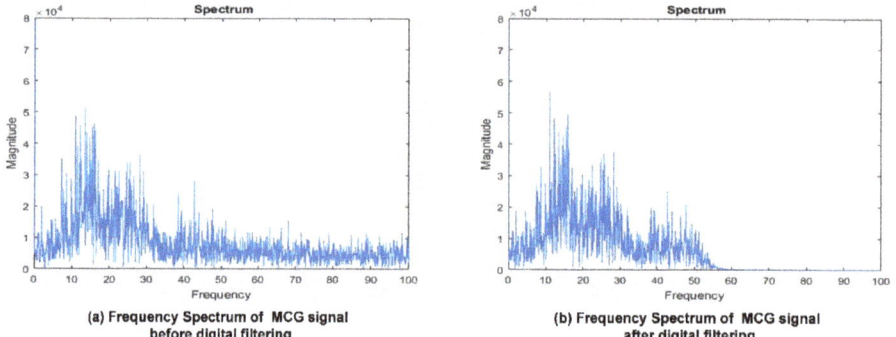

Figure 8. The frequency spectrum comparison of a single channel MCG signal before and after digital filtering in the gateway.

Even though there is a delay of 40 data samples (around 100 ms in this case) after digital filtering, the timing references to the ECG signal still remain the same since both the ECG signal and four-channel MCG signals go through the same digital filtering and suffer the same amount of delay. By aligning the ECG signal and one channel of the MCG signal in the time domain before and after the digital filtering, it is very clear to observe the effect of noise filtering, as shown in Figure 9. In Figure 9, the timing signal before filtering is shown in a black color and after filtering is shown in a red color. Clearly, from the zoom-in portion of the MCG signal, the red line is smoother, i.e., less affected by high frequency noise, after applying the digital filtering on the MCG signal. The ECG signal does not seem to vary a lot before and after digital filtering. This is because the data from the ECG signal for digital filtering were already filtered through the hardware low-pass filter implemented in the AD8232 circuit.

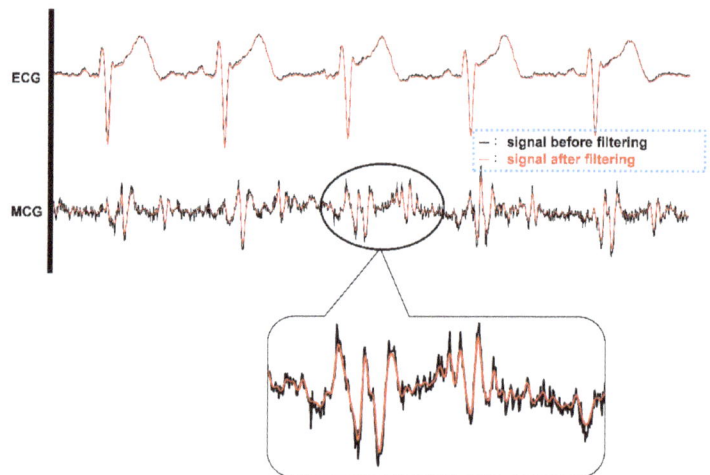

Figure 9. The timing signals of ECG and single channel MCG before (BLACK color) and after (RED color) digital filtering.

3.2. Validations of Multi-Channel MCGs and ECG Smart Monitoring Clothes

Figure 10a shows the picture of a subject wearing the multi-channel MCGs/ECG smart monitoring clothes. The subject also holds an android-based tablet PC running a mobile app for obtaining data received from the smart clothes system wirelessly and performing the identification of feature points automatically. The feature points identified by the mobile app are the newly identified six feature points (FPs) reported in Ref. [8] and other feature points of cardiac activity events reported in Ref. [5]. The waveforms of the data received from these smart monitoring clothes through BlueTooth are shown in Figure 10b, i.e., one ECG waveform and four channels of MCG waveforms. Similar waveforms and features of the signals could be identified visually as in the previous study 8 and it validated the correctness of the multi-channel MCGs and signal-channel ECG measurement with the wireless transmission feature. The sampling rate of the accelerometer was set at 400 Hz. The signals seem to be nosier (lower SNR) than the ones shown in Ref. [24]; however, BCG signals were measured from the vibration of the body, which have bigger amplitudes compared with MCG signals that measure the tiny vibration signals in the chest area caused by cardiac activities. Also, a narrower bandwidth filter (0.5–25 Hz) was used in Ref. [24] and it is more likely to distort the signal waveforms compared to the original ones. Even though the MCG signals acquired from these smart clothes look nosier than the other related works, based on the time-window-based Morphological identification rules proposed previously by the comparison with echocardiography images, all the feature points could be identified accurately by the app, which has the identified rules implemented on the android-based tablet PC.

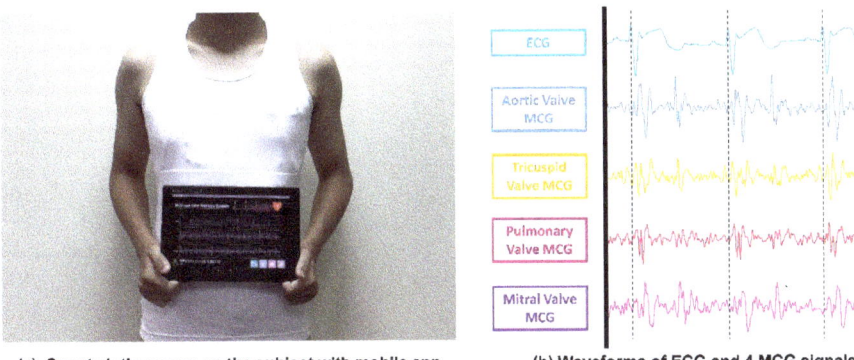

(a) Smart clothes worn on the subject with mobile app for data receiving and feature points identification

(b) Waveforms of ECG and 4 MCG signals received from the smart clothes

Figure 10. (a) Smart clothes worn by a subject with a mobile app for data receiving and auto identification of feature points; (b) the actual measured multi-channel MCGs/ECG signals plotted from the output data transmitted from the smart clothes.

Taking the example of PEP and LVET calculation, the ECG-R, ECG-Q, MCG-MC, MCG-AO, and MCG-AC feature points have to be identified. According to the proposed time-window-based morphological identification rules, these feature points could be identified with the following rules.

a. ECG-R: Use the So-and-Chan detection algorithm [37] to find the ECG-R point.
b. ECG-Q: Find the first valley point, which defines the ECG-Q point, before the time instance of ECG-R point identified in step a.
c. MCG-MC: On the MCG Mitral Valve (MV) channel, find the first peak right before the minimum point within the ECG-Q to ECG-R + 0.04 s time window. The peak defines the MCG-MC point.
d. MCG-AO: On the MCG Aortic Valve (AV) channel, find the first peak right before the minimum point within the time instance of MCG-MC to ECG-R + 0.06 s time window. If no peak can be found, continue searching for the peak backward to ECG-Q. The peak defines the MCG-AO point.
e. MCG-AC: On the MCG Tricuspid Valve (TV) channel, find the first peak, i.e., A point, right before the minimum point within ECG-R + 0.32 s to ECG-R + 0.5 s time window. On the MCG AV channel, find the first peak, which defines the MCG-AC point, backward from the time instance of A point.

Note that, when searching for the local valley points or peak points, if there is more than one data point with the same value, select the first data point from the searching direction as the local valley or local peak point.

Among the identified feature points, i.e., ECG-R, ECG-Q, MCG-MC, MCG-AO, and MCG-AC, of eight randomly selected subjects, 10 continuous heart beat cycles from each of these subjects were chosen randomly to compare with their echocardiography image. Figure 11 illustrates the mapping of an echo image with measured ECG/MCG signals to confirm the accuracy of the identification results in one of the typical cycles. In the figure, ECG-R and ECG-Q were identified correctly on the ECG channel. Then, MCG-MC was identified on the MCG MV channel using the rule described in step c mentioned above and was confirmed with the Mitral Valve of the M-mode echo image, which is now shown in this figure. After that, the MCG-AO and MCG-AC were identified on the MCG AV channel according to the rules described in step d and e and were confirmed with the Aortic Valve M-mode echo image shown in the figure. The time intervals in the second cycle for ECG-R to MCG-MC, ECG-R to MCG-AO, and ECG-R to MCG-AC are also marked in the figure. All identified feature points were found matched with the events corresponding to their echocardiography images. The detailed identified time instances of the feature points compared with the inspection of echocardiography images are provided in the Supplementary Materials.

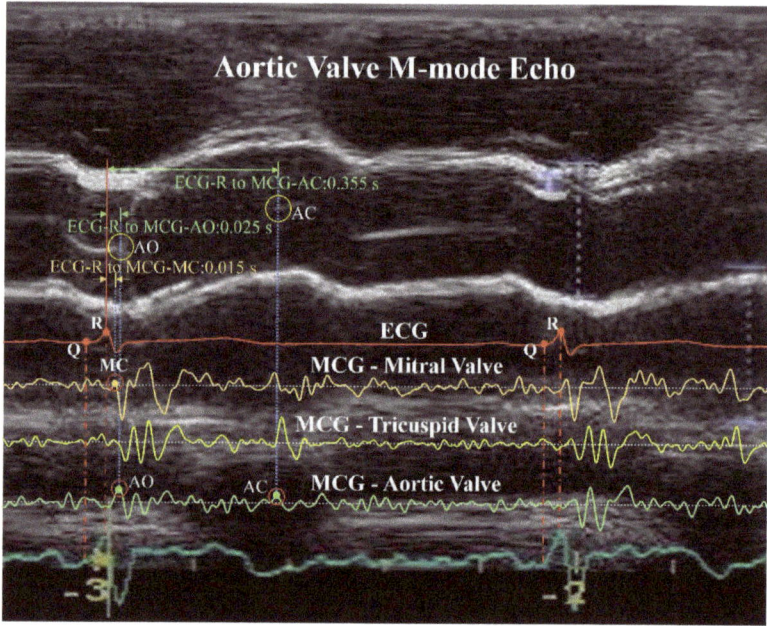

Figure 11. Confirmation of identified ECG-R, ECG-Q, MCG-MC, MCG-AO, and MCG-AC feature points with an Aortic Valve M-mode echocardiography image.

3.3. Data Analysis for Myo-Cardiac Function Interaction

To verify the correlation between CC and LVEF as proposed in Ref. [9], a study which was reviewed and approved by the institutional review board (IRB) of the Chang Gung Memorial Hospital, Taiwan R.O.C., was conducted. Twenty-five HF patients and 15 healthy subjects were enrolled in this study. Each subject wore the smart clothes for 30 min in a supine position and data were collected. These forty subjects were classified into four groups according to their LVEF, as suggested in Ref. [9], and the results are listed in Table 1. The bar charts of PEP, LVET, and PEP/LVET averages of the subjects in these four groups are plotted in Figure 12a and the linear regression of PEP/LVET, i.e., CC, v.s. LVEF, is plotted in Figure 12b. It is very clear that PEP/LVET is inversely proportional to the LVEF with a correlation coefficient of −0.73 and the p value is less than 0.001.

Table 1. Statistics of four groups of subjects and their PEP, LVET, PEP/LVET, and LVEF values.

Groups (LVEF Range)	PEP (ms)	LVET (ms)	PEP/LVET	LVEF (%)
GP1 (<20%)	145.66 ± 11.91	250.83 ± 45.32	0.59 ± 0.10	15.07 ± 4.02
GP2 (21% < LVEF < 30%)	117.76 ± 37.40	251.64 ± 27.42	0.48 ± 0.18	24.91 ± 3.02
GP3 (31% < LVEF < 40%)	93.87 ± 27.84	285.42 ± 51.36	0.33 ± 0.09	34.26 ± 2.47
GP4 (>41%)	73.3 ± 13.47	306.81 ± 43.44	0.24 ± 0.05	59.57 ± 7.58

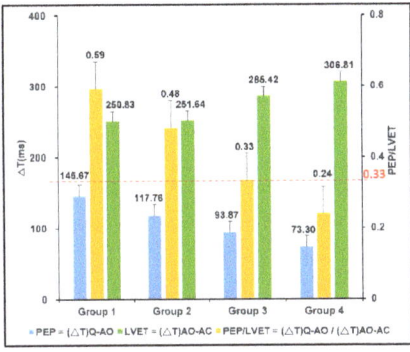
(a) Bar charts of PEP, LVET and PEP/LVET in different groups of subjects

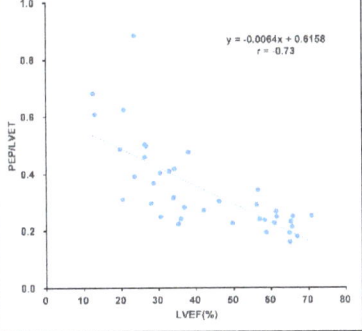
(b) Linear regression of PEP/LVET v.s. LVEF and its correlation coefficient

Figure 12. Analysis of data from multi-channel MCGs/ECG smart monitoring clothes and the myo-cardiac function interpretation. (a) Bar chart comparison in different groups of subjects; (b) linear regression of PEP/LVET, i.e., CC, v.s. LVEF.

By conducting a regression analysis of the tested data, the LVEF value can be derived from the linear equation, as in Equation (2), with the CC value found and calculated from the multi-channel MCGs/ECG smart monitoring clothes.

$$\text{PEP/LVET} = -0.0064 * \text{LVEF} + 0.6158, \text{ and hence,} \\ \text{LVEF} = -156.25 * \text{CC} + 96.219 \qquad (2)$$

According to the grouping of tested subjects shown in Table 1, the subjects in GP1-3 were HF patients, and for the CC value, a threshold value of 0.33 from the statistical analysis using receiver operating characteristic (ROC) curve, as shown by the red-dotted line in Figure 12a, could be set for justification of whether the subject is a HF patient or not. To further analyze the accuracy of the prediction of HF patients according to this threshold, FPs and CTIs from 50 heart beat cycles for HF patients and normal subjects were randomly retrieved from the data for blind testing. The outcomes of the prediction using that threshold are summarized in Table 2. With this analysis, the accuracy rate is 96%, and the positive predictivity rate is 94%, and a sensitivity of 98% and specificity of 94% are achieved. Among this testing, the true positive rate is 98%, false positive rate is 6%, true negative rate is 94%, and false negative rate is only 2%.

Table 2. Accuracy analysis for the prediction of HF patients.

	Predicted Abnormal	Predicted Normal	Total
Actual Abnormal	49	1	50
Actual Normal	3	47	50
Total	52	48	100

3.4. Analysis of the Extended TAM for the Smart Clothes Among Patients with CVD

To analyze the measurement model, Cronbach's alpha and an item-total correlation were first obtained to measure the reliability of the individual items with respect to the corresponding construct variable. The recommended value for Cronbach's alpha should be higher than 0.7, and the value for the item-total correlation is recommended to be higher than 0.3. The composite reliability was also measured, which tests the internal consistency within a construct. The value for composite reliability should be higher than 0.7. The Cronbach's alpha value for all constructs, except for the perceived ease of use, surpassed the recommended value of 0.7. The Cronbach's alpha for PEOU was 0.528, which is lower than 0.7. For the results of the item-total correlation, nearly all of the items had values greater than 0.3, although PEOU3 showed a value of 0.142, which is smaller than 0.3. The results for composite reliability showed that all constructs had values greater than 0.7, indicating a good internal consistency. Factor loading, which reflects how much a factor explains a variable, was also obtained by conducting a confirmatory factor analysis. Because we only included 48 participants in this study, which is considered to be a small sample size, MacCallum et al. [38] advocated that all items in a factor model should have communalities greater than 0.60 to justify the performance of a factor analysis with small sample sizes. The results showed that only PEOU1 had a factor loading of 0.418, while the other items all surpassed the value of 0.6. In terms of validity measures, we tested the construct validity, which included the convergent validity and the discriminant validity. Convergent validity refers to the degree of convergence of the items in the questionnaire in terms of one variable. For convergent validity to be statistically significant, the composite reliability should be higher than the recommended value of 0.7, and the average variance extracted (AVE) of construct variables should be higher than 0.5. Composite reliability has been examined previously, and the results for the AVE showed that only PEOU was smaller than 0.5, while the other constructs had values higher than 0.5. On the other hand, discriminant validity examines the degree to which two constructs that are supposed to be unrelated are distinguishable. To measure discriminant validity, the square root of the AVE of the measured construct should be larger than the correlation coefficient of the other dimensions. The square root of the average change of the construct was larger than the correlation coefficients of the other constructs. In addition to technology anxiety, the other constructs all showed mean values higher than 3. For technology anxiety, the mean value was 2.49, indicating that the participants did not have strong technology anxiety toward smart clothes. In short, the measurement model showed strong results in terms of both reliability and validity. However, perceived ease of use did not meet some of the recommended values in the measurement model.

We conducted a path analysis to test the 10 research hypotheses among eight constructs. The path coefficients and the statistical measurements are shown in Table 3. Eight out of ten hypotheses showed significant results, and two hypotheses were invalid. Hypothesis 1 hypothesized that by using a wearable cardiac health monitoring system, patients with CVD would feel that technology anxiety and perceived usefulness were negatively correlated. The path analysis results showed that $\gamma 1 = -0.39$ ($t = -3.80$, $p < 0.001$). However, the mean value of technology anxiety showed that participants did not perceive the wearable system as anxiety-inducing. Therefore, Hypothesis 1 was not supported. Hypothesis 2 hypothesized that by using a wearable cardiac health monitoring system, patients with CVD would feel that perceived ubiquity and perceived usefulness were positively correlated. The path analysis results showed that $\gamma 2 = 0.62$ ($t = 6.07$, $p < 0.001$). Therefore, Hypothesis 2 was supported. Hypothesis 3 hypothesized that by using a wearable cardiac health monitoring system, patients with CVD would feel that perceived ubiquity and perceived ease of use were positively correlated. The path analysis results showed that $\gamma 3 = 0.54$ ($t = 4.22$, $p < 0.001$). Therefore, Hypothesis 3 was supported. Hypothesis 4 hypothesized that by using a wearable cardiac health monitoring system, patients with CVD would feel that perceived ubiquity and resistance to change were negatively correlated. The path analysis results showed that $\gamma 4 = -0.39$ ($t = -2.86$, $p < 0.01$). Therefore, Hypothesis 4 was supported. Hypothesis 5 hypothesized that by using a wearable cardiac health monitoring system, patients with CVD would feel that perceived ubiquity and attitude were positively correlated. The path analysis results showed that $\gamma 5 = 0.28$ ($t = 2.13$, $p < 0.05$). Therefore, Hypothesis 5 was supported. Hypothesis 6 hypothesized that by using a wearable cardiac health monitoring system, patients with CVD would feel that resistance to change and behavioral intention were negatively correlated. The path analysis results showed that $\gamma 6 = -0.39$ ($t = -3.35$, $p < 0.01$). Therefore, Hypothesis 6 was supported. Hypothesis 7 hypothesized that by using a wearable cardiac health monitoring system, patients with CVD would feel that benefit and behavioral intention were positively correlated. The path analysis results showed that $\gamma 7 = 0.36$ ($t = 2.99$, $p < 0.01$). Therefore, Hypothesis 7 was supported. Hypothesis 8 hypothesized that by using a wearable cardiac health monitoring system, patients with CVD would feel that perceived usefulness and attitude were positively correlated. The path analysis results showed that $\gamma 8 = 0.49$ ($t = 3.65$, $p < 0.05$). Therefore, Hypothesis 8 was supported. Hypothesis 9 hypothesized that by using a wearable cardiac health monitoring system, patients with CVD would feel that perceived ease of use and behavioral intention were positively correlated. The path analysis results showed that $\gamma 9 = -0.20$ ($t = -1.69$, $p > 0.05$). Therefore, Hypothesis 9 was not supported. Hypothesis 10 hypothesized that by using a wearable cardiac health monitoring system, patients with CVD would feel that attitude and behavioral intention were positively correlated. The path analysis results showed that $\gamma 10 = -0.22$ ($t = 1.73$, $p > 0.05$). Therefore, Hypothesis 10 was not supported. Overall, seven hypotheses were supported, and three were invalid. The fit indices of the path analysis are listed in Table 4. All of the fit indices met the recommended values, indicating that the results of the path analysis are appropriate.

Table 3. Summary of the hypothesis results.

	IV	→	DV	Standardized Regression Coefficient	T-Value	p-Value	Support
Hypothesis 1	TA	→	PU	−0.39	−3.80	***	No
Hypothesis 2	PB	→	PU	0.62	6.07	***	Yes
Hypothesis 3	PB	→	PEOU	0.54	4.22	***	Yes
Hypothesis 4	PB	→	RC	−0.39	−2.86	**	Yes
Hypothesis 5	PB	→	AT	0.28	2.13	*	Yes
Hypothesis 6	RC	→	BI	−0.39	−3.35	**	Yes
Hypothesis 7	BF	→	BI	0.36	2.99	**	Yes
Hypothesis 8	PU	→	AT	0.49	3.65	*	Yes
Hypothesis 9	PEOU	→	BI	−0.20	−1.69		No
Hypothesis 10	AT	→	BI	0.22	1.73		No

*** $p < 0.001$, ** $p < 0.01$, * $p < 0.05$.

Table 4. Fit indices for the path analysis.

Measures	Recommended Criteria	Path Analysis
χ^2/df	<3.0	0.7275
GFI	>0.8	0.94
AGFI	>0.8	0.86
NFI	>0.9	0.94
NNFI	>0.9	1.04
CFI	>0.9	1.00
RMSEA	<0.08	0.000

4. Conclusions

In this study, the realization of a wearable cardiac health monitoring and myo-cardiac function interpretation smart clothes with multi-channel MCGs and ECG measurement is presented. To acquire the digital data from multiple accelerometers and to convert the analog data of the ECG signal simultaneously, as well as to provide the capability of wireless data transmission, a platform, i.e., CHAMP, has been designed and implemented. It provides the mobility and capability for real-time data analysis and disease detections, so it is perfectly suitable to integrate the platform into smart clothes.

This work translated the concept of a multi-channel MCG system into a wearable smart clothes for cardiac health monitoring and myo-cardiac function interpretation system, which then can be applied for home-based or clinical usages to detect certain cardiovascular diseases, such as HFs. After the smart clothes delivered continuous real-time multi-channel MCGs/ECG data, data analysis for myo-cardiac function interpretation of this wearable system was validated. A mobile application software has been developed to receive the data from the smart clothes, identify feature points, and calculate CTIs, CC, and LVEF. Also, the relationship between CC and LVEF has been verified in this study. In the system, with the data received from the smart clothes, CC values are calculated and LVEF values are derived from the analyzed data. A highly accurate rate of prediction for HF patients with this system could be achieved. Hence, the developed smart clothes with multi-channel MCGs and ECG for cardiac health monitoring can be applied for long-term and continuous monitoring of myo-cardiac functions.

The usability study of the wearable system is also verified. We extended the technology acceptance model and investigated perceptions of the developed wearable MCG-based cardiac health monitoring system among potential users with CVD. The results of TAM analysis indicated that perceived ubiquity is a crucial construct that can affect participants' perception of intention to use a wearable cardiac sensing technology, such as smart clothes. The perceived benefit of the newly designed wearable system increases participants' willingness to adopt the smart technology. Furthermore, the perceived usefulness of the wearable MCG-based cardiac health monitoring system showed a positive correlation with the participants' attitude toward it. The results of our hypothesized model contribute to the original TAM and the existing research on understanding users' perceptions of wearable sensing technologies in general. In the future, several features of the system can be extended, for example, the application of the system for the prediction of other cardiovascular diseases, such as valvular heart diseases (VHDs), and also the risk assessment of certain heart diseases with expert systems (or machine learning algorithm), cloud computing, and trend analysis for early prediction, etc. Finally, this system can be applied to detect cardiovascular diseases, in particular HF and VHD, for patients and individual users who are self-conscious about their heart health.

In short, unique smart clothes for cardiac health monitoring system is designed and implemented. This is the first wearable system incorporated with multi-channel MCGs and ECG measurement technology which is capable of the long-term and continuous monitoring of cardiac health of the subjects in their daily life. In this work, a mobile application which receives data from the smart clothes, identifies the feature points automatically, and calculates CTIs for deriving the cardiac health-related indices, such as CC and LVEF, in real-time has also been developed. It can help to predict the abnormality of cardiac functions, such as the HFs, for the subjects wearing the clothes, with an accuracy rate of up to 96%. Moreover, the usability study of the smart clothes with proposed extended TAM indicates that people, especially CVD patients, show a positive attitude toward using this wearable MCG-based cardiac health monitoring and early warning system.

Supplementary Materials: The following are available online at http://www.mdpi.com/1424-8220/18/10/3538/s1.

Author Contributions: Conceptualization, W.-Y.L. and M.-Y.L.; Hardware Design, H.-L.K. and W.-C.C.; Software, H.-L.K.; Validation, W.-C.C.; Clinic Analysis, P.-C.C. and M.-Y.L.; Usability Study, T.-H.T.; Writing-Original Draft Preparation, W.-Y.L. and T.-H.T.; Writing-Review & Editing, P.-C.C. and M.-Y.L.; Supervision, M.-Y.L.; Project Administration, W.-Y.L. and M.-Y.L.; Funding Acquisition, M.-Y.L.

Funding: This research was funded by the Ministry of Science and Technology, Taiwan, R.O.C. under Grant No. MOST 104-2221-E-182-013, MOST 105-2627-E-182-001, MOST 106-2627-E-182-001, and MOST 106-2221-E-182-034, as well as CGU fund BMRPC50 and BMRP138. The costs to publish in open access will be covered by Grant MOST 106-2627-E-182-001. The funder had no role in study design, data collection and analysis, decision to publish, or preparation of the manuscript.

Acknowledgments: The authors thank the Biomedical Engineering Research Center (BMERC) of Chang Gung University for providing the resources required for this work. Moreover, without the support of textile technologies from the AiQ, the proposed smart clothes would not have been possible.

Conflicts of Interest: The authors declare no conflict of interest.

References

1. Sarlabous, L.; Torres, A.; Fiz, J.A.; Jane, R. Evidence towards improved estimation of respiratory muscle effort from diaphragm mechanomyographic signals with cardiac vibration interference using sample entropy with fixed tolerance values. *PLoS ONE* **2014**, *9*, e88902. [CrossRef] [PubMed]
2. Salerno, D.M.; Zanetti, J.M.; Green, L.A.; Mooney, M.R.; Madison, J.D.; Van Tassel, R.A. Seismocardiographic changes associated with obstruction of coronary blood flow during balloon angioplasty. *Am. J. Cardiol.* **1991**, *68*, 201–207. [CrossRef]
3. Salerno, D.M.; Zanetti, J. Seismocardiography for monitoring changes in left ventricular function during ischemia. *Chest* **1991**, *100*, 991–993. [CrossRef] [PubMed]
4. Marcus, F.I.; Sorrell, V.; Zanetti, J.; Bosnos, M.; Baweja, G.; Perlick, D.; Ott, P.; Indik, J.; He, D.S.; Gear, K. Accelerometer-derived time intervals during various pacing modes in patients with biventricular pacemakers: Comparison with normal. *Pac. Clin. Electrophysiol.* **2007**, *30*, 1476–1481. [CrossRef] [PubMed]
5. Crow, R.S.; Hannan, P.; Jacobs, D.; Hedquist, L.; Salerno, D.M. Relationship between seismocardiogram and echocardiogram for events in the cardiac cycle. *Am. J. Noninvasive Cardiol.* **1994**, *8*, 39–46. [CrossRef]
6. Stefanadis, C.I. Bioelectronics: The way to discover the world of arrhythmias. *Hellenic J. Cardiol.* **2014**, *55*, 267–268. [PubMed]
7. Zanetti, J.M.; Tavakolian, K. Seismocardiography: Past, present and future. In Proceedings of the Annual International Conference of the IEEE Engineering in Medicine and Biology Society, Osaka, Japan, 3–7 July 2013; pp. 7004–7007.
8. Lin, W.-Y.; Chou, W.-C.; Chang, P.C.; Chou, C.-C.; Wen, M.-S.; Ho, M.-Y.; Lee, W.-C.; Hsieh, M.-J.; Lin, C.-C.; Tsai, T.-H.; et al. Identification of Location Specific Feature Points in a Cardiac Cycle Using a Novel Seismocardiogram Spectrum System. *IEEE J. Biomed. Health Inform.* **2018**, *22*, 442–449. [CrossRef] [PubMed]
9. Reant, P.; Dijos, M.; Donal, E.; Mignot, A.; Ritter, P.; Bordachar, P.; Santos, P.D.; Leclercq, C.; Roudaut, R.; Habib, G.; et al. Systolic time intervals as simple echocardiographic parameters of left ventricular systolic performance: Correlation with ejection fraction and longitudinal two-dimensional strain. *Eur. J. Echocardiogr.* **2010**, *11*, 834–844. [CrossRef] [PubMed]
10. Sahoo, P.K.; Thakkar, H.K.; Lin, W.-Y.; Chang, P.-C.; Lee, M.-Y. On the Design of an Efficient Cardiac Health Monitoring System Through Combined Analysis of ECG and SCG signals. *Sensors* **2018**, *18*, 379. [CrossRef] [PubMed]
11. Mundt, C.W.; Montgomery, K.N.; Udoh, U.E.; Barker, V.N.; Thonier, G.C.; Tellier, A.M.; Ricks, R.D.; Darling, R.B.; Cagle, Y.D.; Cabrol, N.A.; et al. A multiparameter wearable physiologic monitoring system for space and terrestrial applications. *IEEE Trans. Inf. Technol. Biomed.* **2005**, *9*, 382–391. [CrossRef] [PubMed]
12. Wolgast, G.; Helander, J.; Ehrenborg, C.; Israelsson, A.; Johansson, E.; Manefjord, H. Wireless body area network for heart attack detection [Education Corner]. *IEEE Antennas Propag. Mag.* **2016**, *58*, 84–92. [CrossRef]
13. Tanantong, T.; Nantajeewarawat, E.; Thiemjarus, S. False alarm reduction in BSN-based cardiac monitoring using signal quality and activity type information. *Sensors* **2015**, *15*, 3952–3974. [CrossRef] [PubMed]
14. Von Rosenberg, W.; Chanwimalueang, T.; Goverdovsky, V.; Looney, D.; Sharp, D.; Mandic, D.P. Smart helmet: Wearable multichannel ECG and EEG. *IEEE J. Transl. Eng. Health Med.* **2016**, *4*, 2700111. [CrossRef] [PubMed]
15. Heart Force Medical Inc. Cardio Pro. Available online: http://www.heartforce.com/cardio-pro.html (accessed on 10 November 2017).

16. Di Rienzo, M.; Vaini, E.; Castiglioni, P.; Merati, G.; Meriggi, P.; Parati, G.; Faini, A.; Rizzo, F. Wearable seismocardiography: Towards a beat-by-beat assessment of cardiac mechanics in ambulant subjects. *Auton. Neurosci. Basic Clin.* **2013**, *178*, 50–59. [CrossRef] [PubMed]
17. Inan, O.T.; Migeotte, P.F.; Park, K.S.; Etemadi, M.; Tavakolian, K.; Casanella, R.; Zanetti, J.; Tank, J.; Funtova, I.; Prisk, G.K.; et al. Ballistocardiography and Seismocardiography: A Review of Recent Advances. *IEEE J. Biomed. Health Inform.* **2015**, *19*, 1414–1427. [CrossRef] [PubMed]
18. Inan, O.T.; Etemadi, M.; Paloma, A.; Giovangrandi, L.; Kovacs, G.T.A. Non-invasive cardiac output trending during exercise recovery on a bathroom-scale-based ballistocardiograph. *Physiol. Meas.* **2009**, *30*, 261. [CrossRef] [PubMed]
19. Ashouri, H.; Orlandic, L.; Inan, O.T. Unobtrusive Estimation of Cardiac Contractility and Stroke Volume Changes Using Ballistocardiogram Measurements on a High Bandwidth Force Plate. *Sensors* **2016**, *16*, 787. [CrossRef] [PubMed]
20. Starr, I.; Rawson, A.; Schroeder, H.; Joseph, N. Studies on the estimation of cardiac output in man, and of abnormalities in cardiac function, from the heart's recoil and the blood's impacts; the ballistocardiogram. *Am. J. Physiol. Legacy Content* **1939**, *127*, 1–28. [CrossRef]
21. Krug, J.W.; Lusebrink, F.; Speck, O.; Rose, G. Optical Ballistocardiography for gating and patient monitoring during MRI: An initial study. In Proceedings of the Computing in Cardiology 2014, Cambridge, MA, USA, 7–10 September 2014.
22. Shao, D.; Tsow, F.; Liu, C.; Yang, Y.; Tao, N. Simultaneous Monitoring of Ballistocardiogram and Phitiplethysmogram Using a Camera. *IEEE Trans. Biol. Med. Eng.* **2017**, *64*, 1003–1010. [CrossRef] [PubMed]
23. He, D.D.; Winokur, E.S.; Sodini, C.G. An Ear-Worn Vital Signs Monitor. *IEEE Trans. Biol. Med. Eng.* **2015**, *62*, 2547–2552. [CrossRef] [PubMed]
24. Wiens, A.D.; Etemadi, M.; Roy, S.; Klein, L.; Inan, O.T. Towards Continuous, Non-Invasive Assessment of Ventricular Function and Hemodynamics: Wearable Ballistocardiography. *IEEE J. Biomed. Health Inform.* **2015**, *19*, 1435–1442. [CrossRef] [PubMed]
25. Wiens, A.; Etemadi, M.; Klein, L.; Roy, S.; Inan, O.T. Wearable Ballistocardiography: Preliminary Methods for Mapping Surface Vibration Measurements to Whole Body Forces. In Proceedings of the 36th Annual International Conference of the IEEE Engineering in Medicine and Biology Society (EMBC 2014), Chicago, IL, USA, 26–30 August 2014; pp. 5172–5175.
26. Davis, F.D. Perceived usefulness, perceived ease of use, and user acceptance of information technology. *MIS Q.* **1989**, *13*, 319–340. [CrossRef]
27. Chuah, S.H.W.; Rauschnabel, P.A.; Krey, N.; Nguyen, B.; Ramayah, T.; Lade, S. Wearable technologies: The role of usefulness and visibility in smartwatch adoption. *Comput. Hum. Behav.* **2016**, *65*, 276–284. [CrossRef]
28. Kim, K.J.; Shin, D.H. An acceptance model for smart watches: Implications for the adoption of future wearable technology. *Internet Res.* **2015**, *25*, 527–541. [CrossRef]
29. Lunney, A.; Cunningham, N.R.; Eastin, M.S. Wearable fitness technology: A structural investigation into acceptance and perceived fitness outcomes. *Comput. Hum. Behav.* **2016**, *65*, 114–120. [CrossRef]
30. Lin, W.Y.; Chou, W.-C.; Tsai, T.-H.; Lin, C.-C.; Lee, M.-Y. Development of a Wearable Instrumented Vest for Posture Monitoring and System Usability Verification based on the Technology Acceptance Model. *Sensors* **2016**, *16*, 2172. [CrossRef] [PubMed]
31. Guo, X.; Sun, Y.; Wang, N.; Peng, Z.; Yan, Z. The dark side of elderly acceptance of preventive mobile health services in China. *Electron. Mark.* **2013**, *23*, 49–61. [CrossRef]
32. Hsiao, C.-H.; Tang, K.-Y. Examining a model of mobile healthcare technology acceptance by the elderly in Taiwan. *J. Glob. Inf. Technol. Manag.* **2015**, *18*, 292–311. [CrossRef]
33. Demiris, G.; Speedie, S.; Finkelstein, S. A questionnaire for the assessment of patients' impressions of the risks and benefits of home telecare. *J. Telemed. Telecare* **2000**, *6*, 278–284. [CrossRef] [PubMed]
34. Fishbein, M.; Ajzen, I. *Belief, Attitude, Intention, and Behavior: An Introduction to Theory and Research*; Addison-Wesley: Reading, MA, USA, 1977.
35. Ajzen, I. The theory of planned behavior. *Organ. Behave. Hum. Decis. Process.* **1991**, *50*, 179–211. [CrossRef]
36. Venkatesh, V.; Morris, M.G.; Davis, G.B.; Davis, F.D. User acceptance of information technology: Toward a unified view. *MIS Q.* **2003**, *27*, 425–478. [CrossRef]

37. So, H.H.; Chan, K.L. Development of QRS Detection Method for Real-Time Ambulatory Cardiac Monitor. In Proceedings of the 19th International Conference on IEEE/EMBS, Chicago, IL, USA, 30 October–2 November 1997; pp. 289–292.
38. MacCallum, R.C.; Widaman, K.F.; Preacher, K.J.; Hong, S. Sample size in factor analysis: The role of model error. *Multivar. Behav. Res.* **2001**, *36*, 611–637. [CrossRef] [PubMed]

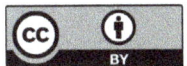

© 2018 by the authors. Licensee MDPI, Basel, Switzerland. This article is an open access article distributed under the terms and conditions of the Creative Commons Attribution (CC BY) license (http://creativecommons.org/licenses/by/4.0/).

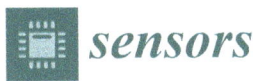

Article

LSTM-Guided Coaching Assistant for Table Tennis Practice

Se-Min Lim [1], Hyeong-Cheol Oh [1,*], Jaein Kim [2], Juwon Lee [3] and Jooyoung Park [3,*]

1. Department of Electronic and Information Engineering, Korea University, 2511 Sejong-ro, Sejong-City 30016, Korea; jaewoong819@korea.ac.kr
2. Department of Mathematics, Korea University, 145 Anam-ro, Anamdong 5-ga, Seoul 02841, Korea; kkjin85@korea.ac.kr
3. Department of Control and Instrumentation Engineering, Korea University, 2511 Sejong-ro, Sejong-City 30016, Korea; saero94j@korea.ac.kr
* Correspondence: ohyeong@korea.ac.kr (H.-C.O.); parkj@korea.ac.kr (J.P.); Tel.: +82-10-6235-1425 (H.-C.O.); +82-10-9003-1810 (J.P.)

Received: 28 October 2018; Accepted: 21 November 2018; Published: 23 November 2018

Abstract: Recently, wearable devices have become a prominent health care application domain by incorporating a growing number of sensors and adopting smart machine learning technologies. One closely related topic is the strategy of combining the wearable device technology with skill assessment, which can be used in wearable device apps for coaching and/or personal training. Particularly pertinent to skill assessment based on high-dimensional time series data from wearable sensors is classifying whether a player is an expert or a beginner, which skills the player is exercising, and extracting some low-dimensional representations useful for coaching. In this paper, we present a deep learning-based coaching assistant method, which can provide useful information in supporting table tennis practice. Our method uses a combination of LSTM (Long short-term memory) with a deep state space model and probabilistic inference. More precisely, we use the expressive power of LSTM when handling high-dimensional time series data, and state space model and probabilistic inference to extract low-dimensional latent representations useful for coaching. Experimental results show that our method can yield promising results for characterizing high-dimensional time series patterns and for providing useful information when working with wearable IMU (Inertial measurement unit) sensors for table tennis coaching.

Keywords: wearable sensors; skill assessment; deep learning; LSTM; state space model; probabilistic inference; latent features

1. Introduction

Wearable technology has drawn intensive interest in the area of human activity recognition (HAR) [1–3]. Using wearable technology, an HAR system can directly receive human activity information from sensors on a human body. The HAR has a variety of application domains including health care and skill assessment. In the domain of health care, problems such as detecting falls while walking [1] have been investigated. In the closely related domain of skill assessment, applications such as personal trainers for coaching fitness or rehabilitation [2,4] have been studied.

Wearable technology can also be useful for people in practicing their sports skills. For example, people may not know enough about the correct or effective exercises in table tennis but want to copy a teacher's skill, in which case an assistant system using wearable sensors can be of great help. This paper uses table tennis as one representative example for sports exercise assistance.

Many prior studies in HAR based on wearable technology use smartphones as data collecting devices. Even though a smartphone is very useful as an everyday monitoring device, its size is too large for attaching to the precise positions at specific points on the human body. Thus, this paper uses IMU sensors attached to the hand and arm of table tennis players. Using the information collected by the IMU sensors, this paper presents a deep learning-based assistant system that can identify which skill and type of player, among those stored in the system, are closest to the skill that the player is exercising and can provide visual information useful for coaching.

Deep learning technology is a promising solution to realizing HAR systems. Convolutional neural networks (CNNs) were used for HAR in [5,6] with a single sensor, and in [7] with multiple sensors. However, the limits on local connectivity in a CNN prevent the network from effectively dealing with lags of unknown duration between certain points in the time series data. Thus, to handle temporal dynamics in an activity more effectively, long short-term memory (LSTM) recurrent neural networks (RNNs) [8] were proposed for adoption in HAR in [3]. In [3], the authors showed that LSTM RNNs worked better than CNNs as well as conventional machine learning technologies, such as random forest and least-square support vector machines, for HAR problems in everyday life, including walking, running, jumping, sitting, sleeping, and so forth. We chose the LSTM RNN because the time and duration of the activities may vary depending on the player and the skill that the player hits. We found that the inference accuracy of a unidirectional regular RNN is significantly (more than 10 %) lower than that of the LSTM RNN for the cases considered in this paper. The number of levels of the network was also determined experimentally. This paper proposes a deep learning-based coaching assistant, which uses a combination of LSTM RNNs along with a deep state space model and probabilistic inference, that can support table tennis practice.

The assistant uses expressive power of LSTM RNNs for efficiently handling high-dimensional sensor data, and resorts to a deep state space model along with probabilistic inference to extract low-dimensional latent representations useful for coaching. For the LSTM RNN component, the unidirectional and bidirectional types [9,10] are both considered for the network. From experiments, we observe that the LSTM RNNs work satisfactorily for the task of classifying high-dimensional sensor data, with and without pruning, and for obtaining meaningful embedding features. We then augment the LSTM RNN network to find latent representations capable of providing assistive coaching information. The augmented network uses a deep state space model for a generative model that can explain the observations with the state and output equations. Also, a probabilistic inference method based on variational inference [11] is used to obtain posterior latent trajectories that can identify the type of user such as a coach or a beginner, and table tennis skills such as forehand stroke, forehand drive, forehand cut, backhand drive, and backhand short. Experimental results show that our method can yield promising results for characterizing high-dimensional time series patterns and providing useful information when working with the wearable IMU sensors for table tennis coaching.

The remainder of this paper is organized as follows. In Section 2, after providing preliminary background on LSTM RNN, we present the state-space-model-based solutions for the problem of characterizing dynamic sequence patterns and providing coaching information while practicing table tennis skills. In Section 3, the effectiveness of the proposed solutions is illustrated by experiments. Finally, in Section 4, the usefulness of the proposed method is discussed, and concluding remarks are provided along with topics for future studies.

2. Methods

The purpose of this paper is to present a deep learning-based coaching assistant method, which can provide useful information in supporting table tennis practice. Our strategy uses a combination of LSTM with a deep state space model and probabilistic inference. More precisely, we use the expressive power of LSTM when handling high-dimensional time series data, and state space model and probabilistic inference to extract low-dimensional latent representations useful for coaching. Detailed steps of the established strategy will be summarized in a table.

2.1. Data Collection

Figure 1 shows the data collection unit set up to develop and evaluate the proposed system. Three IMU sensor modules (MPU-9150s) were attached to the right hand and arm of a player as shown in the figure. The sensors were wired and sent data to a Raspberry Pi 3 model B, which in turn sent data to a notebook through a Bluetooth connection. Using the data collection unit, we collected the sensor data from two table tennis players on five table tennis skills: Forehand stroke, backhand drive, backhand short, forehand cut, forehand drive (Figure 2). Each player struck the ball with each motion skill ten times: seven times for training and three times for testing. Each stroke was sampled at 27 time points. In all our experiments, the observation sequences were obtained from two persons each for 5.4 s with the frequency of 5 Hz. The appropriate size of signal windowing was empirically found. Tri-axial accelerometer data and tri-axial gyro data were collected from each of the three sensor modules. Thus, 2 persons × 5 skills × 7 hits × 3 axes × 2 sensors × 3 modules = 1260 data sequences (27 values per sequence) were used to train the neural networks.

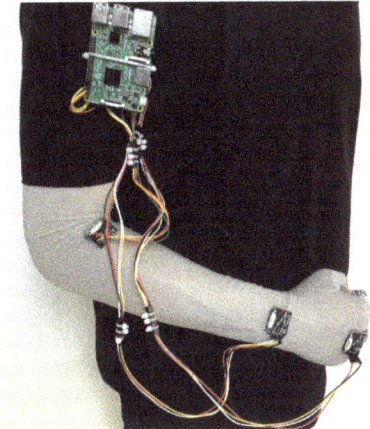

Figure 1. Data collection unit set up.

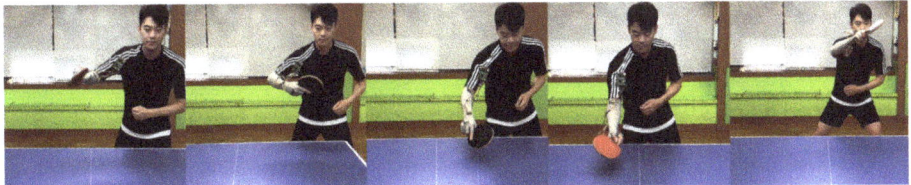

Figure 2. Table tennis motion skills considered in this paper (from left to right): Forehand stroke, backhand drive, backhand short, forehand cut, forehand drive.

2.2. Unidirectional LSTM RNN

The proposed method relies on the expressive power of LSTM RNNs for efficiently handling high-dimensional sensor data. For the LSTM RNN [8] component, the unidirectional and bidirectional types [9,10] are both considered for the network. A cell of an LSTM RNN is modeled as a memory cell. Figure 3 depicts the structure of an LSTM RNN cell, which operates as follows [3]:

$$f_t^{d,l} = \phi_f(W_{xf}^{d,l}, x_t, W_{hf}^{d,l}, h_{t-1}, b_f^{d,l}) \tag{1}$$

$$i_t^{d,l} = \phi_i(W_{xi}^{d,l}, x_t, W_{hi}^{d,l}, h_{t-1}, b_i^{d,l}) \quad (2)$$

$$o_t^{d,l} = \phi_o(W_{xo}^{d,l}, x_t, W_{ho}^{d,l}, h_{t-1}, b_o^{d,l}) \quad (3)$$

$$g_t^{d,l} = \phi_g(W_{xg}^{d,l}, x_t, W_{hg}^{d,l}, h_{t-1}, b_g^{d,l}) \quad (4)$$

$$c_t^{d,l} = f_t^{d,l} \otimes c_{t-1}^{d,l} + g_t^{d,l} \otimes i_t^{d,l} \quad (5)$$

$$h_t^{d,l} = o_t^{d,l} \otimes A(c_t^{d,l}) \quad (6)$$

In Equations (1)–(6), which are defined at time t, d denotes the direction, and l denotes the level of the network where the cell is defined. The operator $\otimes$ denotes the element-wise multiplication operation, while x_t is the input, Ws are the parameter matrices containing the weights of the network connections, and bs are the biases. The functions ϕ_f, ϕ_i, ϕ_o, and ϕ_g are called the *forget gate, input gate, output gate, input modulation gate*, respectively, and defined as follows:

$$\phi_k(W_{xk}, x, W_{hk}, h, b_k) = A(W_{xk}x + W_{hk}h + b_k), \quad (7)$$

where $k = f, i, o,$ or g; and $A(\cdot)$ is an activation function. The *internal state* c_t is used to handle the internal recurrence, while the *hidden state* h_t handles outer recurrences. The block labelled with Δ is a memory element. The current hidden state at time t, h_t, can be considered as the current output.

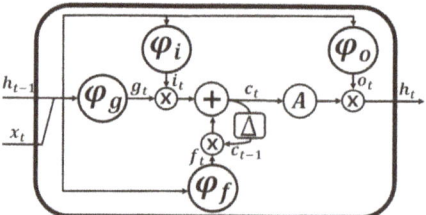

Figure 3. Structure of an LSTM RNN cell.

Unidirectional LSTM RNN [10] is an architecture of LSTM RNN, which connects layers by forward paths only. Thus, d is not defined in Equations (1)–(6). This paper considers a unidirectional LSTM RNN model that consists of two levels ($l = 1, 2$), each of which consists of one LSTM RNN cell. Figure 4 describes the operation performed in the model during three time steps, $t - 1$, t, and $t + 1$.

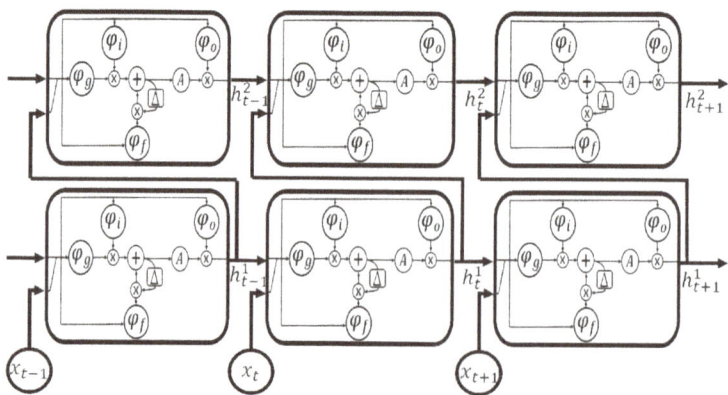

Figure 4. Operation of two-stacked unidirectional LSTM RNN model.

2.3. Bidirectional LSTM RNN

The backward paths are often added to the stacked model in Figure 4, resulting in the bidirectional LSTM RNN. The forward and backward paths are denoted as $d = f$ and $d = b$, respectively, in Equations (1)–(6). Figure 5 describes the operation of the two-stacked bidirectional LSTM RNN considered in this paper, during three time steps, x_{t-1}, x_t, and x_{t+1}. In Figure 5, the cells or levels are denoted as $l = 1$ and $l = 2$. Each block labelled as $LSTM_1$ or $LSTM_2$ represents an LSTM RNN cell, as depicted in Figure 3, that is defined at the level 1 or 2, respectively. At each time step, the model calculates two pairs of hidden states: one for forward paths, h^{f1} and h^{f2}, and the other for backward paths, h^{b1} and h^{b2}.

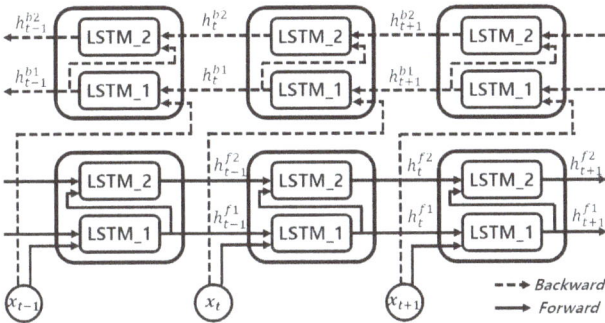

Figure 5. Operation of two-stacked bidirectional LSTM RNN model.

2.4. Pruning Networks

LSTM RNN shows high performance in time series data, but it has large number of learnable parameters due to the four gating functions. This problem of LSTM RNN often leads to over-fitting network and consume large memories [12,13]. The pruning technique tested in this paper begins by creating a pre-trained model, and then removing the non-critical connections by setting a threshold value. A sparse weight matrix is formed due to the weight removed by the desired amount. This matrix is retrained again, and the accuracy is re-measured. Connections that have already been removed are not recreated during the retraining process. Figure 6 shows the pipeline that represents the pruning tested in this paper. Table 1 shows the number of parameters used in the two LSTM RNNs designed as described above.

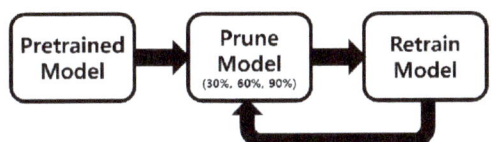

Figure 6. Operation of two-stacked bidirectional & unidirectional LSTM RNN models with pruning.

Table 1. Number of parameters.

The Number of Stacks	Type	Initial Design	After Pruning (30%)	After Pruning (60%)
1	Unidirectional	9.26×10^3	6.48×10^3	3.70×10^3
1	Bidirectional	17.90×10^3	12.53×10^3	7.16×10^3
2	Unidirectional	17.58×10^3	12.30×10^3	7.03×10^3
2	Bidirectional	34.54×10^3	24.18×10^3	13.82×10^3

2.5. Training for Classification

The two models considered for classification were trained in the TensorFlow framework [14], using an Intel i7-7500U CPU and an NVIDIA GeForce 930MX GPU. Among the collected data, 70% were used for training, and 30% were used for testing the models. Supervised learning was used for classification: the dataset and the label corresponding to the dataset were used together in the training phase. The label was represented with one-hot encoding. The weight and bias were randomly initialized and updated to minimize the cost function. The cost function was the mean cross entropy between the ground truth labels and the predicted output labels. The ground truth labels were the true classes. An Adam optimizer was used as the optimization algorithm to minimize the cost function.

Training was performed with data obtained from the accelerometer and gyro sensors after the minmax-scaling by the MinMaxScaler of sklearn [15]. The batch size and the number of hidden units were empirically found after some tuning for better accuracy. Please note that in general, inference using LSTM RNNs is robust to the time variance in time series data [3]. L2 regularization was used to prevent network over-fitting, and the dropout technique was not adopted.

Figure 7 shows the accuracy and cost incurred during the training and testing processes for the bidirectional and unidirectional LSTM RNN models. The accuracy and cost of the testing process are sufficiently close to those of the training process.

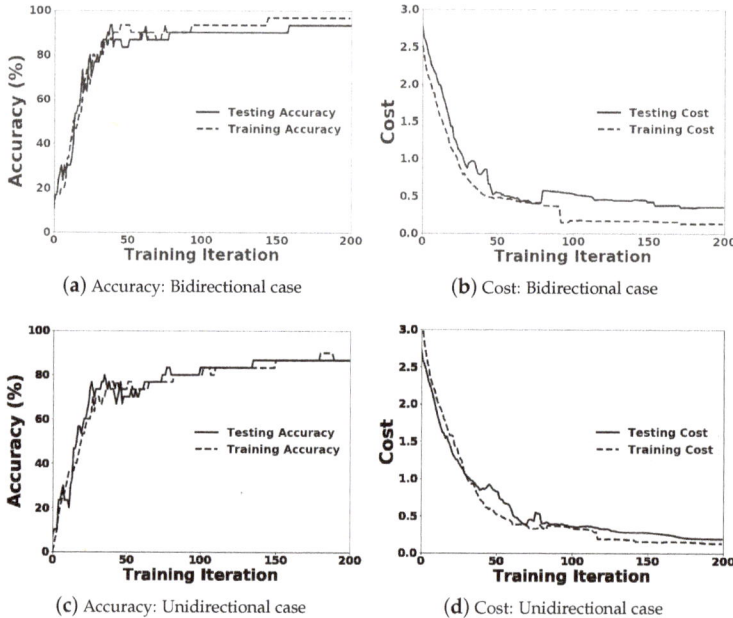

Figure 7. Learning curves on accuracy and cost for the bidirectional and unidirectional LSTM RNN models.

2.6. Network Augmentation for Coaching Information

As mentioned, one of our main goals in this paper is to provide assistive coaching information for table tennis practice. In Sections 2.3–2.5, we focused on how to perform classification tasks over the players (i.e., binary classification of coach vs. beginner) and the motion skills (i.e., multi-class classification of forehand stroke, forehand drive, forehand cut, backhand drive, and backhand short). The resultant LSTM RNN has turned out to be capable of efficiently identifying whether the player is a coach or a beginner and which skills are exercised by the player. In this subsection, we augment the LSTM RNN classifier for the purpose of providing additional coaching information. To fulfill the purpose, the augmented network should satisfy the following criteria:

- The features used for performing the classification tasks should be also used in the augmented network.
- The augmented network should provide some low-dimensional latent representations, which can identify dynamic characteristics of the sensor data and enable visual interactions and/or evaluative feedback between the coach and the beginner concerning skill performance accuracy.
- It should be able to function as a coaching assistant when used in a closed loop with the beginner as the user.

To satisfy the above requirements, we use the embedding of high-dimensional time series of sensor data by the LSTM RNN along with a deep state space model and probabilistic inference (Figure 8). A reasonable framework for modeling the dynamics for the noise-prone high-dimensional data is to use the state equation for low-dimensional latent space along with the output equation. In the framework of the deep probabilistic state space model, one has the following state and output equations:

$$z_{t+1} = f_\theta(z_t), \quad x_t = g_\theta(z_t), \tag{8}$$

where $f_\theta(z_t)$ and $g_\theta(z_t)$ are both random variables indexed by the state vector z_t, and their distributions are implemented by means of deep neural networks with parameters θ. The probabilistic generative model for the state and output Equation (8) can be described as follows:

$$p_\theta(x_{1:T}, z_{1:T}) = p_\theta(x_1|z_1) \prod_{t=2}^{T} p_\theta(x_t|z_t) p_\theta(z_t|z_{t-1}). \tag{9}$$

Based on the variational inference method [11], the true posterior distribution $p(z_{1:T}|x_{1:T})$ can be efficiently approximated by the variational distribution (10):

$$q_\phi(z_t|z_{t-1}, x_{1:T}) = \mathcal{N}(z_{t-1}|\mu(z_{t-1}, x_{t:T}), \Sigma(z_{t-1}, x_{t:T})), \tag{10}$$

where $\mathcal{N}(z|\mu, \Sigma)$ denotes the multivariate Gaussian distribution with the mean vector μ and the covariance matrix Σ. The distributions of q_ϕ are implemented by means of deep neural networks with parameters ϕ. Finally, one can optimize the parameters θ and ϕ by maximizing the variational lower bound $ELBO(\theta, \phi)$ (11) [16,17]:

$$\log p(x_{1:T}) \geq ELBO(\theta, \phi) = E_{z_{1:T} \sim q_\phi(z_{1:T}|x_{1:T})}[\log p_\theta(x_{1:T}|z_{1:T})] - KL(q_\phi(z_{1:T}|x_{1:T}) \parallel p_\theta(z_{1:T})). \tag{11}$$

The above inference and optimization comprise the role of the inference layer of Figure 8.

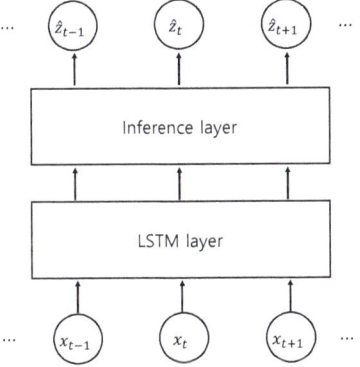

Figure 8. Schematic diagram for the inference network.

3. Experimental Results

In our experiments, we consider two players, one being a table tennis coach and the other being a beginner. For the skills, we consider five motions: forehand stroke, forehand drive, forehand cut, backhand drive, and backhand short. In our continuing study, we will consider more subjects along with a wider class of skills.

In the experiments, we consider a case where the coach and the beginner both use the same table tennis grip. To verify the LSTM RNN models, we use evaluation metrics that are typically used for multi-class classification. In addition, the pruning technique described above is used to remove the weights and then the model is re-evaluated.

3.1. Classifying by LSTM RNNs

Figures 9 and 10 show the confusion matrices of the unidirectional LSTM RNN and bidirectional LSTM RNN for the test set, respectively. Please note that in the confusion matrices in Figures 9 and 10, the sum of the values of a row is the same for every row. Also, Table 2 shows the results of metrics that evaluate the unidirectional LSTM RNN and bidirectional LSTM RNN, respectively. As shown in the figures and tables, all the trained LSTM RNN classifiers yielded satisfactory results for the test dataset.

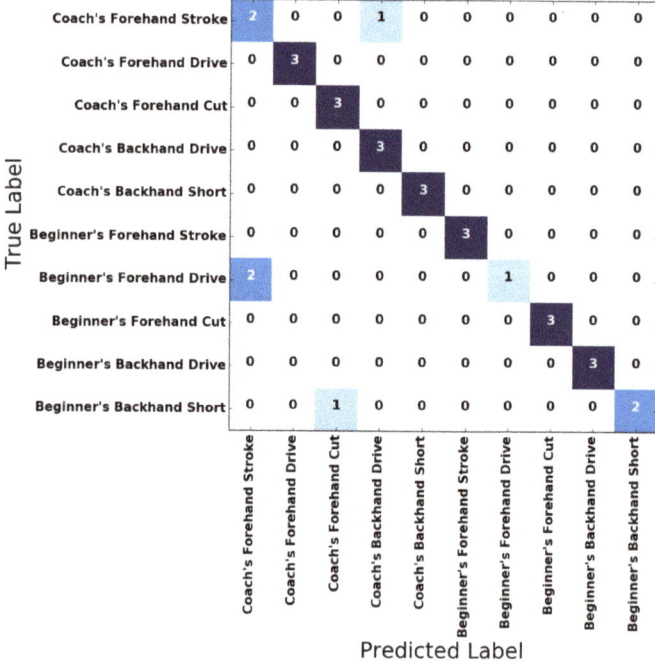

Figure 9. Confusion matrix of the two-stacked unidirectional LSTM RNN model.

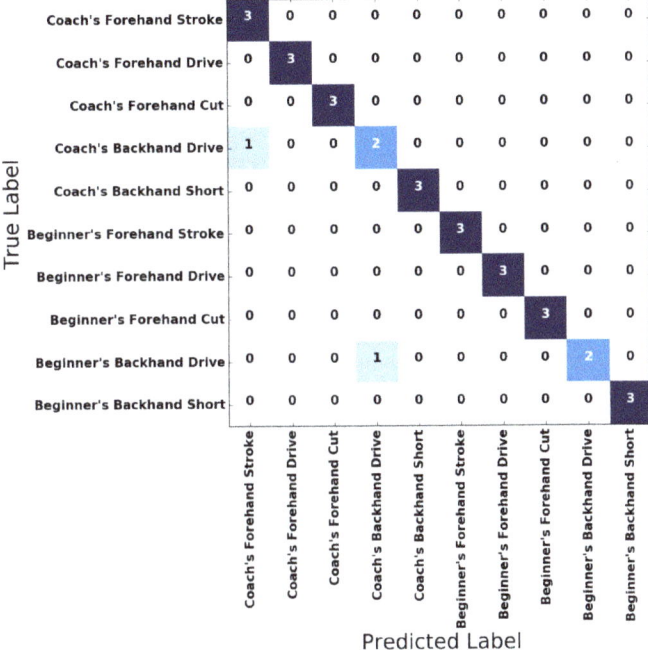

Figure 10. Confusion matrix of the two-stacked bidirectional LSTM RNN model.

Table 2. Classification Performance of the Bidirectional & Unidirectional LSTM RNNs.

Type	Performance
Overall Accuracy (Uni)	86.7%
Average Precision (Uni)	87.5%
Average Recall (Uni)	86.7%
F1 Score (Uni)	86.3%
Overall Accuracy (Bi)	93.3%
Average Precision (Bi)	95.0%
Average Recall (Bi)	93.3%
F1 Score (Bi)	93.1%

3.2. Pruning

Tables 3 and 4 show the results of metrics re-measured through the pruning technique described above. It turns out that the bidirectional LSTM RNN is a stronger network for reasoning than the unidirectional LSTM RNN because it does not have a negative effect on accuracy even after 90% of weights are removed.

Table 3. Performance of Pruning Networks.

Type	Initial Design	After Pruning (30%)	After Pruning (60%)	After Pruning (90%)
Overall Accuracy (Uni)	86.7%	86.7%	86.7%	83.3%
Average Precision (Uni)	87.5%	87.5%	87.5%	84.2%
Average Recall (Uni)	86.7%	86.7%	86.7%	83.3%
F1 Score (Uni)	86.3%	86.3%	86.3%	82.4%
Overall Accuracy (Bi)	93.3%	93.3%	93.3%	93.3%
Average Precision (Bi)	95.0%	95.0%	94.2%	95.0%
Average Recall (Bi)	93.3%	93.3%	93.3%	93.3%
F1 Score (Bi)	93.1%	93.1%	93.3%	93.1%

Table 4. Execution Time of Pruning Networks.

Type	Initial Design	After Pruning (30%)	After Pruning (60%)	After Pruning (90%)
Unidirectional	0.23 s	0.21 s	0.19 s	0.15 s
Bidirectional	0.26 s	0.24 s	0.22 s	0.19 s

3.3. Identifying Latent Patterns

Regarding identifying latent representations, we have two issues in the problem under consideration. The first issue is whether we can find such representations for every player and every skill reliably in the latent space. To examine the first issue, we rely on the holdout cross-validation [18]. For the holdout, we split our sensor dataset into a training set and a test set. We then use the training data for the network training, and check if similar results are observed for the test dataset.

Figures 11 and 12 show a set of the cross-validation results for the coach and the beginner, respectively. The exact meaning of the pictures in the figure is as follows: in the j-th column, which is for the j-th skill, the red solid lines show the latent trajectories obtained for the test dataset, while the blue dashed lines are for the latent trajectories for the training dataset. Figures 11 and 12 show that the proposed method worked reasonably well in characterizing dynamic sequence patterns in the latent space. From the cross-validation results, one can see similarities between the latent trajectory of the test data and that of the training data. This indicates that our approach successfully transformed a high-dimensional time series of sensor data into a time series of low-dimensional latent representations, and the training and test dataset with common characteristics indeed shared same latent representations. We believe that this capability of yielding meaningful latent representations reliably for characterizing high-dimensional time series of sensor data is of significant practical value.

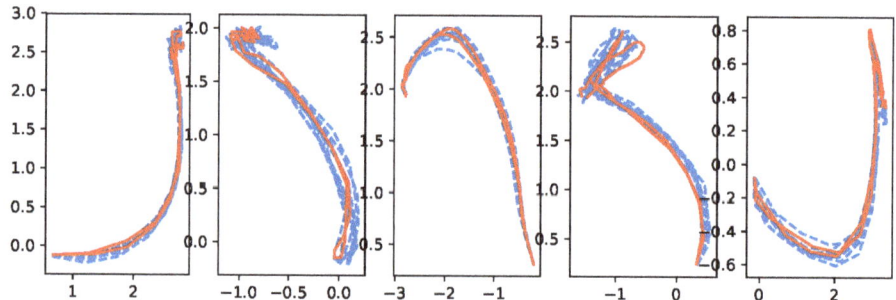

Figure 11. Cross-validation results for the coach's skills (from left to right): Forehand stroke, forehand drive, forehand cut, backhand drive, backhand short.

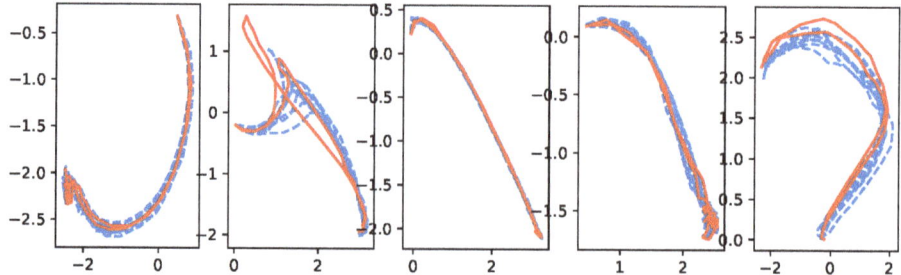

Figure 12. Cross-validation results for the beginner's skills (from left to right): Forehand stroke, forehand drive, forehand cut, backhand drive, backhand short.

The second issue is whether the extracted low-dimensional latent representations are indeed capable of distinguishing the players and the skills well. This capability is crucial in providing the beginner with evaluative feedback, because the beginner can explore and improve skills based on how similar his or her latent trajectories are to the coach's performance. The conceptual diagram for such improvements is shown in Figure 13 along with actual improvements observed for motion skill "forehand drive" when used in a closed loop. Actually, Figures 11 and 12 can also address the second issue well. Since the LSTM RNNs, which provide the embedding of the time series of sensor data for the augmented network, inherit this multi-class classification ability, the training results of the augmented network show an obvious capability for distinguishing players and skills.

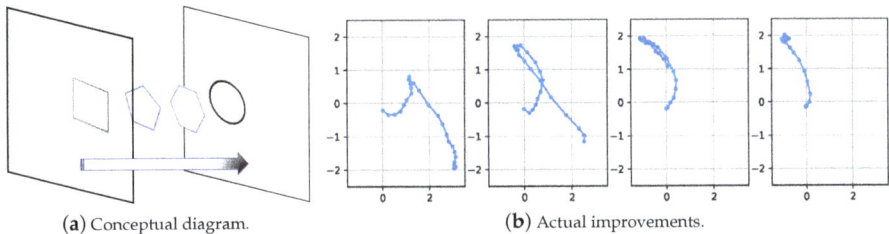

(a) Conceptual diagram. (b) Actual improvements.

Figure 13. Conceptual diagram of the improvement of skills reflected in latent space, along with actual improvements observed for motion skill "forehand drive" when used in a closed loop.

4. Discussion and Conclusions

4.1. Discussion

In this paper, we investigated an LSTM-guided coach assistant for table tennis practice. The proposed method is based on a combination of LSTM with a deep state space model and probabilistic inference, and our experiment results show that the method can yield promising results for characterizing high-dimensional time series patterns and providing useful information when working with the wearable IMU sensors for table tennis coaching. For the assessment of the classification part, we used the cross-entropy loss. More precisely, we used the corresponding method of the TensorFlow library, i.e., `tf.nn.softmax_cross_entropy_with_logits`.

For the probabilistic inference part, the ELBO for the log-likelihood of the data was used, as described in (11). Table 5 reports the training procedure established in this paper.

Table 5. Steps for the established training procedure.

1: Obtain sets of training data for each class of skills, and for each subject (coach or beginner).
2: Obtain sets of test data for each class of skills, and for each subject (coach or beginner).
3: Train the LSTM RNN with the training data for classification purposes, and fix the classifier network.
4: Compose the augmented network by combining the embedding of the LSTM RNN classifiers with inference network, and compute latent trajectories with the training data for each class of skills and each subject (coach or beginner).
5: Check the validity of the obtained latent trajectories via cross-validation using the test dataset. If not satisfactory, repeat the above until satisfactory.
6: Plot the latent trajectories for the coach's skills.
7: In the beginner's practice with the IMU sensors, compute and plot the latent trajectories for skills. When the resultant latent trajectories are not close to the coach's, explore other motion skills and follow the motion yielding more similar latent trajectories.

Our approach is inspired by the deep Markov model (DMM) approach [19]. The most significant difference lies in the way the LSTM RNNs are used in the classification phase: The use of LSTM RNNs as a multi-class classifier as well as a kind of feature extractor in the initial stage is critically important, because it ensures that the augmented network contrasts the latent trajectories of the coach and beginner's skills. Classical machine learning methods can be considered as alternatives to the LSTM RNN, because they often have similar performance in some applications for HAR [3]. However, it was observed in [3] that LSTM RNNs yielded good performance consistently, whereas other classical machine learning method did not. Moreover, data coming from IMU sensors are inherently high-dimensional time series; hence the use of recurrent type neural networks is more natural.

The problem we consider in this paper may also gain some inspirations from the field of imitation learning [20]. More specifically, a policy of an agent (which is not human) is trained to copy the decision-making of an expert in imitation learning. Comparison with imitation learning methods is a worthwhile and attractive subject, e.g., in exploring the challenges of applying guided coaching and machine learning to training actual human subjects. One difference between machine training and human sports skill learning is that humans have previous knowledge of games, and in particular, all types of moves in a ball-based sport. The expert can have difficulty communicating a skill to a beginner, and a beginner may have difficulty understanding an expert's explanations, feedback, or modeling of a skill. Thus, in training an actual human learner from an expert network or trained machine, merely watching an expert and attempting to model its behavior may prove challenging, especially if the expert is unable to convey a conceptual understanding of the task to the learner. We believe that the latent trajectories provided by the propose method can be a significant help in the case.

Currently, we have not covered the issues of C statistics and calibration for the cross-validation. More detailed aspects of cross-validation need to be studied in future works.

Finally, note that overall performance can be maintained, and the execution time can be reduced after a significant amount of pruning as shown in Tables 3 and 4, respectively. These points will be important when dealing with deployment into wearable sensors [21,22].

4.2. Conclusions

In this paper, we presented a deep learning-based coaching assistant method, which can provide useful information in supporting table tennis practice. Our strategy used a combination of LSTM with a deep state space model and probabilistic inference. More precisely, we used the expressive power of LSTM when handling high-dimensional time series data, and state space model and probabilistic inference to extract low-dimensional latent representations useful for coaching. Experimental results showed that the presented method can yield promising results for characterizing high-dimensional time series patterns and for providing useful information when working with wearable IMU sensors for table tennis coaching. Future works include more extensive and comparative studies, which should reveal the strengths and weaknesses of the proposed approach, and further extensions of the method in several directions and with more subjects. Consideration of different kinds of state transition models and applications to other kinds of sports practice are some of the topics to be covered in future research. Issues of embedding the trained coaching assistant into the wearable sensors for training players on real-time are also left for future studies.

Author Contributions: S.-M.L., H.-C.O., and J.P. conceived and designed the methodology of the paper; S.-M.L., J.K., J.L., and J.P. wrote the computer program; S.-M.L. and H.-C.O. performed the experiments with a help from table tennis coaches; and S.-M.L., H.-C.O., and J.P. wrote the paper.

Funding: This research was funded by the National Research Foundation of Korea, grant number 2017R1E1A1A03070652, and a Korea University Grant.

Conflicts of Interest: The authors declare no conflicts of interest.

References

1. Kim, T.; Park, J.; Heo, S.; Sung, K.; Park, J. Characterizing Dynamic Walking Patterns and Detecting Falls with Wearable Sensors Using Gaussian Process Methods. *Sensors* **2017**, *17*, 1172. [CrossRef] [PubMed]
2. Kranz, M.; Möller, A.; Hammerla, N.; Diewald, S.; Plötz, T.; Olivier, P.; Roalter, L. The mobile fitness coach: Towards individualized skill assessment using personalized mobile devices. *Pervasice Mobile Comput.* **2013**, *9*, 203–215. [CrossRef]
3. Murad, A.; Pyun, J.-Y. Deep Recurrent Neural Networks for Human Activity Recognition. *Sensors* **2017**, *17*, 2556. [CrossRef] [PubMed]
4. Bayo-Monton, J.L.; Martinez-Millana, A.; Han, W.; Fernandez-Llatas, C.; Sun, Y.; Traver, V. Wearable Sensors Integrated with Internet of Things for Advancing eHealth Care. *Sensors* **2018**, *18*, 1851. [CrossRef] [PubMed]
5. Zeng, M.; Nguyen, L.T.; Yu, B.; Mengshoel, O.J.; Zhu, J.; Wu, P.; Zhang, J. Convolutional Neural Networks for Human Activity Recognition using Mobile Sensors. In Proceedings of the 6th International Conference on Mobile Computing, Applications and Services, Austin, TX, USA, 6–7 November 2014; pp. 197–205.
6. Chen, Y.; Xue, Y. A Deep Learning Approach to Human Activity Recognition Based on Single Accelerometer. In Proceedings of the 2015 IEEE International Conference on Systems, Man, and Cybernetics, Kowloon, China, 9–12 October 2015.
7. Hessen, H.-O.; Tessem, A.J. Human Activity Recognition with Two Body-Worn Accelerometer Sensors. Master's Thesis, Norwegian University of Science and Technology, Trondheim, Norway, 2015.
8. Hochreiter, S.; Schmidhuber, J. Long Short-term memory. *Neural Comput.* **1997**, *9*, 1735–1780. [CrossRef] [PubMed]
9. Graves, A.; Liwicki, M.; Fernandez, S.; Bertolami, R.; Bunke, H.; Schmidhuber, J. A Novel Connectionist System for Improved Unconstrained Handwriting Recognition. *IEEE Trans. Pattern Anal. Mach. Intell.* **2009**, *31*, 203–215. [CrossRef] [PubMed]
10. Zen, H.; Sak, H. Unidirectional Long Short-term Memory Recurrent Neural Network with Recurrent Output Layer for Low-latency Speech Synthesis. In Proceedings of the IEEE International Conference on Acoustics, Speech, and Signal Processing, Brisbane, Australia, 19–24 April 2015; pp. 4470–4474.
11. Bishop, C. Pattern Recognition and Machine Learning. *J. Korean Soc. Civ. Eng.* **2006**, *60*, 78.
12. Huang, L.; Sun J.; Xu, J.; Yang, Y. An Improved Residual LSTM Architecture for Acoustic Modeling. In Proceedings of the IEEE International Conference on Computer and Communication Systems, Krakow, Poland, 11–14 July 2017; pp. 101–105.
13. Zhu, M.; Gupta, S. To prune, or not to prune: Exploring the efficacy of pruning for model compression. *Mach. Learn.* **2017**, arXiv:1710.01878.
14. Abadi, M.; Barham, P.; Chen, J.; Chen, Z.; Davis, A.; Dean, J.; Devin, M.; Ghemawat, S.; Irving, G.; Isard, M.; et al. TensorFlow: A System for Large-scale Machine Learning. In Proceedings of the 12th USENIX Conference on Operating Systems Design and Implementation, Savannah, GA, USA, 2–4 November 2016; pp. 265–283.
15. Scikit-Learn: Machine Learning in Python. Available online: http://scikit-learn.org/stable/ (accessed on 11 June 2018).
16. Kingma, D.P.; Welling, M. Auto-encoding variational bayes. *Mach. Learn.* **2013**, arXiv:1312.6114.
17. Rezende, D.J.; Mohamed, S.; Wierstra, D. Stochastic backpropagation and approximate inference in deep generative models. *Mach. Learn.* **2014**, arXiv:1401.4082.
18. Raschka, S. *Python Machine Learning*; Packt Publishing Ltd.: Birmingham, UK, 2015.
19. Krishnan, R.G.; Shalit, U.; Sontag, D. Structured Inference Networks for Nonlinear State Space Models. In Proceedings of the Thirty-First AAAI Conference on Artificial Intelligence (AAAI-17), San Francisco, CA, USA, 4–9 February 2017; pp. 2101–2109.
20. Ross, S.; Gordon, G.; Bagnell, D. A reduction of imitation learning and structured prediction to no-regret online learning. In Proceedings of the Fourteenth International Conference on Artificial Intelligence and Statistics, Lauderdale, FL, USA, 11–13 April 2011; pp. 627–635.

21. Table Tennis Terminology. Available online: http://lucioping.altervista.org/English/basicinfo/TT%20terminology.htm (accessed on 12 June 2018).
22. Table Tennis Terminology. Available online: https://www.allabouttabletennis.com/table-tennis-terminology.html (accessed on 12 June 2018).

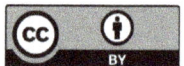

© 2018 by the authors. Licensee MDPI, Basel, Switzerland. This article is an open access article distributed under the terms and conditions of the Creative Commons Attribution (CC BY) license (http://creativecommons.org/licenses/by/4.0/).

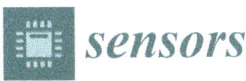

Article

Fusion of Heart Rate, Respiration and Motion Measurements from a Wearable Sensor System to Enhance Energy Expenditure Estimation

Ke Lu [1,*], Liyun Yang [1,2], Fernando Seoane [3,4,5], Farhad Abtahi [1,2], Mikael Forsman [1,2] and Kaj Lindecrantz [2,4]

1. School of Engineering Sciences in Chemistry, Biotechnology and Health, KTH Royal Institute of Technology, Hälsovägen 11C, 141 57 Huddinge, Sweden; liyuny@kth.se (L.Y.); farhad.abtahi@ki.se (F.A.); mikael.forsman@ki.se (M.F.)
2. Institute of Environmental Medicine, Karolinska Institutet, Solnavägen 1, 171 77 Solna, Sweden; kaj.lindecrantz@ki.se
3. Department of Clinical Science, Intervention and Technology, Karolinska Institutet, Hälsovägen 7, 141 57 Huddinge, Sweden; fernando.seoane@ki.se
4. Swedish School of Textiles, University of Borås, Allégatan 1, 501 90 Borås, Sweden
5. Department of Biomedical Engineering, Karolinska University Hospital, 1, 171 76 Solna, Sweden
* Correspondence: kelu@kth.se; Tel.: +46-765-910-501

Received: 17 August 2018; Accepted: 11 September 2018; Published: 14 September 2018

Abstract: This paper presents a new method that integrates heart rate, respiration, and motion information obtained from a wearable sensor system to estimate energy expenditure. The system measures electrocardiography, impedance pneumography, and acceleration from upper and lower limbs. A multilayer perceptron neural network model was developed, evaluated, and compared to two existing methods, with data from 11 subjects (mean age, 27 years, range, 21–65 years) who performed a 3-h protocol including submaximal tests, simulated work tasks, and periods of rest. Oxygen uptake was measured with an indirect calorimeter as a reference, with a time resolution of 15 s. When compared to the reference, the new model showed a lower mean absolute error (MAE = 1.65 mL/kg/min, R^2 = 0.92) than the two existing methods, i.e., the flex-HR method (MAE = 2.83 mL/kg/min, R^2 = 0.75), which uses only heart rate, and arm-leg HR+M method (MAE = 2.12 mL/kg/min, R^2 = 0.86), which uses heart rate and motion information. As indicated, this new model may, in combination with a wearable system, be useful in occupational and general health applications.

Keywords: energy expenditure; wearable device; accelerometer; impedance pneumography; neural network

1. Introduction

The energy expenditure (EE), as an indicator of metabolic state and physical activity level, provides valuable information that can be used for occupational health and safety design [1], exercise, and daily life management, and prevention and treatment of health problems such as obesity and diabetes [2]. Direct measurement methods of EE or oxygen consumption (VO_2), a commonly-used indicator of EE, requires expensive and sophisticated equipment, such as the direct calorimetry using metabolic chamber, the double labeled water method, and indirect calorimetry with a face mask, which are not suitable for daily free-living use [3]. Therefore, indirect measurement techniques using wearable sensors are desired, and have attracted significant attention in the last two decades; consequently, considerable effort has been allocated to the issue [4–32].

Heart rate (HR) monitoring is often used to estimate EE, as it has a good linearity with oxygen consumption in a large range of aerobic work [13,21]. The relationship between HR and EE at an individual level can be established through a calibration procedure, i.e., maximal or submaximal tests performed with a treadmill or cycle ergometer, which requires time and resources [33]. However, the poor relationship between HR and EE in resting and low intensity activities is an important limiting factor [24]. The HR-VO$_2$ relation can vary in different activities [19], e.g., difference has been reported between upper body and lower body activities [34]. In addition, HR is affected by several factors that are not directly related to metabolism e.g., mental stress, emotions, and medication [16].

Accelerometry is also a popular tool to estimate physical activity related EE in free-living conditions. With count-based methods [11,35], the activity count is calculated using acceleration, and then directly linked to EE, while the type of activity being performed is not considered [6]. In activity related methods [4,7,12], firstly, the activity recognition is preformed, then the EE is estimated through a look-up table or by using the activity specified EE model [6]. The acceleration (ACC) measurement directly reflects the movement information. However, it lacks the information about the effort of the movements, which limits its effectiveness for assessing complex activities involving interaction with other objects, such as manual handling. Several methods that utilize HR and ACC have been proposed, which improves the estimation of EE by the sole use of HR or ACC [9,36].

Respiration is another factor that is related to EE [14]. Several studies have demonstrated that pulmonary ventilation (V_E) has better linearity with EE compared to the HR [37,38]. As an accurate V_E measurement requires devices with facemasks or mouthpieces, the real application is very limited in free-living conditions. Recent developments in wearable technologies, such as impedance pneumography (IP), inductive plethysmography, and piezoresistive pneumography integrated in smart clothing [39–43], give new opportunities to use portable respiration measurement devices for EE estimation in a free-living setting, and preliminary studies have been carried out [15,18].

The purpose of this study was to develop and test a method that uses a combination of information from measurements of heart rate, respiration, and accelerations to estimate energy expenditure. The measurements were acquired through a wearable sensor system, and integrated by a model based on neural network. The wearable sensor system was developed under our research projects towards automatic risk assessment at work [44,45]. A lab experiment was implemented to support the development of the model and evaluate the developed system and estimation model. The proposed method was compared with two existing methods: HR-flex [28], a HR based method that uses a bi-linear model to improve the estimation in low intensity, and Arm-Leg HR+M [29,36], a method which uses combined HR and ACC measurements, with independent arm and leg calibration. The results showed improved accuracy over the two existing methods. In addition, the proposed method does not require complex lab calibration, which can dramatically improve the usability of such a system in field settings.

2. Materials and Methods

2.1. The Wearable Sensor System

The wearable sensor system and the sensor placement are shown in Figure 1. The vest, reported in [40,46], includes four textile electrodes made by conductive fabric. One pair of electrodes was used for IP current injection, and the other was used for electric potential sensing for IP and ECG. A compact recorder, ECGZ2 (Z-Health Technologies AB, Borås, Sweden), for ECG and electrical bioimpedance was connected to the vest and placed in a pocket on the shoulder strap of the vest. The frequency of the injection current for impedance measurement was 50 kHz. ECG and IP signals were recorded with sampling rates of 250 Hz and 100 Hz, respectively. Four 3-axis accelerometers (AX3, Axivity Ltd., Newcastle, UK) were placed on both wrists, using rubber wristbands, and on the thighs, using trousers with specially designed pockets to hold the accelerometer units. The acceleration was recorded at 100 Hz.

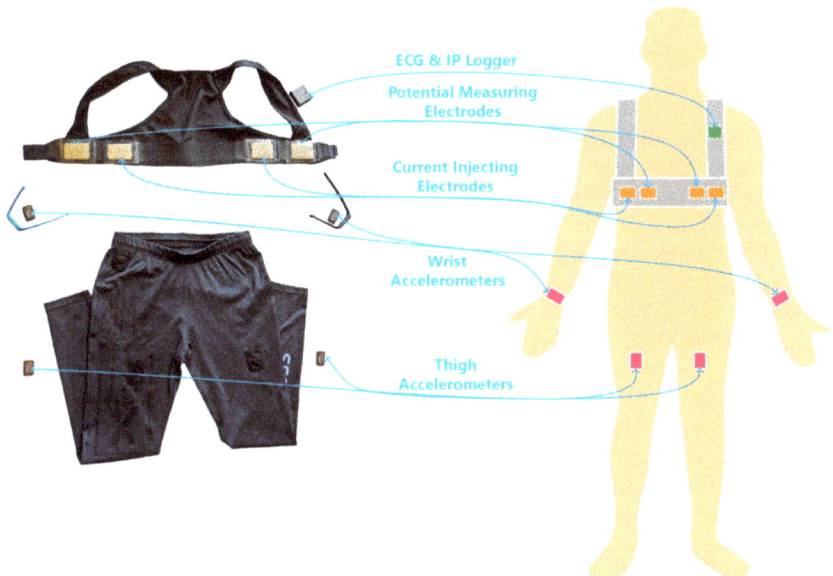

Figure 1. The wearable sensor system and its placement. The system includes a vest with textile electrodes, a wireless ECG and IP recording unit, 4 accelerometers, rubber wristbands, and trousers with specially designed pockets.

2.2. Data Collection

2.2.1. Participants

Nine men and three women participated in the laboratory experiment implemented in GIH, the Swedish School of Sport and Health Sciences, Stockholm, Sweden. The subjects consisted of a homogeneous group with young male subjects, and a heterogeneous group with both male and female participants in different age groups. Data from one subject was removed from the analysis because of the lack of a vest with a suitable size for the participant, which resulted in poor ECG and IP signal quality. The detailed characteristics of the included participants are shown in Table 1. All participants provided written informed consent. Ethical approval for the study was obtained from the Regional Ethical Review Board in Stockholm (Dnr 2016/724-31/5).

Table 1. Characteristics of included participants (median [range]).

	Men (N = 9)	Women (N = 2)	All (N = 11)
Age (year)	27 [21–65]	43 [25–61]	27 [21–65]
Height (cm)	181 [171–199]	169 [165–173]	177 [165–199]
Weight (kg)	77 [51–89]	60 [58–62]	75 [51–89]
BMI (kg/m^2)	22.8 [17.4–25.6]	20.9 [20.7–21.2]	22.6 [17.4–25.6]
VO$_{2\,max}$ (mL/min/kg)	42.9 [32.1–54.6]	35.6 [30.9–40.3]	40.3 [30.9–54.6]

2.2.2. Experiment Protocol

The participants were asked to avoid intense physical activity for 1 day before the experiment, and to refrain from eating, smoking, drinking tea, coffee, or alcohol for at least 2 h beforehand. The experiment process took about 3 h. During the experiment, VO$_2$ was measured by a computerized metabolic system (Jaeger Oxycon Pro, VIASYS Healthcare GmbH, Würzburg, Germany), where a facemask was worn by the participants. The experiment protocol consisted of three categories of activities: resting, simulated working tasks, and submaximal tests. The list of performed tasks and corresponding VO$_2$ levels measured in the experiment is presented in Table 4 under the result section. After each task, the subject had a break for 5 to 25 min, until the HR returned to within 10 percent of the resting HR.

The resting test included resting in three postures: 20 min in lying, 5 min in sitting and 5 min in standing. During the resting test, the resting energy expenditure (REE) was measured. Five different working tasks, with different intensity levels and active muscle groups, were performed afterwards. Each of the tasks lasted 8–10 min. The office work required the participant to type on a computer while sitting beside a table. The painting work required the participant to simulate painting a wall at their own pace using a painting pole. The postal delivery work was performed by cycling at a cycle ergometer with 0.75 kg resistance. The meat cutting work was simulated by pulling a resistance band repetitively. The construction work included arm and whole body lifting tasks. The submaximal tests session consisted of 3 tests. The first was the Chester step test [47], with maximal 5 levels of incremental stepping pace. The second was a walking pace treadmill test as described in [36]. Each level of the treadmill test lasted three minutes. The speed was increased after the first level. From the second level, the inclination was raised by 2% between each stage. The third test was an arm ergometer test with a constant cadence while the resistance increased between each level [36]. All the submaximal tests were terminated when the HR of the subject reached the 80% of the age-predicted maximal HR (220 − age).

2.3. The Model for VO$_2$ Estimation

The process of the estimation is shown in Figure 2. A multilayer perceptron neural network (MLPNN) with four input units, five hidden units, and one output unit was used to construct the model. The activation function of the hidden layer was hyperbolic tangent sigmoid function, and linear function for the output layer. All features and the output are listed in Table 2. All data were analyzed with 15-s non-overlapping windows. Four features were used that represent HR, V$_E$, arm motion and leg motion, respectively. HR, V$_E$, and VO$_2$ were normalized by corresponding individual characteristics before being used as the inputs and output of the MLPNN to train a network with good genericization that learns characteristics at the group level.

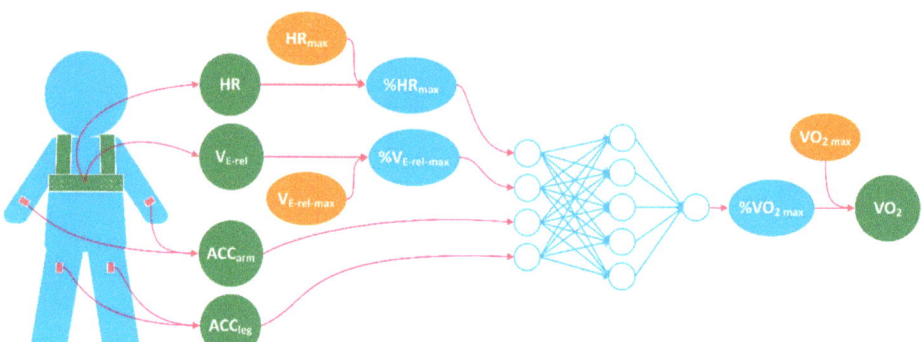

Figure 2. A demonstration of the flow of the oxygen consumption (VO$_2$) process. The input and output are explained in Table 2.

Table 2. Summary of the input features and the output of the neural network.

Input Features	% HR_{max}	HR normalized by age predicted HR_{max}
	% $V_{E\text{-rel max}}$	$V_{E\text{-rel}}$ normalized by estimated $V_{E\text{-rel max}}$
	ACC_{arm}	Mean absolute value of wrist acceleration
	ACC_{leg}	Mean absolute value of thigh acceleration
Output	% $VO_{2\ max}$	VO_2 normalized by estimated $VO_{2\ max}$

The VO_2 measurements were normalized by the individual maximal oxygen uptake ($VO_{2\ max}$), which was estimated through the Chester step test with pre-estimated VO_2 level on each stage [47]. The HR was normalized by individual maximal HR (HR_{max}), calculated by $HR_{max} = 220 - $ age. The relative tidal volume ($V_{T\text{-rel}}$) of each breath was represented by the impedance difference in peak and valley pairs of the filtered IP signal. The relative ventilation ($V_{E\text{-rel}}$) during each 15-s epoch was acquired by the sum of the $V_{T\text{-rel}}$ values in the window. A quadratic relationship between HR and $V_{E\text{-rel}}$ was established for each subject by the least square method using measured HR and $V_{E\text{-rel}}$ during the experiment. The maximal relative ventilation ($V_{E\text{-rel max}}$) was then estimated by applying the HR_{max} to the HR-$V_{E\text{-rel}}$ relationship. $V_{E\text{-rel}}$ was then normalized by the $V_{E\text{-rel max}}$ and fed to the network. The acceleration data was first band pass filtered with a 0.25–6 Hz passband; then, the mean absolute acceleration was computed for each 15-s epoch. For the arm and leg acceleration, the higher value from the right and the left sides of each epoch was picked.

2.4. Model Training and Cross Validation

The so-called Leave one subject out (LOSO) validation method was used. In repeated trials, all data except one subject was used for training the model; the data of that subject was used for testing the model. The LOSO method avoids test results that are overfitted to individual characteristics. The overall performance of the network was evaluated by combining test results from all LOSO cross validation. The training data was split for training and validation set with a ratio of 6:4, and the Levenberg-Marquardt backpropagation was used for the training process.

2.5. Comparision to Published Methods

Results from our method were compared with two published methods, i.e., HR-flex [28], one of the mostly used HR based method in the field, and Arm-Leg HR+M method [29,36], a method showed improved accuracy during occupational tasks in our previous evaluation [48]. The inputs and calibration requirements of all methods are listed in Table 3.

Table 3. A comparison of requirements of input data and personalized measurement among the three methods.

Methods	Input Data	Additional Individualized Measurements
Flex-HR	HR	Flex HR Point REE HR-VO_2 Calibration
Arm-Leg HR+M	HR, ACC_{leg}, ACC_{arm}	REE Leg HR-VO_2 Calibration Arm HR-VO_2 Calibration
Proposed	HR, ACC_{leg}, ACC_{arm}, $V_{E\text{-rel}}$	$VO_{2\ max}$

The flex-HR method [28] considers the nonlinearity in HR-EE relation in low intensity. It uses REE when the HR is below the flex point, and a linear HR-EE relationship when the HR is above the flex point. For the comparison, we chose to use step test data with pre-estimated VO_2 levels on each stage for calibration, as it required the same level of test equipment as the new method. The REE was measured during the resting test. The flex-point was chosen as the average of the highest HR during rest and the lowest HR during walking on treadmill test.

The Arm-Leg HR+M method [29,36] accounts for the difference in HR-EE response between the upper and the lower body. It uses the level of arm and leg ACC and their ratio to determine the arm specified HR-EE equation, the leg specified HR-EE equation, or the REE for EE estimation. We used a treadmill test and arm ergometer test data to establish the arm and leg calibration respectively, together with a simultaneously measured VO_2 level. The calibration requires a treadmill, an arm ergometer, and indirect calorimetry. Thresholds for the ACC level and ratio were re-adapted to our measurement data, as a different accelerometer and acceleration signal processing procedure were used in comparison to the original study.

2.6. Statistics

Estimated VO_2 in 15-s epochs were compared to the criterion measurements. Bias, the mean absolute error (MAE), the root-mean-square-error (RMSE) and the coefficient of determination (R^2) were calculated to evaluate the performance. Paired *t*-tests were performed to compare the absolute errors between the new method and each of the two published methods. Bland-Altman plots with error histograms were plotted to assess the agreement and the error distribution.

3. Results

The mean levels of measured VO_2 for performing each task during the experiment are listed in Table 4.

Table 4. A summary of tasks performed during the experiments and corresponding mean VO_2 level (mL/min/kg) of the 11 subjects.

Group	Task	VO$_2$ Level (Mean ± SD)
Resting	Lying	3.78 ± 0.96
	Sitting	3.82 ± 1.16
	Standing	4.01 ± 0.41
Work Tasks	Office Work	4.01 ± 1.42
	Painting Work	8.51 ± 1.68
	Postal Delivery Work	14.04 ± 2.37
	Meat Cutting Work	7.62 ± 1.89
	Construction Work	12.24 ± 4.56
Submaximal Tests	Step Test	22.23 ± 7.71
	Treadmill Test	22.88 ± 8.05
	Arm Ergometer Test	11.06 ± 4.98

The training and testing results (%$VO_{2\,max}$) on each subject, as well as the averaged results from the LOSO validation, are shown in Table 5. The RMSE and R^2 level from training and testing results were very close, which indicates the method has a good generalization among the participants. The averaged group bias was very low (−0.16%). However, a relatively lager bias (maximal 2.71%) can be found on individual level in few occasions. No strong relationship was found between the estimation errors and the personal characteristics, such as gender, age, and aerobic capacity.

The results of overall performance in VO_2 estimation, measured by individual bias (IB), group bias (GB), MAE, RMSE, and R^2 of three methods, are shown in Table 6. The proposed method showed a more accurate estimation (IB = 0.42 mL/kg/min, GB = −0.01 mL/kg/min, MAE = 1.65 mL/kg/min) compared to the flex-HR method (IB = 1.11 mL/kg/min, GB = 0.69 mL/kg/min, MAE = 2.83 mL/kg/min), where estimation error, individual bias, and group bias were significantly reduced ($p < 0.001$). The proposed method also showed a significant improvement ($p < 0.001$) in estimation error over the arm-leg HR+M method (MAE = 2.12 mL/kg/min).

Table 5. Results of the cross validation of the relative VO$_2$ (%VO$_{2\ max}$) from the neural network.

Gender	Age (Year)	Weight (kg)	Height (cm)	BMI (kg/m^2)	VO$_{2\ max}$ (mL/kg/min)	%VO$_{2\ max}$ Train Bias	RMSE	R^2	Test [1] Bias	RMSE	R^2
M	65	80	188	22.6	32.7	−0.03	5.26	0.92	−2.03	5.74	0.88
M	21	77	176.5	24.7	54.6	0.07	5.54	0.90	−0.35	5.40	0.92
F	61	62	173	20.7	30.9	0.10	5.06	0.92	−1.19	8.03	0.84
F	25	58	165.5	21.2	40.3	−0.01	5.39	0.91	0.11	4.55	0.93
M	27	88.5	199	22.3	47.8	0.04	5.33	0.91	0.18	4.69	0.94
M	27	51	171	17.4	39.6	0.14	5.21	0.92	−0.36	6.61	0.87
M	25	79.8	176.5	25.6	43.6	0.05	5.35	0.91	1.84	4.60	0.93
M	29	88.9	190	24.6	42.9	−0.03	5.54	0.91	−0.51	4.07	0.95
M	42	75	177	23.9	32.1	0.03	5.26	0.92	2.71	5.93	0.88
M	26	75	181.5	22.8	37.2	0.06	5.28	0.91	−0.68	4.86	0.92
M	26	68.5	184	20.2	44.8	0.08	5.30	0.91	−1.47	5.76	0.90
Average Mean (SD)									−0.16 (1.38)	5.47 (1.13)	0.91 (0.03)

[1] In each row, the data for the specific subject was excluded in the training and used for the testing.

Table 6. Comparison of VO$_2$ estimation results among flex-HR, arm-leg HR+M, and proposed method (mL/kg/min).

Methods	Individual Bias [1]	Group Bias	MAE	RMSE	R^2
Flex-HR	1.11	0.69	2.83	4.00	0.75
Arm-Leg HR+M	0.60	−0.09	2.12	2.95	0.86
Proposed	0.42	−0.07	1.65	2.28	0.92

[1] Mean absolute value of individual biases.

The Bland-Altman plots and the error rate histograms of three methods are shown in Figure 3. The proposed method shows a large improvement in the low intensity region. The mean estimation error rate was also reduced (28.1%) compared to the other methods (44.1% and 38.4% respectively).

The errors with each specific activity are shown in Table 7, where for each activity, the worst performance among the three methods is shown in bold and italic. The proposed method has a good overall generalization over different kinds of activities, except that a large bias on the simulated construction work can be found. Comparing to the flex-HR method, the error caused by different HR response to arm and leg activity was reduced in the proposed method by learning from group characteristics without arm calibration, which can be seen from the arm ergometer results, as well as from the top right corner of the Bland-Altman plot in Figure 3.

Table 7. Comparison of task specific errors among three methods (mL/kg/min).

	Resting	Office Work	Painting	Postal Delivery	Meat Cutting	Construction Work	Step	Treadmill	Arm Ergometer
Flex-HR									
Bias	−0.05	−0.29	−0.47	−2.42	*1.84*	1.05	−1.05 [1]	−0.81	4.18
RMSE	0.90	0.84	3.89	4.15	*4.33*	3.90	2.85 [1]	2.92	5.91
Arm-Leg HR+M									
Bias	−1.42	−0.93	−1.90	−1.59	−0.16	−1.09	−0.38	−0.01 [2]	0.00 [2]
RMSE	*2.50*	*2.09*	2.55	2.57	1.56	*4.44*	2.53	1.82 [2]	1.14 [2]
Proposed									
Bias	0.02	0.17	−0.47	−0.46	0.55	*−2.01*	−1.08 [3]	0.44	0.06
RMSE	0.93	0.86	1.69	2.36	1.62	3.88	2.83 [3]	2.71	1.69

The bold and italic numbers indicate the largest error in each activity. [1] Data used for individual calibration, with pre-estimated VO$_2$ level. [2] Data used for individual calibration, with measured VO$_2$ level. [3] Data used for VO$_{2max}$ estimation, with pre-estimated VO$_2$ level.

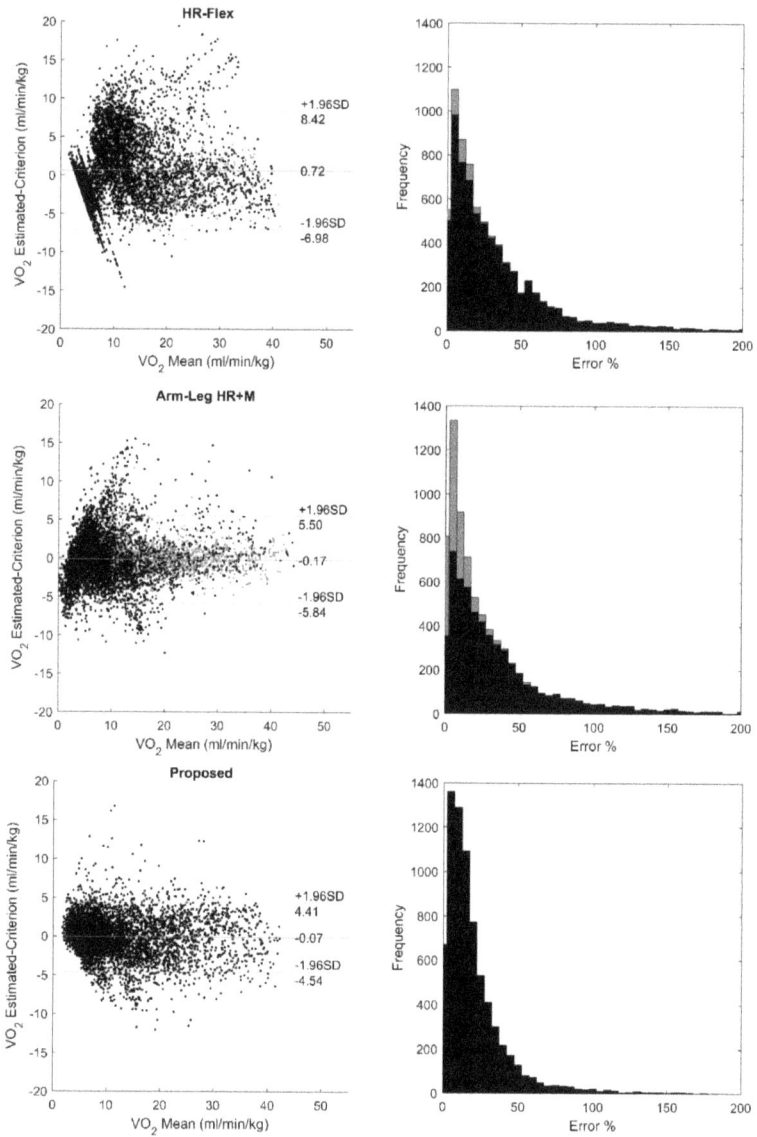

Figure 3. Bland-Altman plots and error rate histograms of flex-HR, arm-leg HR+M, and proposed methods against the criterion measurement. Data used in individual calibration are plotted in grey.

4. Discussion and Conclusions

In this study, we have demonstrated a method for free-living energy expenditure estimation that combines the HR, respiration, and motion information using nonlinear data driven modeling. In the experiment, the method showed improved accuracy over two established methods, based on HR and HR combined with ACC.

The method has also improved the usability by avoiding a complex laboratory calibration. The Chester step test used for $VO_{2\ max}$ estimation only requires a step with designed height, and takes only 6 to 10 min, which can be easily applied in the field. For certain ergonomic applications that use per cent maximum aerobic capacity (%$VO_{2\,max}$) as a measure of physical workload, the output of the network can be used directly without the need of multiplying individual $VO_{2\,max}$ value; hence, no calibration procedure is required. The wearable system used in the study is light-weight and easy to wear, which opens up the possibility for long-term, unobtrusive monitoring in different contexts. However, different contexts will come with different needs regarding number of accelerometers and their placement. The most versatile system would have many accelerometers at different sites on the body, but many sensors will increase the overall price of the system. Obviously, there will be trade-off between versatility, complexity, and cost.

A method using neural network based model to estimate EE from HR has been reported previously in [31,32]. This method uses not only the HR, but also heart rate variability derived respiration rate, and HR 'on and off dynamics' as input features. However, very limited information has been shown about the implementation. Hence, we were not able to compare our method with it.

In previous studies [15,18], which used portable indirect respiration monitoring devices to estimate EE, the measured physical quantities such as transthoracic impedance and thoracic circumference distance were converted into flow or volume through a personal calibration process using a spirometer. In this study, a rough calibration of the personalized impedance level was acquired by using simultaneously-measured HR values. How much data is needed to establish a reliable relationship and the durability of the relationship should be further studied. In the experiment, we found our $V_{E\text{-rel}}$ measurement through IP did not have very high linearity with the V_E measured by the indirect calorimetry. Possible causes for this discrepancy include the configuration of electrode position, posture change that alters the shape of ribcage [49], and motion artifacts. Applying optimized IP electrodes position [50] and advanced processing methods will have the potential to improve the IP measurement hence the EE estimation.

Limitations of this study include a small sample size (11 subjects), and the fact that limited activity types were performed under laboratory condition. The method has not yet been validated for complex real free-living scenarios, and the trained network could be overfitted to the activities that were performed in the experiment. The experiment has not taken into consideration many nonmetabolic-related factors that may alter HR or V_E, such as mental stress and temperature.

Since the new model showed a higher level of agreement with the reference methods compared to two existing methods, this study indicates a high potential for applying information fusion of HR, respiration, and motion data in combination with a nonlinear statistical learning method in the field of unobtrusive energy expenditure estimation. The solution may be used both in occupational and general health applications. Studies with improved respiration monitoring techniques and varied populations with larger size under free-living conditions are suggested in future development.

Author Contributions: L.Y. and K.L. conceived and designed the experiments in collaboration with the other authors; L.Y. and K.L. performed the experiments; K.L. analyzed the data; F.S. contributed with wearables; all authors participated in the discussion of results; K.L. drafted the paper; all authors revised the paper.

Funding: This work was supported by AFA Insurance under Grant Dnr 150039, EIT Health under project no. 18454 "Wellbeing, Health and Safety @ Work", and CSC Scholarship Council.

Conflicts of Interest: Kaj Lindecrantz and Fernando Seoane are co-founders and partial owners of Z-Health Technologies AB, Borås, Sweden. The other authors declare no conflict of interest.

References

1. Wu, H.C.; Wang, M.J. Relationship between Maximum Acceptable Work Time and Physical Workload. *Ergonomics* **2002**, *45*, 280–289. [CrossRef] [PubMed]
2. Colberg, S.R.; Sigal, R.J.; Yardley, J.E.; Riddell, M.C.; Dunstan, D.W.; Dempsey, P.C.; Horton, E.S.; Castorino, K.; Tate, D.F. Physical Activity/Exercise and Diabetes: A Position Statement of the American Diabetes Association. *Diabetes Care* **2016**, *39*, 2065–2079. [CrossRef] [PubMed]
3. Shephard, R.J.; Aoyagi, Y. Measurement of Human Energy Expenditure, with Particular Reference to Field Studies: An Historical Perspective. *Eur. J. Appl. Physiol.* **2012**, *112*, 2785–2815. [CrossRef] [PubMed]

4. Albinali, F.; Intille, S.; Haskell, W.; Rosenberger, M. Using Wearable Activity Type Detection to Improve Physical Activity Energy Expenditure Estimation. In Proceedings of the 12th ACM International Conference on Ubiquitous Computing, Copenhagen, Denmark, 26–29 September 2010.
5. Altini, M.; Penders, J.; Amft, O. Energy Expenditure Estimation Using Wearable Sensors: A New Methodology for Activity-Specific Models. In Proceedings of the Conference on Wireless Health, San Diego, CA, USA, 23–25 October 2012.
6. Altini, M.; Penders, J.; Vullers, R.; Amft, O. Estimating Energy Expenditure Using Body-Worn Accelerometers: A Comparison of Methods, Sensors Number and Positioning. *IEEE J. Biomed. Health Inform.* **2015**, *19*, 219–226. [CrossRef] [PubMed]
7. Bonomi, A.G.; Plasqui, G.; Goris, A.H.; Westerterp, K.R. Improving Assessment of Daily Energy Expenditure by Identifying Types of Physical Activity with a Single Accelerometer. *J. Appl. Physiol.* **2009**, *107*, 655–661. [CrossRef] [PubMed]
8. Bouten, C.V.; Westerterp, K.R.; Verduin, M.; Janssen, J.D. Assessment of Energy Expenditure for Physical Activity Using a Triaxial Accelerometer. *Med. Sci. Sports Exerc.* **1994**, *23*, 21–27. [CrossRef]
9. Brage, S.; Brage, N.; Franks, P.W.; Ekelund, U.; Wong, M.Y.; Andersen, L.B.; Froberg, K.; Wareham, N.J. Branched Equation Modeling of Simultaneous Accelerometry and Heart Rate Monitoring Improves Estimate of Directly Measured Physical Activity Energy Expenditure. *J. Appl. Physiol.* **2004**, *96*, 343–351. [CrossRef] [PubMed]
10. Brage, S.; Westgate, K.; Franks, P.W.; Stegle, O.; Wright, A.; Ekelund, U.; Wareham, N.J. Estimation of Free-Living Energy Expenditure by Heart Rate and Movement Sensing: A Doubly-Labelled Water Study. *PLoS ONE* **2015**, *10*, e0137206. [CrossRef] [PubMed]
11. Crouter, S.E.; Churilla, J.R.; Bassett, D.R. Estimating Energy Expenditure Using Accelerometers. *Eur. J. Appl. Physiol.* **2006**, *98*, 601–612. [CrossRef] [PubMed]
12. Ellis, K.; Kerr, J.; Godbole, S.; Lanckriet, G.; Wing, D.; Marshall, S. A Random Forest Classifier for the Prediction of Energy Expenditure and Type of Physical Activity from Wrist and Hip Accelerometers. *Physiol. Meas.* **2014**, *35*, 2191. [CrossRef] [PubMed]
13. Eston, R.G.; Rowlands, A.V.; Ingledew, D.K. Validity of Heart Rate, Pedometry, and Accelerometry for Predicting the Energy Cost of Children's Activities. *J. Appl. Physiol.* **1998**, *84*, 362–371. [CrossRef] [PubMed]
14. Gastinger, S.; Donnelly, A.; Dumond, R.; Prioux, J. A Review of the Evidence for the Use of Ventilation as a Surrogate Measure of Energy Expenditure. *J. Parenteral Enteral Nutr.* **2014**, *38*, 926–938. [CrossRef] [PubMed]
15. Gastinger, S.; Nicolas, G.; Sorel, A.; Sefati, H.; Prioux, J. Energy Expenditure Estimate by Heart-Rate Monitor and a Portable Electromagnetic-Coil System. *Int. J. Sport Nutr. Exerc. Metab.* **2012**, *22*, 117–130. [CrossRef] [PubMed]
16. Hiilloskorpi, H.; Fogelholm, M.; Laukkanen, R.; Pasanen, M.; Oja, P.; Mänttäri, A.; Natri, A. Factors Affecting the Relation between Heart Rate and Energy Expenditure During Exercise. *Int. J. Sports Med.* **1999**, *20*, 438–443. [CrossRef]
17. Jang, Y.; Jung, M.W.; Kang, J.; Kim, H.C. An Wearable Energy Expenditure Analysis System Based on the 15-Channel Whole-Body Segment Acceleration Measurement. In Proceedings of the 2005 27th Annual International Conference of the Engineering in Medicine and Biology Society, Shanghai, China, 1–4 September 2005.
18. Lu, K.; Yang, L.; Abtahi, F.; Lindecrantz, K.; Rödby, K.; Seoane, F. Wearable Cardiorespiratory Monitoring System for Unobtrusive Free-Living Energy Expenditure Tracking. In Proceedings of the World Congress on Medical Physics and Biomedical Engineering 2018, Prague, Czech Republic, 3–8 June 2018.
19. Li, R.; Deurenberg, P.; Hautvast, J.G. A Critical Evaluation of Heart Rate Monitoring to Assess Energy Expenditure in Individuals. *Am. J. Clin. Nutr.* **1993**, *58*, 602–607. [CrossRef] [PubMed]
20. Lin, C.W.; Yang, Y.T.; Wang, J.S.; Yang, Y.C. A Wearable Sensor Module with a Neural-Network-Based Activity Classification Algorithm for Daily Energy Expenditure Estimation. *IEEE Trans. Inform. Technol. Biomed.* **2012**, *16*, 991–998.
21. Livingstone, M.B. Heart-Rate Monitoring: The Answer for Assessing Energy Expenditure and Physical Activity in Population Studies? *Br. J. Nutr.* **1997**, *78*, 869–871. [CrossRef] [PubMed]

22. Livingstone, M.B.; Prentice, A.M.; Coward, W.A.; Ceesay, S.M.; Strain, J.J.; McKenna, P.G.; Nevin, G.B.; Barker, M.E.; Hickey, R. Simultaneous Measurement of Free-Living Energy Expenditure by the Doubly Labeled Water Method and Heart-Rate Monitoring. *Am. J. Clin. Nutr.* **1990**, *52*, 59–65. [CrossRef] [PubMed]
23. Lu, K.; Yang, L.; Abtahi, F.; Lindecrantz, K.; Rödby, K.; Seoane, F. *Wearable Cardiorespiratory Monitoring System for Unobtrusive Free-Living Energy Expenditure Tracking*; Springer: Singapore, 2019.
24. Luke, A.; Maki, K.C.; Barkey, N.; Cooper, R.; McGEE, D.A. Simultaneous Monitoring of Heart Rate and Motion to Assess Energy Expenditure. *Med. Sci. Sports Exerc.* **1997**, *29*, 144–148. [CrossRef] [PubMed]
25. Meijer, G.A.; Westerterp, K.R.; Koper, H.A. Assessment of Energy Expenditure by Recording Heart Rate and Body Acceleration. *Med. Sci. Sports Exerc.* **1989**, *21*, 343–347. [CrossRef] [PubMed]
26. Montoye, H.J.; Washburn, R.I.; Servais, S.T.; Ertl, A.N.; Webster, J.G.; Nagle, F.J. Estimation of Energy Expenditure by a Portable Accelerometer. *Med. Sci. Sports Exerc.* **1983**, *15*, 403–407. [CrossRef] [PubMed]
27. Murakami, H.; Kawakami, R.; Nakae, S.; Nakata, Y.; Ishikawa-Takata, K.; Tanaka, S.; Miyachi, M. Accuracy of Wearable Devices for Estimating Total Energy Expenditure: Comparison with Metabolic Chamber and Doubly Labeled Water Method. *JAMA Internal Med.* **2016**, *176*, 702–703. [CrossRef] [PubMed]
28. Spurr, G.B.; Prentice, A.M.; Murgatroyd, P.R.; Goldberg, G.R.; Reina, J.C.; Christman, N.T. Energy Expenditure from Minute-by-Minute Heart-Rate Recording: Comparison with Indirect Calorimetry. *Am. J. Clin. Nutr.* **1988**, *48*, 552–559. [CrossRef] [PubMed]
29. Strath, S.J.; Bassett, J.D.; Thompson, D.L.; Swartz, A.M. Validity of the Simultaneous Heart Rate-Motion Sensor Technique for Measuring Energy Expenditure. *Med. Sci. Sports Exerc.* **2002**, *34*, 888–894. [CrossRef] [PubMed]
30. Swartz, A.M.; Strath, S.J.; Bassett, D.R.; O'brien, W.L.; King, G.A.; Ainsworth, B.E. Estimation of Energy Expenditure Using Csa Accelerometers at Hip and Wrist Sites. *Med. Sci. Sports Exerc.* **2000**, *32*, S450–S456. [CrossRef] [PubMed]
31. Pulkkinen, A.; Kettunen, J.; Martinmäki, K.; Saalasti, S.; Rusko, H.K. On-and Off Dynamics and Respiration Rate Enhance the Accuracy of Heart Rate Based Vo2 Estimation. In Proceedings of the 51st Annual Meeting of the American College of Sports Medicine, Indianapolis, IN, USA, 2–5 June 2004.
32. Pulkkinen, A.; Saalasti, S.; Rusko, H.K. Energy Expenditure Can Be Accurately Estimated from Hr without Individual Laboratory Calibration. In Proceedings of the 52nd Annual Meeting of the American College of Sports Medicine, Nashville, TN, USA, 1–4 June 2005.
33. Brage, S.; Ekelund, U.; Brage, N.; Hennings, M.A.; Froberg, K.; Franks, P.W.; Wareham, N.J. Hierarchy of Individual Calibration Levels for Heart Rate and Accelerometry to Measure Physical Activity. *J. Appl. Physiol.* **2007**, *103*, 682–692. [CrossRef] [PubMed]
34. Vokac, Z.H.; Bell, H.; Bautz-Holter, E.; Rodahl, K. Oxygen Uptake/Heart Rate Relationship in Leg and Arm Exercise, Sitting and Standing. *J. Appl. Physiol.* **1975**, *39*, 54–59. [CrossRef] [PubMed]
35. Crouter, S.E.; Kuffel, E.; Haas, J.D.; Frongillo, E.A.; Bassett, D.R., Jr. A Refined 2-Regression Model for the Actigraph Accelerometer. *Med. Sci. Sports Exerc.* **2010**, *42*, 1029. [CrossRef] [PubMed]
36. Strath, S.J.; Brage, S.Ø.; Ekelund, U. Integration of Physiological and Accelerometer Data to Improve Physical Activity Assessment. *Med. Sci. Sports Exerc.* **2005**, *37*, S563–S571. [CrossRef] [PubMed]
37. Gilgen-Ammann, R.; Koller, M.; Huber, C.; Ahola, R.; Korhonen, T.; Wyss, T. Energy Expenditure Estimation from Respiration Variables. *Sci. Rep.* **2017**, *7*, 15995. [CrossRef] [PubMed]
38. Gastinger, S.; Sorel, A.; Nicolas, G.; Gratas-Delamarche, A.; Prioux, J. A Comparison between Ventilation and Heart Rate as Indicator of Oxygen Uptake During Different Intensities of Exercise. *J. Sports Sci. Med.* **2010**, *9*, 110–118. [PubMed]
39. Loriga, G.; Taccini, N.; de Rossi, D.; Paradiso, R. Textile Sensing Interfaces for Cardiopulmonary Signs Monitoring. In Proceedings of the 27th Annual International Conference of the Engineering in Medicine and Biology Society, New York, NY, USA, 31 August–3 September 2006.
40. Seoane, F.; Ferreira, J.; Alvarez, L.; Buendia, R.; Ayllón, D.; Llerena, C.; Gil-Pita, R. Sensorized Garments and Textrode-Enabled Measurement Instrumentation for Ambulatory Assessment of the Autonomic Nervous System Response in the Atrec Project. *Sensors* **2013**, *13*, 8997–9015. [CrossRef] [PubMed]
41. De Rossi, D.; Carpi, F.; Lorussi, F.; Mazzoldi, A.; Paradiso, R.; Scilingo, E.P.; Tognetti, A. Electroactive Fabrics and Wearable Biomonitoring Devices. *AUTEX Res. J.* **2003**, *3*, 180–185.

42. Lanatà, A.; Scilingo, E.P.; Nardini, E.; Loriga, G.; Paradiso, R.; De-Rossi, D. Comparative Evaluation of Susceptibility to Motion Artifact in Different Wearable Systems for Monitoring Respiratory Rate. *IEEE Trans. Inform. Technol. Biomed.* **2010**, *14*, 378–386. [CrossRef] [PubMed]
43. Młyńczak, M.C.; Niewiadomski, W.; Żyliński, M.; Cybulski, G.P. Ambulatory Impedance Pneumography Device for Quantitative Monitoring of Volumetric Parameters in Respiratory and Cardiac Applications. In Proceedings of the Computing in Cardiology Conference (CinC), Cambridge, MA, USA, 7–10 September 2014.
44. Abtahi, F.; Yang, L.; Lindecrantz, K.; Seoane, F.; Diaz-Olivazrez, J.A.; Ke, L.; Eklund, J.; Teriö, H.; Mediavilla Martinez, C.; Tiemann, C. Big Data & Wearable Sensors Ensuring Safety and Health@ Work. In Proceedings of the GLOBAL HEALTH 2017, The Sixth International Conference on Global Health Challenges, Barcelona, Spain, 12–16 November 2017.
45. Yang, L.; Lu, K.; Diaz-Olivares, J.A.; Seoane, F.; Lindecrantz, K.; Forsman, M.; Abtahi, F.; Eklund, J.A. Towards Smart Work Clothing for Automatic Risk Assessment of Physical Workload. *IEEE Access* **2018**, *6*, 40059–40072. [CrossRef]
46. Mohino-Herranz, I.; Gil-Pita, R.; Ferreira, J.; Rosa-Zurera, M.; Seoane, F. Assessment of Mental, Emotional and Physical Stress through Analysis of Physiological Signals Using Smartphones. *Sensors* **2015**, *15*, 25607–25627. [CrossRef] [PubMed]
47. Sykes, K.; Roberts, A. The Chester Step Test—A Simple yet Effective Tool for the Prediction of Aerobic Capacity. *Physiotherapy* **2004**, *90*, 183–188. [CrossRef]
48. Yang, L.; Lu, K.; Forsman, M.; Lindecrantz, K.; Seoane, F.; Ekblom, Ö.; Eklund, J. Development of Smart Wearable Systems for Physiological Workload Assessment Using Heart Rate and Accelerometry. Unpublished work. 2018.
49. Seppa, V.P.; Viik, J.; Hyttinen, J. Assessment of Pulmonary Flow Using Impedance Pneumography. *IEEE Trans. Biomed. Eng.* **2010**, *57*, 2277–2285. [CrossRef] [PubMed]
50. Seppä, V.P.; Hyttinen, J.; Uitto, M.; Chrapek, W.; Viik, J. Novel Electrode Configuration for Highly Linear Impedance Pneumography. *Biomed. Eng.* **2013**, *58*, 35–38. [CrossRef] [PubMed]

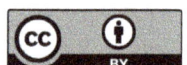

© 2018 by the authors. Licensee MDPI, Basel, Switzerland. This article is an open access article distributed under the terms and conditions of the Creative Commons Attribution (CC BY) license (http://creativecommons.org/licenses/by/4.0/).

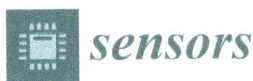

Article

Detection of Talking in Respiratory Signals: A Feasibility Study Using Machine Learning and Wearable Textile-Based Sensors

Andreas Ejupi and Carlo Menon *

Menrva Research Group, Schools of Mechatronic Systems & Engineering Science at Simon Fraser University (SFU), Burnaby, BC V5A 1S6, Canada; andreas@ejupi.at
* Correspondence: cmenon@sfu.ca

Received: 27 June 2018; Accepted: 25 July 2018; Published: 31 July 2018

Abstract: Social isolation and loneliness are major health concerns in young and older people. Traditional approaches to monitor the level of social interaction rely on self-reports. The goal of this study was to investigate if wearable textile-based sensors can be used to accurately detect if the user is talking as a future indicator of social interaction. In a laboratory study, fifteen healthy young participants were asked to talk while performing daily activities such as sitting, standing and walking. It is known that the breathing pattern differs significantly between normal and speech breathing (i.e., talking). We integrated resistive stretch sensors into wearable elastic bands, with a future integration into clothing in mind, to record the expansion and contraction of the chest and abdomen while breathing. We developed an algorithm incorporating machine learning and evaluated its performance in distinguishing between periods of talking and non-talking. In an intra-subject analysis, our algorithm detected talking with an average accuracy of 85%. The highest accuracy of 88% was achieved during sitting and the lowest accuracy of 80.6% during walking. Complete segments of talking were correctly identified with 96% accuracy. From the evaluated machine learning algorithms, the random forest classifier performed best on our dataset. We demonstrate that wearable textile-based sensors in combination with machine learning can be used to detect when the user is talking. In the future, this approach may be used as an indicator of social interaction to prevent social isolation and loneliness.

Keywords: wearable sensors; machine learning; smart textiles; healthcare; talking detection

1. Introduction

Social isolation and loneliness are important health risk factors and known to negatively influence wellbeing. It has been reported that up to 50% of older people suffer from a low level of social interaction [1]. The causes can be diverse including general health issues, disabilities and certain life events such as the loss of a spouse or a change in residence [2,3]. On a positive note, research has shown that social isolation and loneliness can be prevented. Intervention programs such as in-person support activities or phone-mediated groups have shown promising results [3]. However, due to the limited health care resources, it would be warranted to accurately identify people who are in need of targeted interventions. Traditional approaches rely on the self-reports using questionnaires to assess the daily level of social interaction. Self-reports are often described as subjective and influenced by a recall bias [4].

One alternative approach could be to automatically identify people with a low level of social interaction by using technology. Previous work in this area has mainly focused on audio-based systems using a microphone to capture talking throughout the day [5,6]. Previous work has also investigated the use of video-based systems to monitor mouth movements as an indicator of social interaction [7,8].

Both methods look promising in terms of accuracy. However, user acceptance and portability might be a challenge [9].

There is a need for more unobtrusive and portable solutions. We propose to detect if someone is talking by using wearable textile-based sensors, which can be directly integrated into everyday clothing. Our approach does not rely on audio or video recordings; instead, it aims to detect talking by monitoring changes in the respiratory (i.e., breathing) patterns.

1.1. Detection of Talking (Speech Breathing)

Generally, breathing results in an expansion and a contraction of the chest and abdominal region. It has been found that the breathing pattern differs significantly between normal and speech breathing (i.e., talking), with the respiration more rhythmic during normal breathing [10,11]. It has been also reported that the inhalation duration and the ratio between the inhalation and exhalation time are good discriminatory indicators [12,13].

To date, only a few studies have investigated the use of wearable sensors to detect if someone is talking based on respiratory markers [10,12,14]. These studies used inductive plethysmography sensors, which consist of electrical wires embedded in elastic bands usually attached to the chest and abdominal region. By generating a magnetic field and passing it through a sinusoidal arrangement of electrical wires, the self-conductance of the coils, which is proportional to the cross-sectional area surrounded by the band, can be measured [12]. However, these sensors are primarily designed for clinical settings and mainly used for short duration recordings.

1.2. Textile-Based Sensors

In this paper, we investigate the feasibility of wearable textile-based sensors. In particular, we focus on resistive stretch sensors, which are made by a mixture of polymer (e.g., silicone, rubber) and a conductive material (e.g., carbon black). These resistive sensors act like a resistor, which means that any elongation results in a measurable change in electrical resistance. Related work in this field has investigated the use of textile-based stretch sensors in several human applications. For example, Tognetti et al. [15] investigated a textile-based sensor for posture monitoring. Similarly, Mattman et al. [16] integrated sensors into tight-fitting clothing to classify between various body postures. Papi et al. [17] explored the feasibility to discriminate between daily activities (i.e., walking, running, stair climbing) by using a stretch sensor attached to the knee. These studies suggest the preliminary feasibility of textile-based stretch sensors to monitor human motions. To the best of our knowledge, our study is the first to use this type of sensor to detect talking in respiratory signals.

The main aims of this study were to (1) investigate the feasibility of textile-based stretch sensors to monitor breathing patterns, (2) develop an algorithm using machine learning to accurately detect talking and (3) evaluate its performance in a study with 15 participants.

2. Materials and Methods

2.1. Stretch Sensor

In this paper, we investigated the feasibility of a wearable textile-based stretch sensor to detect if someone is talking. The stretch sensor has been fabricated in our research lab (Menrva) at Simon Fraser University, Canada [18], using a mixture of polymer and conductive carbon black. The sensor shows similar properties as the commercially available sensors from Adafruit (New York, NY, USA) [19] and Image SI (Staten Island, NY, USA) [20], but only has a diameter of 0.4 mm, which makes it suitable to integrate into garments (Figure 1). Previous work has shown good results in using machine learning to obtain accurate measurements from these textile-based stretch sensors [21,22] and using them for the monitoring of human movements [15,16,23].

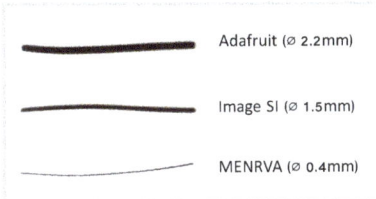

Figure 1. Comparison between the Adafruit, Image SI and Menrva sensors.

2.2. Chest and Abdominal Bands

The approach was to detect talking based on changes in the breathing pattern. As is known from the literature, we can differentiate between chest and abdominal breathing [24,25]. Chest breathing can be described as the drawing of air into the chest area by using the intercostal muscles. This type of breathing is more common during states of exertion. In contrast, abdominal breathing is the expansion of the belly by contracting the diaphragm. This type of breathing is common during phases of relaxation [26].

However, breathing can be quite diverse between people. Some people are more heavily chest breathers, whereas others are more so abdominal breathers [25]. To capture the expansion and contraction of the full torso, we designed three elastic bands with the stretch sensor integrated and positioned them at the abdominal, lower and upper chest region for our study (Figure 2). In the future, the sensor might be directly integrated into the clothing.

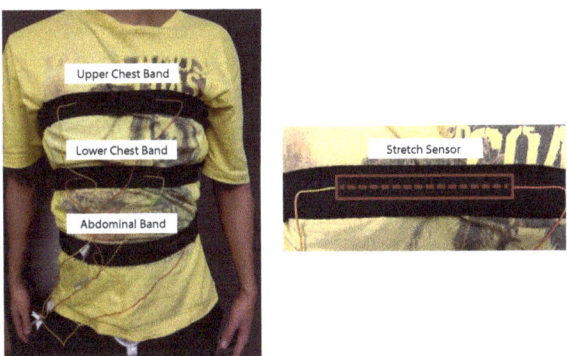

Figure 2. Three custom-made sensor bands to monitor the expansion and contraction of the torso while breathing (and talking). The red dashed line shows the positioning of the sensor.

The bands were made out of two materials. The back and side part were made out of a synthetic knit with medium elasticity. The front piece and attachment of the sensor were made of a fleece material with high elasticity. The intention was to concentrate the stretch during breathing (and talking) primarily on the sensor. Three pieces of the Menrva stretch sensor with a length of 10 cm each were integrated into the front piece of the bands (Figure 2). Sensors were laid out straight and secured with an elastic stitch on top. The wires were connected on both sides with a mixture of rubber glue and conductive ink.

2.3. Data Acquisition Hardware

The three bands were connected to a data acquisition system (Model NI-USB-6009, National Instruments, Austin, TX, USA) using a voltage divider circuit to measure their electrical response by connecting a 5 V DC voltage source and a resistor in series to the sensors. The resistor value was selected to match the base resistance of the stretch sensor (20 kΩ). All data were captured with a sampling rate of 100 Hz.

2.4. Study Protocol

The study protocol included three main parts with a total duration of 1.5 h per participant including the setup time. Participants were asked to wear the three custom-made sensors to monitor the expansion and contraction of the torso while talking. Sensor bands were tightly fitted, but still comfortable, for each participant. The tightness was adjusted based on the user's feedback by explaining that the bands should be similarly tight and comfortable as, for example, a tight-fitting t-shirt, usually used for exercising. Participants were asked to talk while sitting, standing and walking. We selected these activities because they are the most common activities in which people talk in daily life. Each activity lasted for 20 min and included 5 trials with 2 min of non-talking and 2 min of talking. The order of the activities was randomized. To capture sufficient data of talking during each period and activity, we asked the participants to read out the text of a news article. The article included general information about the city of Vancouver, Canada. For the walking part, participants were asked to walk on a treadmill. We used a treadmill for convenience due to the limited length of the wires, which connected the bands with the data acquisition hardware. Talking while walking usually occurs at slower speed, and therefore, we selected 2 mph for this test.

2.5. Participants

Fifteen young adults were asked to participate in this study. Participants were between 19 and 30 years old and were students at Simon Fraser University (SFU), Canada. Table 1 shows the participant characteristics. Written informed consent was obtained from all participants prior to data collection. The study was approved by the Research Ethics Board of SFU.

Table 1. Participant characteristics.

	Study Participants (*n* = 15)
Age (years)	23 (3.8)
Gender (F/M)	6/9
Height (cm)	169.8 (8.9)
Weight (kg)	68.5 (12.1)
BMI (kg/m^2)	23.6 (3.1)

2.6. Talking Detection Algorithm

Our main aim was to detect talking based on changes in the respiratory signals. Before talking, air usually gets inhaled fast and then exhaled slowly while talking. This results in a specific breathing pattern when compared to normal breathing (Figure 3). Our algorithm utilizes this information to detect talking.

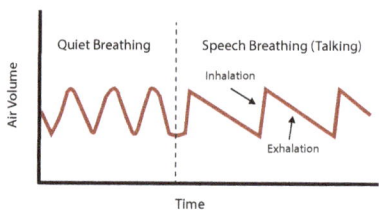

Figure 3. Changes in the air volume while talking.

Our algorithm is based on the following steps of data processing and analysis (Figure 4):

- Data input: The input data to our algorithm were the raw sensor signals (sampled with 100 Hz) of the three bands, which we converted from voltage to resistance values.
- Signal filtering: A healthy adult usually breathes between 12 and 18 times per minute at rest. For older adults, the breathing can vary between 12 and 30 times per minute [27]. We filtered the sensor signals accordingly with a bandpass filter (4th order Butterworth, lower cut-off frequency of 0.1 Hz and higher cut-off of 1.5 Hz) to account for possible drift and reduce the overall level of noise in the sensor signals.
- Breathing detection: Any inhalation of air and consequent expansion of the torso results in a peak of the stretch sensor signal. Our algorithm detects these peaks using MATLAB's peak detection algorithm with an empirically-defined parameter of 5 for the minimum peak prominence setting. The prominence of a peak measures how much the peak stands out due to its intrinsic height and its location relative to other peaks.
- Feature extraction: The detection of a peak triggers the feature extraction process. The algorithm centres a window with an empirically-found length of 3 s on each detected peak. From this time window, a set of predefined features get extracted and used as the input to a machine learning classifier.
- Classification of talking: A machine learning classifier has been trained to detect speech breathing (i.e., talking) based on the extracted features.

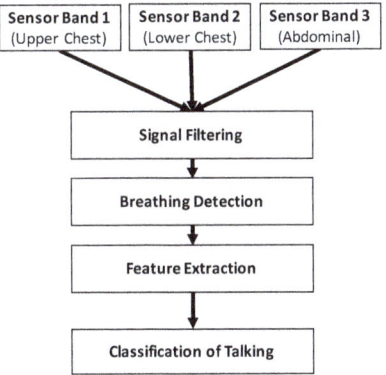

Figure 4. Design of the talking detection algorithm incorporating machine learning.

2.7. Machine Learning Approach

In the first part of the analysis, we were focused on identifying which machine learning algorithm, hyper parameters and features would generally perform best in the task of detecting talking using this kind of technology. In the second part of the analysis, we applied the selected model and calculated the accuracy for each participant.

2.7.1. Model Selection

Four machine learning algorithms have been selected to investigate their feasibility in detecting talking based on our collected data. We have selected these four algorithms because they have been commonly used in health-related machine learning tasks and have achieved promising results in the past. First, random forest is an ensemble method that operates by constructing multiple decision trees at training time and then uses the mean prediction of individual trees to estimate the target values [28]. Second, neural network is a method inspired by the biological neural network system using layers and a number of interconnected nodes to make a prediction [29]. Third, support vector machine operates by constructing a set of hyperplanes in a high- or infinite-dimensional space to estimate the target value [30]. Fourth, linear discriminant analysis uses a linear decision boundary and has been proven to work well in practice due to its low computational costs [31].

The hyper parameters for the machine learning classifiers were empirically identified. To calculate the performance of each model and select the best performing hyper parameters, we used 15-fold cross-validation. This was done on a training dataset that consisted of the first 70% of data of each participant. The model performance was evaluated using the receiver operating characteristics curve (ROC) and the associated area under the curve (AUC) metric.

For the random forest classifier, the best performance was achieved using 200 as the parameter for the number of trees (values tested between 10 and 200). For the support vector machine, the best performance was achieved with gamma set to 0.01 (tested between 0.001 and 1) and C set to 10 (tested between 1 and 100). For the neural network classifier, the best performance was achieved with a network structure of 2 hidden layers (tested from 1 to 2) and 30 neurons in the hidden layers.

2.7.2. Feature Extraction and Selection

Features were extracted with an automated feature extraction approach. Therefore, we used the Python library tsfresh [32], which calculates and tests more than 100 predefined time and frequency-domain features with various parameters. Using this approach, we extracted features from the raw and first derivate of the sensor signals of all three bands. Features were extracted using a sliding window (size of 3 s) approach. For the feature selection, we also applied 15-fold cross-validation and used the same training dataset as for the hyper parameter tuning. A tree-based approach was used to rank the best performing features based on their relevance (i.e., Gini importance [33]) for each run. Only the top 10% features among all runs were selected for the final algorithm to reduce complexity and computation time. For a detailed description of the calculation of these features, see [32]. The majority of significant features were based on the sensor signals of the upper chest and lower chest band. The features included in our final model were:

- Ratio beyond sigma: the ratio of values that are more than $r \times std(x)$ away from the mean of x (with $r = \{1, 2\}$).
- Symmetry looking: the Boolean variable denoting if the distribution of x looks symmetric.
- Continues Wavelet Transform peaks: the number of peaks of the continuous wavelet transform using a Mexican hat wavelet [34].
- Skewness: the sample skewness of x (calculated with the adjusted Fisher–Pearson standardized moment coefficient G1).
- Energy ratio by chunks: the sum of squares of chunk i out of N chunks expressed as a ratio with the sum of squares over the whole (with $N = 10$).
- Augmented Dickey–Fuller: the hypothesis test that checks whether a unit root is present in x [35].
- Count above mean: the number of values in x that are higher than the mean of x.
- Count below mean: the number of values in x that are lower than the mean of x.
- Number of crossings: the number of crossings of x on m (with $m = 0$).
- Fourier coefficients: the coefficients of the one-dimensional discrete Fourier transform [36].
- Welch's spectral density: the cross power spectral density of x [37].
- Sample entropy: the sample entropy of x.
- Autoregressive coefficients: the fit of the unconditional maximum likelihood of an autoregressive $AR(k)$ process.

2.7.3. Performance Evaluation

We integrated the best performing machine learning model, features and parameters into our algorithm and evaluated its performance in detecting talking in an intra-subject analysis. The data of each participant were split into the activities of sitting, standing and walking. For each activity, we trained a model separately and evaluated it using cross-validation.

As sample-based performance metrics, accuracy (*ACC*), true positive rate (*TPR*) and false positive rate (*FPR*) were selected. *TPR* has been defined as the percentage of correctly identified speech breathing patterns. *FPR* has been defined as the percentage of incorrectly identified speech breathing patterns among all other breathing patterns.

$$ACC = \frac{TP + TN}{TP + TN + FP + FN} \quad (1)$$

$$TPR = \frac{TP}{TP + FN} \quad (2)$$

$$FPR = \frac{FP}{FP + TN} \quad (3)$$

Furthermore, the number of correctly identified talking segments was calculated. A talking segment was classified correctly if the majority of prediction labels in this segment predicted talking.

$$ACC_{seg} = \frac{correctly\_classified\_talking\_segments}{total\_number\_of\_talking\_segments} \quad (4)$$

2.8. Software

MATLAB (R2016b) was used for data acquisition, processing of the sensor data and algorithm development. The Python package scikit-learn [38] was used to train and evaluate the machine learning models. The Python package tsfresh [32] was used for automated feature extraction.

3. Results

One hour of sensor data was recorded from each participant with a recording time of 30 min of talking. The entire dataset included 11,924 detected breathings, which were used for further classification. We observed significant differences between normal and speech breathing in the activities of sitting, standing and walking (Figure 5). During the phases of talking, the breathing is less rhythmic with faster inhalations and slower exhalations.

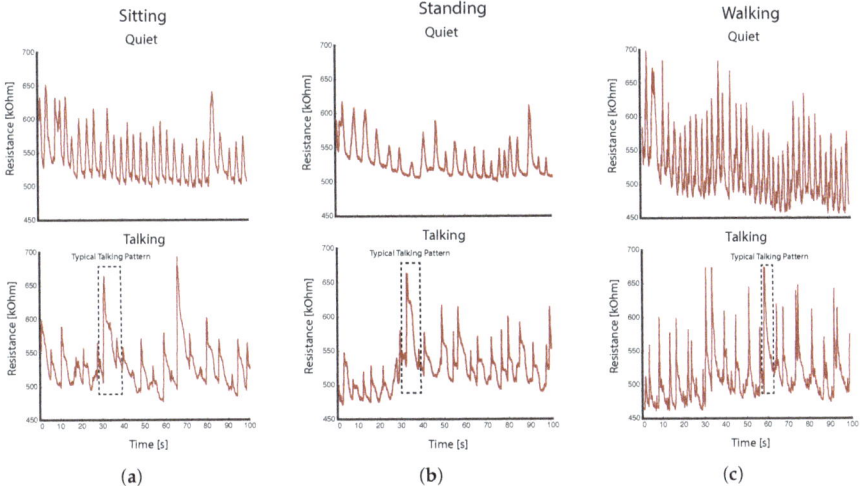

Figure 5. Comparison of the raw sensor signals (upper chest band) between quiet and speech breathing (i.e., talking) for: (**a**) sitting; (**b**) standing; and (**c**) walking.

3.1. Model Selection

Among all tested machine learning algorithms, the random forest (and support vector machine) classifier performed best on our dataset with an AUC value of 0.90, which was slightly higher compared to the performance of the neural network classifier (AUC = 0.89) and linear discriminant analysis (AUC = 0.87) (Figure 6).

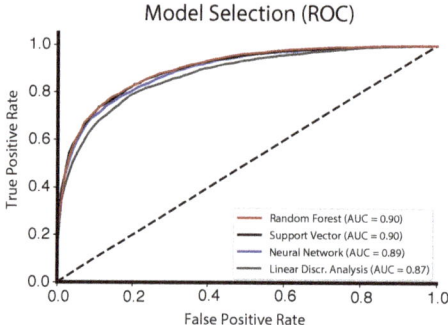

Figure 6. Comparison of the ROC curves (and the associated AUC metric) among the tested machine learning algorithms.

3.2. Accuracy of Talking Detection Algorithm

Among all participants, our algorithm utilizing the random forest classifier detected talking with an average ACC of 85% (TPR: 81.3%, FPR: 12.8%) (Table 2). The highest ACC of 88% was achieved in the sitting task and the lowest ACC of 80.6% in walking. Table 3 shows the results for each participant in detail with the accuracy ranging from 68.8% to 97.5%. Furthermore, segments of talking have been correctly classified with an ACC_{seg} of 96.3%. Figure 7 illustrates the exemplary prediction accuracy of our algorithm on the data of participant P10. The number of misclassifications increased from sitting, standing to walking.

Table 2. Average performance of our algorithm in detecting talking among all participants.

	Average ACC	Average TPR	Average FPR
Sitting	88.0 (5.4)	88.0 (6.1)	12.6 (6.9)
Standing	86.3 (7.3)	84.2 (8.6)	12.5 (7.6)
Walking	80.6 (7.7)	71.8 (12.1)	13.3 (6.5)
Average	85.0 (6.8)	81.3 (8.9)	12.8 (7.0)

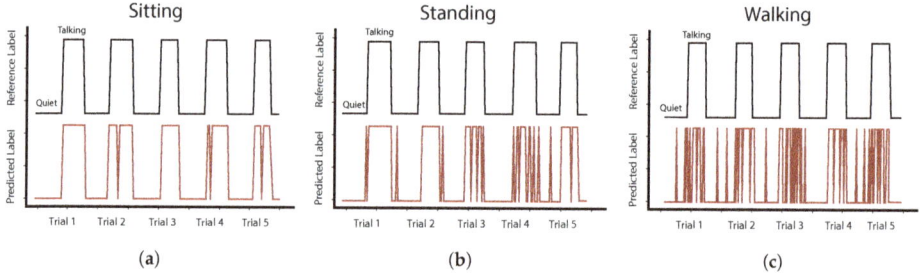

Figure 7. Exemplary detection of talking for participant P10 in activities: (**a**) sitting; (**b**) standing; and (**c**) walking.

Table 3. Performance results of our algorithm in detecting talking for each participant (P).

	P01			P02			P03			P04			P05		
	ACC	TPR	FPR	ACC	TPR	FPR	ACC	TPR	FPR	ACC	TPR	FPR	ACC	TPR	FPR
Sitting	94.3	92.3	3.9	94.8	93.5	4.2	97.5	94.9	0.9	84.9	84.9	15.0	82.9	81.2	15.6
Standing	93.9	92.2	4.4	90.5	90.0	9.1	94.2	91.5	3.7	76.1	73.1	21.3	86.0	79.1	9.9
Walking	79.6	76.4	17.6	85.2	81.0	11.6	90.2	82.4	4.4	68.8	55.3	20.7	87.2	83.6	9.8
	P06			P07			P08			P09			P10		
Sitting	81.6	87.7	24.2	88.6	95.1	20.2	93.7	93.1	5.9	89.3	93.3	14.6	92.0	90.9	7.3
Standing	82.5	79.2	14.7	94.0	94.9	7.1	95.1	92.5	2.9	93.6	96.1	8.9	87.0	81.4	9.1
Walking	71.1	70.5	28.5	87.8	84.7	9.3	95.6	90.8	1.4	79.7	75.4	17.0	81.1	68.2	11.9
	P11			P12			P13			P14			P15		
Sitting	82.7	82.0	16.7	89.8	87.0	7.9	83.5	89.3	22.7	84.3	79.1	12.6	79.3	75.0	16.7
Standing	73.9	73.8	26.1	83.3	70.8	9.0	78.7	76.2	18.8	75.8	79.5	28.2	89.8	93.2	13.9
Walking	68.3	42.5	14.8	79.4	69.4	13.5	73.0	61.3	18.6	81.7	68.2	9.9	80.0	66.9	9.9

4. Discussion

We developed an algorithm that can detect if the user is talking based on respiratory markers. In contrast to previous work, we used textile-based stretch sensors to monitor the expansion and contraction of the torso and achieved a reasonable accuracy by incorporating machine learning into our algorithm.

Previous studies have relied on either audio or video recordings to detect talking. Besides the technical challenges of these approaches, there might be also privacy concerns [9]. The aim of this study was to develop a system that is unobtrusive and portable. We selected a wearable approach, as it would allow quantifying talking throughout the day independent of the user's location. This is in alignment with a recent trend in the development of the wearable technologies for various health applications [39,40].

Our approach uses wearable textile-based sensors to monitor breathing and as a consequence detect if someone is talking. Although there were some studies that have investigated the feasibility of detecting respiratory events in the past, only a few studies have focused on the detection of talking in respiratory signals [10,12,14]. These studies have used inductive plethysmograph sensors. Conventional inductive plethysmograph sensors are primarily designed for the clinical setting and short-term recordings with possible limitations in the size of the electronics and number of sensors that can be used at the same time [41].

In terms of accuracy, Rahman et al. [10] (and Bari et al. [42]) reported 82 to 87% in speech/non-speech classification using inductive plethysmograph sensors. The reported accuracy is in alignment with what we have achieved in this study.

What differentiates this work is the use of textile-based stretch sensors in combination with the developed machine learning-based algorithm. The sensor we used is flexible with a diameter of only 0.4 mm and acts like a resistor, which makes it easy to integrate into garments and to acquire measurements. We proposed an algorithm suitable to detect talking including a comprehensive identified and discriminative set of features upon which future work can build.

What we have observed is that breathing and the corresponding patterns were quite heterogeneous between participants. Breathing was either shallow, normal or deep, and for some participants, the chest expansion was more noticeable, whereas for others, the abdominal region expanded more. We compensated for this behaviour by training our algorithm individually for each participant. In practice, this would suggest that a calibration phase might be needed before the system can be used by an individual. Another factor that might have influenced the accuracy was the sensitivity of the technology to noise due to body movements. Breathing and the corresponding expansion of the torso result in a relatively small elongation of the stretch sensor. What we have observed is that rotational and bending movements of the upper body influenced the measurements. This was especially noticeable in the task of walking, which might explain the lower accuracy in this task. Future work might combine our approach with an accelerometer to filter out the noise due to body movements.

Considering the advantages of the technology, this approach might be suitable for the daily life setting. A future application could be the integration of the sensor (or a series of sensors) into a tight-fitting undershirt. In addition to the sensor, a circuit board and battery would be required. Preliminary results show that the sensor has a power draw of about 1.25 mW (as used in this study). This would allow the monitoring of the user's level of talking throughout the day, and furthermore, this measurement could be used as an indicator of social interaction. Such a system might be used in older adults where social isolation and loneliness are common concerns [1,3]. For example, in an institutionalized setting, such a system could provide the staff daily feedback about the level of social interaction of each resident. Once a significant change in behaviour has been detected, targeted interventions could be started. Similarly, this technology could be used in older people living in the community where a low level of social interaction can lead to more frequent home visits by the healthcare professionals.

We acknowledge certain study limitations. Data were collected in the laboratory setting under fairly controlled conditions with young and healthy adults. Participants were asked to read a text out loud, which might be different from conversational speaking. Future studies are warranted to determine whether this approach can be used in a daily life setting and to investigate the accuracy and user acceptance of this system in the older population.

In summary, we have demonstrated that wearable textile-based sensors in combination with a machine learning-based algorithm can be used to detect when the user is talking. In future, this approach may be used to unobtrusively quantify talking as an indicator of social interaction, and consequently may prevent social isolation and loneliness.

Author Contributions: All authors read and approved the manuscript. Conceptualization, A.E. and C.M. Software, A.E. Validation, A.E. Formal analysis, A.E. Investigation, A.E. Resources, A.E. and C.M. Data curation, A.E. and C.M.; Writing—Original Draft Preparation, A.E.; Writing—Review & Editing, A.E. and C.M. Visualization, A.E. Supervision, C.M. Project administration, C.M. Funding acquisition, C.M.

Funding: This study was supported by operating grants from the Natural Sciences and Engineering Research Council of Canada (NSERC), the Canadian Institutes of Health Research (CIHR) and the Canada Research Chair (CRC) program.

Acknowledgments: The authors would like to thank all participants and individuals who contributed to the data collection.

Conflicts of Interest: The authors declare no conflict of interest.

References

1. Grenade, L.; Boldy, D. Social isolation and loneliness among older people: Issues and future challenges in community and residential settings. *Aust. Health Rev.* **2008**, *32*, 468–478. [CrossRef] [PubMed]
2. Cattan, M.; White, M.; Bond, J.; Learmouth, A. Preventing social isolation and loneliness among older people: A systematic review of health promotion interventions. *Ageing Soc.* **2005**, *25*, 41–67. [CrossRef]
3. Health Quality Ontario. *Social Isolation in Community-Dwelling Seniors: An Evidence-Based Analysis*; Health Quality Ontario: Toronto, ON, Canada, 2008; Volume 8, pp. 1–49.
4. Coughlin, S.S. Recall bias in epidemiologic studies. *J. Clin. Epidemiol.* **1990**, *43*, 87–91. [CrossRef]
5. Choudhury, T.; Pentland, A. Sensing and modeling human networks using the sociometer. In Proceedings of the Seventh IEEE International Symposium on Wearable Computers, White Plains, NY, USA, 21–23 October 2003; pp. 216–222.
6. Wyatt, D.; Choudhury, T.; Bilmes, J.; Kitts, J.A. Inferring colocation and conversation networks from privacy-sensitive audio with implications for computational social science. *ACM Trans. Intell. Syst. Technol.* **2011**, *2*, 1–41. [CrossRef]
7. Cristani, M.; Pesarin, A.; Vinciarelli, A.; Crocco, M.; Murino, V. Look at who's talking: Voice Activity Detection by Automated Gesture Analysis. In Proceedings of the European Conference on Ambient Intelligence, Amsterdam, The Netherlands, 16–18 November 2011; pp. 72–80.

8. Rao, R.R. Cross-modal prediction in audio-visual communication. In Proceedings of the 1996 IEEE International Conference on Acoustics, Speech, and Signal Processing, Atlanta, GA, USA, 9 May 1996.
9. Klasnja, P.; Consolvo, S.; Choudhury, T.; Beckwith, R.; Hightower, J. Exploring privacy concerns about personal sensing. *Lect. Notes Comput. Sci.* **2009**, *5538*, 176–183.
10. Rahman, M.; Ahsan, A.; Plarre, K.; al'Absi, M.; Ertin, E.; Kumar, S. mConverse: Inferring Conversation Episodes from Respiratory Measurements Collected in the Field. In Proceedings of the 2nd Conference on Wireless Health, San Diego, CA, USA, 10–13 October 2011.
11. Fuchs, S.; Reichel, U.D.; Rochet-Capellan, A. Changes in speech and breathing rate while speaking and biking. In Proceedings of the 18th International Congress of Phonetic Sciences (ICPhS 2015), Glasgow, UK, 10–14 August 2015.
12. Wilhelm, F.H.; Handke, E.; Roth, W. Detection of speaking with a new respiratory inductive plethysmography system. *Biomed. Sci. Instrum.* **2003**, *39*, 136–141. [PubMed]
13. Haugh, M. Conversational Interaction. In *The Cambridge Handbook of Pragmatics*; Cambridge University Press: Cambridge, UK, 2012; pp. 251–274.
14. Ramos-Garcia, R.I.; Tiffany, S.; Sazonov, E. Using respiratory signals for the recognition of human activities. In Proceedings of the 2016 38th Annual International Conference of the IEEE Engineering in Medicine and Biology Society (EMBC), Orlando, FL, USA, 16–20 August 2016; pp. 173–176.
15. Tognetti, A.; Bartalesi, R.; Lorussi, F.; De Rossi, D. Body segment position reconstruction and posture classification by smart textiles. *Trans. Inst. Meas. Control* **2007**, *29*, 215–253. [CrossRef]
16. Mattmann, C.; Amft, O.; Harms, H.; Troester, G.; Clemens, F. Recognizing upper body postures using textile strain sensors. In Proceedings of the 2007 11th IEEE International Symposium on Wearable Computers (ISWC), Boston, MA, USA, 11–13 October 2007; pp. 29–36.
17. Papi, E.; Spulber, I.; Kotti, M.; Georgiou, P.; McGregor, A.H. Smart sensing system for combined activity classification and estimation of knee range of motion. *IEEE Sens. J.* **2015**, *15*, 5535–5544. [CrossRef]
18. Ferrone, A.; Maita, F.; Maiolo, L.; Arquilla, M.; Castiello, A.; Pecora, A.; Jiang, X.; Menon, C.; Ferrone, A.; Colace, L.; et al. Wearable band for hand gesture recognition based on strain sensors. In Proceedings of the IEEE RAA/EMBS International Conference on Biomedical Robotics and Biomechatronics, Singapore, 26–29 June 2016; pp. 4–7.
19. Adafruit. Available online: https://www.adafruit.com/ (accessed on 10 June 2018).
20. Images SI. Available online: https://www.imagesco.com/ (accessed on 10 June 2018).
21. Ejupi, A.; Ferrone, A.; Menon, C. Quantification of textile-based stretch sensors using machine learning: An exploratory study. In Proceedings of the IEEE International Conference on Biomedical Robotics and Biomechatronics (BioRob), Twente, The Netherlands, 26–29 August 2018.
22. Gholami, M.; Ejupi, A.; Rezaei, A.; Ferrone, A.; Menon, C. Estimation of Knee Joint Angle using a Fabric-based Strain Sensor and Machine Learning: A Preliminary Investigation. In Proceedings of the IEEE International Conference on Biomedical Robotics and Biomechatronics (BioRob), Twente, The Netherlands, 26–29 August 2018.
23. Rezaei, A.; Ejupi, A.; Gholami, M.; Ferrone, A.; Menon, C. Preliminary Investigation of Textile-Based Strain Sensors for the Detection of Human Gait Phases Using Machine Learning. In Proceedings of the IEEE International Conference on Biomedical Robotics and Biomechatronics (BioRob), Twente, The Netherlands, 26–29 August 2018.
24. Gilbert, R.; Auschincloss, J.H.; Peppi, D. Relationship of rib cage and abdomen motion to diaphragm function during quiet breathing. *Chest* **1981**, *80*, 607–612. [CrossRef] [PubMed]
25. Kaneko, H.; Horie, J. Breathing movements of the chest and abdominal wall in healthy subjects. *Respir. Care* **2012**, *57*, 1442–1451. [CrossRef] [PubMed]
26. Grimby, G.; Bunn, J.; Mead, J. Relative contribution of rib cage and abdomen to ventilation during exercise. *J. Appl. Physiol.* **1968**, *24*, 159–166. [CrossRef] [PubMed]
27. McFadden, J.P.; Price, R.; Eastwood, H.D.; Briggs, R. Raised respiratory rate in elderly patients: A valuable physical sign. *Br. Med. J. (Clin. Res. Ed.)* **1982**, *284*, 626–627. [CrossRef]
28. Liaw, A.; Wiener, M. Classification and Regression by randomForest. *R News* **2002**, *2*, 18–22.
29. Specht, D.F. A general regression neural network. *IEEE Trans. Neural Netw.* **1991**, *2*, 568–576. [CrossRef] [PubMed]

30. Drucker, H.; Burges, C.J.C.; Kaufman, L.; Smola, A.; Vapnik, V. Support vector regression machines. *Adv. Neural Inf. Process. Syst.* **1997**, *1*, 155–161.
31. Mika, S.; Ratsch, G.; Weston, J.; Schölkopf, B.; Muller, K.R. Fisher discriminant analysis with kernels. In Proceedings of the 1999 IEEE Signal Processing Society Workshop (Cat. No. 98TH8468), Madison, WI, USA, 25 August 1999; pp. 41–48.
32. tsfresh. Available online: http://tsfresh.readthedocs.io/ (accessed on 10 June 2018).
33. Breiman, L.; Friedman, J.H.; Olshen, R.A.; Stone, C. *Classification and Regression Trees*; Routledge: Abingdon, UK, 1984; Volume 1.
34. Grossmann, A.; Morlet, J. Decomposition of hardy functions into square integrable wavelets of constant shape. *J. Math. Anal.* **1984**, *15*, 723–736. [CrossRef]
35. Cheung, Y.W.; La, K.S. Lag order and critical values of the augmented dickey-fuller test. *J. Bus. Econ. Stat.* **1995**, *13*, 277–280.
36. Cooley, J.W.; Lewis, P.A.W.; Welch, P.D. The fast fourier transform and its applications. *IEEE Trans. Educ.* **1969**, *12*, 27–34. [CrossRef]
37. Welch, P.D. The use of fast fourier transform for the estimation of power spectra: A method based on time averaging over short, modified periodograms. *IEEE Trans. Audio Electroacoust.* **1967**, *15*, 70–73. [CrossRef]
38. Pedregosa, F.; Varoquaux, G. Scikit-Learn: Machine Learning in Python. *J. Mach. Learn. Res.* **2011**, *12*, 2825–2830.
39. Ejupi, A.; Lord, S.R.; Delbaere, K. New methods for fall risk prediction. *Curr. Opin. Clin. Nutr. Metab. Care* **2014**, *17*, 407–411. [CrossRef] [PubMed]
40. Mukhopadhyay, S.C. Wearable sensors for human activity monitoring: A review. *IEEE Sens. J.* **2014**, *15*, 1321–1330. [CrossRef]
41. Zhang, C.; Tian, Y. RGB-D camera-based daily living activity recognition. *J. Comput. Vis. Image Process.* **2012**, *2*, 12.
42. Bari, R.; Adams, R.J.; Rahman, M.; Parsons, M.B.; Buder, E.H.; Kumar, S. rConverse: Moment by moment conversation detection using a mobile respiration sensor. *Proc. ACM Interact. Mob. Wearable Ubiquitous Technol.* **2018**, *2*, 2:1–2:27. [CrossRef]

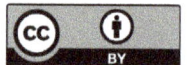

© 2018 by the authors. Licensee MDPI, Basel, Switzerland. This article is an open access article distributed under the terms and conditions of the Creative Commons Attribution (CC BY) license (http://creativecommons.org/licenses/by/4.0/).

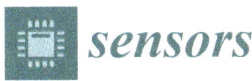

Article

Assessment of Breathing Parameters Using an Inertial Measurement Unit (IMU)-Based System

Ambra Cesareo [1], Ylenia Previtali [1], Emilia Biffi [2,*] and Andrea Aliverti [1]

1 Dipartimento di Elettronica, Informazione e Bioingegneria, Politecnico di Milano, 20133 Milan, Italy; ambra.cesareo@polimi.it (A.C.); ylenia1.previtali@mail.polimi.it (Y.P.); andrea.aliverti@polimi.it (A.A.)
2 Scientific Institute, IRCCS E. Medea, Bioengineering Lab, 23842 Bosisio Parini, Lecco, Italy
* Correspondence: emilia.biffi@lanostrafamiglia.it; Tel.: +39-031-877-862

Received: 24 October 2018; Accepted: 20 December 2018; Published: 27 December 2018

Abstract: Breathing frequency (f_B) is an important vital sign that—if appropriately monitored—may help to predict clinical adverse events. Inertial sensors open the door to the development of low-cost, wearable, and easy-to-use breathing-monitoring systems. The present paper proposes a new posture-independent processing algorithm for breath-by-breath extraction of breathing temporal parameters from chest-wall inclination change signals measured using inertial measurement units. An important step of the processing algorithm is dimension reduction (DR) that allows the extraction of a single respiratory signal starting from 4-component quaternion data. Three different DR methods are proposed and compared in terms of accuracy of breathing temporal parameter estimation, in a group of healthy subjects, considering different breathing patterns and different postures; optoelectronic plethysmography was used as reference system. In this study, we found that the method based on PCA-fusion of the four quaternion components provided the best f_B estimation performance in terms of mean absolute errors (<2 breaths/min), correlation (r > 0.963) and Bland–Altman Analysis, outperforming the other two methods, based on the selection of a single quaternion component, identified on the basis of spectral analysis; particularly, in supine position, results provided by PCA-based method were even better than those obtained with the ideal quaternion component, determined a posteriori as the one providing the minimum estimation error. The proposed algorithm and system were able to successfully reconstruct the respiration-induced movement, and to accurately determine the respiratory rate in an automatic, position-independent manner.

Keywords: principal component analysis; biomedical signal processing; wearable biomedical sensors; wireless sensor network; respiratory monitoring; optoelectronic plethysmography

1. Introduction

Continuous monitoring of respiratory parameters such as breathing frequency (f_B), inspiratory time (T_I) and expiratory time (T_E) could foster early diagnosis of a wide range of respiratory disorders and help to track a patient's condition, discriminating between stable and at-risk patients [1,2]. Conditions of interest could be sleep breathing disorders, sudden infant death syndrome, chronic obstructive pulmonary disease (COPD) and neuromuscular disorders. The current gold standard for measuring f_B is to count the number of breaths in one minute, through auscultation or observation [3,4]. Other methods for breathing function assessment currently used in clinical practice are spirometry or pneumotachograph based on airflow measurement by using mouthpiece or facemask. In overnight polysomnography, breathing activity is assessed both by measuring respiratory flow, through pressure transducer or thermistors near the nostrils, and respiratory efforts (breathing-derived chest-wall movements), by strain-gauge belts. Also, exhaled carbon dioxide sensors, transthoracic inductance and impedance plethysmography and ECG—or PPG—derived f_B have been used to measure breathing signal. Despite their accuracy, these methods are uncomfortable and intrusive, and are not suitable for continuous monitoring in the clinical environment and at home. An emerging area of interest is to use motion sensors to detect the small breathing-derived movements/orientation changes of the chest wall. This method is particularly suitable for long-term breathing monitoring because it is unobtrusive, tolerable, and low-cost. The principle was first presented with a single-axis accelerometer in animal model (dog) using a pressure transducer in the trachea as reference [5]. Starting from this point, a variety of studies demonstrated the feasibility of using one accelerometer placed on the chest wall to derive respiratory signal and/or breathing frequency in different positions [6–14]. Morillo et al. [8] combined a piezoelectric single-axis accelerometer and a polarized capacitive microphone placed on the suprasternal notch to collect information of the cardiac, respiratory, and snoring activities for the screening of patients affected by Sleep Apnea-Hypopnea Syndrome. Measurements were limited to the supine position, that was selected to increase the sensitivity of the single-axis accelerometer, limiting the generality of the findings. The analysis method was based on the estimation of breathing frequency through the identification of the peak of the spectrum or autocorrelation; the main limitation of this approach is that, when the breathing is irregular, a main peak may not exist, and individual breaths must be identified and counted. Hung et al. [7] moved from single-axis to biaxial accelerometers. The aim of their study was to evaluate the reliability of the device in terms of detection of the onsets of expiration and expiration, and to assess the feasibility of differentiating between different breathing patterns (normal breathing, apnea, deep breathing). The signals from both axes (anteroposterior and longitudinal) of the accelerometer were summed, limiting the analysis to the sagittal plane, in sitting and lying positions. An adaptive band-pass filter was applied with a variable passband centered at the detected dominant breathing frequency.

As emerged by these studies, single or dual-axis accelerometers can be used to derive breathing signal when appropriately aligned with the major axis of rotation, which changes when the subject move from a posture to another. Contrarily, the use of a tri-axial accelerometer allows measuring inclination changes due to breathing regardless of orientation. In this case, the problem lies in the identification of the accelerometer axis to consider when posture changes. Bates et al. [13] proposed a method to track the major axis of rotation as it changes, to continuously monitor angular motion due to breathing also when subject change position/orientation. An alternative possibility to the best axis selection is fusing the axes. Jin et al. [12] proposed a posture-independent signal processing method based on three possible algorithms for accelerometer axes fusion. They demonstrated that methods based on Principal Component Analysis (PCA) obtained the highest performance in terms of Signal-to-Noise Ratio (SNR), but no results were provided about breathing rate estimation or validation against a reference method.

With the entry of tri-axial accelerometers new opportunities opened for the monitoring of breathing frequency using inertial sensors, but their use was still confined to static conditions since, when the subject is moving, the degree of the movement-related signal would exceed that due to breathing. One possible approach is to identify non-breathing motion, as proposed by Bates et al [13]. In a successive study, Mann et al. [11] furtherly developed the method proposed by Bates et al. [13], by adding activity tracking, and allowing identification of asymmetric breaths, that was not possible in the original method. An attempt to remove motion artifacts by using signal processing was made by Liu et al. [14]. They proposed an elegant method based on PCA-fusion of the three axes of an accelerometer and on filtering of the first principal component by using an adaptive filter that varied according to the energy expenditure derived by the same accelerometer. To overcome the problems of using a single accelerometer in dynamic conditions, a possibility is to fuse data from accelerometers and from other sensors, such as gyroscopes. Yoon et al. [15] investigated the feasibility of measuring breathing-related motions also during dynamic activities of the subject, by fusing data from a tri-axial accelerometer and a gyroscope and applying Kalman filter. They found that, during dynamic exercises, fusion of accelerometer and gyroscope data provided benefits in terms of reduction of estimation error. Gollee et al. used a more complex system, an inertial measurement unit (IMU) fusing accelerometer, gyroscope and magnetometer but considered only static conditions [16]. Another approach to overcome the problems related to motion artefacts is modularity. Lapi et al. [17] tried to overcome limitations deriving from the use of a single accelerometer by proposing a system based on a couple of 3-axis accelerometers placed bilaterally on the chest. Using two accelerometers permitted to detect respiration-related chest-wall movements regardless of sensor positioning with respect to the gravity vector; secondly, the breathing frequency can be obtained even when one of the two sensors is silenced by postural constraints. Recently, Gaidhani at al. [18] proposed a method that uses two IMUs composed by a 3-axis accelerometer, a 3-axis gyroscope and a 3-axis magnetometer, placed on the anterior and posterior side of the chest to decompose the motions experienced by the two IMUs into trunk movements and breathing actions. This paper presents an automatic processing algorithm to derive breathing frequency and other breathing temporal parameters from quaternion-based orientation signals recorded simultaneously at thoracic and abdominal level by using a modular, wireless, IMU-based device [19]. An important step of the processing algorithm is dimension reduction (DR) that allows the extraction of a single respiratory signal starting from 4-component quaternion data. Three different methods of DR are proposed and compared; two of them are based on the selection of one quaternion component, the third one is based on PCA-fusion of the 4 quaternion components. Results obtained using the IMU-based device, with the three different methods, are validated against optoelectronic plethysmography, an already established method to evaluate ventilation through an external measurement of the chest-wall surface motion [20–25].

2. Materials and Methods

2.1. Device Architecture and Hardware Description

The system used in this study is composed by three IMU-sensor units that communicate via Bluetooth with a smartphone; here data are pre-processed and saved. Two of the three sensor units (peripheral units) are dedicated to the recording of chest-wall respiratory-related movements and are placed on the thorax and on the abdomen to record respiratory information about both the compartments; the third sensor unit (reference central unit) is placed on a body area that is integral with the chest wall, but not involved in respiratory movements (e.g., coccyx or anterior superior iliac crest). The measurement of chest-wall movements, related to both abdominal and thoracic compartments, allows the consideration of the two-degree-of-freedom (DoF) model of chest-wall breathing movements [26], that considers abdomen and rib cage (thorax) as acting independently. Moreover, the compartmental contribution to total chest-wall volume changes according to posture and the breathing strategy adopted by each subject. Thus, the recording of chest-wall movements at different levels provides on the one hand, a more accurate estimation of the breathing signal, and on the other hand allows investigation of asynchronies between compartments, typical of different pathological conditions. The reference central unit, in addition to performing a central role within the Bluetooth piconet, can be used to discriminate between static and dynamic conditions and to map the activity state of the subject. Moreover, it could be used to reduce movement information not linked to breathing by means of frequency domain analysis or by referring orientation change experienced by the peripheral units to the coordinate frame of the reference unit. Each unit is composed by a printed circuit board equipped with a low-power microcontroller, a Bluetooth Low Energy (BLE) module, a 9-DoF IMU (3-axis accelerometer, a 3-axis gyroscope, and a 3-axis magnetometer) and lithium polymer rechargeable battery. A voltage regulator circuit, and Li–Po battery recharge circuit with mini USB port are also included in the design. Differently from the peripheral units, the reference central unit is equipped with a different BLE module, able to support simultaneous central/peripheral role and also brings a Micro Secure Digital (SD) Memory Card Connector for data logging. The dimensions of each peripheral unit, comprehensive of the 3D-printed housing, are 41 mm × 33 mm × 19 mm (LWH), and the weight is 25 g, including the battery, while the reference central unit measures 45 mm × 45 mm × 15 mm (LWH), and weighs 35 g. A prototypal version of this device has been described in [19].

2.2. Quaternion-Based Orientation Estimation and Fusion Algorithm

The final goal is to derive breathing signal by measuring orientation changes during the respiratory movements, both at thoracic and abdominal level. The IMUs provide 3D-acceleration, 3D-magnetic field, and 3D-angular rate. These measures are combined to provide accurate 3D orientation data aboard each unit. The orientation is represented with quaternions [27,28], that even though may suffer from problems of interpretation in terms of meaningfully physical angles, are interesting mathematical entities (four-dimensional complex number (q = [q_0 q_1 q_2 q_3]), since they require less computing time and avoid the singularity problems (i.e., "gimbal lock") typical of other orientation descriptors, e.g., Euler angles. The fusion of the data collected from the sensors is done by using the sensor fusion algorithm proposed by Madgwick et al. [29], based on an analytically derived and optimized gradient descent algorithm enabling levels of accuracy exceeding that of the Kalman-based algorithm, with low computational (277 scalar arithmetic operations each filter update) load and low sampling rates (e.g., 10 Hz); this orientation filter also provides an online magnetic distortion compensation algorithm and gyroscope bias drift compensation. The sensors data were collected at 40 Hz and the fusion algorithm was updated with the same rate, but due to limited buffer of the BLE module and to the stricter timings used for the Bluetooth communication, just one quaternion out of 4 computed is considered (10 Hz); nevertheless, the final sampling rate was considered appropriate given the relative low frequency of the respiratory signal [0.1 ÷ 1 Hz]. Thus, the microprocessor of each unit, receives data from accelerometer, gyroscope and magnetometer that are on board and implements Madgwick fusion filter [29] to compute a quaternion representing the change of orientation of each unit relative to the earth frame ($^{Th}_{Earth}\hat{q}$, $^{Ab}_{Earth}\hat{q}$, $^{Ref}_{Earth}\hat{q}$), or more correctly the change of orientation of the earth relative to each unit frame [29]. In fact, in quaternion form, an arbitrary orientation of a coordinate frame B relative to coordinate frame A, achieved through a rotation of angle θ around an axis $^A\mathbf{r}$ (r_x, r_y, r_z) defined in frame A, is univocally represented through the normalized quaternion $^A_B\hat{q}$ defined by Equation (1):

$$^A_B\hat{q} = [q_0\ q_1\ q_2\ q_3] = \left[\cos\frac{\theta}{2}\ -r_x\sin\frac{\theta}{2}\ -r_y\sin\frac{\theta}{2}\ r_z\sin\frac{\theta}{2}\right] \quad (1)$$

2.3. Quaternion-Derived Breathing Frequency

All the elaborations and computations needed to extract breathing parameters from data collected by the device were performed offline using MATLAB, the processing took on average 1.027 ± 0.129 seconds for the analysis of signals of 1071 ± 270 samples. A signal processing procedure was designed to extract the breathing frequency starting from quaternions representing the change of orientation of each unit relative to the earth frame ($^{Th}_{Earth}\hat{q}$, $^{Ab}_{Earth}\hat{q}$, $^{Ref}_{Earth}\hat{q}$). The block diagram of the signal processing part is presented in Figure 1. The algorithm is divided into 4 main blocks: (i) pre-processing, (ii) DR, (iii) spectrum analysis, and (iv) processing.

Pre-processing block includes the preliminary steps that leads to chest-wall respiratory-related orientation change signals. The orientations changes of thoracic and abdominal units were referred to the reference unit frame (that in turn represents orientation changes of trunk) applying Equations (2) and (3) respectively:

$$^{Th}_{Ref}\hat{q} = {^{Th}_{Earth}\hat{q}} \otimes {^{Ref}_{Earth}\hat{q}^*} = {^{Th}_{Earth}\hat{q}} \otimes {^{Earth}_{Ref}\hat{q}}, \quad (2)$$

$$^{Ab}_{Ref}\hat{q} = {^{Ab}_{Earth}\hat{q}} \otimes {^{Ref}_{Earth}\hat{q}^*} = {^{Ab}_{Earth}\hat{q}} \otimes {^{Earth}_{Ref}\hat{q}}, \quad (3)$$

These two quaternions represent the outputs of the pre-processing block and the input of the DR block.

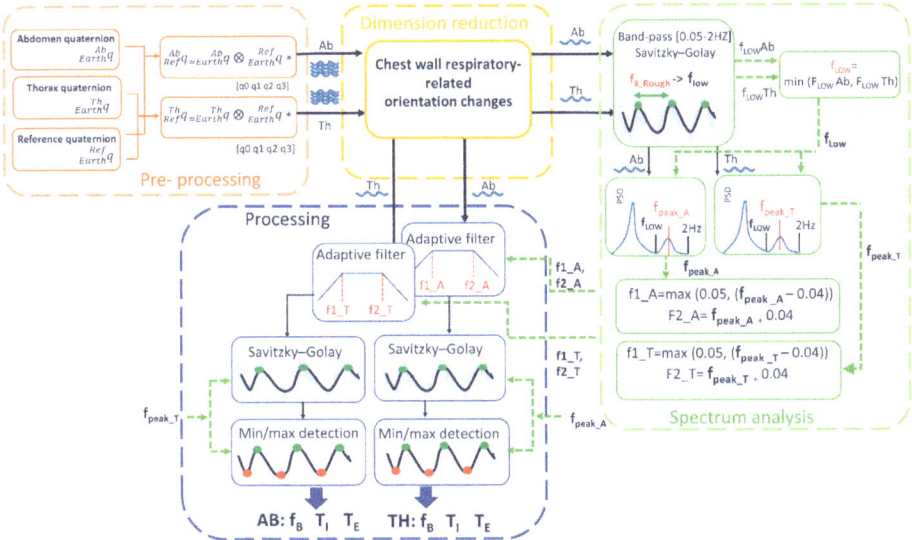

Figure 1. Block Diagram of the Analysis algorithm that allows derivation of breathing temporal parameters (f_B, T_I, T_E) from quaternion-based orientation change signals recorded on Thorax, Abdomen and Reference point.

Dimension-reduction block takes the quaternions obtained from Equations (2) and (3), that are composed by 4 components each, and provides as output 2 single-component signals (1 for the abdomen and 1 for the thorax) representing chest-wall respiratory-related orientation change signals. These two signals represent the input of the power spectrum block and of the processing block. To reduce dimension from 4 components to 1, two possibilities were investigated as shown in Figure 2:

(i). Best quaternion component selection
(ii). PCA-based fusion of the quaternion components

To select the best component among the 4 components representing the orientation quaternion, two different methods were proposed, both based on spectrum analysis. The idea was to choose the component with the highest breathing information, computing the power spectral density estimate (PSD) between 0.5–2 Hz for each component and selecting the component with: (1) maximum PSD peak ("Peak" method) or (2) maximum area under the PSD ("Area" method). To assess the goodness of these two methods in predicting the best quaternion component, the ideal component ("Ideal") was determined a posteriori, case by case, based on minimum breathing frequency estimation error (see Section 2.5).

Since more than one quaternion component is supposed to convey breathing information, the possibility to maximize this information fusing the 4 components of the quaternion by means of PCA was investigated. PCA is a mathematical procedure that transforms an original set of correlated variables into a (smaller) number of uncorrelated variables by determining a set of orthogonal vectors called principal components, which are defined by a linear combination of the original variables [30,31]. To do this, the directions in the data with the most variation, i.e., the eigenvectors corresponding to the largest eigenvalues of the covariance matrix, are computed and the data are projected onto these directions. To compute the eigenvectors, data were arranged into a two-dimensional matrix $\mathbf{X}(m \times n)$, where m was the number of observations of the time series and n the number of variables (quaternion components). Then, the univariate means were subtracted from the n columns, to center the data. Singular Value Decomposition (SVD) was used to compute the eigenvectors ($\mathbf{V} = [v_1, v_2, v_3, v_4]$) and corresponding eigenvalues ($\lambda_1, \lambda_2, \lambda_3, \lambda_4$). Original data were finally projected in the new coordinate system ($\mathbf{Y} = \mathbf{XV}$) and the first principal component, accounting for the largest possible variance, was selected and passed to other blocks [30,31].

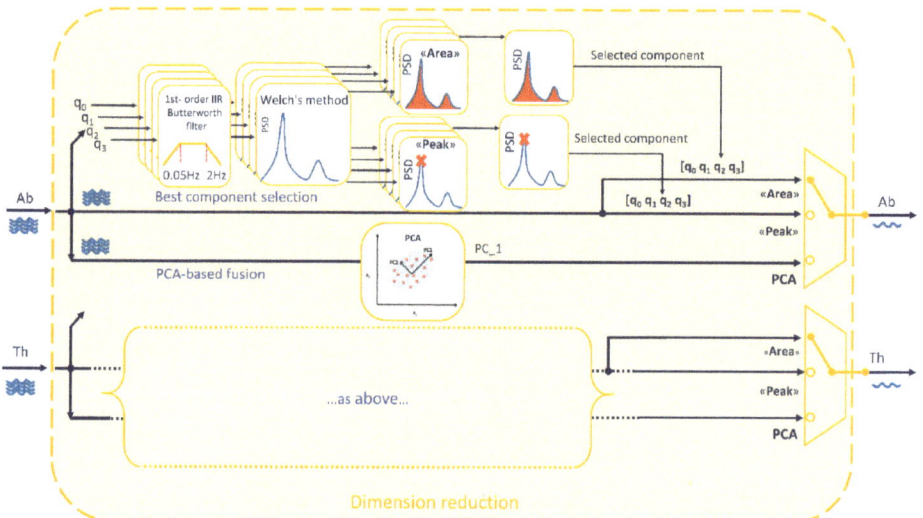

Figure 2. Dimension-reduction block in detail. Starting from the 4 components [q_0, q_1, q_2, q_3] of each quaternion (Abdominal: Ab and Thoracic: Th), three methods are applied to obtain a single-component signal: two methods based on best quaternion component selection ("Area" and "Peak") and one method based on the fusion of the 4 components through Principal Component Analysis (PCA). "Area" method selects the quaternion component with the larger area under the Power Spectral Density (PSD) estimate, while "Peak" method selects the quaternion component with the highest PSD's peak. PCA-fusion method selects the first principal component (PC_1) that accounts for the largest variance in the data.

Spectrum Analysis block include a set of steps needed to optimize the subsequent processing phase. The two signals representing chest-wall (abdominal and thoracic) respiratory-related orientation obtained downstream of the dimension-reduction block underwent the following steps (Figure 1):

(i). A low-frequency threshold (f_{LOW}) was determined based on a first estimate of the breathing frequency (f_B). The rough estimate of f_B was done by identifying maxima points of the signal and computing the f_B, breath by breath, as reciprocal of the temporal distance between consecutive maxima points. Then, the mean (f_{B_Rough}) and the standard deviation ($f_{B\_Rough\_SD}$) of the f_B over the entire trial were computed. To facilitate maxima points identification, signals were at first band-pass filtered using a first-order infinite impulse response (IIR) Butterworth filter [0.05 Hz–2 Hz] and smoothed with a third-order Savitzky–Golay [32] finite impulse response (FIR) filter (fixed window length = 31 samples). Low thresholds $f_{LOW}Ab$ and $f_{LOW}Th$ were determined for the abdominal and thoracic signals respectively as difference $f_{B\_Rough} - f_{B\_Rough\_SD}$. Then the minimum value between $f_{LOW}Ab$ and $f_{LOW}Th$ was chosen as final low-frequency threshold, named f_{LOW}, and it was used in the next step.

(ii). PSD estimate (Welch's method, Hamming window size: 300 samples, overlapping: 50 samples) was computed and the spectrum frequency corresponding to the breathing rate was identified, both for the thorax (f_{peak_T}) and the abdomen (f_{peak_A}), by looking for the local peak of the PSD within the window [$f_{LOW} \div 2$ Hz]. The use of a low threshold, based on a rough estimate of the breathing frequency, supports the selection of the PSD peak linked to breathing rate and avoid selecting wrong peaks, often related to low-frequency oscillation artifacts.

(iii). The breathing frequency derived by the spectrum was used to set an adaptive band-pass filter, as proposed in a previous study [7], centered on f_{peak} frequency. For the abdomen, upper (f_U) and lower (f_L) cut-off frequency points for the band-pass filter were defined, by applying Equations (4) and (5) respectively [7]:

$$f_{U\_A} = f_{peak\_A} + 0.04, \tag{4}$$

$$f_{L\_A} = \max(0.05, (f_{peak\_A} - 0.04)), \tag{5}$$

For the thorax, Equations (6) and (7) were applied:

$$f_{U\_T} = f_{peak\_T} + 0.04, \tag{6}$$

$$f_{L\_T} = \max(0.05, (f_{peak\_T} - 0.04)), \tag{7}$$

Moreover, based on f_{peak}, a set of parameters was selected to optimize subsequent smoothing and minima/maxima detection phases of the processing block.

Processing block includes all the steps needed to extract breathing frequency and temporal parameters from the signals obtained downstream of the dimension-reduction block. Chest-wall respiratory-related orientation change signals (abdominal and thoracic) underwent the following steps:

(i). Adaptive band-pass filter. The signals were band-pass filtered (first-order IIR Butterworth filter), with f_U and f_L cut-off frequency points determined within the spectrum analysis block.

(ii). Smoothing. Filtered signals were furtherly smoothed (third-order Savitzky–Golay FIR filter) to simplify subsequent identification of maxima and minima points. The level of smoothing (window length) was automatically selected based on f_{peak}, i.e., increasing window length for decreasing f_{peak}. Relation between optimal window length values and f_{peak} values has been determined empirically.

(iii). Minima and maxima points detection. A set of optimized parameters (i.e., minimum peak distance (MPD) and minimum prominence threshold (MPT)) was automatically selected based on f_{peak} to optimize recognition of minima and maxima points of the smoothed signals. Optimal MPD and MPT values depending on f_{peak} were experimentally determined.

(iv). Breathing frequency extraction. Breath by breath, inspiratory time (T_I) was computed as the temporal distance between a minimum point (m_i) and the consecutive maximum point (M_i); Expiratory time (T_E) was computed as the temporal distance between the maximum point (M_i) and the consecutive minimum point ($m_i + 1$); total time (T_{TOT}) was computed as $T_{TOT} = T_I + T_E$ [s], duty cycle (DC) was computed as $\frac{T_I}{T_{TOT}} \times 100$ [%] and breathing frequency was computed as $\frac{60}{(T_{TOT})}$ [breaths/minute]. A mean value for each of the above-mentioned parameter was computed for each trial (~3 min).

2.4. Experimental Setup

To evaluate the capability of the device and of the proposed methods to correctly estimate breathing frequency (and temporal parameters) 8 healthy volunteers (4 males, 4 females) were enrolled. All subjects gave their informed consent for inclusion before they participated in the study. The study was conducted in accordance with the Declaration of Helsinki, and the protocol (Project identification code n° 534) was approved by the Ethics Committee of Scientific Institute IRCCS Medea (date of approval: 25 January 2018). Chest-wall movements during breathing, in seated and supine position, were measured using the proposed device and optoelectronic plethysmography (OEP) simultaneously. OEP [21] is a technique based on a similar functioning principle of the proposed device; in fact, it allows assessment of ventilatory and breathing pattern by measuring chest-wall movements related to breathing, by using motion capture principles. The system is composed of eight infrared video cameras working at a sampling rate of 60 Hz. It can compute the 3D coordinates of retro-reflective markers positioned on the chest wall in specific anatomic points. From the three-dimensional coordinates of the markers, it is possible to obtain the volume enclosed by the chest-wall surface, by applying the Gauss's theorem. The chest wall is modelled by a bicompartmental model, composed of rib cage and abdomen, and thus it is possible to investigate the contribution of both the compartments. This is an advantage for the validation of the proposed device, in fact, using OEP as reference method it is possible to compare the data recorded with the thoracic and abdominal units of the device with those obtained by using OEP for the thoracic and abdominal compartments, respectively. OEP has been widely validated against spirometer, in healthy subjects, in different conditions and positions, also during submaximal and maximal exercise on cycle ergometer, obtaining discrepancies in tidal volume measurements always <5% [22–24,33,34].

The subjects were prepared, placing the reflective markers according to the 89-marker protocol (previously described in [24,35]) used for seated position and the 52-marker protocol (previously described in [36,37]) used for supine position or, more generally, when a back support is present. Then peripheral IMU-units were placed on the thorax and on the abdomen, while reference IMU-unit was placed on the coccyx in seated position, and on the bed in supine position (Figure 3).

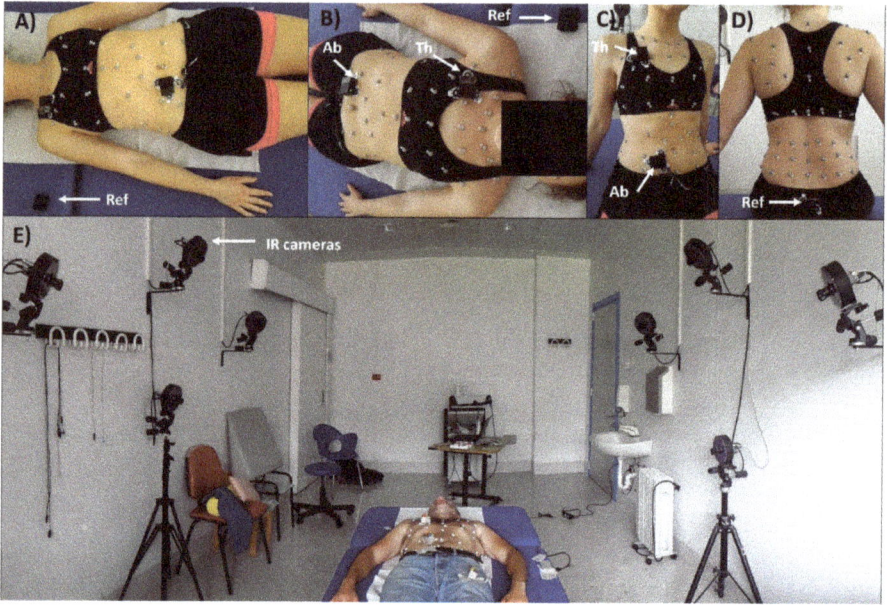

Figure 3. Experimental setup. Retroreflective-marker configuration for optoelectronic plethysmography (OEP) and IMU-unit (Ab: Abdomen, Th: Thorax, Ref: Reference) placement in supine (A and B panels) and seated (C and D panels) positions. Panel E shows the experimental setup and the OEP Lab; Infrared cameras of the motion capture system are also noticeable.

Subjects were then asked to seat or lie on a bed and were invited to perform a slow vital capacity maneuver (SVC) and then to start breathing with the following patterns: (I) quiet breathing (QB), (II) increasing f_B but same tidal volume of QB ($\uparrow f_B$, V_T=), (III) increasing f_B and reducing tidal volume ($\uparrow f_B$, $V_T \downarrow$), (IV) decreasing f_B with the same tidal volume of QB ($\downarrow f_B$, V_T=), (V) decreasing f_B increasing tidal volume of QB ($\downarrow f_B$, $V_T \uparrow$). QB trial was repeated two times, thus, each subject performed 6 trials of the duration of 3 min each. The SVC maneuver was used to align OEP signal and device signals during data analysis, since it is generally recognizable with respect to QB. In fact, SVC requires a maximal inspiration followed by a complete expiration without forced or rapid effort.

The subjects were asked to maintain the same breathing pattern (namely, QB, ↑f_B, V_T=, ↑f_B, V_T↓, ↓f_B, V_T=, ↓f_B, V_T↑) until the end of the trial; in case of fatigue they were asked to perform a second SVC before returning to QB. This procedure was repeated in seated position and in supine position.

2.5. Statistical Analysis

For each trial, mean values of f_B, T_I, T_E and DC were extracted from the best quaternion components identified online by using "Area" and "Peak" methods, and from the signal obtained with the PCA-based fusion method, both for the thoracic and abdominal tracings. Moreover, to evaluate the performance of the selection methods ("Area" and "Peak") and their ability to select the best component, the same parameters were obtained for all the quaternion components (q_0, q_1, q_2, q_3) and compared with those obtained by OEP, on the abdominal and thoracic compartment, respectively. The "Ideal" quaternion component was identified a posteriori, trial by trial, as the one providing the minimum estimation error of the breathing frequency. Obviously, the "Ideal" component cannot be identified during online analysis, or when a reference method is not present. Thus, for each trial, 5 sets of parameters were available:

- f_{B_OEP}, T_{I_OEP}, T_{E_OEP} and $DC_{\_OEP}$
- f_{B_Peak}, T_{I_Peak}, T_{E_Peak} and $DC_{\_Peak}$
- f_{B_Area}, T_{I_Area}, T_{E_Area} and $DC_{\_Area}$
- f_{B_PCA}, T_{I_PCA}, T_{E_PCA} and $DC_{\_PCA}$
- f_{B_Ideal}, T_{I_Ideal}, T_{E_Ideal} and $DC_{\_Ideal}$

Among the entire set of trials, those with f_{B_OEP} < 6 breaths/minute or f_{B_OEP} > 60 breaths/minute were discarded. Then, the absolute (Equation (8)) and relative (Equation (9)) errors of estimation in static conditions (supine and seated position) were computed for each parameter:

$$Absolute\ Error\ (E) = |Device - OEP|, \quad (8)$$

$$Relative\ Error\ (E\%) = \frac{|Device - OEP|}{OEP} \times 100 \quad (9)$$

For all the dimension-reduction methods ("Area", "Peak", "PCA"), mean and standard deviation (SD) were computed for E and E% considering all the subjects and all the trials, for the supine and seated position and compared with those obtained considering the "Ideal" component. The error obtained with the "Ideal" component, identified a posteriori, is thus the minimum error obtainable using a single quaternion component, and represents the performance that the other methods ("Area", "Peak", and PCA-fusion) should achieve or beat. For E% obtained in f_B and DC estimation, non-parametric alternative to the one-way Analysis of variance (ANOVA) with repeated measures (Friedman test) was performed to assess if significant differences between methods ("Area", "Peak", "PCA") and "Ideal" component occurred, "Ideal"); post-hoc analysis was done performing Wilcoxon signed-rank tests on the different combinations of related methods, applying the correction for multiple comparisons using false discovery rate (FDR) method [38,39].

For f_B, T_I, T_E, linear regression analysis and correlation analysis (Pearson's product-moment correlation r_P, or Spearman's rank-order correlation r_S, if data were not normally distributed) were performed between measurements obtained with the device and measurements obtained with the OEP, for the supine and seated position, respectively.

To assess the agreement between measurements obtained with the device and with the OEP, Bland–Altman analysis was performed plotting the difference of the two paired measurements (device–OEP) against the mean of the two measurements [40–42]. Mean of the differences (d) and limits of agreement (LOA: from d − (1.9 × SD) to d + (1.9 × SD)) were calculated. The presence of heteroscedasticity was always examined to assess the presence of proportional biases and/or the correlation between differences and mean values. As proposed by Brehm et al. [43], to determine if data were heteroscedastic a visual inspection of Bland–Altman plots was performed at first. If the errors (y-axes: absolute differences) increased with increasing measured values (x-axes: mean), the data were suspected of being heteroscedastic. Then Kendall's tau (τ) correlation between the absolute differences and the corresponding means was computed to assess the degree of heteroscedasticity. Data were denoted heteroscedastic when a positive, significant correlation ($\tau > 0.1$ and p-value < 0.05) was found, for other cases data were considered homoscedastic [43].

When heteroscedasticity was present the "classical" 95% confidence and tolerance limits cannot be constructed, thus the approach based on the construction of V-shaped limits was applied: the regression line (ordinary least squares (OLS) best fit) was constructed for differences on mean values and the V-shaped confidence limits (upper confidence limit: UCL, lower confidence limit: LCL) were constructed modelling the variability in the SD of the differences directly as a function of the level of the measurement, using a method based on absolute residuals from a fitted regression line [44,45].

3. Results

3.1. Breathing Patterns

Table 1 presents the mean and SD of breathing rate for each breathing pattern (QB_1 e QB_2, ↑f_B, V_T=, ↑f_B, V_T↓, ↓f_B, VT=, ↓f_B, V_T↑) estimated with OEP and device, using "PCA", "Area", and "Peak" methods and the "Ideal" component, for all subjects, in supine and seated position. Sample size (n) of each condition is reported in Table 1 for the breathing pattern ↑f_B, V_T↓, just one thoracic tracing was available for seated position (n = 1). It can be noticed that each subject demonstrated a different breathing frequency for each breathing pattern and SD in the forced breathing patterns is higher than those obtained for QB, meaning that subjects interpreted the required speed differently.

Table 1. Breathing frequencies for different breathing patterns.

Supine		QB 1		↑f_B, V_T=		↓f_B, V_T=		↑f_B, V_T↓		↓f_B, V_T↑		QB 2	
		AB (n = 8)	TH (n = 7)	AB (n = 8)	TH (n = 8)	AB (n = 6)	TH (n = 6)	AB (n = 3)	TH (n = 2)	AB (n = 5)	TH (n = 6)	AB (n = 8)	TH (n = 8)
OEP		17.13 ± 2.23	17.62 ± 2.21	39.49 ± 10.26	39.48 ± 10.25	11.17 ± 2.64	11.14 ± 2.63	48.11 ± 13.29	47.66 ± 13.95	8.38 ± 2.40	8.61 ± 2.24	15.29 ± 4.34	15.24 ± 4.48
Device	Area	17.20 ± 2.15	18.53 ± 3.96	39.19 ± 10.84	38.16 ± 14.67	15.52 ± 8.14	19.29 ± 9.42	34.47 ± 34.58	30.01 ± 25.52	10.11 ± 3.91	10.62 ± 4.44	21.28 ± 8.14	16.55 ± 3.62
	Peak	17.20 ± 2.15	16.63 ± 2.29	38.92 ± 11.12	38.96 ± 13.01	15.52 ± 8.14	16.97 ± 9.59	34.47 ± 34.58	53.39 ± 7.55	10.11 ± 3.91	9.32 ± 2.12	21.25 ± 8.15	16.55 ± 3.62
	PCA	17.23 ± 2.09	17.03 ± 1.98	40.06 ± 9.22	40.63 ± 8.45	11.51 ± 2.59	11.56 ± 3.04	48.61 ± 12.64	49.93 ± 11.94	8.61 ± 2.19	8.95 ± 2.06	15.11 ± 4.82	15.23 ± 3.79
	Ideal	17.57 ± 2.52	16.34 ± 2.00	39.81 ± 10.50	40.94 ± 9.97	12.11 ± 1.99	13.60 ± 2.61	49.53 ± 12.31	48.12 ± 13.89	9.34 ± 3.33	8.83 ± 2.06	17.74 ± 4.70	15.37 ± 3.82

Seated		QB 1		↑f_B, V_T=		↓f_B, V_T=		↑f_B, V_T↓		↓f_B, V_T↑		QB 2	
		AB (n = 8)	TH (n = 8)	AB (n = 8)	TH (n = 7)	AB (n = 8)	TH (n = 8)	AB (n = 2)	TH (n = 1)	AB (n = 6)	TH (n = 5)	AB (n = 7)	TH (n = 6)
OEP		16.99 ± 2.65	16.94 ± 2.77	42.74 ± 10.97	46.49 ± 7.58	14.57 ± 13.40	14.49 ± 13.41	33.20 ± 16.01	22.01	10.04 ± 3.56	10.05 ± 3.81	18.47 ± 4.32	18.47 ± 4.49
Device	Area	17.15 ± 2.86	15.78 ± 3.62	43.06 ± 11.22	40.71 ± 13.59	15.71 ± 13.52	17.06 ± 13.05	32.63 ± 12.87	27.62	10.83 ± 2.93	12.58 ± 4.08	19.80 ± 5.15	17.04 ± 2.09
	Peak	16.48 ± 3.58	16.27 ± 3.76	43.06 ± 11.22	40.71 ± 13.59	16.53 ± 13.50	17.15 ± 12.99	32.63 ± 12.87	27.62	10.83 ± 2.93	12.58 ± 4.08	17.23 ± 2.19	16.54 ± 1.95
	PCA	16.54 ± 3.01	16.58 ± 2.10	42.26 ± 11.38	45.31 ± 8.56	16.07 ± 13.07	14.91 ± 13.39	33.79 ± 14.50	27.27	10.76 ± 2.90	11.35 ± 3.73	16.59 ± 2.17	15.47 ± 1.69
	Ideal	16.68 ± 2.59	16.61 ± 2.34	42.64 ± 11.21	45.42 ± 7.98	15.29 ± 13.33	11.07 ± 2.36	33.38 ± 13.92	24.53	10.40 ± 3.53	10.29 ± 3.66	19.06 ± 4.89	18.73 ± 5.04

Across subject mean ± SD of the breathing frequency (f_B, [breaths/minute]) measurements with OEP and the device, using best component-selection methods ("Area" and "Peak"), PCA-fusion method and "Ideal" component, for the requested patterns. Data are reported for the supine and seated positions, subdivided in abdominal and thoracic contributions.

3.2. Accuracy Errors

Relative errors of estimation in supine and seated position computed for best component-selection methods ("Peak", "Area"), for PCA-fusion method and for the "Ideal" quaternion component for f_B and DC are presented in Figure 4. For what concerns f_B estimation in supine position, relative errors obtained using PCA were similar or even better than those provided by the "Ideal" component; on the contrary, both component-selection methods, namely "Area" and "Peak", provided errors higher than 10%, both for the abdominal and the thoracic compartments. Errors obtained with PCA resulted significantly lower than those obtained with the "Area" method, both for the abdominal (Wilcoxon post-hoc test FDR-adjusted, p = 0.038) and thoracic compartment (Wilcoxon post-hoc test FDR-adjusted, p = 0.015); also, PCA was significantly better than "Peak" method considering abdominal compartment (Wilcoxon post-hoc test FDR-adjusted, p = 0.038). Errors obtained with "Ideal" component resulted significantly lower than those obtained with the component-selection methods both for the abdominal (Wilcoxon post-hoc test FDR-adjusted, Ideal vs. Area p = 0.038, Ideal vs. Peak p = 0.038) and thoracic (Wilcoxon post-hoc test FDR-adjusted, Ideal vs. Area p = 0.000, Ideal vs. Peak p = 0.020) compartments.

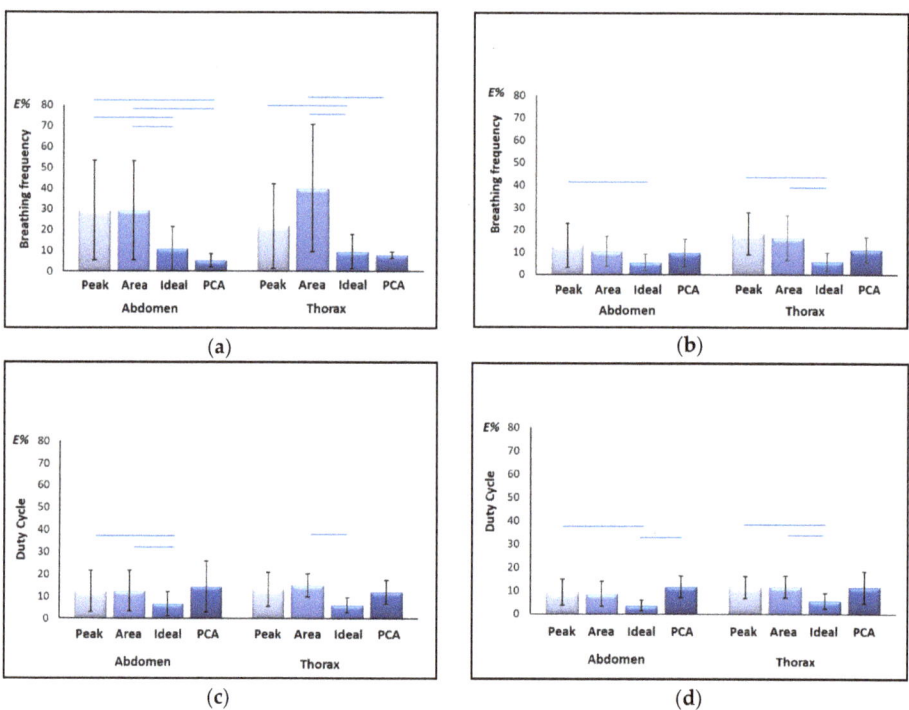

Figure 4. Relative errors (E%) of estimation of breathing frequency (**a**,**b**) and Duty Cycle (**c**,**d**) in supine (**a**,**c**) and seated (**b**,**d**) positions, computed for each method (Peak, Area and PCA) and for the "Ideal" component with respect to the reference (OEP). Errors are computed both for the Thoracic and abdominal compartments. Horizontal blue lines indicate statistical significance of difference (post-hoc analysis, Wilcoxon test FDR corrected).

In seated position, f_B estimation errors obtained with component-selection methods were lower on average than those obtained in supine position, while PCA performances declined. This led to a sort of equalization effect, confirmed also by the statistical analysis: significant differences remained only for comparisons "Ideal" vs. "Area" method (Wilcoxon post-hoc test FDR-adjusted, AB: p = 0.102,

TH: p = 0.015) and "Ideal" vs. "Peak" method (Wilcoxon post-hoc test FDR-adjusted, AB: p = 0.006, TH: p = 0.015).

Regarding duty cycle, relative errors of estimation obtained with the different methods are comparable, with exception of those provided by "Ideal" component that are on average lower, both in supine (Wilcoxon post-hoc test FDR-adjusted, AB: Ideal vs. Peak p = 0.042, Ideal vs. Area p = 0.042; TH: Ideal vs. Area p = 0.006) and seated position (Wilcoxon post-hoc test FDR-adjusted, AB: Ideal vs. Peak p = 0.015, Ideal vs. PCA p = 0.006; TH: Ideal vs. Area p = 0.015, Ideal vs. Peak p = 0.015, Ideal vs. PCA p = 0.05).

Absolute estimation errors of f_B, T_I and T_E obtained with the device using different methods (Area, Peak, Ideal, PCA) relative to OEP are reported in Table 2.

Table 2. Absolute errors of breathing frequency (E_f_B), Inspiratory time (E_T_I) and expiratory time (E_T_E) obtained for the device with respect to OEP, using best component-selection methods ("Area" and "Peak"), PCA-fusion method and "Ideal" component.

			Area	Peak	PCA	Ideal
E_f_B [breaths/minute]	supine	AB	3.64 ± 7.46	3.64 ± 7.46	1.00 ± 1.24	1.39 ± 2.76
		TH	5.46 ± 8.89	3.17 ± 4.92	1.55 ± 1.51	1.56 ± 1.96
	seated	AB	2.19 ± 2.49	2.12 ± 2.74	1.71 ± 2.25	1.04 ± 1.24
		TH	3.35 ± 5.68	3.31 ± 5.69	1.79 ± 2.04	0.96 ± 0.22
E_T_I [s]	supine	AB	0.48 ± 0.73	0.48 ± 0.73	0.33 ± 0.51	0.20 ± 0.38
		TH	0.43 ± 0.52	0.41 ± 0.49	0.47 ± 0.67	0.17 ± 0.25
	seated	AB	0.33 ± 0.58	0.36 ± 0.56	0.46 ± 0.71	0.16 ± 0.27
		TH	0.43 ± 0.48	0.44 ± 0.49	0.42 ± 0.35	0.17 ± 0.25
E_T_E [s]	supine	AB	0.58 ± 0.82	0.58 ± 0.82	0.43 ± 0.58	0.29 ± 0.52
		TH	0.79 ± 0.94	0.67 ± 0.92	0.46 ± 0.63	0.36 ± 0.71
	seated	AB	0.43 ± 0.56	0.43 ± 0.56	0.43 ± 0.55	0.22 ± 0.31
		TH	0.56 ± 0.66	0.56 ± 0.66	0.39 ± 0.41	0.24 ± 0.36

Data are reported as mean ± SD, in supine and seated position for thoracic (TH) and abdominal (AB) compartments.

3.3. Linear Regression and Correlation Analysis

Scatter plots showing the relationship between measurements obtained with the OEP and with the device, using "Area", "Peak", "Ideal" components, and PCA-fusion respectively are presented for f_B (Figure 5), T_I (Figure 6) and T_E (Figure 7). For each scatter plot the regression line is computed, both for thorax and abdomen, and the relative equations are reported.

Correlation coefficients for the comparisons Device vs. OEP are reported in Table 3. Regarding the main parameter, f_B, results obtained with correlation analysis confirmed what emerged from estimation error analysis: in supine position, PCA exhibited the best performances in terms of correlation with OEP measurements both in terms of regression line and correlation coefficient. In seated position, "Ideal" component was the one with the highest correlation with OEP measurements, followed by PCA.

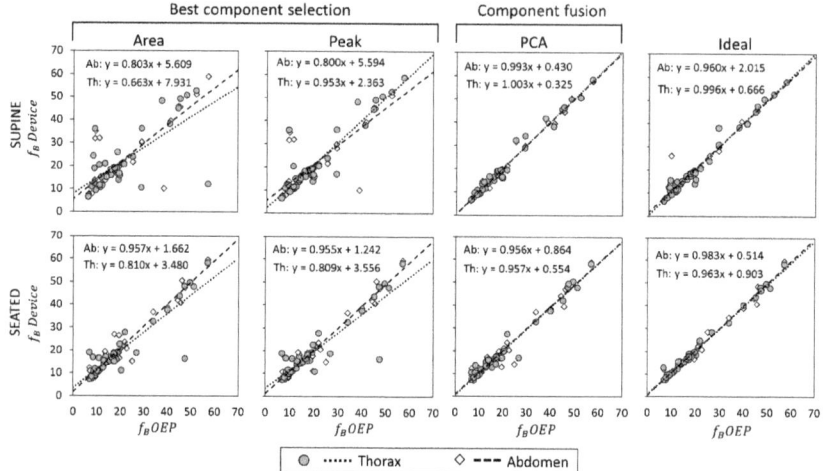

Figure 5. Comparisons of breathing frequency (f_B expressed as breaths/minuteute) measurements by using the proposed device and by using Optoelectronic plethysmography (OEP) presented as regression analysis, in supine (top panels) and seated (bottom panels) positions. For what concerns f_B measurements obtained with the IMU-device, three dimension-reduction methods were considered: Area, Peak and PCA-fusion. The performance obtained by using these three methods is benchmarked against that obtained with the Ideal quaternion component determined a posteriori based on the minimum estimation error. The regression line between measurements done by OEP and the proposed device is plotted, and the relative equation presented, both for the thorax and the abdomen.

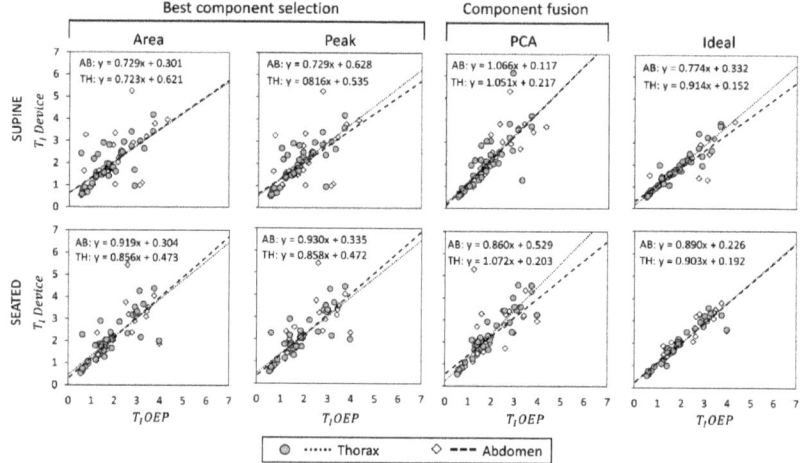

Figure 6. Comparisons of inspiratory time (T_I expressed as seconds) measurements by using the proposed device and by using Optoelectronic plethysmography (OEP) presented as regression analysis, in supine (top panels) and seated (bottom panels) positions. For what concerns T_I measurements obtained with the IMU-device, three dimension-reduction methods were considered: Area, Peak and PCA-fusion. The performance obtained by using these three methods is benchmarked against that obtained with the Ideal quaternion component determined a posteriori based on the minimum estimation error. The regression line between measurements done by OEP and the proposed device is plotted, and the relative equation presented, both for the thorax and the abdomen.

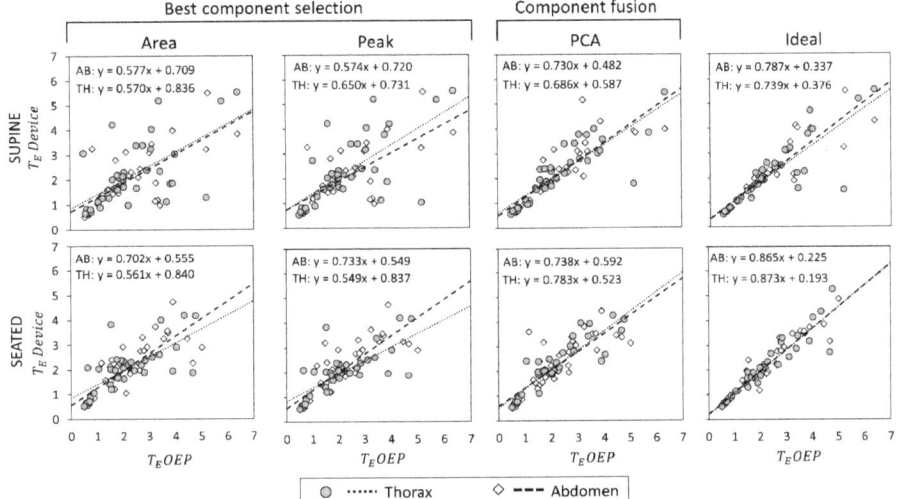

Figure 7. Comparisons of expiratory time (T_E, expressed as seconds) measurements by using the proposed device and by using Optoelectronic plethysmography (OEP) presented as regression analysis, in supine (top panels) and seated (bottom panels) positions. Regarding T_E measurements obtained with the IMU-device, three dimension-reduction methods were considered. Area, Peak and PCA-fusion. The performance obtained by using these three methods is benchmarked against that obtained with the Ideal quaternion component determined a posteriori based on the minimum estimation error. The regression line between measurements done by OEP and the proposed device is plotted, and the relative equation presented, both for the thorax and the abdomen.

Table 3. Correlation outcomes across subjects and breathing patterns. Coefficient of correlation (r) between measurements obtained using Device vs. OEP are reported for f_B, T_I and T_E using best component-selection methods ("Area" and "Peak"), PCA-fusion method and "Ideal" component, in supine (Thorax: n = 37. Abdomen: n = 37) and seated (Thorax: n = 35. Abdomen: n = 39) position.

		Supine		Seated	
		Thorax	Abdomen	Thorax	Abdomen
f_B	Area	0.580 $	0.706 $	0.748 $	0.915 $
	Peak	0.833 $	0.706 $	0.759 $	0.861 $
	PCA	**0.963** $	**0.985** $	0.953 $	0.924 $
	Ideal	0.935 $	0.931 $	**0.974** $	**0.977** $
T_I	Area	0.727 #	0.665 $	0.812 #	0.812 #
	Peak	0.785 #	0.659 $	0.809 #	0.824 #
	PCA	0.783 #	**0.874** #	0.926 #	0.731 #
	Ideal	**0.943** #	0.862 $	**0.951** #	**0.948** #
T_E	Area	0.600 $	0.713 #	0.682 #	0.818 #
	Peak	0.687 $	0.712 #	0.723 #	0.835 #
	PCA	**0.891** #	0.864 #	0.888 #	0.824 #
	Ideal	0.874 #	**0.966** $	**0.938** #	**0.951** #

Correlations are all significant (p-value < 0.001). $ Spearman correlation coefficient; # Pearson correlation coefficient; Bold: best correlation result.

With reference to T_I estimation in supine position, "Ideal" component provided the best performances, followed by PCA method; "Peak" and "Area" methods provided comparable, poor performances. In seated position, measurements of T_I provided by component-selection methods were on average more correlated with OEP measurements than measurements obtained using PCA-fusion method. The "Ideal" component presented the best results, followed by "Area" and "Peak" methods; PCA provided the worst performance considering the abdominal compartment, while correlation between measurements obtained with the thoracic unit and OEP measurements was good.

Estimation of T_E was on average more problematic. In terms of regression lines in fact, slope values were far from the unity for all the considered methods, highlighting a proportional error leading to an overestimation for low values of expiratory time and an underestimation at high expiratory times, as shown in Figure 7. For what concerns supine position, correlation coefficients were good both for "Ideal" component and PCA-fusion method; on the contrary, correlation coefficients were low both for "Area" and "Peak" methods. Also, in seated position correlation coefficients provided by "Ideal" and PCA-fusion method were higher than those provided by "Area" and "Peak" methods, especially with respect to the thoracic compartment.

3.4. Bland–Altman Analysis

Bland–Altman plots representing the agreement between measurements obtained with the OEP and with the device, using "Area", "Peak", "Ideal" components, and PCA-fusion respectively are presented for f_B (Figure 8), T_I (Figure 9) and T_E (Figure 10). In Bland–Altman plots, the difference of the two paired measurements (device−OEP) is plotted against the mean of the two measurements (device+OEP)/2. Results of agreement analysis, including evaluation of heteroscedasticity (Kendall's τ correlation and relative p-value) are reported in Table 4. As shown there, for homoscedastic data, the mean of the differences representing the fixed bias, and LOAs were computed. On the other hand, for heteroscedastic data, OLS line of best fit representing the proportional bias and upper and lower 95% V-shape confidence limits (UCL and LCL) are reported.

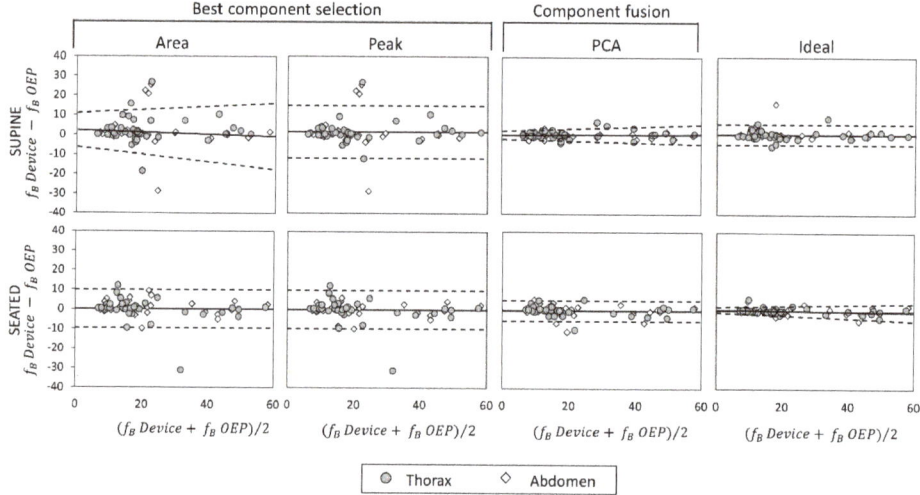

Figure 8. Agreement analysis between OEP and the IMU-based device for breathing frequency (f_B, expressed as breaths/minuteute) measurements, in supine (top panels) and seated (bottom panels) position. In each Bland–Altman plot the differences between measurements of f_B obtained by using the IMU-based device and by using OEP are plotted against the mean of the two measurements. For homoscedastic data, the mean of the differences (bias: —) and limits of agreement (black dotted line) from mean − 1.96 s to mean + 1.96 s are represented by lines parallel to the X axis. For heteroscedastic data, the proportional bias (—) is represented by the ordinary least squares (OLS) line of best fit for the difference on mean values; V-shaped upper and lower 95% confidence limits (- - -) are calculated according to Bland [44].

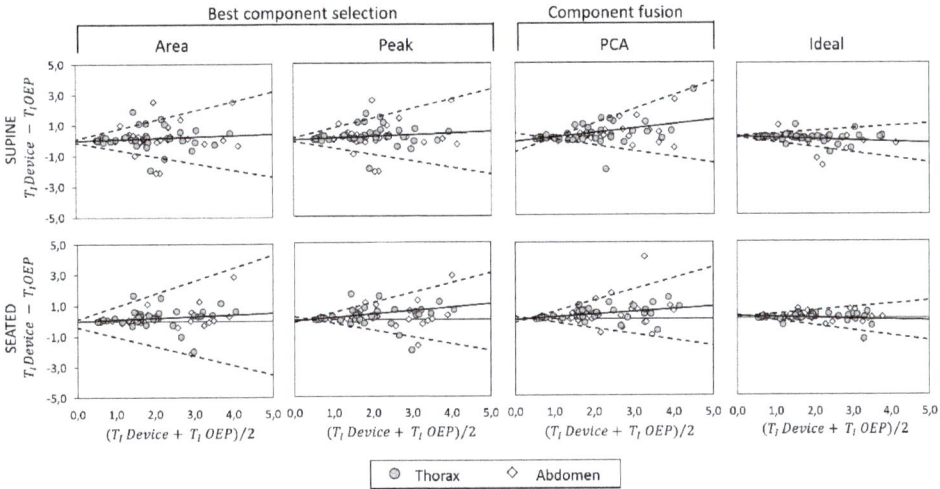

Figure 9. Agreement analysis between OEP and the IMU-based device for inspiratory time (T_I, [s]) measurements, in supine (top panels) and seated (bottom panels) position. In each Bland–Altman plot the differences between measurements of T_I obtained by using the IMU-based device and by using OEP are plotted against the mean of the two measurements. For homoscedastic data, the mean of the differences (bias: —) and limits of agreement (- - -) from mean − 1.96 s to mean + 1.96 s are represented by lines parallel to the X axis. For heteroscedastic data, the proportional bias (—) is represented by the OLS line of best fit for differences on mean values; V-shaped upper and lower 95% confidence limits (- - -) are calculated according to Bland [44].

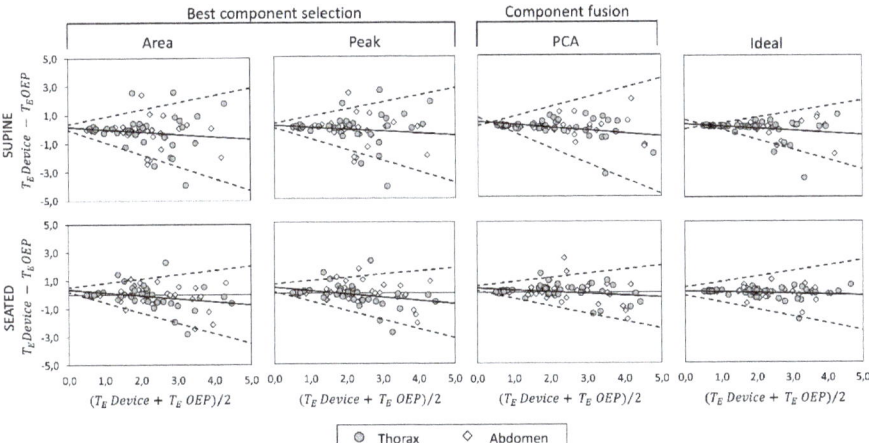

Figure 10. Agreement analysis between OEP and the IMU-based device for expiratory time (T_E, [s]) measurements, in supine (top panels) and seated (bottom panels) position. In each Bland–Altman plot the differences between measurements of T_E obtained by using the IMU-based device and by using OEP are plotted against the mean of the two measurements. For homoscedastic data, the mean of the differences (bias: —) and limits of agreement (- - -) from mean − 1.96 s to mean + 1.96 s are represented by lines parallel to the X axis. For heteroscedastic data, the proportional bias (—) is represented by the OLS line of best fit for differences on mean values; V-shaped upper and lower 95% confidence limits (- - -) are calculated according to Bland [44].

Table 4. Agreement analysis outcomes across subjects and different breathing patterns. Bland and Altman plot statistics for measurements of f_B, T_I and T_E using best component-selection methods ("Area" and "Peak"), PCA-fusion method and "Ideal" component and, in supine (n = 74) and seated (n = 74) position.

		τ	p-Value	Heteroscedastic?	Fixed Bias [a]/OLS	LOA [c]/V-Shape Limits [d]
f_B supine	Area	0.159	0.045	Yes	y = −0.054x + 2.316 [b]	UCL: y = 0.085x + 10.907 [d] LCL: y = −0.192x − 6.275
	Peak	0.142	0.074	No	1.380 [a]	From −11.95 to 14.72 [c]
	PCA	0.211	0.008	Yes	y = 0.008x + 0.130 [b]	UCL: y = 0.054x + 2.299 [d] LCL: y = −0.038x − 2.039
	Ideal	0.038	0.631	No	0.884 [a]	From −4.171 to 5.940 [c]
f_B seated	Area	0.142	0.074	No	0.084 [a]	From −9.635 to 9.803 [c]
	Peak	0.132	0.096	No	−0.121 [a]	From −9.931 to 9.688 [c]
	PCA	0.108	0.174	No	−0.23 [a]	From −5.474 to 5.010 [c]
	Ideal	0.196	0.014	Yes	y = −0.021x + 0.597 [b]	UCL: y = 0.028x + 2.057 [d] LCL: y = −0.071x − 0.864
T_I supine	Area	0.302	0.000	Yes	y = 0.084x − 0.019 [b]	UCL: y = 0.618x + 0.095 [d] LCL: y = −0.450x − 0.132
	Peak	0.334	0.000	Yes	y = 0.104x − 0.021 [b]	UCL: y = 0.638x + 0.093 [d] LCL: y = −0.430x − 0.135
	PCA	0.375	0.001	Yes	y = 0.283x − 0.175 [b]	UCL: y = 0.926x − 0.840 [d] LCL: y = −0.390x + 0.354
	Ideal	0.292	0.000	Yes	y = −0.090x + 0.121 [b]	UCL: y = 0.158x + 0.163 [d] LCL: y = −0.338x + 0.078
T_I seated	Area	0.430	0.000	Yes	y = 0.1022x − 0.0141 [b]	UCL: y = 0.834x + 0.112 [d] LCL: y = −0.618x − 0.409
	Peak	0.422	0.000	Yes	y = 0.220x − 0.075 [b]	UCL: y = 0.642x − 0.173 [d] LCL: y = −0.438x + 0.197
	PCA	0.489	0.000	Yes	y = 0.171x − 0.0332 [b]	UCL: y = 0.7182x − 0.226 [d] LCL: y = −0.377x + 0.160
	Ideal	0.313	0.000	Yes	y = −0.059x + 0.129 [b]	UCL: y = 0.211x + 0.069 [d] LCL: y = −0.329x + 0.189
T_E supine	Area	0.421	0.000	Yes	y = −0.170x + 0.166 [b]	UCL: y = 0.508x + 0.358 [d] LCL: y = −0.847x − 0.026
	Peak	0.405	0.000	Yes	y = −0.138x + 0.144 [b]	UCL: y = 0.496x + 0.306 [d] LCL: y = −0.771x − 0.017
	PCA	0.522	0.000	Yes	y = −0.209x + 0.328 [b]	UCL: y = 0.667x + 0.037 [d] LCL: y = −1.084x + 0.620
	Ideal	0.484	0.000	Yes	y = −0.153x + 0.148 [b]	UCL: y = 0.3987x − 0.185 [d] LCL: y = −0.705x + 0.481
T_E seated	Area	0.384	0.000	Yes	y = −0.216x + 0.364 [b]	UCL: y = 0.303x + 0.532 [d] LCL: y = −0.735x + 0.197
	Peak	0.396	0.000	Yes	y = −0.231x + 0.413 [b]	UCL: y = 0.226x + 0.666 [d] LCL: y = −0.657x + 0.101
	PCA	0.422	0.000	Yes	y = −0.127x + 0.320 [b]	UCL: y = 0.284x + 0.498 [d] LCL: y = −0.538x + 0.142
	Ideal	0.316	0.000	Yes	y = −0.058x + 0.054 [b]	UCL: y = 0.383x + 0.337 [d] LCL: y = −0.500x − 0.228

τ: Kendall's τ correlation coefficient and relative p-value (heteroscedasticity test). [a] Fixed Bias. obtained as the mean of differences (device − OEP). for homoscedastic data. [b] OLS: ordinary least squares line of best fit (proportional bias) for heteroscedastic data. [c] LOA: limits of agreement. computed as mean difference ± 1.96SD (for homoscedastic data). [d] V-shape limits: UCL and LCL 95% confidence limits. calculated according to Bland [44].

With respect to the main parameter (f_B), agreement between OEP and the device is very strong when the "Ideal" component or the PCA-fusion are used, both in supine and seated position. In relation to time estimation, the agreement decreases for all the methods considered. In particular, for what concerns inspiratory times, a significant relationship between errors and mean value emerged, with a general increase of the difference (device–OEP) at higher time values (overestimation of the device), both in supine and seated position. Also, for expiratory times absolute errors increased with increasing time values, but in this case the device underestimated at high time values (negative slope of the OLS).

3.5. Quaternion Component Selection

Considering the quaternion components selected by the "Area" and "Peak" methods as best component or identified as "Ideal" component, a clear rule did not emerge. In fact, there was not a quaternion component that was selected as best component with a considerable frequency. Relative frequencies of quaternion component selection with the different methods are presented in Figure 11. It is interesting to notice that quaternion component q_0 was never selected by "Area" and "Peak" methods, while the "Ideal" component was q_0 in 14.86 % of cases (n = 74) in supine position and 6.76% of cases (n = 74) in seated position. In seated position, the component q_1 was selected more frequently as best component both by using "Area" (44.59) and "Peak" (39.19%) methods. In contrast, in supine position, the components q_2 ("Area" 51.35%, "Peak": 41.89) and q_3 ("Area": 39.19% and "Peak": 40.54%) were selected more frequently.

Excluding q_0 component, that was clearly less selected, the other quaternion components were almost equally selected as "Ideal" component considering all the trials, both in supine position (q_0: 14.86%, q_1: 22.97%, q_2: 32.43%, q_3: 29.73%), and seated position (q_0: 6.76%, q_1: 33.78, q_2: 22.97%, q_3: 36.49%).

In regard to the ability of the two component-selection methods ("Area" and "Peak") to identify the "Ideal" component, i.e., the component providing the minimum f_B estimation error, in supine position, the "Area" method was able to identify the "Ideal" component in 45.94% of the cases (relative frequency for the event "the component selected by "Area" method and the "Ideal" component corresponded"), the "Peak" method identified the "Ideal" component in 52.70% of the cases, while for the 45.94% of the cases neither the "Area" method nor the "Peak" method were able to identify the "Ideal" component. In 44.59% of cases, "Area" method and "Peak" method selected the same quaternion component, that was also identified as "Ideal" component.

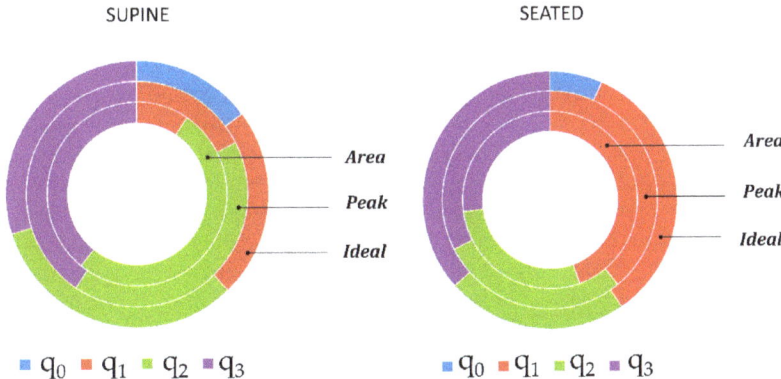

Figure 11. Relative frequencies of quaternion component (q_0, q_1, q_2, q_3) selection using Area and Peak methods and of quaternion component selection as Ideal component, in supine and seated position. Each portion of the rings represents the ratio between the number of times that each quaternion component has been selected (by Area and Peak methods or as Ideal component respectively) and the total number of trials (n = 74).

4. Discussion

In this study, we presented an automatic, position-independent processing algorithm to derive breathing signal, and subsequently breathing temporal parameters, from chest-wall orientation changes acquired using an IMU-based device previously developed by our group [19], composed of three sensor units. Even if the modular configuration of the device was designed to reduce non-breathing movements, the aim of this work was neither to demonstrate the effectiveness of this approach nor to support the presence of the reference unit. On the contrary the focus is on the analysis algorithm, which uses quaternion form to represent orientation, avoiding singularity problem that affects Euler representation; thus, thoracic and abdominal orientation change signals are 4-dimensional entities. The proposed algorithm includes therefore a dimension-reduction block to obtain a 1-dimension signal representing chest-wall orientation changes due to breathing activity.

Another aim of this study was, therefore, to compare three different dimension-reduction methods. The first two methods ("Peak" and "Area") are based on the selection of the quaternion component with the highest breathing information. The third method is based on the fusion of the 4 components of the quaternion using PCA.

The PCA-fusion method performed better than the best component-selection methods ("Peak" and "Area") as regards breathing frequency estimation, both in supine and seated position. In supine position, it provided better results than "Ideal" component, while in seated position it provided closer performances to those obtained by using the "Ideal" component with respect to "Area" and "Peak" methods.

About estimation of other temporal parameters (T_I, T_E and duty cycle), "Ideal" component provided the best results, while PCA-fusion method gave results comparable to the best component-selection methods. Thus, a quaternion component providing the best performance exists, the problem lies in its a priori identification. In fact, both "Area" and "Peak" methods failed to identify it on the basis of spectral analysis (in 45.94% of the cases neither the "Area" method nor the "Peak" method were able to identify the "Ideal" component), and no quaternion component emerged as the most selected as "Ideal" component (supine q_0:14.86%, q_1: 22.97%, q_2: 32.43%, q_3: 29.73%; seated q_0: 6.76%, q_1: 33.78, q_2: 22.97%, q_3: 36.49%).

Geometrical or morphological considerations to determine which quaternion component is more involved in breathing movement are problematic when considering quaternions, and are position- and IMU-placement dependent, thus not suitable in dynamic conditions. On the contrary, PCA-fusion method represents an interesting solution to this problem because it fuses the information of the four quaternion components regardless the position of the subject or the IMUs placement, avoiding the necessity to select a best component/axes, as reported in previous studies [7,11,13].

In this study, we found that PCA-fusion method provided the best f_B estimation performance in terms of mean absolute errors (<2 breaths/minute), correlation (r > 0.963) and agreement (see Table 4) with the reference method. Comparing our results in terms of accuracy errors with those obtained by previous studies is difficult because in most cases only relative errors were reported, but these errors depend on the breathing frequency adopted. Liu et al. [14] reported a mean absolute error of 15.45 breaths/minute (thus about 7 times higher than the error obtained in this study) during quiet sitting. Bates et al. [13] obtained an RMS error of 0.38 breaths/minute and a peak error of 3 breaths/minute in a postoperative patient during sleep. Considering comparable conditions (abdominal compartment in supine position) we obtained an RMS error of 1.51 breaths/minute, using PCA-fusion method, but in our study different, forced, breathing patterns were included, leading to higher mean error.

Regarding correlation between f_B measurements obtained with the proposed method and OEP, our results are comparable to those obtained by Bates et al. [13] that reported a correlation coefficient equal to 0.985 between measurements of f_B obtained with the accelerometer and nasal cannula. Mann et al. [11] obtained a correlation coefficient of 0.97 between measurements of f_B obtained with a tri-axial accelerometer and with a system based on oxygen consumption measurement (Oxycon Mobile). In both cases [11,13], breath-by-breath analysis was not possible. Liu et al. [14] reported correlation coefficients lower than 0.6 between f_B computed with a 3-axis accelerometer and with the reference (Airflow CO_2 analysis).

There are few studies in the literature that performs Bland–Altman analysis to assess the agreement between breathing frequency measurements obtained by using inertial sensors and other validated methods. In the study from Morillo et al. [8] agreement analysis using Bland Altman plots was done against PSG thermistor. The authors reported a mean difference (fixed bias) of 0.02 (SD = 1.09) breaths/minute and LOAs from -3.05 to $+2.11$ breaths/minute in the range $\sim 12 \div 35$ breaths/minute. In that case, the use of a single-axis accelerometer, prevent the use of that method during postural changes. Dehkrodi et al. [9] used a tri-axial accelerometer placed on the suprasternal notch extending the validation presented in [8] to different sleeping positions and breathing conditions (Deep: 13.5 ± 4.3, Normal: 16.5 ± 5.2 and Shallow: 39.7 ± 30.3 breath/minute). They reported a mean difference (fixed bias) of 0.042 breaths/minute and LOAs from -0.65 to 0.74 breaths/minute. Lapi et al. [17] performed agreement analysis with Bland Altman plots for measurements of breathing frequency (range $12 \div 26$ breaths/minute) obtained with the accelerometer and with the standard method (counting breaths by visual inspection), in supine position. They reported a mean difference (fixed bias) of 0.33 breaths/minute and LOA from -1.92 to 2.60 with 3.2% of data outside that range. For all the above-mentioned studies heteroscedasticity of data was not considered or reported making it difficult compare them directly with our results. In fact, taking into account heteroscedasticity of data, for f_B in supine position, we built Bland–Altman plot with proportional bias (OLS: $y = 0.008x + 0.130$, thus going from 0.18 (at $x = 6$ breaths/minute) to 0.61 (at $x = 60$ breaths/minute) breaths/minute) and V-shaped limits (LCL: $y = -0.038x - 2.039$ thus the lower limit goes from -2.26 (at $x = 6$ breaths/minute) to -4.32 (at $x = 60$ breaths/minute) breath/minute; UCL: $y = 0.054x + 2.299$; thus the upper limit goes form 2.62 (at $x = 6$ breaths/minute) to 5.539 (at $x = 60$ breaths/minute) breaths/minute)). Thus, considering comparable breathing frequency ranges our results are closer to those obtained by Morillo et al. [8] and Lapi et al. [17]. On the contrary, Dehkrodi et al. [9] obtained better results; unfortunately, the steps to obtain the acceleration derived respiratory (ADR) signal are not described in detail.

For the best of our knowledge, this is the first study that provides a detailed analysis of respiratory timing measurements obtained by using inertial sensor systems, validating them against an established method.

5. Conclusions

PCA-fusion method provided overall best performances with respect to selecting the best quaternion component identified based on spectrum analysis. In supine position results obtained fusing the 4 quaternion components were even better than those obtained with the "Ideal" component, identified a posteriori considering the minimum breathing frequency estimation error. Performance in seated position were worse than those obtained in supine position, probably because subjects were seated without the back support and some oscillations of the trunk were more likely to occur. This could particularly affect PCA-based method where the first principal component selected for further analysis is the one with the largest variance, and thus more subject to larger body motions. This must be taken into account in dynamic conditions; signal baseline removal prior to PCA-fusion should be considered in this case.

The analysis algorithm proposed in this work, applying PCA-fusion as dimension-reduction method, can be used to analyze further data. In fact, an extended validation of the proposed device and method is needed also in dynamic conditions, during daily activities, considering not only healthy subjects but also patients that could particularly take advantage of this system (e.g., COPD, neuromuscular patients, sleep apnea, etc.). This would also allow study of asynchronies of thoraco-abdominal compartments taking advantage of the modular configuration of the device. Another key step will be the adaptation of our method, currently implemented as an offline analysis, to online monitoring, moving the computation process aboard the smartphone. This enhancement could allow immediate computation of an average breathing frequency over a certain period (e.g., 60 s) directly aboard the smartphone, fostering the use of the device in other applications such as sport and fitness, exercise testing, breathing training to use different respiratory muscles, rehabilitation protocols and treatment evaluation where respiratory assessment could be of great interest.

6. Patents

The present work is partially described in the International Patent application n° PCT/IB2018/054956, priority date 11 July 2017, title "A wearable device for the continuous monitoring of the respiratory rate". Inventors: Ambra Cesareo, Andrea Aliverti, Assignee: Politecnico di Milano.

Author Contributions: A.C. and A.A. contributed IMU circuit design and fabrication; A.C. conceived and designed the experiments; A.C. and Y.P. performed the experiments and analyzed the data; A.C. and E.B. prepared the original draft; E.B. and A.A. reviewed the paper; E.B. and A.A. supervised the project and contributed to funding acquisition.

Funding: This research received no external funding.

Acknowledgments: This work was supported by "FoRST -Fondazione per la Ricerca Scientifica Termale".

Conflicts of Interest: The authors declare no conflict of interest.

References

1. Subbe, C.; Davies, R.; Williams, E.; Rutherford, P.; Gemmell, L. Effect of Introducing the Modified Early Warning Score on Clinical Outcomes, cardio-pulmonary Arrests and Intensive Care Utilisation in Acute Medical Admissions. *Anaesthesia* **2003**, *58*, 797–802. [CrossRef] [PubMed]
2. Cretikos, M.A.; Bellomo, R.; Hillman, K.; Chen, J.; Finfer, S.; Flabouris, A. Respiratory Rate: The Neglected Vital Sign. *Med. J. Aust.* **2008**, *188*, 657.
3. World Health Organization. *Acute Respiratory Infections in Children: Case Management in Small Hospitals in Developing Countries, a Manual for Doctors and Other Senior Health Workers*; World Health Organization: Geneva, Switzerland, 1990.
4. Karlen, W.; Gan, H.; Chiu, M.; Dunsmuir, D.; Zhou, G.; Dumont, G.A.; Ansermino, J.M. Improving the Accuracy and Efficiency of Respiratory Rate Measurements in Children using Mobile Devices. *PLoS ONE* **2014**, *9*, e99266. [CrossRef] [PubMed]
5. Torres, A.; Fiz, J.; Galdiz, B.; Gea, J.; Morera, J.; Jané, R. Assessment of Respiratory Muscle Effort Studying Diaphragm Movement Registered with Surface Sensors. Animal Model (Dogs). In Proceedings of the 26th Annual International Conference of the IEEE Engineering in Medicine and Biology Society (IEMBS'04), San Francisco, CA, USA, 1–4 September 2004; pp. 3917–3920.
6. Reinvuo, T.; Hannula, M.; Sorvoja, H.; Alasaarela, E.; Myllyla, R. Measurement of Respiratory Rate with High-Resolution Accelerometer and EMFit Pressure Sensor. In Proceedings of the 2006 IEEE Sensors Applications Symposium, Houston, TX, USA, 7–9 February 2006; pp. 192–195.
7. Hung, P.; Bonnet, S.; Guillemaud, R.; Castelli, E.; Yen, P.T.N. Estimation of Respiratory Waveform using an Accelerometer. In Proceedings of the 5th IEEE International Symposium on Biomedical Imaging: From Nano to Macro (ISBI 2008), Paris, France, 14–17 May 2008; pp. 1493–1496.
8. Morillo, D.S.; Ojeda, J.L.R.; Foix, L.F.C.; Jiménez, A.L. An Accelerometer-Based Device for Sleep Apnea Screening. *IEEE Trans. Inf. Technol. Biomed.* **2010**, *14*, 491–499. [CrossRef] [PubMed]
9. Dehkordi, P.K.; Marzencki, M.; Tavakolian, K.; Kaminska, M.; Kaminska, B. Validation of Respiratory Signal Derived from Suprasternal Notch Acceleration for Sleep Apnea Detection. In Proceedings of the 2011 Annual International Conference of the IEEE Engineering in Medicine and Biology Society (EMBC), Boston, MA, USA, 30 August–3 September 2011; pp. 3824–3827.
10. Fekr, A.R.; Janidarmian, M.; Radecka, K.; Zilic, Z. A Medical Cloud-Based Platform for Respiration Rate Measurement and Hierarchical Classification of Breath Disorders. *Sensors* **2014**, *14*, 11204–11224. [CrossRef] [PubMed]
11. Mann, J.; Rabinovich, R.; Bates, A.; Giavedoni, S.; MacNee, W.; Arvind, D. Simultaneous Activity and Respiratory Monitoring using an Accelerometer. In Proceedings of the 2011 International Conference Body Sensor Networks (BSN), Dallas, TX, USA, 23–25 May 2011; pp. 139–143.
12. Jin, A.; Yin, B.; Morren, G.; Duric, H.; Aarts, R.M. Performance Evaluation of a Tri-Axial Accelerometry-Based Respiration Monitoring for Ambient Assisted Living. In Proceedings of the Annual International Conference of the IEEE Engineering in Medicine and Biology Society (EMBC 2009), Minneapolis, MN, USA, 2–6 September 2009; pp. 5677–5680.

13. Bates, A.; Ling, M.J.; Mann, J.; Arvind, D. Respiratory Rate and Flow Waveform Estimation from Tri-Axial Accelerometer Data. In Proceedings of the 2010 International Conference on Body Sensor Networks (BSN), Singapore, 7–9 June 2010; pp. 144–150.
14. Liu, G.; Guo, Y.; Zhu, Q.; Huang, B.; Wang, L. Estimation of Respiration Rate from Three-Dimensional Acceleration Data Based on Body Sensor Network. *Telemed. e-Health* **2011**, *17*, 705–711. [CrossRef] [PubMed]
15. Yoon, J.; Noh, Y.; Kwon, Y.; Kim, W.; Yoon, H. Improvement of Dynamic Respiration Monitoring through Sensor Fusion of Accelerometer and Gyro-Sensor. *J. Electr. Eng. Technol.* **2014**, *9*, 334–343. [CrossRef]
16. Gollee, H.; Chen, W. Real-Time Detection of Respiratory Activity using an Inertial Measurement Unit. In Proceedings of the 29th Annual International Conference of the IEEE Engineering in Medicine and Biology Society (EMBS 2007), Lyon, France, 23–26 August 2007; pp. 2230–2233.
17. Lapi, S.; Lavorini, F.; Borgioli, G.; Calzolai, M.; Masotti, L.; Pistolesi, M.; Fontana, G.A. Respiratory Rate Assessments using a Dual-Accelerometer Device. *Respir. Physiol. Neurobiol.* **2014**, *191*, 60–66. [CrossRef]
18. Gaidhani, A.; Moon, K.S.; Ozturk, Y.; Lee, S.Q.; Youm, W. Extraction and Analysis of Respiratory Motion using Wearable Inertial Sensor System during Trunk Motion. *Sensors* **2017**, *17*, 2932. [CrossRef]
19. Cesareo, A.; Gandolfi, S.; Pini, I.; Biffi, E.; Reni, G.; Aliverti, A. A Novel, Low Cost, Wearable Contact-Based Device for Breathing Frequency Monitoring. In Proceedings of the 2017 39th Annual International Conference of the IEEE Engineering in Medicine and Biology Society (EMBC), Seogwipo, Korea, 11–15 July 2017; pp. 2402–2405.
20. Romei, M.; Mauro, A.L.; D'angelo, M.; Turconi, A.; Bresolin, N.; Pedotti, A.; Aliverti, A. Effects of Gender and Posture on Thoraco-Abdominal Kinematics during Quiet Breathing in Healthy Adults. *Respir. Physiol. Neurobiol.* **2010**, *172*, 184–191. [CrossRef]
21. Aliverti, A.; Pedotti, A. Opto-electronic plethysmography. In *Mechanics of Breathing*; Springer: Milano, Italy, 2002; pp. 47–59.
22. Aliverti, A.; Dellacà, R.; Pelosi, P.; Chiumello, D.; Gattinoni, L.; Pedotti, A. Compartmental Analysis of Breathing in the Supine and Prone Positions by Optoelectronic Plethysmography. *Ann. Biomed. Eng.* **2001**, *29*, 60–70. [CrossRef] [PubMed]
23. Aliverti, A.; Dellaca, R.; Pelosi, P.; Chiumello, D.; Pedotti, A.; Gattinoni, L. Optoelectronic Plethysmography in Intensive Care Patients. *Am. J. Respir. Crit. Care Med.* **2000**, *161*, 1546–1552. [CrossRef] [PubMed]
24. Cala, S.; Kenyon, C.; Ferrigno, G.; Carnevali, P.; Aliverti, A.; Pedotti, A.; Macklem, P.; Rochester, D. Chest Wall and Lung Volume Estimation by Optical Reflectance Motion Analysis. *J. Appl. Physiol.* **1996**, *81*, 2680–2689. [CrossRef] [PubMed]
25. Ferrigno, G.; Carnevali, P.; Aliverti, A.; Molteni, F.; Beulcke, G.; Pedotti, A. Three-Dimensional Optical Analysis of Chest Wall Motion. *J. Appl. Physiol.* **1994**, *77*, 1224–1231. [CrossRef] [PubMed]
26. Konno, K.; Mead, J. Measurement of the separate volume changes of rib cage and abdomen during breathing. *J. Appl. Physiol.* **1967**, *22*, 407–422. [CrossRef] [PubMed]
27. Hamilton, W.R. XI. On Quaternions; Or on a New System of Imaginaries in Algebra. *Lond. Edinb. Dublin Philos. Mag. J. Sci.* **1848**, *33*, 58–60. [CrossRef]
28. Rosenfeld, B. *The History of Non-Euclidean Geometry: Evolution of the Concept of a Geometrical Space*; Springer-Verlag: Berlin, Germany, 1988.
29. Madgwick, S.O.; Harrison, A.J.; Vaidyanathan, R. Estimation of IMU and MARG Orientation using a Gradient Descent Algorithm. In Proceedings of the 2011 IEEE International Conference on Rehabilitation Robotics (ICORR), Zurich, Switzerland, 29 June–1 July 2011; pp. 1–7.
30. Pearson, K. LIII. On Lines and Planes of Closest Fit to Systems of Points in Space. *Lond. Edinb. Dublin Philos. Mag. J. Sci.* **1901**, *2*, 559–572. [CrossRef]
31. Hotelling, H. Analysis of a Complex of Statistical Variables into Principal Components. *J. Educ. Psychol.* **1933**, *24*, 417. [CrossRef]
32. Savitzky, A.; Golay, M.J. Smoothing and Differentiation of Data by Simplified Least Squares Procedures. *Anal. Chem.* **1964**, *36*, 1627–1639. [CrossRef]
33. Kenyon, C.M.; Cala, S.J.; Yan, S.; Aliverti, A.; Scano, G.; Duranti, R.; Pedotti, A.; Macklem, P.T. Rib cage mechanics during quiet breathing and exercise in humans. *J. Appl. Physiol.* **1997**, *83*, 1242–1255. [CrossRef]
34. Layton, A.M.; Moran, S.L.; Garber, C.E.; Armstrong, H.F.; Basner, R.C.; Thomashow, B.M.; Bartels, M.N. Optoelectronic plethysmography compared to spirometry during maximal exercise. *Respir. Physiol. Neurobiol.* **2013**, *185*, 362–368. [CrossRef] [PubMed]

35. LoMauro, A.; Cesareo, A.; Agosti, F.; Tringali, G.; Salvadego, D.; Grassi, B.; Sartorio, A.; Aliverti, A. Effects of a Multidisciplinary Body Weight Reduction Program on Static and Dynamic Thoraco-Abdominal Volumes in Obese Adolescents. *Appl. Physiol. Nutr. Metab.* **2016**, *41*, 649–658. [CrossRef] [PubMed]
36. Lo Mauro, A.; D'Angelo, M.G.; Romei, M.; Motta, F.; Colombo, D.; Comi, G.P.; Pedotti, A.; Marchi, E.; Turconi, A.C.; Bresolin, N.; et al. Abdominal Volume Contribution to Tidal Volume as an Early Indicator of Respiratory Impairment in Duchenne Muscular Dystrophy. *Eur. Respir. J.* **2010**, *35*, 1118–1125. [CrossRef] [PubMed]
37. Cesareo, A.; LoMauro, A.; Santi, M.; Biffi, E.; D'Angelo, M.G.; Aliverti, A. Acute Effects of Mechanical Insufflation-Exsufflation on the Breathing Pattern in Stable Subjects with Duchenne Muscular Dystrophy. *Respir. Care* **2018**. [CrossRef] [PubMed]
38. Benjamini, Y.; Hochberg, Y. Controlling the False Discovery Rate: A Practical and Powerful Approach to Multiple Testing. *J. R. Stat. Soc. Ser. B Methodol.* **1995**, *57*, 289–300. [CrossRef]
39. Benjamini, Y.; Yekutieli, D. The Control of the False Discovery Rate in Multiple Testing Under Dependency. *Ann. Stat.* **2001**, 1165–1188.
40. Altman, D.G.; Bland, J.M. Measurement in Medicine: The Analysis of Method Comparison Studies. *Statistician* **1983**, 307–317. [CrossRef]
41. Bland, J.M.; Altman, D. Statistical Methods for Assessing Agreement between Two Methods of Clinical Measurement. *Lancet* **1986**, *327*, 307–310. [CrossRef]
42. Bland, J.M.; Altman, D.G. Measuring Agreement in Method Comparison Studies. *Stat. Methods Med. Res.* **1999**, *8*, 135–160. [CrossRef]
43. BREHM, M.; Scholtes, V.A.; Dallmeijer, A.J.; Twisk, J.W.; Harlaar, J. The Importance of Addressing Heteroscedasticity in the Reliability Analysis of ratio-scaled Variables: An Example Based on Walking energy-cost Measurements. *Dev. Med. Child Neurol.* **2012**, *54*, 267–273. [CrossRef]
44. Bland, J. How Do I Estimate Limits of Agreement When the Mean or SD of Differences Is Not Constant? Available online: https://www-users.york.ac.uk/~{}mb55/meas/glucose.htm (accessed on 4 October 2018).
45. Ludbrook, J. Confidence in Altman–Bland Plots: A Critical Review of the Method of Differences. *Clin. Exp. Pharmacol. Physiol.* **2010**, *37*, 143–149. [CrossRef] [PubMed]

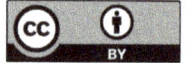

© 2018 by the authors. Licensee MDPI, Basel, Switzerland. This article is an open access article distributed under the terms and conditions of the Creative Commons Attribution (CC BY) license (http://creativecommons.org/licenses/by/4.0/).

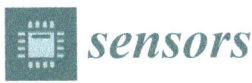

Article

Physical Workload Tracking Using Human Activity Recognition with Wearable Devices

Jose Manjarres *, Pedro Narvaez, Kelly Gasser, Winston Percybrooks and Mauricio Pardo

Department of Electrical and Electronics Engineering, Universidad del Norte, Barranquilla 081001, Colombia; pjnarvaez@uninorte.edu.co (P.N.); kgasser@uninorte.edu.co (K.G.); wpercyb@uninorte.edu.co (W.P.); mpardo@uninorte.edu.co (M.P.)
* Correspondence: jemanjarres@uninorte.edu.co

Received: 14 November 2019; Accepted: 13 December 2019; Published: 19 December 2019

Abstract: In this work, authors address workload computation combining human activity recognition and heart rate measurements to establish a scalable framework for health at work and fitness-related applications. The proposed architecture consists of two wearable sensors: one for motion, and another for heart rate. The system employs machine learning algorithms to determine the activity performed by a user, and takes a concept from ergonomics, the Frimat's score, to compute the corresponding physical workload from measured heart rate values providing in addition a qualitative description of the workload. A random forest activity classifier is trained and validated with data from nine subjects, achieving an accuracy of 97.5%. Then, tests with 20 subjects show the reliability of the activity classifier, which keeps an accuracy up to 92% during real-time testing. Additionally, a single-subject twenty-day physical workload tracking case study evinces the system capabilities to detect body adaptation to a custom exercise routine. The proposed system enables remote and multi-user workload monitoring, which facilitates the job for experts in ergonomics and workplace health.

Keywords: human activity recognition; physical workload; wearable systems for healthcare; machine learning for real-time applications

1. Introduction

According to the World Health Organization (WHO), the amount of workload can be a hazard at the workplace leading to work-related stress [1]. Having too much or too little to do at work is often an indication of bad time management that results on mental stress [1,2]. Mental stress affects the heart rate (HR) that in turns spreads its effects to other parts of the body [3]. Workload is a key factor in ergonomics to determine the adequate length and number of rest breaks for a given job, helping to reduce work-related stress [4]. However, the amount of physical workload is not necessarily determined by the length of a particular task, but by the quantity of energy required to complete it, and can also be reflected on the HR [5].

In consequence, works like [5] describe the importance of HR tracking in physical workload assessment. The authors of [5] perform a comparison between using absolute cardiac cost (ACC) and relative cardiac cost (RCC) to evaluate physical workload based on HR values during resting periods between activities. Similarly, Solé proposes in [6] an standardization for workload values based on RCC using the Chamoux [7] and Frimat [8] criteria, where the numeric workload scores are mapped into categories going from *extremely hard* to *very light*. These criteria allow a qualitative assessment of workload using only HR measurements.

A common element among the physical effort assessment systems is HR tracking. HR has a well-known relation with mental stress, as evidenced in [9–12]. The methods to obtain information about heart activity must be reliable and must allow their implementation using non-invasive devices to be relevant in practice. In [13], a comparison of HR signals coming from an electrocardiography (ECG) and a photoplethysmography (PPG) sensor establishes the reliability of PPG to obtain HR information. Additionally, the authors of [14] validate the use of a commercial HR monitor, which employs PPG to track HR waveforms during rest. A similar conclusion is found in [15] with a smartwatch. This validation of PPG-based HR tracking has led to developments that seek to strengthen HR monitoring on environments where sensor signals can be corrupted by body movements [16]. Despite of such possible corruption, other systems have been built with PPG sensors under movement conditions and have not displayed issues regarding performance [17–19].

Regarding physical workload, several methods for continuous track of the physical effort can be found in literature where qualitative data are not provided. For example, in [20] Jovanov et al. use a wireless body area network (WBAN) to monitor motion from on-body accelerometer and electrocardiography (ECG) sensors. Such a system intends to keep track of the physical activity and health status with non-invasive technology. Other works like [21–24] propose manually initiated recording of activities with data from HR trackers to measure the physical workload of a given population. Such a method is tested in [21–24] with salsa dancers, dockers, nurses and porters, respectively. Complementary, Jovanov et al. introduce real-time HR monitoring and step counting to track the work stress in nurses in [12]. Our previous work in [19] improves the method proposed in [21] by developing a mobile application that computes the workload during each activity performed by janitorial staff. In the case of [19] the system is manually initiated, as in [21–24], and allows only local monitoring, which requires the presence of an expert next to the worker. In most real-life scenarios, having an ergonomics expert all over the workplace is unfeasible.

To follow the tendencies on mobile-health applications, it is necessary to address the problem of workload assessment from a real-time perspective as suggested by [12]. Therefore, HR tracking must be integrated with real-time human activity recognition (HAR) or online HAR (according to [25]) to achieve workload assessment without requiring manual intervention to indicate the start and end of an activity. Some works have shown efforts to achieve this integration. For example, [26–28] exhibit systems that combine HR tracking and online HAR using on-body sensors and an integration device to receive and display the sensors information. The integration device, typically a smartphone, can take the place of a movement sensor [29]. Accordingly, [30–32] describe smartphone-based HAR systems along with their corresponding challenges regarding feature extraction and selection. However, these systems are highly dependent on the on-body location of the smartphone. On the other hand, accelerometer-based HAR architectures present robust performance regardless the sensor location and allow to distinguish among a wider range of activities compared to smartphone-based systems [26,33–35].

The robustness and reliability of HAR with accelerometers is reflected in the variety of the e-health applications where it is found. For example, [36] employs accelerometer-based HAR for posture recognition which helps to monitor falls in elderly people. Such an approach is also present in [37–39], which demonstrates the rising popularity of this application. Moreover, some developments related with sports and fitness complemented with HAR are shown in [40,41].

Thus from these previous works, it can be concluded that HAR is suitable as a key component for workload tracking. Nevertheless, the need of relevant implementations that integrate HR and HAR tracking and take it a step further to qualitative workload assessment remains a challenge from an ergonomic point-of-view. Consequently, the work described in this article presents a solution that embraces wearable technology and machine learning algorithms to compute physical workload in real-time. Our solution here combines the HAR and HR tracking to achieve a workload assessment that is linked automatically with the performed activity. Compared to our previous work in [19], this new system eliminates the need of an expert next to every single worker that is being tracked, since it enables remote and multi-user monitoring.

The rest of the paper is organized as follows. Section 2 describes the characteristics of the wearable devices implemented in this system, details the workflow of the mobile application, and displays how the system classifies the workload. Section 3 shows the development of the online HAR component and presents two cases of study to evaluate the online HAR performance and the physical workload assessment. Sections 4 and 5 contain the discussion and conclusions regarding the results, respectively.

2. Materials and Methods

2.1. Wearable Devices and Mobile Application

The hardware for HAR comprises of an ultra-low power (ULP) microcontroller unit (MCU) with Bluetooth low energy (BLE) capability, an ULP MEMS (Micro Electro-Mechanical Systems) based accelerometer and a small Li-ion battery. The HAR hardware is displayed in Figure 1. The selected ULP MCU is the Lilypad Simblee, as used in [26]. The advantages of this device include small footprint (50 mm diameter), embedded BLE radio, and a battery charge controller. A 100 mAh Li-ion battery powers the Lilypad Simblee and can be recharged through a USB controller module [42]. This MCU samples the signal from a tri-axial accelerometer at a 20 Hz rate, as recommended in [25]. The accelerometer selection also follows the hardware used in [26], which is the ADXL335. This sensor allows us to obtain information from movement and inclination with a sampling frequency up to 50 Hz and an acceleration up to 2 g [43].

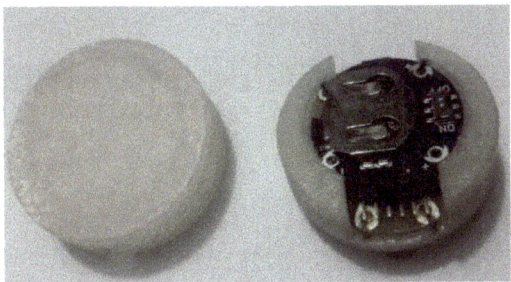

Figure 1. Human activity recognition hardware. The case allows the system to be worn on the hip.

For the HR tracking, a Microsoft Band performs HR sampling with a built-in PPG sensor [44]. This wearable enables the tracking of other fitness-related variables such as sweating, arm movement and step counting, among others [44]. This device has been validated by different authors for HR monitoring [45,46]. For this work, we only required the HR sensor; and therefore, other sensors are deactivated to save energy. A specialized Software Development Kit (SDK) for Android devices permits the control of the Microsoft Band. This SDK can be found in [47]. We develop a mobile application that connects automatically to both sensors and has two operating modes: training mode and testing mode.

In training mode, the user interface (UI) asks for the activity that the user is going to perform from a list of predefined exercises (jogging, squatting, doing push-ups and doing crunches) and the average HR at rest to use it as a reference parameter for workload estimation. A 1-minute timer is used to standardize the length of the training sessions for the classification algorithms. The UI for this operation mode is displayed in Figure 2a. The application stores the incoming data from both sensors in a JSON (JavaScript Object Notation) array, expecting to have 20 samples of each accelerometer axis, the average HR within one second and a label representing the activity. Every second, the JSON array containing the sensor samples is sent to a cloud server for storage in a database. After taking training samples from nine subjects, a Python script retrieves the stored data along with its corresponding activity labels and trains a classification model using the scikit-learn library [48]. The details regarding training and validation are explained in the Section Results. Once the model is validated, the mobile application can function in the testing mode. In this mode, the sampling process from the sensors remains the same as in the training mode; however, the UI does not have any time restriction. Therefore, an array containing the samples from the tri-axial accelerometer is taken by a feature-computing function followed by the classification model and the average HR during activity passes through a workload estimator. Figure 2b shows the UI for the testing mode.

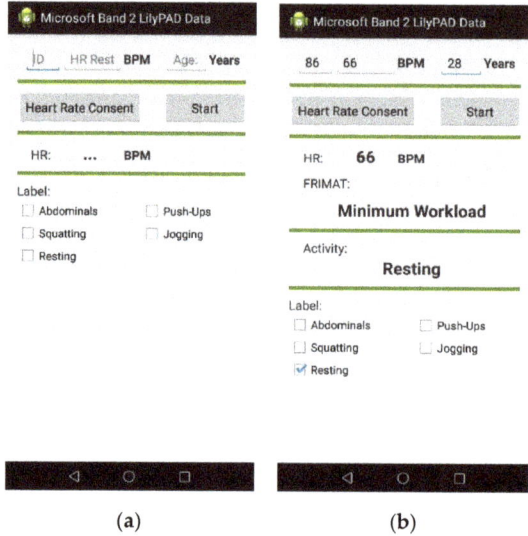

(a)   (b)

Figure 2. User interface of the mobile application. (**a**) Training mode. (**b**) Testing mode.

2.2. Physical Workload Computation

As [6] mentions, physical workload can be computed using metabolic consumption tables, oxygen consumption tables and HR measurements. However, HR measurements are the only non-invasive method, which allows the integration of wearable technology. In the literature, there are two criteria to evaluate HR-based workload: Frimat's [8] and Chamoux's [7]. In one hand, the Frimat's criterion estimates workload on short work times or on specific activities; while, on the other hand, the Chamoux criterion computes the workload of a full workday (at least 8 h) [19]. For this work, the Frimat's criterion is chosen since the target are fitness-related activities. The methodology used for physical workload computation is the same as in [19].

The selected method requires the computation of some cardiac indicators. The first one is the absolute cardiac cost (ACC) as defined by Equation (1),

$$ACC = HR_{activity} - HR_{rest}, \tag{1}$$

where $HR_{activity}$ refers to the average heart rate during the activity and HR_{rest} is the statistical mode of the HR values measured during resting periods. ACC allows the estimation of intensity for a given task. Another indicator, the relative cardiac cost (RCC) is derived from the ACC as shown in Equation (2).

$$RCC = \frac{ACC}{HR_{max} - HR_{rest}} \times 100. \tag{2}$$

RCC indicates the adaptation of the body to an activity.

In Equation (2), HR_{max} stands for the maximum achievable HR by a subject. The exact value of HR_{max} should be found in a stress test. However, [6] provides a theoretical definition, which can have up to 5% of error compared to the actual value. Such definition for HR_{max} depends on the subject age as stated in Equation (3),

$$HR_{max} = 220 - Age. \tag{3}$$

Frimat's criterion also needs the calculation of the cardiac acceleration (ΔHR) defined in Equation (4), and the mean heart rate ($\overline{HR}$) within an arbitrary time window.

$$\Delta HR = HR_{max} - \overline{HR}. \tag{4}$$

Thus, once the five variables for Frimat's criterion (ACC, RCC, HR_{max}, $\overline{HR}$ and ΔHR) are computed, each one of them is mapped into a corresponding Frimat's coefficient, which takes an integer value between 1 and 5. Table 1 details the relation between the values of each indicator and their respective Frimat's coefficient.

Table 1. Relation between Frimat's coefficients and cardiac indicators.

Frimat's Coeffs. Value	Variable Ranges				
	ACC (bpm)	RCC (bpm)	HR_{max} (bpm)	$\overline{HR}$ (bpm)	ΔHR (bpm)
1	10–14	0.10–0.14	110–119	90–94	20–24
2	15–19	0.15–0.19	120–129	95–99	25–29
3	20–24	0.20–0.24	130–139	100–104	30–34
4	25–29	0.25–0.29	140–149	105–109	35–39
5	>30	>0.30	>150	>110	>40

Then, the method requires to take the Frimat's coefficient from each input variable and add them up to obtain a Frimat's score, which ranges between 5 and 25. This score is the value that determines the level of physical workload of an activity. Following the ranking presented in [6], an activity can be ranked as shown in Table 2. During the implementation of the workload computation, the system takes the resting HR that must be previously measured and compares it with the average HR within one-second time windows to compute the five cardiac indicators needed to obtain the Frimat's Score. This score was mapped to its corresponding category according to Table 2, accompanied with the label of the most recent activity.

Table 2. Ranking of an activity according to its Frimat's score.

Frimat's Score Values	Ranking
25	Extremely hard
24	Very hard
22–23	Hard
20–21	Distressing
18–19	Bearable
14–17	Light
12–13	Very light
≤10	Minimum workload

3. Results

3.1. Training and Validation of the Activity Classifier

The implementation of the online HAR subsystem requires three critical steps: data collection, training and validation. To perform a reliable data collection, the selected activities must be clearly distinguishable from the sensor point-of-view and they should be related to a common set of tasks. For the sake of test subject availability, we selected a fitness routine, which includes jogging, doing crunches, push-ups and squatting. These activities are among the most common exercises performed by the local population. Since the workload assessment requires us to track the resting periods, standing still is also an activity into consideration. Additionally, to increase the system generalization capabilities, data collection must be done from heterogeneous sources, i.e., subjects with different anatomic characteristics and different styles to perform exercises. Thus, nine volunteer subjects (six men and three women) performed the four mentioned exercises during the same amount of time. The ages of the volunteers ranged between 19 and 32 years. At least four hours before each exercise session, volunteers did not drink substances that alter HR, such as: caffeine, alcohol, nicotine, etc. Five subjects exercise four times a week, while the other four subjects only exercise once in a week. Data was collected between Monday and Friday in the evening (18:00–20:00). Since exercises like push-ups and crunches are generally more physically demanding than jogging and squatting, we designed the sessions of the experiments to consist of one-minute part of exercise and three-minute part of resting. Hence, each volunteer performs at least four different sessions, one per exercise. To avoid unexpected short pauses during the exercising part of each session, hydration needs of the subjects are attended as required. These unexpected pauses would represent noise on the motion signals and can introduce undesired glitches in the training and validation datasets. Such glitches are unavoidable in the practice, but to guarantee the correct labeling of data, we asked subjects to reduce the pauses during exercises. Thus, to overcome this issue, subjects with better physical condition were asked to participate in more than one experiment. By the end of collection, the dataset for training and validation contained over 118,000 three-dimensional samples taken at 20 Hz from the hip-placed accelerometer.

Consequently, the dataset must be converted to a multidimensional space of features. The considered feature set was the same as in the previous work [26]. Thus, it is shown that the most relevant features are those summarized in Table 3.

Table 3. Features considered for training.

Feature name	Symbol per axis	Meaning
Mean	$\bar{x}, \bar{y}, \bar{z}$	Statistical tendency of a group of samples from the same axis
Standard deviation	std(x), std(y), std(z)	Measure of variability of a group of samples from the same axis
Variance	var(x), var(y), var(z)	Measure of variability of the squares of a group of samples from their corresponding mean
Mean absolute deviation	MAD(x), MAD(y), MAD(z)	Measure of variability of a group of samples from their corresponding mean
Difference of means	$\bar{x} - \bar{y}, \bar{y} - \bar{z}, \bar{x} - \bar{z}$	Difference between means of two different axes

This preselected feature set is the product of an extensive literature review about online HAR systems and the engineering process carried out in [26]. Table 3 describes each considered feature along with their corresponding symbol and meaning. Each one of the 15 mentioned features must be computed from a group of samples, and each array forms a feature vector; therefore, the sample-group size becomes a concern. The group size is named time-window size, since the number of samples required to calculate a feature vector is directly related to the amount of time that the system takes to gather the samples. From the real-time implementation perspective, this time-window size is critical to determine the system latency. Hence, the selected time-window size is one second considering that the perception of activity changes for different users is not immediate and there is the need of gathering enough data within a time window to allow a clear distinction between activities. Thus, the minimum delay for the classifier to detect a change of activities was one second, and each feature vector was computed using 20 samples, due to the sensor 20 Hz sampling frequency.

After setting the time-window size, the dataset was reduced to 5900 feature vectors approximately, each one associated to their respective activity label. Next, classification algorithms to train with this dataset were needed. According to [25], random forest (RF) and k-nearest neighbors (kNN) are the most common choices for online HAR applications. In the present work, both algorithms were used in order to compare their performance to select one for implementation.

RF algorithm is an estimator that separates the training dataset into subsets for a custom number of decision trees. These trees decide over their respective samples and then the estimator averages their decisions. On the other hand, kNN algorithm maps the feature vectors into a multidimensional space and separates them according to their labels. Then, an incoming sample was compared to its closest training samples (or neighbors), determined by an internal distance measure, and the incoming sample was assigned to the class of most of its neighbors.

Collected data from the volunteers was separated by assigning 70% to a training subset and 30% for a validation subset, following a proper data randomization to avoid underfitting. Then, RF estimators were trained varying the number of trees from 2 to 100, and kNN with the number of neighbors from 2 to 50. These values are chosen after noticing that there was not a significant improvement on overall accuracy by increasing the number of trees or neighbors, respectively. Best results show an overall accuracy of 97.7% for RF with 63 trees and 95.2% for kNN with five neighbors. The normalized confusion matrices for both algorithms are displayed in Figure 3. These confusion matrices evince the difference in the overall accuracies by exhibiting less confusion in crunches, push-ups and squatting for the RF algorithm compared to kNN. Such results were obtained using the validation subset. Consequently, optimization efforts were conducted towards RF.

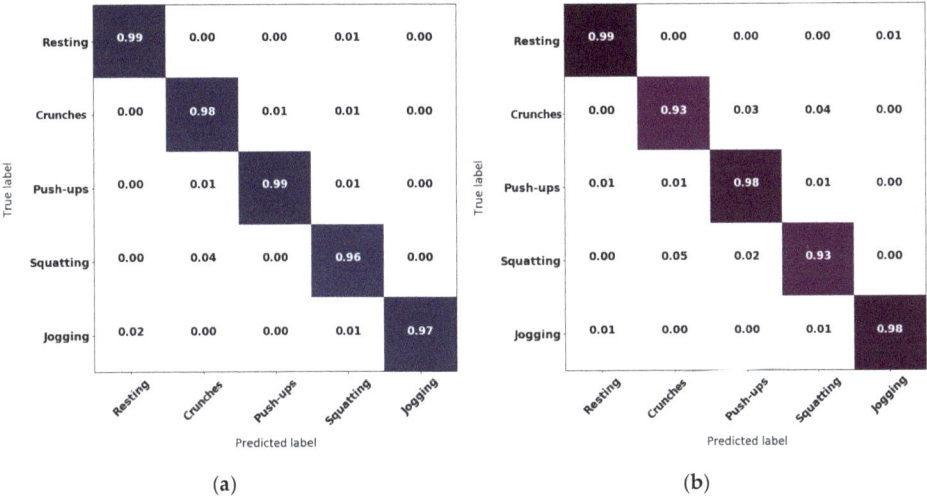

Figure 3. Normalized confusion matrices for: (**a**) random forest (RF) classifier and (**b**) k-nearest neighbor (kNN) classifier.

A classifier optimization process is required to reduce dimensionality and, in the case of RF, reduce the number of decision trees. After such a process, validation of the optimized classifier should not show significant reduction on the performance metrics (overall accuracy and confusion matrix).

For dimensionality reduction, the level of importance that each feature has during training was analyzed. The importance levels considered here were equivalent to Gini importance, which is described in [49]. This importance was computed considering the decrease in average accuracy for the trained trees when a feature value was varied randomly. Thus, significant accuracy detriments point to the significant importance for a feature. In the case of the scikit-learn library, the feature importance levels are normalized. Figure 4 displays a bar graph of the feature importance. As observed, it was clear that $\bar{y}$, MAD(y), MAD(z) and $\bar{x} - \bar{y}$ were the features with the lower significance; and therefore, we proceeded to remove them from the feature vectors. Even though further reduction in the number of features reduced the code size that would be embedded in the mobile application; extra reductions could also compromise the classifier performance. Thus, we decided to work with the new feature set of 11 features; but therefore, the model needs to be retrained with this new set.

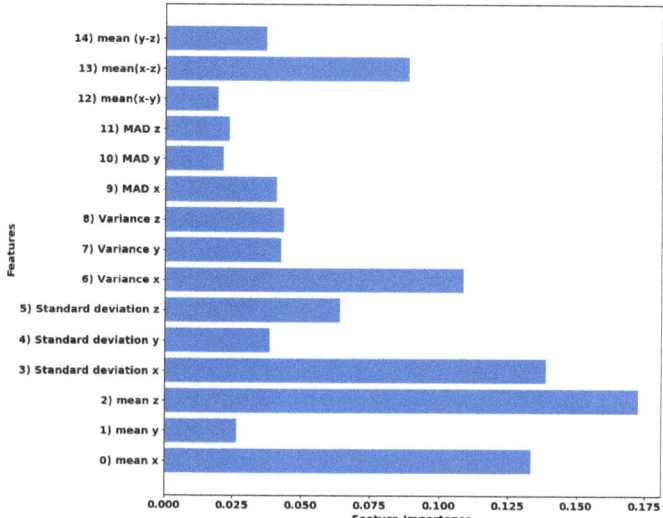

Figure 4. Bar graph of the importance of the features in RF classifier.

Figure 5 shows the variation of classifier accuracy with respect to the number of trees, along with a dashed tendency line. According to the accuracy tendency line, after 20 trees, the classifier trended to a stable behavior. Consequently, the number of trees could be reduced to a value above 20 trees without sacrificing performance. In our tests, the overall accuracy with the validation subset changed from 97.7% with 63 trees to 97.5% with 24 trees, but with lower computational cost. Figure 6 exhibits the confusion matrix of this new model, where it could be observed that there was no performance compromise, which facilitated performing the classification directly on the mobile application.

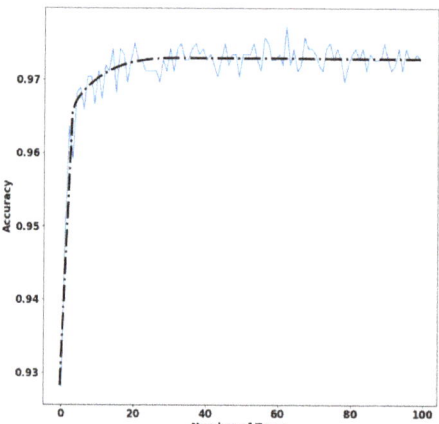

Figure 5. Variation of the overall accuracy with the number of trees in the RF classifier.

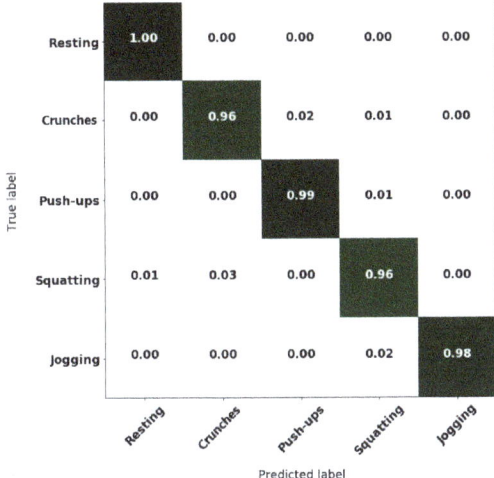

Figure 6. Confusion matrix of the optimized RF classifier.

The resulting model was exported from Python to Java using the Porter tool described in [50] given the requirements of the Android environment. Thus, the model converted into a Java class contains the mathematical description of the 24 decision trees and computes the average decision among them to estimate the corresponding activity. The mobile application includes a testing mode where it reports the true label of the activity performed during the experiment and the labels detected by the model, along with a user identification number and the time stamps of the samples. Thus, this working mode was used for the remaining tests described next.

3.2. Online HAR Performance

Once the classifier model was embedded in the mobile application, the model was tested in a real-time environment. For the test, 20 people, different from the nine volunteers who participated in the training data collection, were asked to participate in a new set of experiments. This time, people registered their age on the application along with the average heart rate obtained from the smartwatch on a preliminary 30-seconds resting period. Then, they wore the HAR device on the hip and performed the following exercise routine: push-ups, resting, jogging, resting, squatting, resting, crunches and resting. Each of these activities had a fixed duration of 30 s, which was set seeking a limitation of physical demand to avoid unexpected resting moments. Planned, 30-second resting moments were situated between exercises to help subjects to fulfill the routine without extreme fatigue. Along with each routine, a researcher manipulated the application to set the activity label manually as the subjects shifted from one activity to another. Meanwhile, the system reported to a cloud-stored database the labels obtained from the model, the labels entered manually, a system-custom user identification number and the time stamp.

After this data collection stage, the detected labels were compared against the manual labels to obtain the accuracy rate per activity and per user. Table 4 resumes the statistics of the accuracies from the testing stage. Figure 7 also shows the confusion matrix from online HAR testing. Although the validation accuracy was reported to be 97.5%, real-time tests had an average accuracy between 86% and 92% due to unexpected movements that induced noise for the classifier. Further details regarding the results of Table 4 and Figure 7 are given in the Section Discussion.

Table 4. Representative statistics of the online human activity recognition (HAR) testing.

Statistical Parameter	Accuracy Percentages per Activity					
	Resting	Crunches	Push-ups	Squatting	Jogging	Overall accuracy
Average	92.26%	86.11%	87.01%	86.71%	87.82%	89.53%
Standard deviation	3.34%	7.89%	4.90%	7.53%	6.47%	3.19%
Maximum	96.92%	100.00%	96.81%	98.76%	100.00%	95.13%
Minimum	84.22%	65.95%	75.24%	70.73%	76.96%	82.69%

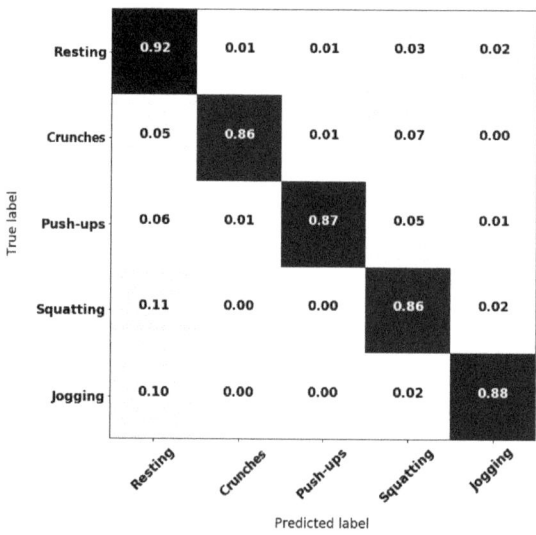

Figure 7. Confusion matrix from testing data.

3.3. Case Study: Physical Workload Evolution on an Individual

This second case study set its focus on testing the workload estimator reliability. For this purpose, a 27-year-old healthy male subject volunteered to participate in a twenty-day experiment. The subject performed the same exercise routine every day, and its physical workload was recorded. In our system, the collection of workload data was linked to the activity recognition function in order to provide meaningful insights of physical performance. Then, the tests set-up implies that the subject must wear both devices during each session. Figure 8 shows how the subject wears the devices and evinces that they do not represent major discomfort. Before the first session, a preliminary exercising round reveals that crunches do not represent significant physical effort for the subject. Thus, the routine for each day is defined as follows: 15 s of resting to find the reference HR for workload estimation, followed by 60 s of push-ups, 60 s of jogging, 60 s of squatting and 60 s of resting. Then, the one-minute rounds are repeated three times.

The subject did not exercise regularly, which led to the expectation of high levels of workload on the first session and a progressive decline on the physical exigency on successive sessions, as the body adjusts to the exercise routine. The performance of the online HAR was also expected to be steady along the sessions, since the system was used by the same person. Due to the methodology of workload estimation, several Frimat's scores can be obtained during a one-minute exercise round given the HR variations. However, the system maps those scores into the eight categories, reducing information sensitivity. After each session, a Python script retrieves the classified activities and the true label of activities for HAR assessment, and the workload categories for each activity. Consequently, this script found the statistical mode of the workload categories for an activity and set it as the estimated physical workload.

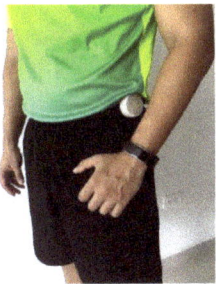

Figure 8. Subject wearing the devices before exercising.

Figure 9 displays the resulting mean HR for push-ups, squatting and jogging, during each daily session. Figure 10 shows the Frimat's score values assessment during the resting rounds at the end of each session. These workload values reflect the overall perception of the body of the subject after all the exercising rounds. Complementary, Table 5 resumes the online HAR performance for each session.

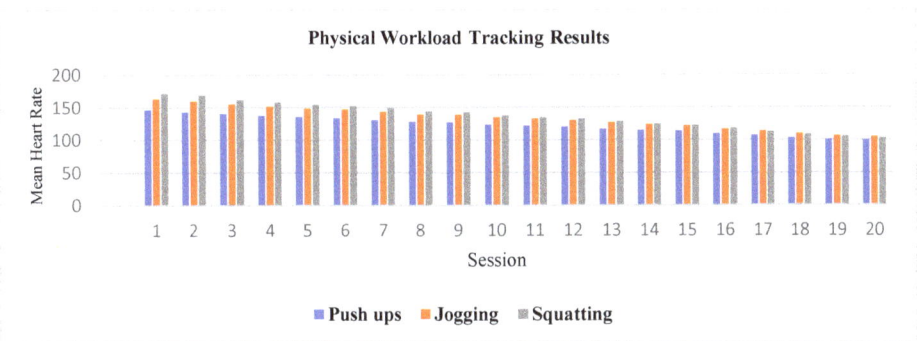

Figure 9. Physical workload tracking results for an individual after 20 days.

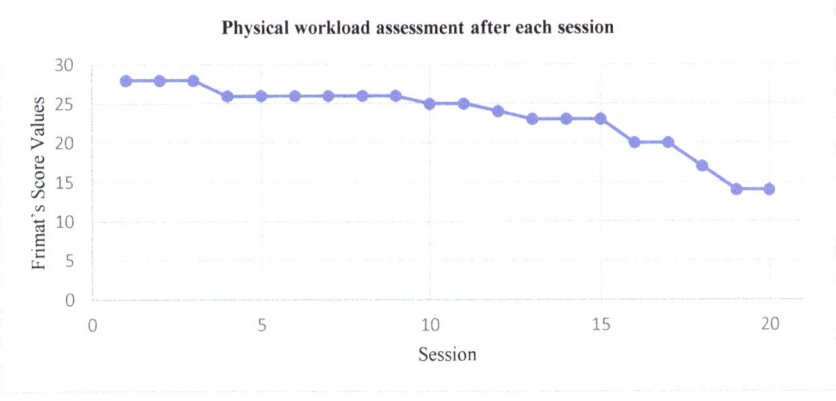

Figure 10. Physical workload assessment after each session.

Table 5. Average accuracies of online HAR for the second case study.

Session	Activity Classification Accuracy		
	Push-ups	Jogging	Squatting
1	94.53%	90.36%	91.38%
2	94.24%	93.83%	89.76%
3	93.03%	91.73%	88.53%
4	92.86%	89.77%	87.76%
5	89.53%	84.20%	90.73%
6	88.50%	87.83%	92.53%
7	88.95%	89.17%	92.67%
8	89.73%	90.13%	91.44%
9	90.64%	90.13%	91.43%
10	91.78%	92.60%	90.14%
11	92.13%	91.27%	90.74%
12	92.16%	90.66%	91.03%
13	91.06%	90.46%	92.80%
14	89.73%	90.36%	90.03%
15	92.63%	90.93%	91.56%
16	92.36%	91.43%	91.03%
17	91.66%	89.43%	92.23%
18	91.23%	90.44%	90.26%
19	90.96%	91.27%	89.43%
20	89.66%	90.13%	93.03%
Average	91.37%	90.31%	90.93%

4. Discussion

This work introduced a system that combines real-time activity monitoring and physical workload estimation to allow remote tracking of workers in physically demanding jobs (as in our previous case study in [19]) and athletes for work health and fitness purposes, respectively. For a comprehensive assessment of system performance, two case studies were presented. The first one embraces the training, validation and real-time testing with 20 subjects of the human activity recognition component. The second case shows the evolution of physical workload for an individual over twenty days.

The training and validation results stood above 95% for overall classification accuracy, compared to previous studies, which also employed wearable devices as shown in Table 6. Critical parameters regarding real-time implementation were considered for comparison such as number of sensors, number of activities and accuracy.

Table 6. Online HAR comparison with previous studies.

Article	Number of Wearable Sensors	Number of Activities	Validation Accuracy
[26]	1	10	98.7%
[27]	5	9	94.8%
[28]	1	5	95.7%
[30]	Smartphone	3	98.6%
[51]	1	9	94.8%
[52]	1	8	95%
This work	1	5	97.5%

The comparison in Table 6 allows us to locate the present work with an overall accuracy that is only surpassed by a system that only considers three activities and by our previous work in [26]. However, the only work from Table 6 that displays results of real-time tests is [30]. There, tests are 10 s long, compared to the 30 s tests of the present work. Reference [30] considers six test subjects, while our case study considered twenty. Hence, such a length and subject quantity difference can lead to errors in movement data, which makes the results shown in Table 4 generalizable to expected performance during real use.

Additionally, results in Table 4 and Figure 7 containing the average accuracy per activity and their respective standard deviation evinced the tendency of the system to keep a classification exactitude above 85%. However, tests on the first case study were carried by people who do not know the system nor where intensively introduced to its use. Instead, the explanation of the experiment was held short and they were asked to perform the exercises in the most natural way for them. Thus, there were some cases where the subjects took unexpected pauses or just trembled during the exercise, which introduced noise on the one-second time-windows of sampling and reflects on a reduction of the overall accuracy. Nevertheless, by observing at the maximum values, there was also evidence of cases where classification of the embedded model shows no incorrect estimations.

Regarding the second case study, it helps us to validate the reliability of the workload computation in real-time. This approach differs from other workload-related works like [21–24] where there is no real-time feedback. Instead, authors from [21–24] take activity and HR data manually and then compute the workload and categorize it. The proposed system does all this process automatically, facilitating the relationship between activity and physical effort, which takes relevance at the application field. The subject considered for the twenty-day experiment of the second case study performed a physically demanding routine that was evaluated as extremely hard at the end of the first ten days, according to Frimat's criteria. However, a remarkable evolution in the perception of each activity by the subject is shown in Figure 9. In the first sessions, the system evaluated that each type of exercise was extremely hard for the subject, obtaining an average HR of 150 bpm, then in the last session these activities were classified as a light workload, obtaining an average HR of 95 bpm. As expected, the first exercise of the routine (push-ups) displayed the lowest workload amounts, since the body started to adapt to the routine. However, as the exercising round advances, the HR started to increase, which was reflected in higher workloads. Another evidence of the assimilation of the exercising routine was the change from Frimat's scored values in the resting periods at the end of each session, as shown in Figure 10. Considering that the subject always performed the same exercise routine for twenty sessions (that is, there was no increase or variation in the load), a principle of adaptation is presented in the physical state of the subject [53–55]. As can be seen in Figures 9 and 10, at the beginning of the sessions, the physical capacity of the subject was not enough for the established load, but as the exercise sessions increased, the body managed to adapt to that load.

Additionally, Table 5 shows the performance stability of the online HAR component during the second case study. The accuracies stood around 90% for the three activities, considering the fatigue effect on the subject movements. It also must be noticed that these experiments were longer than in the first case study and exhibited higher average accuracy; this is due to the lack of heterogeneity, which leads the system to be exposed to more similar movements each session. Thus, these results confirmed the reliability of the two components of our system for workload tracking purposes.

Finally, the contributions of this work are highlighted as follows:

1. We described the development of a smart physical workload tracking system that allows health and fitness professionals to monitor several people simultaneously and remotely, which is critical in manufacturing and sport industries. To the best of our knowledge, this solution integrating the physical workload concept has not been explored before.
2. We included a well-known concept from ergonomics (Frimat's criteria) into a real-time e-health application. We achieved this by embedding the workload computation and activity classification on a mobile application, which integrates the signal from a hip-placed accelerometer and a wrist-placed PPG sensor. To the best of our knowledge, this approach has not been presented before.
3. We displayed tests with 20 people performing the same exercise routine. We trained the classification algorithms with data sampled from chosen volunteers; and then tested with a different set of subjects using the devised wearable device during an exercise routine, which

comprises crunches, push-ups, squatting and jogging. The accuracy of the classifier was above 85% during real-time testing.
4. We showed the physical progress of a volunteer by tracking his/her physical workload for twenty days while he/she performed the same routine. This case study evidenced that Frimat's score could provide enough information to determine the level of fitness progress of a person that intends to train using physically demanding exercises.

5. Conclusions

A physical workload tracking using human activity recognition and HR measurements with wearable devices was presented. The system used a hip-placed motion sensor and a wrist-placed photoplethysmography sensor for HR. The information from both sensors was gathered by a mobile application through BLE connections; then, performed activity recognition with a trained random forest model and computed physical workload using Frimat's method. The activity classifier displayed a 97.5% accuracy during validation, and 92% accuracy during real-time tests with 20 subjects. In addition, a twenty-day experiment with a single subject who performed a custom exercise routine shows that the system could recognize the body adaptation to the physically demanding activities.

Future research directions point to a further study of the information relating physical workload and the activities performed. Given the reliability of the wearable-based activity classifier and the workload estimation method, new developments combining ergonomics and machine learning can be carried to predict the amount of physical effort that an activity can represent for a subject. Hence, this could lead to an injury prevention environment powered by historical information on a workplace or physically/mentally demanding tasks.

Author Contributions: Conceptualization, P.N. and J.M.; methodology, P.N.; hardware, J.M.; software, K.G., P.N. and J.M.; validation, J.M., and P.N.; writing—original draft preparation, J.M.; writing—review and editing, W.P. and M.P.; supervision, W.P.; project administration, M.P and W.P. All authors have read and agreed to the published version of the manuscript.

Funding: This work was supported in part by Departamento Administrativo de Ciencia, Tecnología e Innovación (809-2018).

Conflicts of Interest: The authors declare no conflict of interest. The funders had no role in the design of the study; in the collection, analyses, or interpretation of data; in the writing of the manuscript, or in the decision to publish the results.

References

1. World Health Organization. *Work Organisation and Stress*; Protecting Workers Health Series; World Health Organization: Geneva, Switzerland, 2003; pp. 1–27.
2. Caplan, R.D.; Jones, K.W. Effects of work load, role ambiguity, and type A personality on anxiety, depression, and heart rate. *J. Appl. Psychol.* **1975**, *60*, 713–719. [CrossRef] [PubMed]
3. Taelman, J.; Vandeput, S.; Spaepen, A.; Van Huffel, S. Influence of mental stress on Heart Rate and Heart Rate Variability. In Proceedings of the 4th European conference of the international federation for medical and biological engineering (IFMBE), Antwerp, Belgium, 23–27 November 2008; pp. 1366–1369.
4. Dababneh, A.J.; Swanson, N.; Shell, R.L. Impact of added rest breaks on the productivity and well being of workers. *Ergonomics* **2001**, *44*, 164–174. [CrossRef] [PubMed]
5. De la Iglesia, A.; Gómez, J.; Sáenz, R.; Ruiz, C. Carga de trabajo físico y costo cardiaco: La freuencia cardiaca de referencia. *Rev. Salud y Trab.* **1994**, *106*, 16–21.
6. Solé, M.D. NTP 295: Valoración de la carga física mediante la monitorización de la frecuencia cardiaca. *Cent. Nac. de Cond. de Trab.* **1991**, *1*, 1–6.
7. Frimat, P.; Amphoux, M.; Chamoux, A. Interprétation et mesure de la fréquence cardiaque. *Rev. de Med. du Trav. XV* **1988**, *147*, 165.
8. Frimat, P.; Furon, D.; Cantineau, A.; Delepine, P.; Six, F.; Luez, G. Le travail à la chaleur (verrerie). Etude de la charge de travail par ECG dynamique. Applications de la Méthode de VOGT. *Arch. Mal. Prof* **1979**, *40*, 191.

9. Föhr, T.; Pietilä, J.; Helander, E.; Myllymäki, T.; Lindholm, H.; Rusko, H.; Kujala, U.M. Physical activity, body mass index and heart rate variability-based stress and recovery in 16 275 Finnish employees: A cross-sectional study. *BMC Public Health* **2016**, *16*, 701. [CrossRef]
10. Choi, J.; Ricardo, G.O. Using heart rate monitors to detect mental stress. In Proceedings of the 2009 6th International Workshop on Wearable and Implantable Body Sensor Networks (BSN 2009), Berkeley, CA, USA, 3–5 June 2009; pp. 219–223.
11. Rosa, B.M.G.; Yang, G.Z. Smart wireless headphone for cardiovascular and stress monitoring. In Proceedings of the 2017 IEEE 14th International Conference on Wearable and Implantable Body Sensor Networks (BSN), Eindhoven, The Netherlands, 9–12 May 2017; pp. 75–78.
12. Jovanov, E.; Frith, K.; Anderson, F.; Milosevic, M.; Shrove, M.T. Real-time monitoring of occupational stress of nurses. In Proceedings of the 2011 Annual International Conference of the IEEE Engineering in Medicine and Biology Society, Boston, MA, USA, 30 August–3 September 2011; pp. 3640–3643.
13. Bolanos, M.; Nazeran, H.; Haltiwanger, E. Comparison of heart rate variability signal features derived from electrocardiography and photoplethysmography in healthy individuals. In Proceedings of the Annual International Conference of the IEEE Engineering in Medicine and Biology, New York, NY, USA, 30 August–3 September 2006; pp. 4289–4294.
14. Gamelin, F.X.; Berthoin, S.; Bosquet, L. Validity of the polar S810 Heart rate monitor to measure R-R intervals at rest. *Med. Sci. Sports Exerc.* **2006**, *38*, 887–893. [CrossRef]
15. Hendrikx, J.; Ruijs, L.S.; Cox, L.G.; Lemmens, P.M.; Schuijers, E.G.; Goris, A.H. Clinical Evaluation of the Measurement Performance of the Philips Health Watch: A Within-Person Comparative Study. *JMIR mHealth uHealth* **2017**, *5*, e10. [CrossRef]
16. Khan, E.; Al Hossain, F.; Uddin, S.Z.; Alam, S.K.; Hasan, M.K. A Robust Heart Rate Monitoring Scheme Using Photoplethysmographic Signals Corrupted by Intense Motion Artifacts. *IEEE Trans. Biomed. Eng.* **2016**, *63*, 550–562. [CrossRef]
17. Asada, H.H.; Shaltis, P.; Reisner, A.; Rhee, S.; Hutchinson, R.C. Mobile Monitoring with Wearable Photoplethysmographic Biosensors. *IEEE Eng. Med. Biol. Mag.* **2003**, *22*, 28–40. [CrossRef] [PubMed]
18. Aileni Raluca, M.; Pasca, S.; Strungaru, R. Heart rate monitoring by using non-invasive wearable sensor. In Proceedings of the E-Health and Bioengineering Conference (EHB), Sinaia, Romania, 22–24 June 2017; pp. 587–590.
19. Narváez, P.; Manjarrés, J.; Percybrooks, W.; Pardo, M.; Calle, M. Assessing the Level of Physical Activity in the Workplace: A Case Study With Wearable Technology. *Int. J. Interdiscip. Telecommun. Netw.* **2019**, *11*, 44–56. [CrossRef]
20. Jovanov, E.; Milenkovic, A.; Otto, C.; de Groen, P.C.; Johnson, B.; Warren, S.; Taibi, G. A WBAN System for Ambulatory Monitoring of Physical Activity and Health Status: Applications and Challenges. In Proceedings of the 2005 IEEE Engineering in Medicine and Biology 27th Annual Conference, Shanghai, China, 17–18 January 2005; pp. 4–7.
21. Arana, T.; Velásquez, J.; Carvajal, R. Determinación de la capacidad y la carga física de trabajo en bailarines de una escuela de baile de la ciudad de Cali. *Cienc. Salud* **2013**, *1*, 11–16.
22. Zapata, H.; Arango, G.L.; Estrada, L.M. Valoración de carga física en estibadores de una cooperativa de trabajo asociado. *Rev. Fac. Nac. Salud Pública* **2011**, *29*, 53–64.
23. Romero, M.; Fernández, C.; Ballesteros, A. Evaluación de la carga física de trabajo, mediante la monitorización de la frecuencia cardíaca, en auxiliares de Enfermería de una residencia geriátrica municipal. *Rev. Enfermería del Trab.* **2011**, *1*, 193–202.
24. Castillo, J.A.; Cubillos, Á. Using Pulse Rate in Estimating Workload: Evaluating a Load Mobilizing Activity. *Rev. Cienc. la Salud* **2014**, *12*, 27–43.
25. Lara, O.D.; Labrador, M.A. A survey on human activity recognition using wearable sensors. *IEEE Commun. Surv. Tutor.* **2013**, *15*, 1192–1209. [CrossRef]
26. Manjarrés, J.; Russo, V.; Peñaranda, J.; Pardo, M. Human Activity and Heart Rate Monitoring System in a Mobile Platform. In Proceedings of the 2018 Congreso Internacional de Innovación y Tendencias en Ingenieria (CONIITI), Bogota, Colombia, 3–5 October 2018; pp. 1–6.
27. Wang, Z.; Zhao, C.; Qiu, S. A system of human vital signs monitoring and activity recognition based on body sensor network. *Sens. Rev.* **2014**, *34*, 42–50. [CrossRef]

28. Lara, Ó.D.; Prez, A.J.; Labrador, M.A.; Posada, J.D. Centinela: A human activity recognition system based on acceleration and vital sign data. *Pervasive Mob. Comput.* **2012**, *8*, 717–729. [CrossRef]
29. Labrador, M.A.; Lara, O.D. *Human Activity Recognition: Using Wearable Sensors and Smartphones*, 1st ed.; CRC Press: Boca Raton, FL, USA, 2013; ISBN 3-540-30506-8.
30. Jongprasithporn, M.; Yodpijit, N.; Srivilai, R.; Pongsophane, P. A smartphone-based real-time simple activity recognition. In Proceedings of the 2017 3rd International Conference on Control, Automation and Robotics (ICCAR), Nagoya, Japan, 24–26 April 2017; pp. 539–542.
31. Prabowo, O.M.; Mutijarsa, K.; Supangkat, S.H. Missing Data Handling using Machine Learning for Human Acitivity Recognition on Mobile Device. In Proceedings of the 2016 International Conference on ICT For Smart Society, Surabaya, Indonesia, 20–21 July 2016; pp. 20–21.
32. Quiroz, J.C.; Banerjee, A.; Dascalu, S.M.; Lau, S.L. Feature Selection for Activity Recognition from Smartphone Accelerometer Data. *Intell. Autom. Soft Comput.* **2017**, 1–9. [CrossRef]
33. Yazdansepas, D.; Niazi, A.H.; Gay, J.L.; Maier, F.W.; Ramaswamy, L.; Rasheed, K.; Buman, M.P. A Multi-featured Approach for Wearable Sensor-Based Human Activity Recognition. In Proceedings of the 2016 IEEE International Conference on Healthcare Informatics (ICHI), Chicago, IL, USA, 4–7 October 2016; pp. 423–431.
34. Bulling, A.; Blanke, U.; Schiele, B. A tutorial on human activity recognition using body-worn inertial sensors. *ACM Comput. Surv.* **2014**, *46*, 1–33. [CrossRef]
35. Long, X.L.X.; Yin, B.Y.B.; Aarts, R.M. Single-accelerometer-based daily physical activity classification. In Proceedings of the 2009 Annual International Conference of the IEEE Engineering in Medicine and Biology Society, Minneapolis, MN, USA, 3–6 September 2009; pp. 6107–6110.
36. Babu, A.; Dube, K.; Mukhopadhyay, S.; Ghayvat, H.; Mukhopadhyay, P.S. Accelerometer based human activities and posture recognition. In Proceedings of the 2016 International Conference on Data Mining and Advanced Computing (SAPIENCE), Medellín, Colombia, 16–18 May 2016; pp. 367–373.
37. Liu, X.; Liu, L.; Simske, S.J.; Liu, J. Human Daily Activity Recognition for Healthcare Using Wearable and Visual Sensing Data. In Proceedings of the 2016 IEEE International Conference on Healthcare Informatics (ICHI), Chicago, IL, USA, 4–7 October 2016; pp. 24–31.
38. Uddin, M.Z.; Hassan, M.M. Activity Recognition for Cognitive Assistance Using Body Sensors Data and Deep Convolutional Neural Network. *IEEE Sens. J.* **2018**, *19*, 8413–8419. [CrossRef]
39. Lau, S.L.; König, I.; David, K.; Parandian, B.; Carius-Düssel, C.; Schultz, M. Supporting patient monitoring using activity recognition with a smartphone. In Proceedings of the 2010 7th International Symposium on Wireless Communication Systems (ISWCS'10), York, UK, 19–22 September 2010; pp. 810–814.
40. Ahmadi, A.; Mitchell, E.; Richter, C.; Destelle, F.; Gowing, M.; O'Connor, N.E.; Moran, K. Toward automatic activity classification and movement assessment during a sports training session. *IEEE Internet Things J.* **2015**, *2*, 23–32. [CrossRef]
41. Albinali, F.; Intille, S.; Haskell, W.; Rosenberger, M. Using wearable activity type detection to improve physical activity energy expenditure estimation. In Proceedings of the 12th ACM International Conference on Ubiquitous Computing, Copenhagen, Denmark, 26–29 September 2010; pp. 311–320.
42. Simblee Corp. Simblee User Guide. 2016. Available online: https://cdn.sparkfun.com/datasheets/IoT/Simblee%20User%20Guide%20v2.05.pdf (accessed on 16 December 2019).
43. Analog Devices ADXL335 Datasheet. 2009. Available online: https://www.analog.com/media/en/technical-documentation/data-sheets/ADXL335.pdf (accessed on 2 September 2019).
44. Microsoft Microsoft Band Features. Available online: https://www.microsoft.com/microsoft-band/en-us/features (accessed on 30 August 2017).
45. Stahl, S.E.; An, H.-S.; Dinkel, D.M.; Noble, J.M.; Lee, J.-M. How accurate are the wrist-based heart rate monitors during walking and running activities? Are they accurate enough? *BMJ Open Sport Exerc. Med.* **2016**, *2*, e000106. [CrossRef]
46. Shcherbina, A.; Mattsson, C.M.; Waggott, D.; Salisbury, H.; Christle, J.W.; Hastie, T.; Wheeler, M.T.; Ashley, E.A. Accuracy in wrist-worn, sensor-based measurements of heart rate and energy expenditure in a diverse cohort. *J. Pers. Med.* **2017**, *7*, 3. [CrossRef]
47. Microsoft Microsoft Band-Developers. Available online: https://developer.microsoftband.com/bandsdk (accessed on 2 September 2019).

48. Pedregosa, F.; Varoquaux, G.; Gramfort, A.; Michel, V.; Thirion, B.; Grisel, O.; Blondel, M.; Prettenhofer, P.; Weiss, R.; Dubourg, V.; et al. Scikit-learn: Machine Learning in Python. *J. Mach. Learn. Res.* **2011**, *12*, 2825–2830.
49. Breiman, L.; Friedman, J.; Stone, C.J.; Olshen, R.A. *Classification and Regression Trees*; The Wadsworth and Brooks-Cole statistics-probability series; Taylor & Francis: Abingdon, UK, 1984; ISBN 9780412048418.
50. Morawiec, D. Sklearn-Porter: Transpile Trained Scikit-Learn Estimators to C, Java, JavaScript and Others. Available online: https://github.com/nok/sklearn-porter (accessed on 2 April 2019).
51. Wu, Y.; Qi, S.; Hu, F.; Ma, S.; Mao, W.; Li, W. Recognizing activities of the elderly using wearable sensors: A comparison of ensemble algorithms based on boosting. *Sens. Rev.* **2019**, *39*, 743–751. [CrossRef]
52. Bhat, G.; Tuncel, Y.; An, S.; Lee, H.G.; Ogras, U.Y. An Ultra-Low Energy Human Activity Recognition Accelerator for Wearable Health Applications. *ACM Trans. Embed. Comput. Syst.* **2019**, *18*, 49. [CrossRef]
53. Bellido, D.C. *Teoría y Práctica del Entrenamiento Deportivo*; Universidad de León: León, Spain, 2006.
54. Bompa, T.O.; Buzzichelli, C. *Periodization: Theory and Methodology of Training*; Human Kinetics: Stanningley, UK, 2018.
55. Crossley, J. *Personal Training: Theory and Practice*; Routledge: Abingdon, UK, 2013.

© 2019 by the authors. Licensee MDPI, Basel, Switzerland. This article is an open access article distributed under the terms and conditions of the Creative Commons Attribution (CC BY) license (http://creativecommons.org/licenses/by/4.0/).

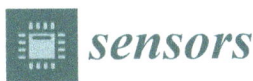

Article

Inertial Measurement Unit Based Upper Extremity Motion Characterization for Action Research Arm Test and Activities of Daily Living

Hyung Seok Nam [1,2], Woo Hyung Lee [1], Han Gil Seo [2], Yoon Jae Kim [3], Moon Suk Bang [2,4,*] and Sungwan Kim [1,5,*]

1. Department of Biomedical Engineering, Seoul National University College of Medicine, Seoul 03080, Korea; ignite31@snu.ac.kr (H.S.N.); v3night9@snu.ac.kr (W.H.L.)
2. Department of Rehabilitation Medicine, Seoul National University Hospital, Seoul 03080, Korea; hangilseo@snu.ac.kr
3. Interdisciplinary Program for Bioengineering, Seoul National University Graduate School, Seoul 08826, Korea; kyj182731@naver.com
4. Department of Rehabilitation Medicine, Seoul National University College of Medicine, Seoul 03080, Korea
5. Institute of Medical and Biological Engineering, Seoul National University, Seoul 03080, Korea
* Correspondence: msbang@snu.ac.kr (M.S.B.); sungwan@snu.ac.kr (S.K.)

Received: 18 March 2019; Accepted: 12 April 2019; Published: 14 April 2019

Abstract: In practical rehabilitation robot development, it is imperative to pre-specify the critical workspace to prevent redundant structure. This study aimed to characterize the upper extremity motion during essential activities in daily living. An IMU-based wearable motion capture system was used to access arm movements. Ten healthy subjects performed the Action Research Arm Test (ARAT) and six pre-selected essential daily activities. The Euler angles of the major joints, and acceleration from wrist and hand sensors were acquired and analyzed. The size of the workspace for the ARAT was 0.53 (left-right) × 0.92 (front-back) × 0.89 (up-down) m for the dominant hand. For the daily activities, the workspace size was 0.71 × 0.70 × 0.86 m for the dominant hand, significantly larger than the non-dominant hand ($p \leq 0.011$). The average range of motion (RoM) during ARAT was 109.15 ± 18.82° for elbow flexion/extension, 105.23 ± 5.38° for forearm supination/pronation, 91.99 ± 0.98° for shoulder internal/external rotation, and 82.90 ± 22.52° for wrist dorsiflexion/volarflexion, whereas the corresponding range for daily activities were 120.61 ± 23.64°, 128.09 ± 22.04°, 111.56 ± 31.88°, and 113.70 ± 18.26°. The shoulder joint was more abducted and extended during pinching compared to grasping posture ($p < 0.001$). Reaching from a grasping posture required approximately 70° elbow extension and 36° forearm supination from the initial position. The study results provide an important database for the workspace and RoM for essential arm movements.

Keywords: inertial measurement unit; upper extremity; motion; action research arm test; activities of daily living

1. Introduction

In the last decade, there have been dramatic improvements in rehabilitation robots and kinematic analyses of the upper extremities. Many types of multi-axis exoskeletons have been developed, as well as relatively simple end-effector type robots [1–5]. Exoskeletons are commonly defined as having a structure in which the robot joints correspond to human joints, whereas end-effector type robot structures do not correspond to human anatomical structures [1,6]. However, even in exoskeletons, the angular movements of human and robot joints do not exactly match. This discrepancy comes from the fundamental difference in that exoskeleton joints have mechanical joint axes with their corresponding motors, whereas human joints consist of bones, muscle and tendons, and soft tissues [7]. Therefore, the goal of exoskeleton rehabilitation robot development should not focus on perfectly resembling the human arm joint and structure, but rather on designing a modified structure based on a better understanding of human kinematics.

Many types of sensors are used for a motion analysis of the upper extremities including electromagnetic sensors, mechanical sensors, optical sensors, and inertial sensors. Aizawa et al. [8] reported the range of motions (RoM) of the major upper extremity joints during selected activities of daily living (ADL), using a commercial electromagnetic sensor system. Gates et al. [9] also quantified the RoM of the upper extremities during eight ADLs using reflective sensors. Kim et al. [10] conducted a kinematic analysis of drinking movements using reflective markers. Chen and Lum [11] used a spring-operated exoskeleton to compare the RoM with and without robotic assistance during the given tasks, where the angles were evaluated using mechanical sensors within the robot. Perez et al. [12] introduced a portable motion analysis for the upper limbs using inertial measurement unit (IMU) sensors. A recent review showed that accelerometers and IMUs are most frequently used devices for an analysis of upper limb motion [13]. Although many of these reports present quantitative angular values during specific ADL tasks, assessments focusing on clinically relevant applications of the motion data remain scarce.

To minimize the size and complexity of neurorehabilitation robots, the number of axes and the workspace of a robotic hand or end-effector should be minimized; at the same time, however, essential tasks need to be performable during daily activities. From the viewpoint of performing a specific task, although the human performance using an arm may seem similar to the actuation of a robot, when considering the mechanism of the performance, they are significantly different. Moreover, it is possible to state that biological and engineering mechanisms are in significant opposition [7]. It is important to have a database on the position and joint angles while performing essential daily activities; however, the movement patterns in healthy subjects and stroke patients differ significantly, and the exoskeleton cannot be actuated in exactly the same manner as a human limb. It is necessary to create a design that patients may not only wear but also actuate in an appropriate manner to help the movement of a paralyzed limb and induce neuroplasticity.

The purpose of this study was to provide a database on the dimensions of the essential workspace and the RoM of the major upper extremity joints during the normal motion of healthy subjects from clinical and practical perspectives.

2. Materials and Methods

In this section, we present the IMU-based motion capture system used in this study with validation protocol, followed by participants information and task protocols. Detailed information on extracted parameters and statistical methods are also provided.

2.1. Upper Extremity Motion Capture System and Its Validation

For motion capture of the upper extremities, Perception Neuron® (Noitom Ltd., Beijing, China), a wearable multi-IMU based modular motion capture system was used. In this study, we utilized 25 IMU sensors for the upper body assessment; three sensors for the body axis, four sensors for each arm, and seven sensors for each hand including the fingers (Figure 1). User-interface software, Axis Neuron (Noitom Ltd., Beijing, China), was applied for motion recording and data extraction. The sampling rate of the data was set to 60 Hz.

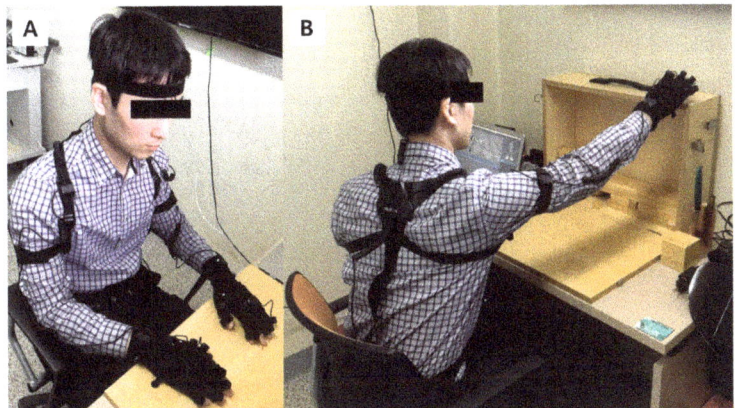

Figure 1. (**A**) A volunteer subject is wearing the IMU-based upper extremity motion capture system. (**B**) The subject is performing a task in the Action Research Arm Test.

To validate the accuracy and consistency of the system, root mean square error (RMSE) analyses for the elbow flexion/extension and wrist dorsiflexion/volarflexion axes were performed using an electro-goniometer as a reference. During real motion with the system worn on the body, it is not possible to isolate single joint movements in a single plane with all other joint being fixed. Therefore, coefficient of variation (CoV) analyses for forearm supination/pronation and elbow flexion/extension for the angles from a gyrosensor, and the z-axis (up-down) and y-axis (front-back) distances from accelerometers in the forearm and hand sensors were conducted using the data collected during the tasks.

2.2. Participants

Ten healthy volunteers (six males, four females) were recruited for this study, and participated after providing written informed consent. Their mean age was 29.3 ± 4.7 years (age range: 23–35).

2.3. Tasks and Procedure

All subjects wore the IMU sensor based motion capture system on both upper extremities. After sensor calibration, they performed all 19 test items of the Action Research Arm Test (ARAT) with using both their right and left hands alternatively [14]. ARAT consists of four domains: domain 1 includes six grasp and reaching tasks with various size of wooden blocks, ball, or a stone; domain 2 consists of four grip activities such as pouring water from glass to glass or putting a hollow tube through a stick; domain 3 includes six pinch and reaching tasks using various size of marbles using different fingers; and domain 4 consists of four gross movements placing the hand on three different parts of the head [14]. They also performed six pre-specified ADL tasks: (1) opening a water bottle and drinking, (2) peeling off a banana, (3) buttoning and unbuttoning a shirt, (4) combing their hair, (5) squeezing toothpaste from a tube and brushing their teeth, and (6) turning a door knob. These pre-specified ADL tasks were selected from the survey results from our previous study which evaluated the practical needs of stroke patients owing to their hemiplegia [15]. During the ADL tasks, the subjects were instructed to perform the task in the most natural way possible, without specifying which hand to use to hold or manipulate the object.

2.4. Extracted Parameters

Using Axis Neuron (Noitom Ltd., Beijing, China) software, acceleration and position data of the wrist and hand sensors from the accelerometer, and the Euler angles for the sensors of all major joints with reference to their proximal segment sensors during the ARAT and ADL tasks, were extracted. For each ARAT domain and ADL task, the size of the workspace in three orthogonal coordinates and the angular position and RoM for each upper extremity joint were calculated. For a sub-analysis, grasping/pinching and reaching movements when conducting the tasks in ARAT domains 1 and 3 were additionally analyzed regarding the initial grasping/pinching position and RoM during a reaching movement.

2.5. Statistical Analysis

For validation purposes, the intra-subject covariance and inter-subject covariance were both calculated for repetitive grasping/pinching and reaching tasks. Paired t tests were conducted to compare the workspace dimensions and RoM between dominant and non-dominant arms. Paired t tests were also conducted for a comparison of the major joint angles in the grasping/pinching position and reaching position, the initial position between grasping and pinching, and the reaching position from grasping and pinching. The statistical program SPSS ver. 25 (SPSS Inc., Chicago, IL, USA) was used for analysis. A p value of less than 0.05 was considered statistically significant.

3. Results

The validation results followed by data analysis on movement characteristics are provided in this section.

3.1. Validation of Upper Extremity Motion Capture System

The range of RMSE for the elbow flexion/extension angle ranged from 2.11° to 4.75° (3.61 ± 1.32°), and 0.42° to 1.22° (0.85 ± 0.40°) for wrist dorsiflexion/volarflexion angle. During the reaching task, the mean change in forearm supination/pronation was 36.65 ± 6.98°, with an intra-subject CoV of 17.29% and inter-subject CoV of 19.05%. The change in elbow flexion/extension was 69.96 ± 16.89°, and intra-subject and inter-subject CoV was 11.67% and 24.14%, respectively. Distance data extracted from the sensors during the reaching tasks were evaluated and then compared with the real movement distance. Regarding the accelerometer on the forearm sensor, the average of calculated movement distance was 34.14 ± 4.15 cm in the z-axis, and 33.54 ± 4.79 cm in the y-axis, where the measured distance in each direction was 34.0 cm and 33.5 cm, respectively. Data calculated from hand sensors were 36.78 ± 3.09 cm and 32.35 ± 4.64 cm), respectively. The intra-subject CoV ranged from 5.5% to 9.5%, whereas the inter-subject CoV ranged from 8.4% to 14.3%. The complete results are shown in Table 1.

Table 1. Coefficient of variation (CoV) for major movements [a].

Sensor Type	Axis	Average Change during Task (Across Subjects)	Intra-Subject CoV Average	Inter-Subject CoV	Estimated Real Distance *
Gyrosensor	Forearm supination/pronation	36.65 ± 6.98°	17.29%	19.05%	-
	Elbow flexion/extension	69.96 ± 16.89°	11.67%	24.14%	-
Accelerometer (forearm sensor)	z-axis distance (up/down)	34.14 ± 4.15 cm	6.18%	12.17%	34.0 cm
	y-axis distance (front/back)	33.54 ± 4.79 cm	7.16%	14.28%	33.5 cm
Accelerometer (hand sensor)	z-axis distance (up/down)	36.78 ± 3.09 cm	5.56%	8.41%	34.0 cm
	y-axis distance (front/back)	32.35 ± 4.64 cm	9.49%	14.33%	33.5 cm

[a] Tasks performed by 10 normal subjects, six trials per reaching. * Estimated distance between initial object position and target position is approximately 33.5 cm for y-axis and 34.0 cm for z-axis. Note that this is the distance regarding common position of the forearm and hand sensors during the task and it varies by trials and subjects.

3.2. Workspace and RoM in Basic Upper Extremity Movements

All ten subjects were right-handed. For an orthogonal coordination, the axes were defined as follows: left-right direction for the x-axis, front-right direction for the y-axis, and up-down direction for the z-axis. For ARAT tasks, the size of the workspace for the right hand with reference to the sensor on the dorsum of the hand was 0.53 ± 0.11 m for the x-axis, 0.92 ± 0.08 m for the y-axis, and 0.89 ± 0.10 m for the z-axis. For the left side, the average workspace size was 0.62 × 0.80 × 0.86 m (in x, y, z-axis order). For pre-specified ADL tasks, the workspace for the dominant hand was 0.71 ± 0.22 m, 0.70 ± 0.17 m, and 0.86 ± 0.11 m (in x, y, z-axis order). The workspace of the non-dominant hand was significantly smaller, with an average size of 0.52 × 0.53 × 0.65 m ($p = 0.001, 0.011$, and 0.001 for the x-, y-, and z-axes, respectively). For the RoM in the major upper extremity joints, the angular ranges were similar between the right and left sides. The elbow flexion/extension and forearm supination/pronation showed the highest RoM in both ARAT and ADL for the dominant arm. The mean RoM values were 109.15 ± 18.82° and 105.23 ± 15.38° (elbow flexion/extension and forearm supination/pronation, respectively) for ARAT tasks, and 120.61 ± 23.64° and 128.09 ± 22.04° for ADL tasks. The RoM of the dominant side was significantly greater than on the non-dominant side for all joint directions except for the wrist dorsiflexion/volarflexion, which showed similar values (mean 113.70 ± 18.26° versus 110.08 ± 12.16°; right versus left, $p = 0.526$). All workspaces and RoM data during the ARAT and ADL tasks are shown in Table 2.

Table 2. Range of motion angle between right and left upper extremities during ARAT and ADL tasks.

	Axis	Right	Left	p [a]
ARAT	x-axis (left-right, hand sensor)	0.53 ± 0.11 m	0.62 ± 0.07 m	0.082
	y-axis (front-back, hand sensor)	0.92 ± 0.08 m	0.80 ± 0.11 m	0.049 *
	z-axis (hand sensor)	0.89 ± 0.10 m	0.86 ± 0.08 m	0.224
	Shoulder abduction/adduction	50.16 ± 11.14°	55.34 ± 13.48°	0.249
	Shoulder flexion/extension	79.52 ± 19.34°	75.71 ± 21.56°	0.478
	Elbow flexion/extension	109.15 ± 18.82°	106.89 ± 12.83°	0.705
	Forearm supination/pronation	105.23 ± 15.38°	108.64 ± 12.64°	0.426
	Shoulder IR/ER	91.99 ± 20.98°	84.44 ± 44.75°	0.584
	Wrist dorsiflexion/volarflexion	82.90 ± 22.52°	81.26 ± 11.16°	0.833
ADL tasks	x-axis (left-right, hand sensor)	0.71 ± 0.22 m	0.52 ± 0.13 m	0.001 *
	y-axis (front-back, hand sensor)	0.70 ± 0.17 m	0.53 ± 0.15 m	0.011 *
	z-axis (hand sensor)	0.86 ± 0.11 m	0.65 ± 0.13 m	0.001 *
	Shoulder abduction/adduction	58.84 ± 14.53°	35.43 ± 10.09°	<0.001 *
	Shoulder flexion/extension	68.41 ± 17.56°	40.49 ± 18.54°	0.002 *
	Elbow flexion/extension	120.61 ± 23.64°	102.53 ± 19.51°	0.044 *
	Forearm supination/pronation	128.09 ± 22.04°	108.00 ± 16.23°	0.027 *
	Shoulder IR/ER	111.56 ± 31.88°	77.04 ± 21.28°	0.030 *
	Wrist dorsiflexion/volarflexion	113.70 ± 18.26°	110.08 ± 12.16°	0.526

[a] p value for paired t test between right and left side; * p value less than 0.05 considered statistically significant.

3.3. Characteristics of Grasping/Pinching and Reaching

The upper extremity postures during grasping/pinching and reaching were analyzed as a subset analysis of the motion data extracted from grasping/pinching and reaching tasks in ARAT domains 1 and 3. Comparing grasping and pinching postures, the shoulder was more significantly abducted during pinching (19.39 ± 7.84°) compared to grasping (15.33 ± 6.91°, $p = 0.040$) and more extended during pinching (29.12 ± 12.33°) than grasping (22.99 ± 10.63°, $p = 0.038$). Elbow flexion/extension, forearm supination/pronation, and shoulder internal/external rotation did not significantly differ between the two postures. While reaching after grasping, the elbow was extended for an average of 87.87 ± 25.18° from the initial flexed posture, and pronated for an average of 36.65 ± 6.98° from the initial posture. The degrees of elbow extension and forearm pronation while reaching after pinching were similar ($p = 0.849$ and 0.294, respectively). The full results are shown in Table 3.

Table 3. Major joint angle position and change during grasping/pinching and reaching.

Axis	Grasping Initial Position	ROM during Reaching	p	Pinching Initial Position	ROM during Reaching	p	Grasp-Pinch p [a]	Reaching Difference p [b]
Shoulder abduction/adduction	15.33 ± 6.91° (abduction)	22.48 ± 19.81° (toward abduction)	0.006 *	19.39 ± 7.84° (abduction)	23.67 ± 13.35° (toward abduction)	<0.001 *	0.040 *	0.015 *
Shouler flexion/extension	22.99 ± 10.63° (extension)	47.80 ± 17.70° (toward flexion)	<0.001 *	29.12 ± 12.33° (extension)	41.83 ± 13.69° (toward flexion)	<0.001 *	0.038 *	0.948
Elbow flexion/extension	87.87 ± 25.18° (near fully flexed)	69.96 ± 16.89° (toward extension)	<0.001 *	84.82 ± 20.25° (near fully flexed)	67.91 ± 14.16° (toward extension)	<0.001 *	0.543	0.849
Forearm supination/pronation [c]	34.37 ± 11.07° (supinated)	36.65 ± 6.98° (toward pronation)	<0.001 *	30.98 ± 13.71° (supinated)	36.02 ± 12.44° (toward pronation)	<0.001 *	0.181	0.294
Shoulder IR/ER	0.68 ± 23.56° (inward direction)	16.55 ± 23.02° (toward external rotation)	0.049 *	2.01 ± 13.74° (inward direction)	18.10 ± 13.02° (toward external rotation)	0.002 *	0.794	0.860
Wrist deviation	8.94 ± 12.12° (to thumb side)	−1.76 ± 10.21° (to finger side)	0.599	1.05 ± 8.19° (to thumb side)	4.81 ± 8.85° (to thumb side)	0.120	0.004 *	0.522
Wrist rotation	4.59 ± 7.35° (toward palm down)	7.12 ± 4.59° (toward palm up)	0.001 *	0.80 ± 5.25° (toward palm down)	4.75 ± 4.05° (toward palm up)	0.005 *	0.023 *	0.385
Wrist dorsiflexion/volarflexion	18.79 ± 16.35° (dorsiflexed)	6.79 ± 6.00° (toward volarflexion)	0.006 *	11.30 ± 13.90° (dorsiflexed)	7.28 ± 11.22° (toward volarflexion)	0.070	0.166	0.123

[a] Comparison between grasping and pinching posture by paired t test; [b] Comparison between RoM change during reaching after grasping and pinching by paired t test; [c] Full pronation: 0°, full supination: 180°; * p value less than 0.05 considered statistically significant.

4. Discussion

The purpose of this study was to provide clinically relevant information regarding the workspace and major joint angle range while performing essential ADLs or important movements. By identifying these factors, it is possible to limit the extent of exoskeleton movements and, therefore, modify the design of the robot such that it can move within the designated workspace with a relatively simpler structure. In this study, we evaluated the RoM and workspace while conducting ARAT tasks, which is a common functional evaluation tool used in the clinics, because it is well known to significantly correlate with the patients' functional status or recovery state [16–18]. ARAT consists of four domains: domain 1 and 3 tasks consist of the grasping and pinching of various sized objects and reaching afterwards. Domain 2 mainly involves moving items on a table focusing on the grip function, and domain four items are gross movement tasks that require lifting the arm to the head or face [19].

Validation of the IMU-based motion analysis system used in this study showed that the accuracy and reliability of the sensors themselves are very high regarding angles. However, in the form of wearable multi-sensor system, it is impossible to isolate a single joint movement, because all joints systemically move in three dimensions, including body trunk and contralateral upper extremity. Intra-subject covariance and inter-subject covariance were calculated for the forearm supination/pronation and elbow flexion/extension angles to evaluate the system reliability, and the range was deemed acceptable when considering that the reaching tasks were not completely identical. For the position data from the accelerometers, we compared the calculated data in the y and z directions using the estimated real movement distance. The calculated distance data were similar to the measured data, and the variability was considered acceptable. In addition, the calculated workspace and RoM during ARAT tasks were similar between the two extremities with no significant difference (Table 2). This may also support the reliability of the system-derived parameter values. Although it is difficult to state that the system provides a completely accurate measurement, it seems to provide consistent and meaningful data.

The workspaces of the right and left hands were mostly similar, because ARAT repeats the same tasks with both hands alternatively. The slight difference between both sides is likely due to the difference in posture and orientation based on the limb dominance. During the ADL tasks, the workspace of the dominant hand, right hand for all subjects, was significantly larger than that of the non-dominant side by up to nearly 20 cm for all directions. In the view of stroke rehabilitation, most of the patients demonstrated hemiplegia of up to 80% or more [20], which means that their intact limb should be able to perform all normal functions. Patients with hemiplegia will use their intact hand as their dominant hand and, therefore, in certain occasions, the exoskeleton may only need to cover a smaller workspace than the dominant side.

The RoMs of the major upper extremity joints during essential daily activities are presented in Table 2. The forearm supination/pronation and elbow flexion/extension showed the highest values for the dominant side. The RoM for the forearm supination/pronation was 128.09° and 108.00° on average for the right and left sides, respectively, during all ADL tasks. In a study using a reflective marker-based motion capture system, the whole RoM calculated by overlapping all 95% confidential interval range during various ADL tasks was approximately 92° [9]. Another study applied using an electromagnetic sensor system reported that the maximal supination angle from full pronation was 110° while glass drinking and 75° while combing their hair [8]. In a study by van Andel et al. [21], four selected ADL tasks were evaluated using an optic marker-based system, and their reported RoM for forearm supination/pronation was approximately 130°. Regarding elbow flexion/extension RoM, other studies also showed similar results. Aizawa et al. [8] reported a RoM of approximately 120° to 130° during various tasks, and Gates et al. [9] showed that the peak flexion angle of the elbow joint was 121° on average when drinking from a cup, which was the highest value among the evaluated tasks. Another study reported a RoM of around 140° from full extension [21]. Wrist dorsiflexion/volarflexion RoM was also similar with other studies, which ranged from 90° to 130°, whereas it was 113.70° and 110.08° for right and left side, respectively, in our study. It is important to ensure a sufficient

RoM for elbow flexion/extension, forearm supination/pronation, and wrist dorsiflexion/volarflexion movements during rehabilitation, because such joint movements are essential for conducting ADL tasks, while recovery for distal joints are relatively slow and insufficient for a large portion of stroke patients [22–24].

The angular changes in the major joints when reaching after a grasping/pinching motion are evaluated because such actions are the fundamental movements for conducting any kind of tasks [25,26], and most of the activities are performed within the spatial range of these actions. Pinching was performed at a slightly but significantly more abducted and flexed posture of the shoulder joint, and showed a significant difference in fine tuning movements of the wrist joint.

In contrast to a simple pure reaching movement, a reaching movement associated with a task may differ significantly regarding the arm postures, grasping position, and orientation [27,28]. The human motor system has high redundancy in terms of a multi-degree-of-freedom control system, and while task-relevant factors are specifically controlled, task-irrelevant variables are given relatively high variability [27]. In this study, the shoulder joint angles showed significantly different postures between grasping and pinching, which reflects different positions of the elbow joint while conducting a task. The wrist deviation and rotation angles also showed a significant difference, reflecting the difference in the fine motor posture and movements. Given the difference in posture, the main components of the reaching movement, elbow flexion/extension and forearm supination/pronation, did not differ significantly between the two types of tasks. This result may be applied to the swivel angle model suggested by Li et al. [27], where the shoulder joint angles can be simplified to a swivel angle regarding the orientation and posture, and the other distal joint angles account for essential reaching movements. In regular stroke rehabilitation, proximal muscle power recovery occurs in the early stage and more sufficiently compared to distal muscles [22–24] and, thus, it will be reasonable to motivate the patient to practice taking an appropriate posture for providing the right orientation of the upper extremity using the proximal muscles voluntarily, with the help of a gravity support system if applicable, whereas the individual robot joint actuation should focus on the essential distal joint movements such as elbow, forearm, and wrist movements.

Based on the current study dataset and the analysis, the workspace of the end-effector and its corresponding elbow or forearm position workspace, along with the essential elbow flexion/extension and forearm supination/pronation, may provide minimal structural requirements for the rehabilitation robot to maintain basic grasping, pinching, and reaching movements which are necessary to perform daily activities. This may be applied in both neurorehabilitation exoskeletons and assistive exoskeletons. These results may have helpful applications in virtual reality rehabilitation systems, especially in developing games or tasks which are clinically relevant.

This study has several limitations. To generalize the findings of the motion analysis, the number of subjects was relatively small. However, the statistical analyses provided minimal requirements regarding the validity and reliability and the data pattern for each subject was nearly identical especially during the structured movements (ARAT). Still, further studies with advanced protocol are necessary to verify and generalize the study results. In addition, gender and age factors could not be investigated sufficiently due to small number of subjects. Nevertheless, we have performed non-parametric tests to compare the major sensor-based parameters between men and women, and because the age range for this study was relatively in the young age, they were compared with additional dataset of the intact limb of the older people with hemiplegia. Most of the parameters did not show statistically significant difference according to the gender or age, except that older people tend to perform tasks within a smaller workspace during free ADL tasks and that women tend to abduct the shoulder more than men during pinching. IMU-based sensors basically have their own inevitable limitations, which include drift phenomenon in both the position and angular values, which may affect the values of the outcome measures [29]. In addition, a gimbal-lock phenomenon regarding the shoulder joint angles in particular may have occurred during the data measurements [8]. In this regard, the data may not be accurate in terms of the absolute values; however, because the data are sufficiently consistent, it seems that the general pattern of the data is reliable.

5. Conclusions

These study results provide the essential workspace and RoM of the major upper extremity joints during ARAT and ADL tasks in healthy subjects, which will serve as a basis in designing a practical and simple upper extremity exoskeleton robot. Further motion analyses on stroke patients are necessary to characterize upper extremity movements in neurological disorders and determine the key features in the stroke recovery process, which will be important in extracting the clinically relevant movement characteristics for designing new exoskeletons for neurorehabilitation purposes.

Author Contributions: Conceptualization: H.S.N., H.G.S., M.S.B. and S.K.; data curation: H.S.N. and W.H.L.; formal analysis: H.S.N.; funding acquisition: M.S.B. and S.K.; investigation: H.S.N., M.S.B. and S.K.; methodology: H.G.S.; software: Y.J.K.; supervision: S.K.; validation: W.H.L. and Y.J.K.; writing—original draft, H.S.N.; writing—review and editing: H.S.N., W.H.L., H.G.S., Y.J.K., M.S.B. and S.K.

Funding: This research was supported by the Brain Research Program through the National Research Foundation of Korea (NRF) funded by the Ministry of Science, ICT and Future Planning (2016M3C7A1904984).

Acknowledgments: This study was approved by the Institutional Review Board of Seoul National University Hospital (IRB No. 1505-017-668).

Declaration: This manuscript is a revision of part of the first author's (Nam HS) Ph. D. thesis from Seoul National University.

Conflicts of Interest: The authors declare no conflict of interest.

References

1. Bertani, R.; Melegari, C.; De Cola, M.C.; Bramanti, A.; Bramanti, P.; Calabro, R.S. Effects of robot-assisted upper limb rehabilitation in stroke patients: A systematic review with meta-analysis. *Neurol. Sci.* **2017**, *38*, 1561–1569. [CrossRef]
2. Mehrholz, J.; Pohl, M.; Platz, T.; Kugler, J.; Elsner, B. Electromechanical and robot-assisted arm training for improving activities of daily living, arm function, and arm muscle strength after stroke. *Cochrane Database Syst. Rev.* **2015**. [CrossRef] [PubMed]
3. Ren, Y.; Kang, S.H.; Park, H.S.; Wu, Y.N.; Zhang, L.Q. Developing a multi-joint upper limb exoskeleton robot for diagnosis, therapy, and outcome evaluation in neurorehabilitation. *IEEE Trans. Neural Syst. Rehabil. Eng.* **2013**, *21*, 490–499. [CrossRef] [PubMed]
4. Klamroth-Marganska, V.; Blanco, J.; Campen, K.; Curt, A.; Dietz, V.; Ettlin, T.; Felder, M.; Fellinghauer, B.; Guidali, M.; Kollmar, A.; et al. Three-dimensional, task-specific robot therapy of the arm after stroke: A multicentre, parallel-group randomised trial. *Lancet Neurol.* **2014**, *13*, 159–166. [CrossRef]
5. Fasoli, S.E.; Krebs, H.I.; Stein, J.; Frontera, W.R.; Hogan, N. Effects of robotic therapy on motor impairment and recovery in chronic stroke. *Arch. Phys. Med. Rehabil.* **2003**, *84*, 477–482. [CrossRef] [PubMed]
6. Lo, H.S.; Xie, S.Q. Exoskeleton robots for upper-limb rehabilitation: State of the art and future prospects. *Med. Eng. Phys.* **2012**, *34*, 261–268. [CrossRef] [PubMed]
7. Valero-Cuevas, F.J.; Santello, M. On neuromechanical approaches for the study of biological and robotic grasp and manipulation. *J. Neuroeng Rehabil.* **2017**, *14*, 101. [CrossRef]
8. Aizawa, J.; Masuda, T.; Koyama, T.; Nakamaru, K.; Isozaki, K.; Okawa, A.; Morita, S. Three-dimensional motion of the upper extremity joints during various activities of daily living. *J. Biomech.* **2010**, *43*, 2915–2922. [CrossRef]
9. Gates, D.H.; Walters, L.S.; Cowley, J.; Wilken, J.M.; Resnik, L. Range of Motion Requirements for Upper-Limb Activities of Daily Living. *Am. J. Occup. Ther.* **2016**, *70*, 7001350010p1–7001350010p10. [CrossRef]
10. Kim, K.; Song, W.K.; Lee, J.; Lee, H.Y.; Park, D.S.; Ko, B.W.; Kim, J. Kinematic analysis of upper extremity movement during drinking in hemiplegic subjects. *Clin. Biomech. (Bristol, Avon)* **2014**, *29*, 248–256. [CrossRef] [PubMed]
11. Chen, J.; Lum, P.S. Pilot testing of the spring operated wearable enhancer for arm rehabilitation (SpringWear). *J. Neuroeng. Rehabil.* **2018**, *15*, 13. [CrossRef] [PubMed]

12. Perez, R.; Costa, U.; Torrent, M.; Solana, J.; Opisso, E.; Caceres, C.; Tormos, J.M.; Medina, J.; Gomez, E.J. Upper limb portable motion analysis system based on inertial technology for neurorehabilitation purposes. *Sensors* **2010**, *10*, 10733–10751. [CrossRef] [PubMed]
13. Wang, Q.; Markopoulos, P.; Yu, B.; Chen, W.; Timmermans, A. Interactive wearable systems for upper body rehabilitation: A systematic review. *J. Neuroeng Rehabil.* **2017**, *14*, 20. [CrossRef] [PubMed]
14. Lyle, R.C. A performance test for assessment of upper limb function in physical rehabilitation treatment and research. *Int. J. Rehabil. Res.* **1981**, *4*, 483–492. [CrossRef] [PubMed]
15. Nam, H.S.; Seo, H.G.; Leigh, J.H.; Kim, Y.J.; Kim, S.; Bang, M.S. External Robotic Arm vs Upper Limb Exoskeleton: What Do the Potential Users Need? Unpublished.
16. Hsieh, C.L.; Hsueh, I.P.; Chiang, F.M.; Lin, P.H. Inter-rater reliability and validity of the action research arm test in stroke patients. *Age Ageing* **1998**, *27*, 107–113. [CrossRef] [PubMed]
17. Koh, C.L.; Hsueh, I.P.; Wang, W.C.; Sheu, C.F.; Yu, T.Y.; Wang, C.H.; Hsieh, C.L. Validation of the action research arm test using item response theory in patients after stroke. *J. Rehabil. Med.* **2006**, *38*, 375–380. [CrossRef]
18. Chen, H.F.; Lin, K.C.; Wu, C.Y.; Chen, C.L. Rasch validation and predictive validity of the action research arm test in patients receiving stroke rehabilitation. *Arch. Phys. Med. Rehabil.* **2012**, *93*, 1039–1045. [CrossRef]
19. Yozbatiran, N.; Der-Yeghiaian, L.; Cramer, S.C. A standardized approach to performing the action research arm test. *Neurorehabil. Neural Repair* **2008**, *22*, 78–90. [CrossRef]
20. Parker, V.M.; Wade, D.T.; Langton Hewer, R. Loss of arm function after stroke: Measurement, frequency, and recovery. *Int. Rehabil. Med.* **1986**, *8*, 69–73. [CrossRef]
21. Van Andel, C.J.; Wolterbeek, N.; Doorenbosch, C.A.; Veeger, D.H.; Harlaar, J. Complete 3D kinematics of upper extremity functional tasks. *Gait Posture* **2008**, *27*, 120–127. [CrossRef]
22. Krakauer, J.W. Arm function after stroke: From physiology to recovery. *Semin. Neurol.* **2005**, *25*, 384–395. [CrossRef] [PubMed]
23. Shelton, F.N.; Reding, M.J. Effect of lesion location on upper limb motor recovery after stroke. *Stroke* **2001**, *32*, 107–112. [CrossRef] [PubMed]
24. Brunnstrom, S. Motor testing procedures in hemiplegia: Based on sequential recovery stages. *Phys. Ther.* **1966**, *46*, 357–375. [CrossRef] [PubMed]
25. Shumway-Cook, A.; Woollacott, M.H. *Motor Control: Translating Research into Clinical Practice*, 5th ed.; Wolters Kluwer: Philadelphia, PA, USA, 2017; pp. 465–489.
26. Guccione, A.A.; Wong, R.; Avers, D. *Geriatric Physical Therapy*, 3rd ed.; Elsevier: Louis, MO, USA, 2012.
27. Li, Z.; Milutinovic, D.; Rosen, J. From reaching to reach-to-grasp: The arm posture difference and its implications on human motion control strategy. *Exp. Brain Res.* **2017**, *235*, 1627–1642. [CrossRef] [PubMed]
28. Scharoun, S.M.; Scanlan, K.A.; Bryden, P.J. Hand and Grasp Selection in a Preferential Reaching Task: The Effects of Object Location, Orientation, and Task Intention. *Front. Psychol.* **2016**, *7*, 360. [CrossRef] [PubMed]
29. Luinge, H.J.; Veltink, P.H. Measuring orientation of human body segments using miniature gyroscopes and accelerometers. *Med. Biol. Eng. Comput.* **2005**, *43*, 273–282. [CrossRef]

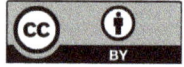

© 2019 by the authors. Licensee MDPI, Basel, Switzerland. This article is an open access article distributed under the terms and conditions of the Creative Commons Attribution (CC BY) license (http://creativecommons.org/licenses/by/4.0/).

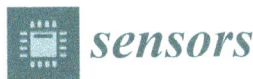

Article

Complexity of Daily Physical Activity Is More Sensitive Than Conventional Metrics to Assess Functional Change in Younger Older Adults

Wei Zhang [1,*], Michael Schwenk [2,3], Sabato Mellone [4], Anisoara Paraschiv-Ionescu [1], Beatrix Vereijken [5], Mirjam Pijnappels [6], A. Stefanie Mikolaizak [2], Elisabeth Boulton [7], Nini H. Jonkman [6], Andrea B. Maier [6,8], Jochen Klenk [2,9], Jorunn Helbostad [5], Kristin Taraldsen [5] and Kamiar Aminian [1]

1. Laboratory of Movement Analysis and Measurement, Ecole Polytechnique Federale de Lausanne, 1015 Lausanne, Switzerland; anisoara.ionescu@epfl.ch (A.P.-I.); kamiar.aminian@epfl.ch (K.A.)
2. Robert Bosch Foundation for Medical Research, 70376 Stuttgart, Germany; michael.schwenk@rbk.de (M.S.); stefanie.mikolaizak@rbk.de (A.S.M.); jochen.klenk@rbk.de (J.K.)
3. Network Aging Research, Heidelberg University, 69115 Heidelberg, Germany
4. Department of Electrical, Electronic and Information Engineering, University of Bologna, 40136 Bologna, Italy; sabato.mellone@unibo.it
5. Department of Neuromedicine and Movement Science, Norwegian University of Science and Technology, 7491 Trondheim, Norway; beatrix.vereijken@ntnu.no (B.V.); jorunn.helbostad@ntnu.no (J.H.); kristin.taraldsen@ntnu.no (K.T.)
6. Department of Human Movement Sciences, Vrije Universiteit Amsterdam, Amsterdam Movement Sciences, 1081BT Amsterdam, The Netherlands; m.pijnappels@vu.nl (M.P.); n.h.jonkman@vu.nl (N.H.J.); andrea.maier@mh.org.au (A.B.M.)
7. School of Health Sciences, Faculty of Medicine, Biology and Health, University of Manchester, and Manchester Academic Health Science Centre, Manchester M13 9PL, UK; elisabeth.boulton@manchester.ac.uk
8. Department of Medicine and Aged Care, @AgeMelbourne, Royal Melbourne Hospital, University of Melbourne, Melbourne 3050, Australia
9. Institute of Epidemiology and Medical Biometry, Ulm University, 89081 Ulm, Germany
* Correspondence: w.zhang@epfl.ch; Tel.: +41-21-6937606

Received: 18 May 2018; Accepted: 21 June 2018; Published: 25 June 2018

Abstract: The emerging mHealth applications, incorporating wearable sensors, enables continuous monitoring of physical activity (PA). This study aimed at analyzing the relevance of a multivariate complexity metric in assessment of functional change in younger older adults. Thirty individuals (60–70 years old) participated in a 4-week home-based exercise intervention. The Community Balance and Mobility Scale (CBMS) was used for clinical assessment of the participants' functional balance and mobility performance pre- and post- intervention. Accelerometers worn on the low back were used to register PA of one week before and in the third week of the intervention. Changes in conventional univariate PA metrics (percentage of walking and sedentary time, step counts, mean cadence) and complexity were compared to the change as measured by the CBMS. Statistical analyses (21 participants) showed significant rank correlation between the change as measured by complexity and CBMS ($\rho = 0.47$, $p = 0.03$). Smoothing the activity output improved the correlation ($\rho = 0.58$, $p = 0.01$). In contrast, change in univariate PA metrics did not show correlations. These findings demonstrate the high potential of the complexity metric being useful and more sensitive than conventional PA metrics for assessing functional changes in younger older adults.

Keywords: wearable sensors; multivariate analysis; longitudinal study; functional decline; exercise intervention

1. Introduction

The aging process is often accompanied by functional decline and increased risk of chronic diseases [1]. However, functional ability varies between older adults, depending on individual health condition and lifestyles. Physical inactivity is one of the known risk factors that can lead to morbidity and mortality [2]. The transition from work to retirement, which often occurs between 60 and 70 years of age, can involve a significant change in structured daily activities, with physical activity declining. A study on the Dutch population found that retirement introduces a reduction in physical activity from work-related transportation that is not compensated for by an increase in sports participation or an increase in non-sports leisure-time physical activity [3]. Thus, this population is of particular importance for addressing maintenance of their functional status.

In recent years, mobile health (mHealth) applications, incorporating wearable sensing technologies with modern mobile communication devices, are emerging. From the early adoption in younger populations for fitness tracking in particular, mHealth has been continuously developing and diversifying its applications for different populations [1,4]. The scalability of mHealth technologies enables data collection in diverse geographic locations over prolonged time periods [5]. This provides a new perspective in studying physical activities in real life and allows new analytical tools to be developed to analyze and present the data.

An earlier systematic review on body-worn, accelerometer-based physical activity monitoring revealed the challenge of achieving consensus on the reporting and the interpretation of the measurements provided by various mHealth applications [6]. Furthermore, the review pointed out that energy expenditure, walking time, and total activity are most frequently reported and are comparable variables across studies. In addition, several variables, such as walking time, number of steps, and cadence are the most widely adopted variables in research [5,7,8] to characterize walking pattern, the most common daily physical activity across all age groups. Descriptive statistics (e.g., mean, maximum values) are applied to the above walking parameters for analysis. Detrended fluctuation analysis proposed by Hausdorff et al. is used to quantify the stride-to-stride variability in supervised walking tasks [9]. However, physical activity involves multiple components and has more than one dimension. Different types of activities in daily life, as well as the quantity and the quality (performance) of each activity jointly determine a person's functional status. Thus, a variable that models a person's physical activity behaviour based on these aspects is warranted.

Complexity analysis as introduced by Paraschiv-Ionescu et al. [10] aims at combining both the quantity and quality dimensions of multiple, commonly performed daily activities into one metric to describe physical activity behaviour. This complexity metric has demonstrated discriminative power to distinguish groups of patients suffering from chronic pain [11,12]. Besides analyzing accelerometry-derived activities, the metric has been validated also for analyzing activity behaviour of older adults using an application based on wearable pressure insoles [13].

While several cross-sectional studies exist for clinical validation of complexity metrics, the sensitivity of those metrics for detecting changes in physical function over time has not yet been determined. Therefore, we aimed to examine the ability of the aforementioned complexity metric to detect change in a longitudinal intervention study conducted in younger older adults in comparison to conventionally applied univariate physical activity metrics. Within this context, we further explored the impact of smoothing sensor-based physical activity data on the complexity metric.

2. Materials and Methods

2.1. Study Protocol

The study is part of the larger PreventIT project [1], developing and testing an ICT-based mHealth system that enables early identification of risk for age-related functional decline, and engenders behavioural change in younger older adults (aged 60–70 years) in order to adopt a healthy, active lifestyle.

Thirty participants, aged between 60 and 70 years, were recruited at three different sites, Trondheim (Norway), Amsterdam (the Netherlands), and Stuttgart (Germany), to participate in a 4-week pre-post pilot intervention study. All participants were instructed by an experienced physical therapist or exercise therapist to follow an adapted Lifestyle-integrated Functional Exercise (aLiFE) programme specifically developed for improving balance and strength and increasing physical activity in younger older adults [14]. aLiFE was taught during four weekly home visits, and the participants were asked to integrate the aLiFE activities into everyday routines. Pre and post intervention, the participants completed a balance and mobility assessment using the Community Balance and Mobility Scale (CBMS). The scale has been validated to capture high-level balance, gait, and mobility performances in healthy active younger older adults based on the quality of performing the tasks [15]. CBMS assessments were performed in the research hospital or university by trained assessors. In addition, daily physical activity (PA) of each participant was measured twice for one week with wearable sensors. The participants were instructed to wear an inertial sensor (DynaPort, MoveMonitor, McRoberts, The Hague, The Netherlands) at their lower back at the level of L5 using an elastic belt during the day and night. The sensor needed to be removed when showering or during any water activity and needed to be put back on afterwards. The sensor did not need to be recharged during the one week measurement. All sensors were collected at the end of the measurement and raw sensor data was downloaded for offline data analysis. The first measurement was prior to the start of the intervention period. The measurement was repeated during the third week of the pilot study to capture the change of daily activity patterns during the intervention.

2.2. Sensor Data Processing

The sensor consists of a 3D accelerometer with sampling frequency of 100 Hz. The recording start time of each sensor was registered on the device by manual insertion of a timestamp. A non-commercial activity classification software was used to extract quantitative as well as qualitative features of PA from raw sensor data. The software is an outcome of the FARSEEING EU project (FP7/2007–2013, grant agreement 288940). It has been applied in studies with dementia patients [16] and older people residing in independent-living retirement homes [17]. The software has been further developed based on two datasets of elderly subjects. The first one is the ADAPT dataset [18], where video recording was performed using ceiling-mounted cameras in lab settings and an action camera in free-living conditions. The second dataset is from the University of Auckland [17], where subjects performed both scripted and unscripted activities of daily living collected in a free-living environment. First, the algorithm estimates Metabolic Equivalents (METs); signals are filtered and processed as described in [19]. An interval is labelled as 'sedentary', if associated energy expenditure is below or equal to 1.5 MET [20]. Otherwise, the interval is labelled as 'active'. 'Sedentary' intervals with a mean angle between the vertical axis and the medio-lateral or the anterior–posterior direction of the trunk below 30° are labelled as 'lying'. The 'active' intervals, where steps are detected are labelled as 'walking'. Step detection is based on [21]. Each interval is then characterized by the category (label), the duration, and the activity counts (counts/minute) from which METs are estimated [19]. In addition, number of steps and the cadence (steps/minute) are extracted for each 'walking' bout. Data is labelled as 'non-wearing', if the sensor is detected lying flat with very low variance in acceleration signals for longer than half an hour.

The classified activities were sorted into natural days based on the registered timestamp. Days with less than 16 h of measurements (i.e., the first and the last day of the measurement) were excluded from further processing and analysis. Given the high resolution (1 s) of the PA output data, bouts of one activity may be interspersed with short episodes of other activities. For example, short breaks of a few seconds are often present during one walking bout due to environmental factors (e.g., walking episodes whiles shopping in a supermarket), which may lead to a string of several walking episodes rather than one continuous walking bout. Such short breaks during an activity introduce artificial changes in the dynamics of the PA time series, which are not relevant to one's physical behaviour. Therefore, a smoothing technique was devised to filter such artefacts and to aggregate bouts in the original PA output belonging to the same PA category based on the following steps, as illustrated in Figure 1. First, we applied a moving forward sliding window of 30 s without overlap to smooth the PA time series [22]. The activity category of these 30 s was replaced by the activity with the highest density (counts) within the window. Second, the process was repeated for K folds. At each fold, the smoothing starts with a random shift between 1 and 30 s at the beginning of the time series. Third, the activity category of each second in the aggregated time series was determined by the majority vote of the K-fold smoothing. The sliding window length was chosen according to the 'barcode' design (explained in the later section Complexity analysis), where 30-s is the threshold of activity duration corresponding to indoor walking.

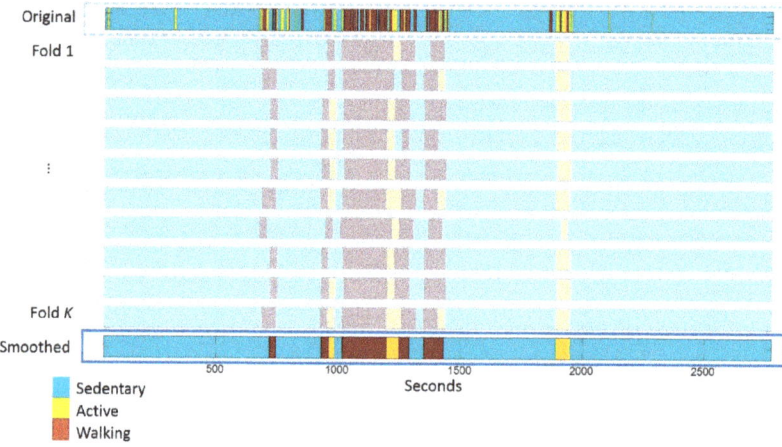

Figure 1. Smoothing activity classification output to aggregate activity bouts in a measurement time series of 45 min. The top bar shows the original PA sequence and the bottom bar shows the smoothed sequence.

2.3. Univariate Analysis

For each activity bout, its duration and activity counts per minute ('ActiCount') were estimated. In addition, the total number of steps and the average cadence (steps/min) were provided for each classified walking bout. PA was characterized by various univariate metrics including the percentage of time being sedentary, the percentage of time spent walking, the number of steps normalized to the measurement duration (in hours), and the mean cadence of walking bouts of each day. The univariate metrics were computed based on the original and the smoothed PA time series.

2.4. Complexity Analysis

Complexity was introduced in order to analyze the variability of biological and physiological time series data [23,24]. The technique was subsequently adapted and applied to analyze ambulatory activity patterns [25]. Paraschiv-Ionescu et al. proposed complexity analysis on a multivariate PA pattern ('barcode') derived from wearable sensor data [10]. The 'barcode' is constructed for the analyzed period based on the classified activity category, the duration and the intensity. The entropy rate of the resulting multi-state 'barcode' represents complexity. In the analysis of the pilot data, an adapted 'barcode' was used, where the 'ActiCount' was modeled according to a validation study presented in [19]. Entropy rate of the 'barcode' was computed in terms of Lempel-Ziv complexity based on the method described in [26]. (Additional materials are presented in Appendix A.1). Complexity of the 'barcode' generated from both the original and the smoothed time series of PA were computed to analyze the influence of activity classification on the calculated complexity.

2.5. Statistical Analysis

For each participant, the univariate metrics and the complexity metric of PA were analyzed for each day. The average value of each metric over the one-week measurement before (Week0) and during (Week3) the pilot study was calculated. According to study [27], participants having more than two days' sensor data during the one-week measurement, in both Week0 and Week3, were included for statistical analysis. The changes in PA metrics between Week0 and Week3 were computed. The change in CBMS score pre and post the pilot study was calculated. The primary analysis was to examine the correlations between the change in PA metrics and the change in CBMS score. Given the small sample size and ordinal data type (CBMS scores), spearman coefficient (ρ) was used to analyse the strength of correlation. In addition, a non-parametric effect size calculator, Cliff's Delta, was applied to measure the degree of overlap between the distribution of various variables extracted pre- and during/post interventions [28]. Cliff's Delta approaching 1 or −1 indicates absence of overlap, whereas 0 indicates overlap completely. Wilcoxon signed rank test was applied to examine the statistical significance of the change. Changes with a p value < 0.05 was considered statistically significant. The secondary analysis consisted of the impact of PA time series smoothing on the conventional metrics and the complexity metric. The analysis compared the aforementioned statistical outcomes before and after smoothing. Additional analyses on Week0 data compared the distributions of the length of sedentary and walking bouts before and after smoothing. The coefficients of variance (CV) of the daily complexity value of the original and the smoothed PA time series were compared.

3. Results

In total, 30 participants were included in the pilot study with 10 participants at each trial site. Due to technical problems with the sensor devices (no data could be retrieved), eight participants were excluded from further data processing and analysis (n = 5 in Week0 and n = 3 in Week3). One participant's CBMS score was not available at the baseline assessment and was excluded from further data analysis leaving 21 participants for statistical analyses. All participants in statistical analysis had minimum 3 days of data in Week0 and Week3. Table 1 summarizes the descriptive statistics of PA metrics and CBMS score for the included participants (n = 21, except the CV of complexity, where n = 25 from Week0 were analyzed) in the pilot study. The included participants were not significantly different from the excluded participants in CMBS scores at the pre- (Willcoxon ranksum test, p = 0.14) or the post- (p = 0.23) intervention assessment. To illustrate, Figure 2 shows one participant's barcode (based on smoothed PA time series) in Week0 (left) and Week3 (right). The barcode in Week3 shows richer colours filled in throughout several days of measurements, which was reflected by the higher mean complexity score of 0.120 compared to 0.111 in Week0.

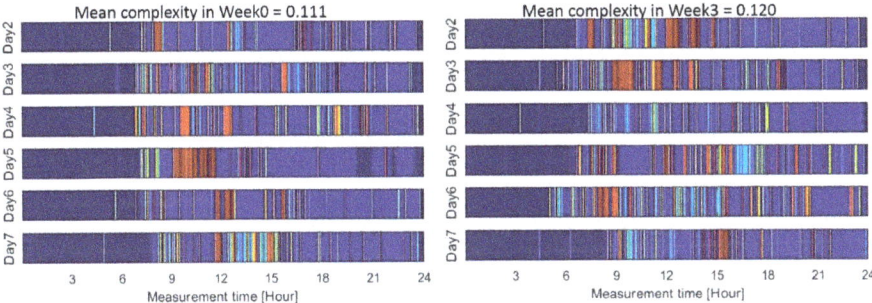

Figure 2. Barcode and mean complexity of one-week PA time series of Week0 (**left**) and Week3 (**right**) in one participant.

Table 1. Descriptive statistics of PA metrics, complexity, and CBMS scores in pre- and post- intervention assessments. PA metrics and complexity based on original and smoothed PA time series are compared with CMBS scores.

	Week0 or Pre Pilot (Mean ± SD) Original/Smoothed	Week3 or Post Pilot (Mean ± SD) Original/Smoothed	Association (ρ) with CBMS Original/Smoothed	Effect Size (Cliff's Delta) Original/Smoothed
Percentage of sedentary time (%)	44.9 ± 6.0/47.7 ± 6.5	44.4 ± 5.6/47.5 ± 6.0	−0.35/−0.28	−0.12/−0.08
Percentage of walking time (%)	9.1 ± 2.0/9.1 ± 2.2	9.9 ± 3.0/10.0 ± 3.3	0.05/−0.01	0.13/0.15 [a]
Normalised nr. of steps (steps/hour)	489 ± 123/361 ± 111	532 ± 182/395 ± 160	0.02/−0.17	0.11/0.08
Mean cadence (steps/minute)	78 ± 5/52 ± 8	78 ± 6/51 ± 7	−0.25/−0.33	0/−0.13
Complexity	0.178 ± 0.024/0.101 ± 0.006	0.185 ± 0.024/0.103 ± 0.007	0.47 [a]/0.58 [a]	0.18/0.15
CV of complexity [b]	0.11 ± 0.05/0.07 ± 0.02			
CBMS score	66.4 ± 12.8	70.2 ± 12.9		0.20 [a]

[a] Statistically significant ($p < 0.05$), [b] based on 25 participants' data at Week0.

For the primary analysis, scatter plots in Figure 3 show the correlations. Spearman correlations between changes in PA metrics (based on original PA time series) and CBMS score (between the change in CBMS score and the changes measured by various conventional univariate metrics and the complexity metric) are based on original PA time series. Changes in univariate metrics had no significant association with the change as measured by the CBMS score. In contrast, complexity had a significant positive correlation ($\rho = 0.47$, $p = 0.03$) with the change in CBMS. Complexity was higher after intervention with an effect size of 0.18, which was comparable to the effect size as measured by the CBMS score (0.20). Despite an increase in complexity post intervention, the change was not statistically significant. Changes in univariate metrics had smaller effect size and were not statistically significant (see Table 1).

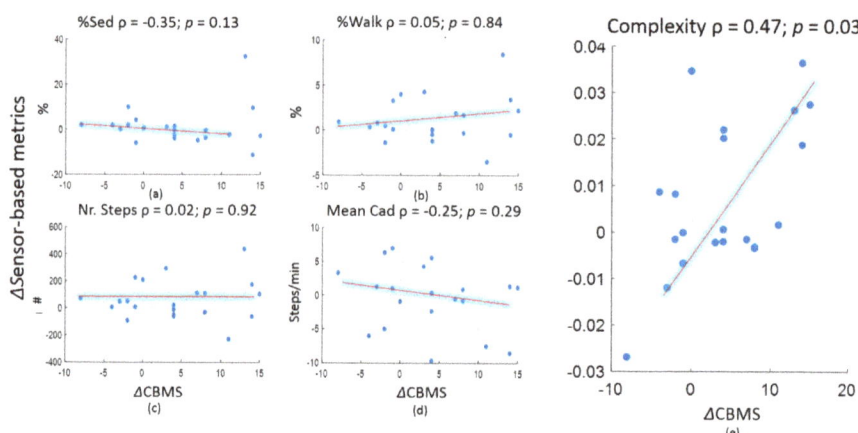

Figure 3. Spearman correlations between changes in PA metrics (based on original PA time series) and CBMS score. (**a**) Change in percentage of sedentary time vs. change in CBMS. (**b**) Change in percentage of walking time vs. change in CBMS. (**c**) Change in normalized number of steps vs. change in CBMS. (**d**) Change in mean cadence vs. change in CBMS. (**e**) Change in complexity vs. change in CBMS.

For the secondary analysis, after smoothing the PA time series, multiple very short sedentary bouts were merged into one longer bout. Similarly, multiple walking bouts with short interruptions were concatenated to form a continuous walking bout (see Appendix A.2). Comparison of mean values of various univariate metrics presented in Table 1 indicated that smoothing had little impact on the percentage of sedentary time and the percentage of walking time, whereas the total number of steps and mean cadence were reduced. The value of complexity for the smoothed PA time series was smaller, compared to the original complexity. The change in complexity for the smoothed PA time series resulted in a stronger association with the change in CBMS score ($\rho = 0.58, p = 0.01$ as shown in Figure 4. Association between complexity change and CBMS score change after smoothing PA time series.). Moreover, the mean CV of complexity of the participants in Week0 decreased from 0.11 to 0.07 after smoothing the PA time series (see Appendix A.2).

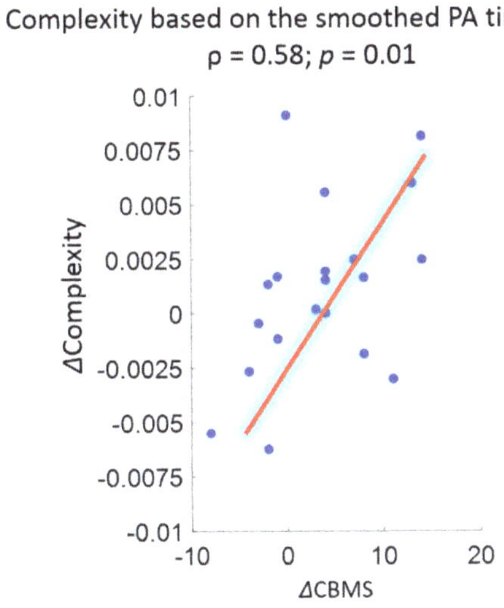

Figure 4. Association between complexity change and CBMS score change after smoothing PA time series.

4. Discussion

Authors should discuss the results and how they can be interpreted from the perspective of previous studies and of the working hypotheses. The findings and their implications should be discussed in the broadest context possible. Future research directions may also be highlighted. The primary analysis of this study focused on the relevance of various conventional PA metrics and the complexity in the assessment of functional change after an exercise intervention in younger older adults. In addition, we analyzed the impact of smoothing PA time series data on the calculation of various PA metrics and the complexity metric. Despite a very short intervention, the change in complexity was significantly correlated with the change as measured by the CBMS score, whereas, the changes in conventional PA metrics did not show significant correlation with the change as measured by the clinical assessment. Moreover, smoothing the PA time series, to aggregate short activity bouts, improved the complexity metric in terms of stronger correlation with functional change as measured by a clinical assessment and higher measurement reproducibility as quantified by the CV of one-week measurements.

These results revealed that complexity is a useful and a more sensitive metric than conventionally applied univariate PA metrics in the assessment of functional change in younger older adults. Conventional PA metrics derived from wearable sensors, step counts, or cadence, might not be sensitive enough to capture the functional change after short interventions. Metrics characterizing one aspect of daily physical activity, such as the time spent walking or being sedentary, do not provide a comprehensive picture of the determinants of functional status. The complexity metric of physical behaviour, on the other hand, characterizes the quantity, the quality, and the dynamic changes between different activities and different performances while doing the same activity (such as a change in cadence) in the 'barcode'. Further, the entropy rate increases while the number of sub-patterns in the 'barcode' increases as illustrated in Figure 2. Since it captures more aspects of physical behaviour simultaneously, the complexity metric has the potential to capture the underlined important aspect in the aging process that the variety and dimension of activities decreases due to functional decline [29,30].

The 'barcode', as defined in Table A1 and illustrated in Figure 2, is constructed with generic activity features derived from the wearable sensors. This makes complexity a generic metric for PA data analysis in principle without constraints in specific sensor configuration or wearing position. The activity features required by the 'barcode', such as walking time and number of steps, are universally recognized by the state-of-the-art wearable sensors [10,12,25]. Selection of activity features to be included in barcode construction is a topic worth separate investigation. For example, efficacy and sensitivity to wearing position of a 'barcode' that states sensor-derived activity levels (sedentary, light, and moderate-to-vigorous) can be analyzed [31].

The complexity metric analyses the entropy rate of the 'barcode'. Changes in 'barcode' states depend on the richness of the activity performed but is also influenced by the resolution of the activity features. The higher the resolution, the more detailed the features in the activity performed can be described; however, the resolution becomes less resistant to noise in the activity data. As demonstrated in Figure 1, the original PA time series (the top bar) has second-by-second feature resolution, which shows frequent fast changes between sedentary and walking activities (for example, see between 1000 and 1250 s). In the original PA time series, almost all sedentary bouts were shorter than five minutes, and less than 5% of walking continued for more than one minute in all participants (see distribution of PA activity data before and after smoothing in Figure A1). It is plausible that very short bouts were artifacts of the activity features due to the noise in the accelerometry signal acquired at the waist. The complexity metric aims to capture the dynamic change of real activity patterns that are encoded in the 'barcode' rather than the signal noise. Thus, a pre-processing method to remove the noise, or smooth the activity features before barcoding for complexity analysis is necessary and important. We proposed a smoothing method in this study to remove the noise. As shown in the secondary analysis, the resulting complexity value was lower than the complexity of the original PA time series, indicating that there was less frequent change in the activities after smoothing. The smoothing method improved the reproducibility of the complexity metric, which implies that the smoothing removed irrelevant noise existing in the original PA time series. However, it preserved the clinically relevant activity patterns as shown in the significant correlation with the clinical outcome. We observed a decrease in step counts and mean cadence after smoothing, which was likely due to the procedure, where steps in very short walking bouts were removed, but no step was inserted in the concatenated walking bouts.

There are some limitations in the study presented in this manuscript. First, the sample size was relatively small. Due to missing data, only 21 participants were included in the statistical analyses. Even though, there was no significant difference in functional status as measured by the CBMS score between the included and the excluded subject, the strength of association and effect size of change measured in this pilot study will need to be confirmed in a larger cohort of comparable participants. Secondly, the assessment of daily activity with wearable sensors during the intervention (Week3) was collected one week prior to the post-intervention assessment of CBMS. For the short intervention pilot, this time discrepancy might have introduced bias. This bias likely has made our estimates of pre- or post-intervention change in PA metrics to be more conservative. Lastly, the window of 30 s chosen for the smoothing method is based on the lowest threshold for walk analysis in the 'barcode' design. Conceptually, this threshold corresponds to most indoor walking activities [7,10]. However, future research should conduct a systematic evaluation to confirm the optimized activity feature resolution for complexity analysis.

In the context of PreventIT project, the on-going multi-national randomized controlled trial (RCT) study will provide a larger cohort data of 180 participants with comparable demographic and health profile as studied in this pilot. The RCT will assess the participant's CBMSs and monitor their PAs using a similar sensor configuration at baseline, 6-month, and 12-month follow-up. Correlation between the change in complexity and the change in CBMS will be validated after the longer intervention. Analyses on the association between complexity and CBMS at baseline will be conducted. In addition, relationship between complexity and each individual balance and mobility components assessed in CBMS will be analyzed.

5. Conclusions

This study demonstrated the clinical relevance of using a multivariate metric for physical behavioural complexity to capture change in functional status in a longitudinal study in younger older adults. The complexity metric showed higher sensitivity to functional change than conventionally applied univariate PA metrics such as sedentary time and step count. Complexity can be applied as a generic metric to analyze the daily life activity patterns derived from wearable sensors. A meaningful resolution of sensor-derived activity features is important for reliable complexity analysis. The complexity metric is a useful metric to be further developed for the outcome measure of the feasibility and the effectiveness of PreventIT interventions.

Author Contributions: Conceptualization, B.V., M.P., A.B.M., J.H. and K.A.; Methodology, W.Z., M.S., A.P.-I. and K.A.; Software, W.Z., S.M. and A.P.I.; Data Analysis, W.Z. and M.S.; Data Curation, A.S.M., N.H.J. and K.T.; Writing-Original Draft Preparation, W.Z.; Writing-Review & Editing, all authors.

Funding: This research was funded by European Union's Horizon 2020 research and innovation programme grant number 689238.

Acknowledgments: We thank ADAPT project for providing dataset for technical development of the activity classification algorithm. We thank all PreventIT consortium partners for the inspiring discussions in project meetings. We are grateful to all participants, therapists and trainers in the aLiFE study.

Conflicts of Interest: The authors declare no conflict of interest.

Appendix

Appendix A.1 Adapted Barcode Design and Complexity Computation

A 'barcode' state was assigned to each second of the time series according to Table A1. The definition was modified for the type 'active' from the original design presented in [10] that applied the absolute value of acceleration. As acceleration is sensitive to the sensor wearing location, the acceleration based threshold was replaced by the 'ActiCount' in this study. The 'ActiCount' thresholds are determined based on a validation study presented in [19]. Complexity computation was according to Equation (A1), where 'nrPattern' is the total number of sub-patterns found in the 'barcode'. 'nBC' is the total number of 'barcode' states. In our analysis, nBC = 18. N is the total length of PA time series in seconds.

$$\text{Complexity} = \frac{\text{nrPattern} * (\frac{\log_{10}(\text{nrPattern})}{\log_{10}(\text{nBC})} + 1)}{N} \quad (A1)$$

Table A1. Definition of barcode state according to PA category, intensity and duration.

Category	Intensity	Duration	State
Lying			1
Sedentary			2
Active	ActiCounts $\leq$ 3500 (counts/minute)		3
	3500 < ActiCounts $\leq$ 7000		4
	7000 < ActiCounts $\leq$ 10000		5
	ActiCounts > 10000		6
Walking	Cadence $\leq$ 60 (steps/minute)	Duration $\leq$ 30 s	7
	60 < Cadence $\leq$ 90		8
	90 < Cadence $\leq$ 140		9
	Cadence > 140		10
	Cadence $\leq$ 60	30 < Duration $\leq$ 120	11
	60 < Cadence $\leq$ 90		12
	90 < Cadence $\leq$ 140		13
	Cadence > 140		14
	Cadence $\leq$ 60	Duration > 120	15
	60 < Cadence $\leq$ 90		16
	90 < Cadence $\leq$ 140		17
	Cadence > 140		18

Appendix A.2 Effect of Smoothing on the Duration of Activity Bouts and Reliability of Complexity

Figure A1 shows that, after smoothing, 90% of the sedentary bouts lasted up to 15 min, whereas only 10% of the walking bouts were longer than two and half minutes before a stop. Figure A2 compares the mean and standard deviation of daily complexity in one-week measurement before and after smoothing. Smoothing lowered the mean values and the CV of the complexity.

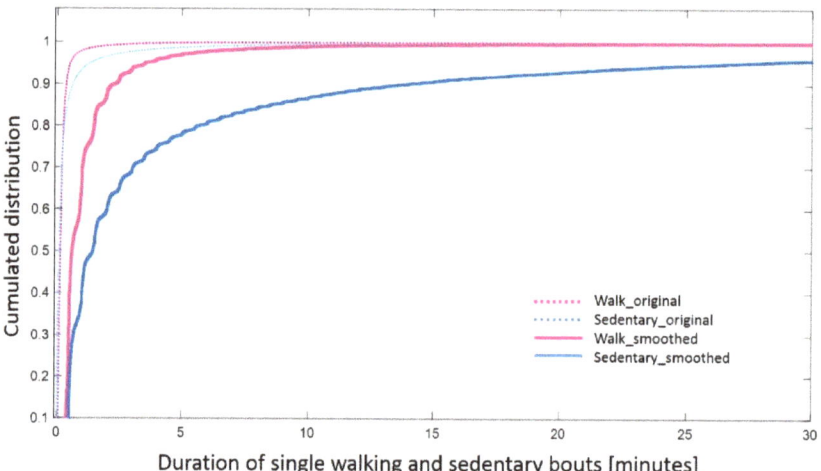

Figure A1. Comparison of cumulated distribution of walking and sedentary bouts before and after smoothing of activity classification output.

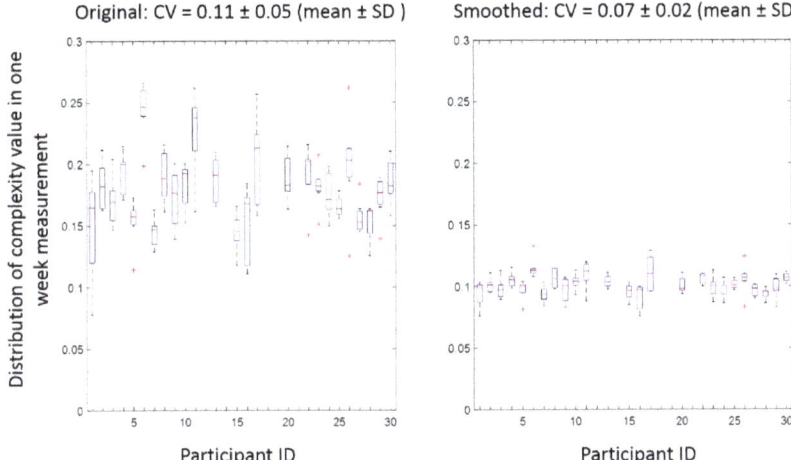

Figure A2. CV before and after smoothing PA time series.

References

1. Helbostad, J.L.; Vereijken, B.; Becker, C.; Todd, C.; Taraldsen, K.; Pijnappels, M.; Aminian, K.; Mellone, S. Mobile Health Applications to Promote Active and Healthy Ageing. *Sensors* **2017**, *17*, 622. [CrossRef] [PubMed]
2. World Health Organization. *Global Health Risks: Mortality and Burden of Disease Attributable to Selected Major Risks*; World Health Organization: Geneva, Switzerland, 2009.
3. Slingerland, A.S.; van Lenthe, F.J.; Jukema, J.W.; Kamphuis, C.B.M.; Looman, C.; Huisman, M.; Narayan, K.M.; Mackenbach, J.P.; Brug, J. Aging, Retirement, and Changes in Physical Activity: Prospective Cohort Findings from the GLOBE Study. *Am. J. Epidemiol.* **2007**, *165*, 1356–1363. [CrossRef] [PubMed]
4. Bort-Roig, J.; Gilson, N.D.; Puig-Ribera, A.; Contreras, R.S.; Trost, S.G. Measuring and influencing physical activity with smartphone technology: A systematic review. *Sports Med.* **2014**, *44*, 671–686. [CrossRef] [PubMed]
5. Althoff, T.; Sosič, R.; Hicks, J.L.; King, A.C.; Delp, S.L.; Leskovec, J. Large-scale physical activity data reveal worldwide activity inequality. *Nature* **2017**, *547*, 336–339. [CrossRef] [PubMed]
6. Taraldsen, K.; Chastin, S.F.M.; Riphagen, I.I.; Vereijken, B.; Helbostad, J.L. Physical activity monitoring by use of accelerometer-based body-worn sensors in older adults: A systematic literature review of current knowledge and applications. *Maturitas* **2012**, *71*, 13–19. [CrossRef] [PubMed]
7. Brodie, M.A.; Lord, S.R.; Coppens, M.J.; Annegarn, J.; Delbaere, K. Eight-Week Remote Monitoring Using a Freely Worn Device Reveals Unstable Gait Patterns in Older Fallers. *IEEE Trans. Biomed. Eng.* **2015**, *62*, 2588–2594. [CrossRef] [PubMed]
8. Ahlrichs, C.; Samà, A.; Lawo, M.; Cabestany, J.; Rodríguez-Martín, D.; Pérez-López, C.; Sweeney, D.; Quinlan, L.R.; Laighin, G.Ò.; Counihan, T.; et al. Detecting freezing of gait with a tri-axial accelerometer in Parkinson's disease patients. *Med. Biol. Eng. Comput.* **2016**, *54*, 223–233. [CrossRef] [PubMed]
9. Hausdorff, J.M. Gait Dynamics, Fractals and Falls: Finding Meaning in the Stride-To-Stride Fluctuations of Human Walking. *Hum. Mov. Sci.* **2007**, *26*, 555–589. [CrossRef] [PubMed]
10. Paraschiv-Ionescu, A.; Perruchoud, C.; Buchser, E.; Aminian, K. Barcoding Human Physical Activity to Assess Chronic Pain Conditions. *PLoS ONE* **2012**, *7*, e32239. [CrossRef] [PubMed]
11. Paraschiv-Ionescu, A.; Perruchoud, C.; Rutschmann, B.; Buchser, E.; Aminian, K. Quantifying dimensions of physical behavior in chronic pain conditions. *J. Neuroeng. Rehabil.* **2016**, *13*, 85. [CrossRef] [PubMed]
12. Paraschiv-Ionescu, A.; Buchser, E.; Aminian, K. Unraveling dynamics of human physical activity patterns in chronic pain conditions. *Sci. Rep.* **2013**, *3*, 2019. [CrossRef] [PubMed]

13. Moufawad el Achkar, C.; Lenoble-Hoskovec, C.; Paraschiv-Ionescu, A.; Major, K.; Büla, C.; Aminian, K. Physical Behavior in Older Persons during Daily Life: Insights from Instrumented Shoes. *Sensors* **2016**, *16*, 1225. [CrossRef] [PubMed]
14. ISRCTN—ISRCTN37750605: Feasibility of the Adapted LiFE (aLiFE) Intervention—A pilot Study. Available online: http://www.isrctn.com/ISRCTN37750605 (accessed on 16 February 2017).
15. Balasubramanian, C.K. The community balance and mobility scale alleviates the ceiling effects observed in the currently used gait and balance assessments for the community-dwelling older adults. *J. Geriatr. Phys. Ther.* **2015**, *38*, 78–89. [CrossRef] [PubMed]
16. Fleiner, T.; Haussermann, P.; Mellone, S.; Zijlstra, W. Sensor-based assessment of mobility-related behavior in dementia: Feasibility and relevance in a hospital context. *Int. Psychogeriatr.* **2016**, *28*, 1687–1694. [CrossRef] [PubMed]
17. Chigateri, N.; Kerse, N.; MacDonald, B.; Klenk, J. Validation of Walking Episode Recognition in Supervised and Free-living Conditions Using Triaxial Accelerometers. In Proceedings of the 2017 World Congress of International Society for Posture & Gait Research, Fort Lauderdale, FL, USA, 25–29 June 2017; pp. 289–290.
18. Bourke, A.K.; Ihlen, E.A.F.; Bergquist, R.; Wik, P.B.; Vereijken, B.; Helbostad, J.L. A Physical Activity Reference Data-Set Recorded from Older Adults Using Body-Worn Inertial Sensors and Video Technology—The ADAPT Study Data-Set. *Sensors* **2017**, *17*, 559. [CrossRef] [PubMed]
19. Sasaki, J.E.; John, D.; Freedson, P.S. Validation and comparison of ActiGraph activity monitors. *J. Sci. Med. Sport* **2011**, *14*, 411–416. [CrossRef] [PubMed]
20. Mansoubi, M.; Pearson, N.; Clemes, S.A.; Biddle, S.J.; Bodicoat, D.H.; Tolfrey, K.; Edwardson, L.; Yates, T. Energy expenditure during common sitting and standing tasks: Examining the 1.5 MET definition of sedentary behaviour. *BMC Public Health* **2015**, *15*, 516. [CrossRef] [PubMed]
21. Ryu, U.; Ahn, K.; Kim, E.; Kim, M.; Kim, B.; Woo, S.; Chang, Y. Adaptive Step Detection Algorithm for Wireless Smart Step Counter. In Proceedings of the 2013 International Conference on Information Science and Applications (ICISA), Suwon, Korea, 24–26 June 2013; pp. 1–4.
22. Razjouyan, J.; Grewal, G.S.; Rishel, C.; Parthasarathy, S.; Mohler, J.; Najafi, B. Activity Monitoring and Heart Rate Variability as Indicators of Fall Risk: Proof-of-Concept for Application of Wearable Sensors in the Acute Care Setting. *J. Gerontol. Nurs.* **2017**, *43*, 53–62. [CrossRef] [PubMed]
23. Orlov, Y.L.; Potapov, V.N. Complexity: An internet resource for analysis of DNA sequence complexity. *Nucleic Acids Res.* **2004**, *32*, W628–W633. [CrossRef] [PubMed]
24. Seely, A.J.; Macklem, P.T. Complex systems and the technology of variability analysis. *Crit. Care* **2004**, *8*, R367. [CrossRef] [PubMed]
25. Cavanaugh, J.T.; Kochi, N.; Stergiou, N. Nonlinear Analysis of Ambulatory Activity Patterns in Community-Dwelling Older Adults. *J. Gerontol. Ser. A* **2010**, *65A*, 197–203. [CrossRef] [PubMed]
26. Lempel, A.; Ziv, J. On the Complexity of Finite Sequences. *IEEE Trans. Inf. Theory.* **1976**, *22*, 75–81. [CrossRef]
27. De Bruin, E.D.; Najafi, B.; Murer, K.; Uebelhart, D.; Aminian, K. Quantification of everyday motor function in a geriatric population. *J. Rehabil. Res. Dev.* **2007**, *44*, 417–428. [CrossRef] [PubMed]
28. Macbeth, G.; Razumiejczyk, E.; Ledesma, R.D. Cliff's Delta Calculator: A non-parametric effect size program for two groups of observations. *Univ. Psychol.* **2011**, *10*, 545–555.
29. Lipsitz, L.A. Physiological Complexity, Aging, and the Path to Frailty. *Sci. Aging Knowl. Environ.* **2004**, *2004*, pe16. [CrossRef] [PubMed]
30. Vaillancourt, D.E.; Newell, K.M. Changing complexity in human behavior and physiology through aging and disease. *Neurobiol. Aging.* **2002**, *23*, 1–11. [CrossRef]
31. Razjouyan, J.; Naik, A.D.; Horstman, M.J.; Kunik, M.E.; Amirmazaheri, M.; Zhou, H.; Sharafkhaneh, A.; Najafi, B. Wearable Sensors and the Assessment of Frailty among Vulnerable Older Adults: An Observational Cohort Study. *Sensors* **2018**, *18*, 1336. [CrossRef] [PubMed]

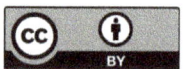

© 2018 by the authors. Licensee MDPI, Basel, Switzerland. This article is an open access article distributed under the terms and conditions of the Creative Commons Attribution (CC BY) license (http://creativecommons.org/licenses/by/4.0/).

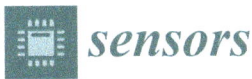

Article

Design of a Wearable 12-Lead Noncontact Electrocardiogram Monitoring System

Chien-Chin Hsu [1,2], Bor-Shing Lin [3], Ke-Yi He [4] and Bor-Shyh Lin [4,*]

1. Department of Emergency Medicine, Chi Mei Medical Center, Tainan 710, Taiwan; nych2525@gmail.com
2. Department of Biotechnology, Southern Taiwan University of Science and Technology, Tainan 71005, Taiwan
3. Department of Computer Science and Information Engineering, National Taipei University, New Taipei 23741, Taiwan; bslin@mail.ntpu.edu.tw
4. Institute of Imaging and Biomedical Photonics, National Chiao Tung University, Tainan 711, Taiwan; nctukeyiho@gmail.com
* Correspondence: borshyhlin@gmail.com; Tel.: +886-6-3032121-57835

Received: 19 February 2019; Accepted: 25 March 2019; Published: 28 March 2019

Abstract: A standard 12-lead electrocardiogram (ECG) is an important tool in the diagnosis of heart diseases. Here, Ag/AgCl electrodes with conductive gels are usually used in a 12-lead ECG system to access biopotentials. However, using Ag/AgCl electrodes with conductive gels might be inconvenient in a prehospital setting. In previous studies, several dry electrodes have been developed to improve this issue. However, these dry electrodes have contact with the skin directly, and they might be still unsuitable for patients with wounds. In this study, a wearable 12-lead electrocardiogram monitoring system was proposed to improve the above issue. Here, novel noncontact electrodes were also designed to access biopotentials without contact with the skin directly. Moreover, by using the mechanical design, this system allows the user to easily wear and take off the device and to adjust the locations of the noncontact electrodes. The experimental results showed that the proposed system could exactly provide a good ECG signal quality even while walking and could detect the ECG features of the patients with myocardial ischemia, installation pacemaker, and ventricular premature contraction.

Keywords: electrocardiogram; conductive gels; noncontact electrode; myocardial ischemia; pacemaker; ventricular premature contraction

1. Introduction

The standard 12-lead electrocardiogram (ECG) is an important tool to assist the diagnosis of myocardial ischemia and arrhythmia. In particular, for the diagnosis of myocardial infarction, 12-lead ECG provides important and meaningful information. The timely treatment of occluded coronary artery is critical to reduce myocardial injury and mortality. In order to save the ischemia myocardium, a 12-lead ECG of the patient must be obtained in emergency or prehospital settings. Myocardial infarction must be identified as early as possible and the patient must be taken to a hospital with a cardiac cath lab. In general, the conventional Ag/AgCl ECG electrodes with conductive gels are used to measure ECG signals. The use of conductive gels can effectively improve the conductivity of the skin electrode interface to acquire a better ECG signal quality [1]. However, the use of conductive gels usually encounters the dying issue of long-time measurement or the dislodgement of electrodes due to wet skin.

In order to improve the above issue of the conventional ECG electrodes, several novel dry electrodes have been proposed in previous studies. Some studies applied the technique of microelectromechanical systems (MEMS) in the development of novel dry electrodes [2]. However, the manufacturing cost and process of these MEMS-based dry electrodes is relatively expensive and complex. Moreover, the measuring method of these MEMS-based dry electrodes are semi-invasive, and this also increases the risk of a skin allergy. Several conductive fabrics, conductive materials, or metals are also used for the development of dry electrodes [3–15]. In 2013, Zhou et al. proposed microstructure-array metal dry electrodes [16]. In 2012, Jung et al. developed carbon nanotube (CNT)/polydimethylsiloxane (PDMS) composite flexible dry electrodes for ECG measurement [17]. The above dry electrodes are also semi-invasive and could provide a good signal quality in a hairless site. In 2011, Lin et al. proposed a novel foam dry electrode [18,19] to acquire biopotentials without conductive gels. However, the abovementioned dry electrodes have to contact the skin directly and may be unsuitable for measuring biopotentials in a hairy site due to the fact that the hair layer might increase the impedance of the skin-electrode interface.

Different from the above dry electrodes which have to contact with the skin directly, the noncontact dry electrode was developed in recent years. In general, the design of dry electrodes has to minimize the impedance of the skin-electrode interface. Different from other skin-electrode models of other dry electrodes, the skin-electrode interface model of a noncontact dry electrode can be viewed as a coupling capacitance. In 2013, Lin et al. successfully applied the technique of noncontact electrode to acquire a lead I ECG signal [20,21]. Based on our experience of the noncontact electrode design, a wearable 12-lead ECG monitoring system with noncontact electrodes was proposed in this study. By using the properties of the noncontact electrode technique, ECG signal can be measured across thin clothes to avoid contacting a wound of the subject. Moreover, by using the wearable mechanical design, the proposed system can be easily worn and taken off, and the locations of noncontact electrodes can be quickly and easily adjusted. Finally, the performance of the proposed noncontact electrode has also be validated and applied in the detection of myocardial ischemia, installation pacemaker, and ventricular premature contraction.

2. Materials and Methods

2.1. Fundamental Theory of Noncontact Electrode

The electrode-skin interface models of conventional Ag/AgCl electrode and noncontact electrode are shown in Figure 1a,b. In general, conductive gel has to be applied in the conventional Ag/AgCl electrode to form a conductive layer between the electrode and skin and to reduce the impedance of the electrode-skin interface. Therefore, the equivalent circuit of the conductive gel layer can be simply viewed as a resistor. The skin layer can be viewed as a plate, and its equivalent circuit can be presented as a resistance and a capacitor in parallel. Therefore, the measurement of a biopotential by using the conventional Ag/AgCl electrode has to pass through these equivalent impedances, such as the skin layer, the conductive gel layer, and the metal electrode.

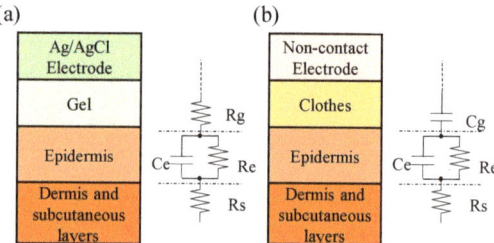

Figure 1. The skin-electrode interface models of (**a**) an Ag–AgCl electrode and (**b**) a noncontact dry electrode.

In the electrode-skin interface model of a noncontact electrode, the skin layer and the metal electrode can be viewed as two parallel plates, and the clothes can be viewed as an isolation layer. Therefore, the electrode-skin interface model of a noncontact electrode can be viewed as a capacitor.

Figure 2a shows the basic scheme of the designed noncontact electrode. Its major parts contain a metal electrode; an impedance converter, which is used to provide an ultrahigh input impedance to reduce the influence of the variation of the skin-electrode interface impedance; and a high-impedance pathway, which is used to reduce the influence of the bias variation of the unit buffer to ensure it works within the active region. Here, the metal electrode was coated with an isolated layer of solder mask. Figure 2b shows the equivalent electrical model of the used noncontact electrodes. Let V_i and V_o denote the ECG signal source of the human body and the output of the noncontact electrode, respectively, C_g denote the coupling capacitance formed by the skin and the metal electrode plate, R_g be the equivalent impedance of the bias pathway, and R_i and C_i denote the equivalent resistance and the equivalent capacitance of the used operational amplifier, respectively. Therefore, the transfer function of the used noncontact electrode can be expressed as followings.

$$\frac{V_o(S)}{V_i(S)} = \frac{R_g // R_i // \frac{1}{SC_i}}{\frac{1}{SC_g} + R_g // R_i // \frac{1}{SC_i}} = \frac{SC_g R_g R_i}{SC_g R_g R_i + SC_i R_g R_i + R_g + R_i} \quad (1)$$

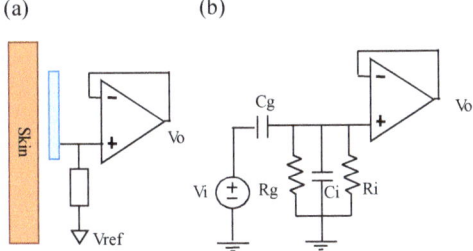

Figure 2. (**a**) A basic scheme and (**b**) the equivalent electrical model of a used noncontact electrode.

From the above formula, it showed that decreasing C_i could provide the larger amplitude response when C_g, R_g, and R_i are large enough. In the design of the noncontact electrode, R_i and C_i are decided by the selection of the used operational amplifier. C_g is a coupling capacitor, formed by the metal plate of the noncontact electrode and the skin. In order to increase the value of C_g, the electrode surface area has to be increased or the distance between the skin and the electrode has to be decreased.

2.2. Measurement of Standard 12-Lead Electrocardiogram

The standard 12-lead ECG system is used to collect 12 different ECG signals from different locations simultaneously to completely estimate the vector of electrocardiogram. The measurement of 12-lead ECG system can be simply classified into three parts, including three bipolar limb leads (LeadI, LeadII, and LeadIII), three unipolar limb leads (aVR, aVL, and aVF), and six unipolar chest leads (V1–V6). The measurement of LeadI–LeadIII uses three electrodes placed on the left arm (LA), the right arm (RA), and the left leg (LL) respectively. These unipolar limb leads can be represented as Equations (2)–(4).

$$aVR = RA - \frac{1}{2}(LA + LL) = -\frac{1}{2}(LeadI + LeadII) \quad (2)$$

$$aVL = LA - \frac{1}{2}(RA + LL) = LeadI - \frac{1}{2}LeadII \quad (3)$$

$$aVF = LL - \frac{1}{2}(RA + LA) = LeadII - \frac{1}{2}LeadI \quad (4)$$

The six unipolar chest leads (V1 to V6) represent the voltage difference between the chest voltage and the average voltages of LA, RA, and LL, and they can be expressed by

$$V_k = \text{Chest}_k - \frac{1}{3}(\text{RA} + \text{LL} + \text{LA}) \tag{5}$$

where V_k and Chest_k denote the *k*th chest leads and the voltage of the *k*th chest electrode, respectively.

3. Design and Implementation of Wearable 12-Lead ECG Monitoring System

The system architecture and photograph of the proposed system is shown in Figure 3, and it mainly contains a wearable mechanical design, a wireless 12-lead ECG acquisition module, and a back-end host system. The wireless 12-lead ECG acquisition module is designed to measure ECG signals and can be embedded into the wearable mechanical design. The wearable mechanical design is designed to be worn easily in daily life and can provide a suitable pressure to avoid the sliding of the wireless 12-lead ECG acquisition module to acquire a good ECG signal quality. Finally, the acquired ECG signal will be transmitted to the back-end host system wirelessly via Bluetooth.

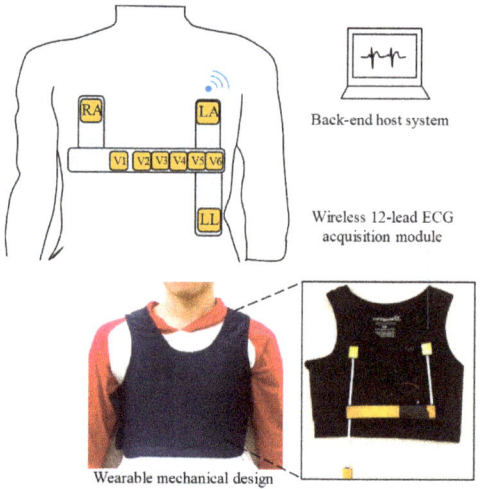

Figure 3. A basic scheme and photograph of the wearable 12-Lead electrocardiogram (ECG) monitoring system.

The block diagram of the wireless 12-lead ECG acquisition module is shown in Figure 4, and it mainly consists of several parts: noncontact dry electrodes, multiplexers, a summing amplifier, a front-end amplifier, a microprocessor, and a wireless transmission circuit. First, the biopotentials would be acquired by these noncontact dry electrodes. In order to measure the six unipolar chest leads, the reference signal, combined from the voltages of RA, LL, and LA, has to be obtained. Here, the summing amplifier is used to obtain the combination of the RA, LL, and LA voltages. According to the definition of the 12-lead ECG system, nine dry electrodes would be switched by two multiplexers and, then, would be inputted into the front-end amplifier to obtain the 12-lead ECG signals. The front-end amplifier contains an instrumentation amplifier (AD620, Analog Devices, Norwood, MA, USA; gain = 20), a band-pass filter (gain = 20, and frequency band = 0.1 Hz–150 Hz), and a notch filter of 60 Hz. Then, the preprocessed ECG signals would be digitized by an analog-to-digital converter built into the microprocessor with the sampling rate of 500 Hz and, then, would be sent to the wireless transmission circuit to transmit to the back-end host system. The wearable mechanical design mainly consists of an elastic chest vest and Velcros. By using these Velcros, the designed wireless 12-lead ECG acquisition module could be easily embedded on the elastic chest vest, and it also allows the adjustment of the positions of the noncontact electrodes to reduce the influence of the individual body size difference.

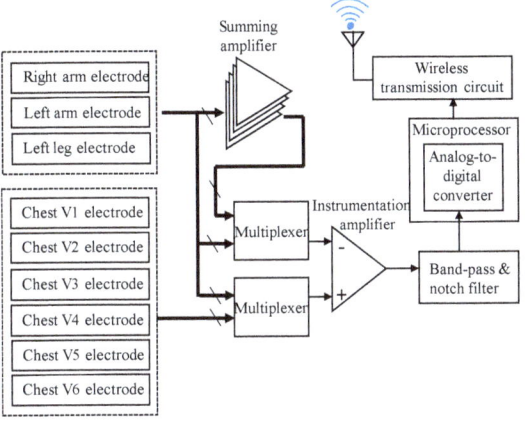

Figure 4. A block diagram of the wearable 12-Lead ECG acquisition module.

In this system, a commercial tablet was used as the platform for the host system, and a 12-lead ECG monitoring program was also designed to continuously monitor the 12-lead ECG signals. This program would first build the graphical user interface to allow the user operating and setting the program parameters. When clicking the start button, it would call the Bluetooth application programming interface (API) to search the wireless 12-lead ECG acquisition module and to make a connection with this module. After connecting with this module, the thread of DataREC would receive the 12-lead ECG signals, store them into the program buffer, real-time display them on the screen, and store the raw data into the local files.

4. Results

4.1. Electrical Specifications of Noncontact Electrodes

In this section, the electrical specifications of the designed noncontact electrodes were first investigated. Figure 5a,b shows the magnitude response and phase response of the designed noncontact electrodes. Here, a function generator was used to generate a 1 voltage p-p sine wave with varying frequency (from 0.1 Hz to 1000 Hz), and it was connected to a copper plate coated with an insulation tape as the input of the noncontact electrode. From the experimental results, the magnitude response of the noncontact electrode at the frequency range between 1 Hz and 1000 Hz is stable and flat, and its phase response is also almost linear. Figure 5c shows the referred noise spectrum of the noncontact electrode. In this test, the input of the noncontact electrode was connected to the ground. It showed that the referred noise spectrum of the noncontact electrode in higher frequency would be slightly decayed, and the whole referred noise is almost below 10^{-5} V/Hz.

Next, the ECG signal quality obtained by the proposed noncontact electrode was compared with that of the conventional ECG electrode with conductive gels. In this experiment, the noncontact electrodes were placed across the chest through a thin T-shirt, and their locations were close to that of these conventional ECG electrodes. Figure 6a–c shows the comparisons between the lead II, aVL, and V6 ECG signals randomly selected from 12-lead ECG signals of different ECG electrodes and their spectra. Here, the ECG machine (PageWriter TC30, Philips, Amsterdam, Netherlands) with Ag/AgCl electrodes in Chi Mei Medical Center, Taiwan was used, and the function of the linear correlation coefficient in the Matlab software was used to estimate the difference between the ECG signal qualities obtained by different ECG electrodes. It showed that the correlation between ECG signals obtained by different electrodes was over 0.95 and that the correlation for the ECG spectra was over 0.99. The ECG signal quality obtained by the proposed noncontact electrodes across a T-shirt was exactly similar to that of the conventional ECG electrodes with conductive gels.

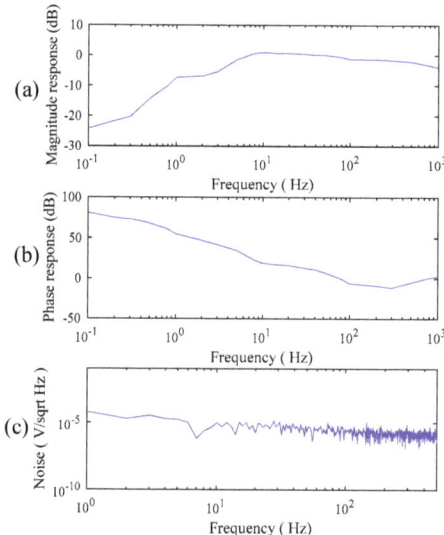

Figure 5. (**a**) The magnitude response, (**b**) phase response, and (**c**) referred noise spectrum of the proposed noncontact electrode.

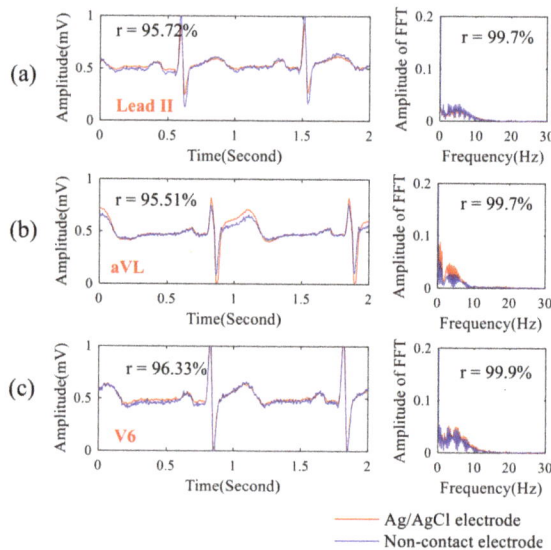

Figure 6. Comparisons between the ECG signals and their spectra obtained by different electrodes: (**a**) lead II, (**b**) aVL, and (**c**) V6.

4.2. ECG Signal Quality of Wearable 12-Lead ECG Monitoring System under Different Conditions

In this section, the influence of motion artifact on the ECG signal quality of the proposed system was first investigated. Figure 7a,b shows the ECG signals obtained by the proposed system while sitting and walking respectively. While walking, the motion artifact of walking causes the slight baseline swinging of the ECG signals, but its signal quality is still similar to that while sitting. Next, the ECG signals of patients in the emergency room were measured by the proposed system. Figure 8a–c shows the ECGs signal obtained from the patients with myocardial ischemia, installation pacemaker, and ventricular premature contraction, respectively. From the experimental results, the ECG features of Lead III T-wave inversion and the V6 ST-wave depression for myocardial ischemia [22] were measured by the proposed system. In Figure 8b, the pulse waves generated by installation pacemaker [23] in the front of each ECG cycle were also measured. For ventricular premature contraction, its ECG features can be reflected on the broadening QRS wave and the lack of P-wave [24], and the ECG signal in Figure 8c could also present these ECG features of ventricular premature contraction. Next, the effect of the cloth material, the effect of the thickness, and the influence of sweating on the ECG signal quality of the proposed system was also investigated. Figure 9a–d shows the ECG signal measured under different cloth conditions, including materials, thicknesses, and humidity. It shows that the amplitude of the ECG signal is slightly attenuated when the cloth thickness increased. In this experiment, the effect of selecting the cloth material on the ECG signal quality was unobvious. Moreover, the effect of sweating could improve the ECG signal quality.

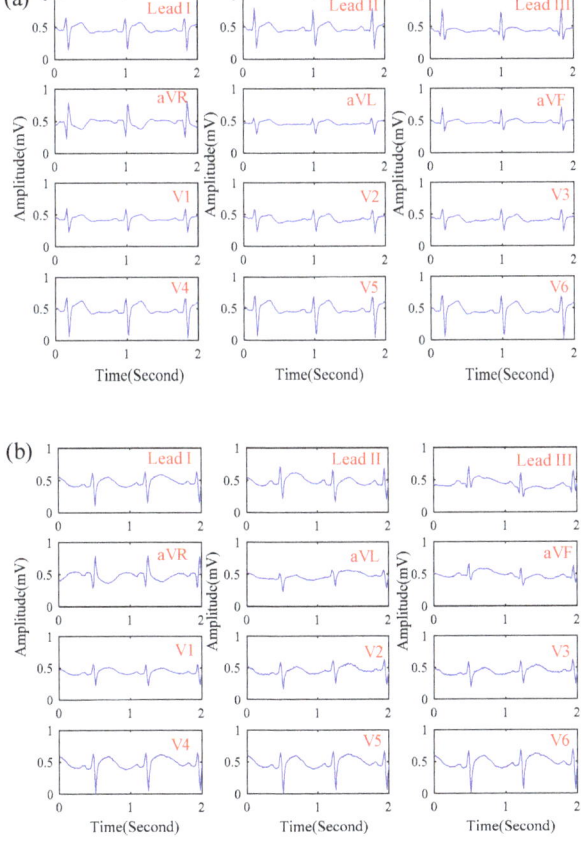

Figure 7. The 12-lead ECG signals obtained by the proposed system when (**a**) sitting and (**b**) walking.

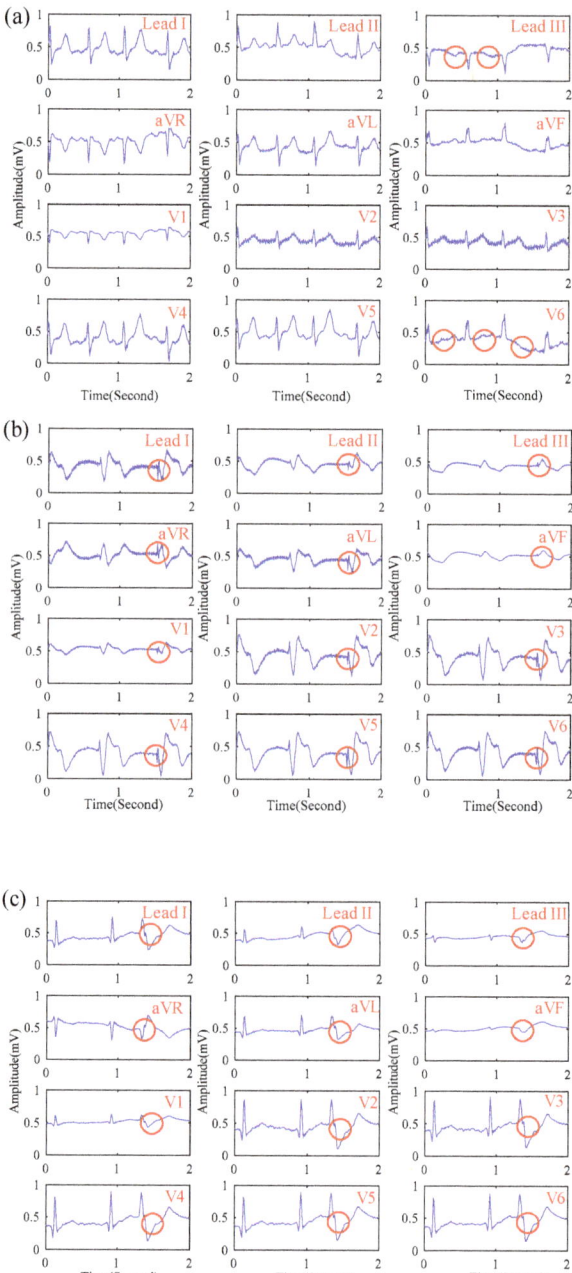

Figure 8. The ECG signal of patients with (**a**) myocardial infarction, (**b**) installation pacemaker, and (**c**) ventricular premature contraction obtained by the proposed system.

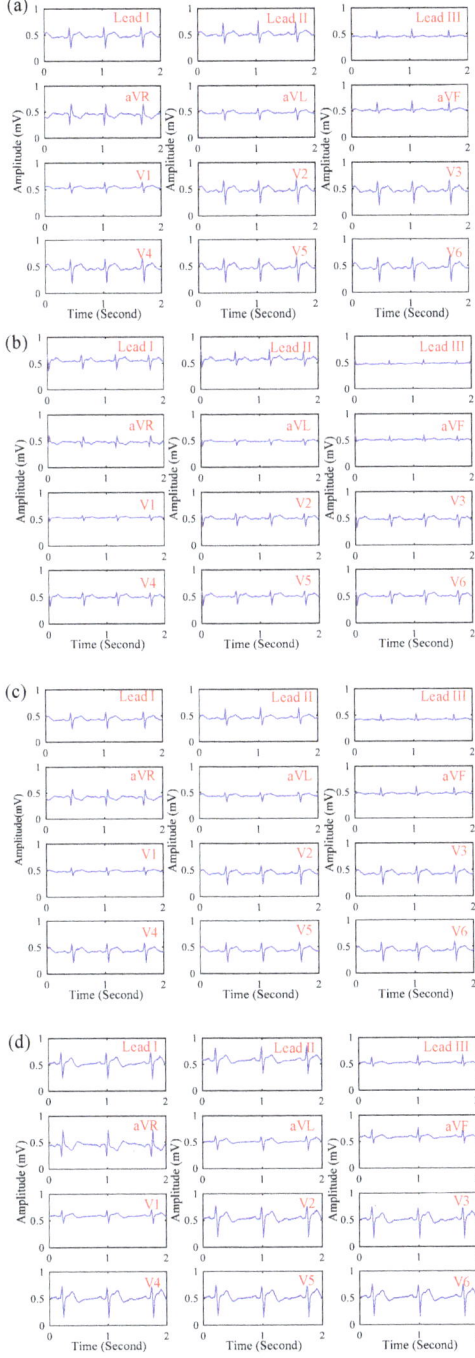

Figure 9. The 12-lead ECG signals obtained by the proposed system under different cloth conditions: (**a**) material: 100% cotton, thickness: 0.8 mm, dry; (**b**) material: 100% cotton, thickness: 1.4 mm, dry; (**c**) material: 80% cotton and 20% polyester, thickness: 0.8 mm, dry; (**d**) material: 100% cotton, thickness: 0.8 mm, sweating.

5. Discussion

In Figure 5a–c, in the frequency range between 0.1 Hz and 1000 Hz, the amplitude response of the proposed noncontact electrode is stable, and its phase response is linear. The whole referred noise of the proposed electrode is less than 10^{-5} V/Hz. From the above electrical specifications, the proposed noncontact electrode is suitable for measuring biopotentials, such as ECG, EEG, etc. In Figure 6a–c, the correlations between the EEG signals and spectra obtained by the proposed noncontact electrode and the conventional electrode with conductive gels are high. The influence of motion artifact on measuring the ECG signal was also investigated. The experimental results showed that the ECG signal quality was also good while walking, due to the fact that the flexibility of the wearable mechanical design might provide a suitable pressure to reduce the shifting of the noncontact electrodes. Moreover, the ECG features of myocardial ischemia, installation pacemaker, and ventricular premature contraction were also measured by the proposed system. Therefore, the reliability and practicability of the proposed system on measuring ECG were good. Moreover, the effect of the cloth condition on the ECG signal quality was also investigated. In Figure 9 a–d, it shows the amplitude of the ECG signal would be attenuated when the cloth thickness increased. Moreover, the effect of sweating could improve the ECG signal quality. This can be explained by the value of C_g in Equation (1) which would increase when the distance between the electrode and skin decreased or the humidity increased, due to the increase in dielectric.

Several dry and noncontact electrodes have been proposed in previous studies, and their specification comparison is summarized in Table 1. In 2013, Zhang et al. proposed a microneedle array (MNA) electrode [25]. The size of this MNA electrode was about 12×12 mm^2. Its substrate and microneedles were made of polydimethylsiloxane (PDMS) and silicon respectively, and finally, the MNA electrode was coated with poly-3,4-ethylenedioxythiophene/polystyrene sulfonate (PEDOT/PPS). This MNA electrode contained the properties of excellent flexibility, good conductivity, and semi-invasive measurement. The MNA electrode could directly penetrate the human stratum corneum to reduce the impedance of the skin-electrode interface and the electrode movement caused from the body friction. However, the manufacturing procedure of the MNA electrode is relatively complex, and its cost is also expensive. Under strenuous exercise, sweating might cause the falling off of the PEDOT/PSS coating, increase the skin-electrode interface impedance, and further affect the signal quality. In 2015, Weder et al. proposed an embroidered electrode [26]. The size of this embroidered electrode was about 70×20 mm^2. Here, polyethylene terephthalate (PET) yarn was used as the electrode substrate, and then, it was coated with silver/titanium (Ag/Ti) to provide a good biocompatibility and good conductivity. However, body hair might easily affect the measurement of this embroidered electrode. In 2011, Liao et al. proposed a spring probe dry electrode [27]. The size of this spring probe dry electrode was about 13×13 mm^2. A 13-mm-diameter copper piece was used as the substrate, and 17 gold-plated spring probes were soldered on the copper piece. The electrode was also coated with silicone. The comb telescopic structure of this electrode allowed it to pass through the hair layer and contact the skin directly. However, the skin-electrode interface impedance might be still higher and affect the signal quality [11]. In 2018, Castro et al. proposed a four-channel contactless capacitively coupled electrocardiography (ccECG) system for the extraction of sleep apnea features [28]. The ccECG system has the advantage of long-term physiological monitoring but the disadvantage of a high variation in the quality of the acquired signals due to its high sensitivity to motion artefacts. This system was only used in sleep apnea; it was not verified and did not guarantee a good performance of the ECG measurement under motion. Different from the above dry and noncontact electrodes, the proposed noncontact electrode could access biopotentials across the clothes without contacting the skin directly. Moreover, a flexible printed circuit board (PCB) was used as the substrate of the proposed electrode. The proposed electrode could easily be embedded into the clothes, and its flexibility could fit the body contour to provide a stable and good signal quality even under motion.

Table 1. The specification comparisons between different dry and noncontact electrodes and the proposed noncontact electrode.

	Zhang et al. [25]	Weder et al. [26]	Liao et al. [27]	Castro et al. [28]	Proposed Electrode
Area of electrode (cm^2)	1.44	14	1.69	-	6.16
Frequency band (Hz)	0.5–50	-	-	0.5–40	0.1–100
Input-referred noise (V/Hz)	-	-	-	-	6×10^{-5}
Electrode material	PEDOT/PSS	Ag/Ti	Gold, copper	Ag/AgCl	Copper
Noncontact electrode	No	No	No	Noncontact	Noncontact
Advantages	Excellent flexibility and conductivity, measurement under motion	Good biocompatibility and conductivity	Measurement in hairy site	Good measurement under slight motion (e.g., sleep)	Excellent flexibility, noncontact measurement under motion
Affecting factors	Influence of sweating	Influence of body hairs	Poor skin-electrode interface impedance	Not verified and guaranteed under motion	Thickness of clothing

In previous studies, several wearable 12-lead ECG systems have also been designed, and a comparison between the proposed system and other systems is listed in Table 2. In 2016, Boehm et al. proposed a 12-lead ECG T-Shirt [29], and its system size was about 70 × 65 mm^2. Ten active electrodes were embedded in a T-Shirt to greatly improve the convenience of use. However, it might be difficult to fit the body closely to affect the signal quality under motion. In 2015, Yasunori Tada et al. proposed a 12-lead ECG smart shirt [30], and its system size was about 90 × 28 mm^2. The system contained 10 dry foam electrodes, and conductive ink lines were also used as the ECG leads. The flexibility of the compressed shirt could help these foam electrodes contact the skin well to provide a good ECG signal quality, even under motion. However, these foam electrodes still have to contact the skin directly to acquire a biopotential, and body hairs might affect their measuring performance. In this study, the size of the proposed system was about 25 × 65 mm^2, and it contains 9 noncontact electrodes. Different from the above 12-lead ECG system, the flexible PCB was used as the substrate of the proposed noncontact electrodes and a wearable mechanical design was also designed to closely fit the body and provide a suitable pressure to reduce transversal motion and lateral motion. Thus, the proposed system could provide a good ECG signal quality under motion. Moreover, different from other wearable ECG monitoring systems, the proposed systems could access biopotentials across the clothes without contacting with the skin directly.

Table 2. The specification comparisons between the proposed 12-Lead ECG monitoring system and other systems.

	Anna Boehm et al. [29]	Yasunori Tada et al. [30]	Proposed System
Operation voltage	3.3 V	-	3.3 V
Amplifier gain	-	-	400 V/V
System of size	70 × 65 mm^2	90 × 28 mm^2	25 × 65 mm^2
Signal resolution	24 bits	-	12 bits
Frequency band (Hz)	2–20 Hz	-	0.1–100 Hz
Wireless transmission	-	XBee	Bluetooth
Power consumption	260 mW	-	150 mW
Advantages	Wearability, long-term monitoring	Wearability, measurement under motion	Wearability, noncontact measurement under motion
Affecting factors	Influence of motion	Influence of body hairs	Thickness of clothing

6. Conclusions

In this study, a wearable 12-lead noncontact electrocardiogram monitoring system was proposed and successfully applied in measuring the ECG signals of patients with myocardial ischemia and arrhythmia. From the experimental results, the magnitude and phase responses of the designed noncontact electrodes were suitable for measuring ECG signal, and its referred noise was less than 10^{-5} V/Hz. The proposed system could provide a good signal quality even while walking. Moreover, the ECG features of myocardial ischemia, installation pacemaker, and ventricular premature contraction could be measured by the proposed system. The properties of the noncontact electrode technique can effectively avoid contacting the wound of the subject. Moreover, the positions of the noncontact electrodes can be easily adjusted to reduce the influence of the individual body size difference. Therefore, the proposed system might be usefully applied in the applications of mobile ECG monitoring in the future.

Author Contributions: B.-S.L. (Bor-Shyh Lin) and B.-S.L. (Bor-Shing Lin) conceived the study idea, designed the framework and system architecture in this study, and modified the manuscript. K.-Y.H. implemented the system, collected data, analyzed the collected data, and wrote the draft. C.-C.H. provided conceptual advice, the design of the wearable device, and the domain knowledge of cardiology.

Funding: This research was partly supported by the Ministry of Science and Technology in Taiwan, under grants MOST 107-2221-E-009-017 and MOST 107-2221-E-305-014. This research was also partly supported by the University System of Taipei Joint Research Program, under grant USTP-NTPU-TMU-107-02, and by the Faculty Group Research Funding Sponsorship by National Taipei University, under grant 2018-NTPU-ORDA-04. This work was also supported by the Higher Education Sprout Project of the National Chiao Tung University and Ministry of Education (MOE), Taiwan.

Conflicts of Interest: The authors declare no conflict of interest.

References

1. Searle, A.; Kirkup, L. A direct comparison of wet, dry and insulating bioelectric recording electrodes. *Physiol. Meas.* **2000**, *21*, 271–283. [CrossRef]
2. Griss, P.; Enoksson, P.; Tolvanen-Laakso, H.K.; Merilainen, P.; Ollmar, S.; Stemme, G. Micromachined electrodes for biopotential measurements. *J. Microelectromech. Syst.* **2001**, *10*, 10–16. [CrossRef]
3. Oh, T.I.; Yoon, S.; Kim, T.E.; Wi, H.; Kim, K.J.; Woo, E.J.; Sadleir, R.J. Nanofiber web textile dry electrodes for long-term biopotential recording. *IEEE Trans. Biomed. Circuits Syst.* **2013**, *7*, 204–211. [PubMed]
4. Taji, B.; Shirmohammadi, S.; Groza, V.; Batkin, I. Impact of skin–electrode interface on electrocardiogram measurements using conductive textile electrodes. *IEEE Trans. Instrum. Meas.* **2014**, *63*, 1412–1422. [CrossRef]
5. Yokus, M.A.; Jur, J.S. Fabric-based wearable dry electrodes for body surface biopotential recording. *IEEE Trans. Biomed. Eng.* **2016**, *63*, 423–430. [CrossRef]
6. Abu-Saude, M.J.; Morshed, B.I. Patterned Vertical Carbon Nanotube Dry Electrodes for Impedimetric Sensing and Stimulation. *IEEE Sensors J.* **2015**, *15*, 5851–5858. [CrossRef]
7. Wang, L.-F.; Liu, J.-Q.; Yang, B.; Yang, C.-S. PDMS-based low cost flexible dry electrode for long-term EEG measurement. *IEEE Sensors J.* **2012**, *12*, 2898–2904. [CrossRef]
8. Chen, Y.; Atnafu, A.D.; Schlattner, I.; Weldtsadik, W.T.; Roh, M.-C.; Kim, H.J.; Lee, S.-W.; Blankertz, B.; Fazli, S. A high-security EEG-based login system with RSVP stimuli and dry electrodes. *IEEE Trans. Inf. Forensics Secur.* **2016**, *11*, 2635–2647. [CrossRef]
9. Ueno, A.; Akabane, Y.; Kato, T.; Hoshino, H.; Kataoka, S.; Ishiyama, Y. Capacitive sensing of electrocardiographic potential through cloth from the dorsal surface of the body in a supine position: A preliminary study. *IEEE Trans. Biomed. Eng.* **2007**, *54*, 759–766. [CrossRef]
10. Pei, W.; Zhang, H.; Wang, Y.; Guo, X.; Xing, X.; Huang, Y.; Xie, Y.; Yang, X.; Chen, H. Skin-potential variation insensitive dry electrodes for ECG recording. *IEEE Trans. Biomed. Eng.* **2017**, *64*, 463–470. [CrossRef]
11. Huang, Y.-J.; Wu, C.-Y.; Wong, A.M.-K.; Lin, B.-S. Novel active comb-shaped dry electrode for EEG measurement in hairy site. *IEEE Trans. Biomed. Eng.* **2015**, *62*, 256–263. [CrossRef] [PubMed]
12. Laferriere, P.; Lemaire, E.D.; Chan, A.D. Surface electromyographic signals using dry electrodes. *IEEE Trans. Instrum. Meas.* **2011**, *60*, 3259–3268. [CrossRef]

13. Ribeiro, D.M.D.; Fu, L.S.; Carlos, L.A.D.; Cunha, J.P.S. A novel dry active biosignal electrode based on an hybrid organic-inorganic interface material. *IEEE Sensors J.* **2011**, *11*, 2241–2245. [CrossRef]
14. Chi, Y.M.; Jung, T.-P.; Cauwenberghs, G. Dry-contact and noncontact biopotential electrodes: Methodological review. *IEEE Rev. Biomed. Eng.* **2010**, *3*, 106–119. [CrossRef]
15. Yang, B.; Yu, C.; Dong, Y. Capacitively coupled electrocardiogram measuring system and noise reduction by singular spectrum analysis. *IEEE Sensors J.* **2016**, *16*, 3802–3810. [CrossRef]
16. Zhou, W.; Song, R.; Pan, X.; Peng, Y.; Qi, X.; Peng, J.; Hui, K.; Hui, K. Fabrication and impedance measurement of novel metal dry bioelectrode. *Sens. Actuators A Phys.* **2013**, *201*, 127–133. [CrossRef]
17. Jung, H.-C.; Moon, J.-H.; Baek, D.-H.; Lee, J.-H.; Choi, Y.-Y.; Hong, J.-S.; Lee, S.-H. CNT/PDMS composite flexible dry electrodesfor long-term ECG monitoring. *IEEE Trans. Biomed. Eng.* **2012**, *59*, 1472–1479. [CrossRef]
18. Lin, C.-T.; Liao, L.-D.; Liu, Y.-H.; Wang, I.-J.; Lin, B.-S.; Chang, J.-Y. Novel dry polymer foam electrodes for long-term EEG measurement. *IEEE Trans. Biomed. Eng.* **2011**, *58*, 1200–1207.
19. Tseng, K.C.; Lin, B.-S.; Liao, L.-D.; Wang, Y.-T.; Wang, Y.-L. Development of a wearable mobile electrocardiogram monitoring system by using novel dry foam electrodes. *IEEE Syst. J.* **2014**, *8*, 900–906. [CrossRef]
20. Lin, B.-S.; Chou, W.; Wang, H.-Y.; Huang, Y.-J.; Pan, J.-S. Development of novel non-contact electrodes for mobile electrocardiogram monitoring system. *IEEE J. Transl. Eng. Health Med.* **2013**, *1*. [CrossRef]
21. Chen, Y.-C.; Lin, B.-S.; Pan, J.-S. Novel noncontact dry electrode with adaptive mechanical design for measuring EEG in a hairy site. *IEEE Trans. Instrum. Meas.* **2015**, *64*, 3361–3368. [CrossRef]
22. De Winter, R.J.; Tijssen, J.G. Non–ST-Segment Elevation Myocardial Infarction. *JACC Cardiovasc. Interv.* **2012**, *5*, 903–905. [CrossRef] [PubMed]
23. Murray, A.; Jordan, R.S.; Gold, R.G. Pacemaker assessment in the ambulant patient. *Heart* **1981**, *46*, 531–538. [CrossRef]
24. Talbi, M.L.; Charef, A. PVC discrimination using the QRS power spectrum and self-organizing maps. Comput. *Methods Programs. Biomed.* **2009**, *94*, 223–231. [CrossRef] [PubMed]
25. Zhang, H.; Pei, W.; Chen, Y.; Guo, X.; Wu, X.; Yang, X.; Chen, H. A motion interference-insensitive flexible dry electrode. *IEEE Trans. Biomed. Eng.* **2016**, *63*, 1136–1144. [CrossRef] [PubMed]
26. Weder, M.; Hegemann, D.; Amberg, M.; Hess, M.; Boesel, L.F.; Abächerli, R.; Meyer, V.R.; Rossi, R.M. Embroidered electrode with silver/titanium coating for long-term ECG monitoring. *Sensors* **2015**, *15*, 1750–1759. [CrossRef]
27. Liao, L.-D.; Wang, I.-J.; Chen, S.-F.; Chang, J.-Y.; Lin, C.-T. Design, fabrication and experimental validation of a novel dry-contact sensor for measuring electroencephalography signals without skin preparation. *Sensors* **2011**, *11*, 5819–5834. [CrossRef]
28. Castro, I.D.; Varon, C.; Torfs, T.; Huffel, S.V.; Puers, R.; Hoof, C.V. Evaluation of a multichannel non-contact ECG system and signal quality algorithms for sleep apnea detection and monitoring. *Sensors* **2018**, *18*, 577. [CrossRef]
29. Boehm, A.; Yu, X.; Neu, W.; Leonhardt, S.; Teichmann, D. A novel 12-lead ECG T-shirt with active electrodes. *Electronics* **2016**, *5*, 75. [CrossRef]
30. Tada, Y.; Amano, Y.; Sato, T.; Saito, S.; Inoue, M. A smart shirt made with conductive ink and conductive foam for the measurement of electrocardiogram signals with unipolar precordial leads. *Fibers* **2015**, *3*, 463–477. [CrossRef]

© 2019 by the authors. Licensee MDPI, Basel, Switzerland. This article is an open access article distributed under the terms and conditions of the Creative Commons Attribution (CC BY) license (http://creativecommons.org/licenses/by/4.0/).

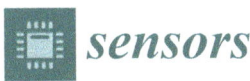

Article

Comparing Clothing-Mounted Sensors with Wearable Sensors for Movement Analysis and Activity Classification

Udeni Jayasinghe *,†, William S. Harwin † and Faustina Hwang †

Biomedical Engineering, School of Biological Sciences, University of Reading, Reading RG6 6AY, UK; w.s.harwin@reading.ac.uk (W.S.H.); f.hwang@reading.ac.uk (F.H.)
* Correspondence:u.kankanipathirage@pgr.reading.ac.uk
† These authors contributed equally to this work.

Received: 15 November 2019; Accepted: 18 December 2019; Published: 21 December 2019

Abstract: Inertial sensors are a useful instrument for long term monitoring in healthcare. In many cases, inertial sensor devices can be worn as an accessory or integrated into smart textiles. In some situations, it may be beneficial to have data from multiple inertial sensors, rather than relying on a single worn sensor, since this may increase the accuracy of the analysis and better tolerate sensor errors. Integrating multiple sensors into clothing improves the feasibility and practicality of wearing multiple devices every day, in approximately the same location, with less likelihood of incorrect sensor orientation. To facilitate this, the current work investigates the consequences of attaching lightweight sensors to loose clothes. The intention of this paper is to discuss how data from these clothing sensors compare with similarly placed body worn sensors, with additional consideration of the resulting effects on activity recognition. This study compares the similarity between the two signals (body worn and clothing), collected from three different clothing types (slacks, pencil skirt and loose frock), across multiple daily activities (walking, running, sitting, and riding a bus) by calculating correlation coefficients for each sensor pair. Even though the two data streams are clearly different from each other, the results indicate that there is good potential of achieving high classification accuracy when using inertial sensors in clothing.

Keywords: actigraph; body worn sensors; clothing sensors; cross correlation analysis; healthcare movement sensing; wearable devices

1. Introduction

In many countries, a significant increase can be seen in the number and proportion of older adults year on year. The population of people over 60 years old is projected to increase in Europe, Northern and Latin America, Asia and Africa from the year 2015 to 2030 [1]. The number of people who have noncommunicable diseases is also projected to increase significantly by 2030 [2]. Generally older people are more prone to noncommunicable diseases [2] resulting in high care costs in each country. In OECD (Organisation for Economic Co-operation and Development) countries, an annual increment of 4.8% of the cost allocated for long-term monitoring from 2005 to 2011 was seen. It is predicted that this cost will double in the period from 2015 to 2060 [3].

Home-based monitoring potentially offers a cost-effective mechanism for prevention of disease and promotion of healthier lifestyles. A number of factors have to be taken into account when using a long-term monitoring system, such as whether these systems are reliable for measuring real time data, are safe to use with patients, have high power efficiency, and provide clinically useful data. Wearable sensors have the capability to provide efficient monitoring of daily routines for a long period in a cost effective way [4].

A growing interest in health monitoring has led to the commercial availability of a number of wearable sensors for self-monitoring. Consumer products for self-monitoring generally comprise a single device, often wrist worn, which may hinder the accuracy of the data analysis and classification. In contrast, in research work, multiple sensor devices are often used in order to achieve a higher accuracy in activity classification. However, there are feasibility issues with the wearing of multiple sensors on a daily basis in a residential environment. There are also challenges in maintaining a consistent sensor orientation and approximate location with respect to the body during the data collection periods. Further, in healthcare the patient or research participant may not have the patience, or abilities to attach multiple sensors each day. Embedding sensors into the clothing may, to some extent, address both issues of wearing multiple sensors every day and managing the sensor orientation and approximate location.

This study considers the quality of data that would arise from inertial sensors embedded into clothes that people wear on a daily basis.

It examines whether these sensor devices would be able to provide data as accurate as that collected by sensors attached to the person. In particular, can the data be used to predict the actions and behaviour of the individual and allow activity classification?

The aim of this research is to investigate and quantify to what extent the data obtained from the clothing sensors can be used in characterising activities, as compared with body worn sensor data. To achieve this, sensor data were collected from body worn sensors and sensors attached to three different clothing types, across a range of daily activities. The correlation coefficients were calculated between the clothing-embedded and worn data to check how much they agree with each other across a range of daily activities and different styles of clothes.

2. Related Work

Research relating to the use of wearable sensors with older adults has largely been in three areas – indoor tracking, activity classification and real-time vital sign monitoring [5]. Activity classification using body worn inertial sensor data in long-term monitoring is a well-established approach [6]. Accelerometers are being used as the key instrument, while gyroscopes and barometric pressure sensors are also used in some studies. Out of those studies some are using a single sensor while others are using multiple sensors for activity recognition. For example, a single sensor, i.e., a sensor only on the waist, thigh, lower-back and thigh, in activity classification of the whole body can be seen respectively in [7–10]. Other studies, using multiple sensors, investigate the accuracy of activity classification compared across placement of the sensors on the wrist, hip, neck, knee, chest, lower arm, lower back, upper arm and ankle. Montoye et al. [11] observed high accuracy in activity classification for three levels of physical activities, i.e., SB (sedentary behaviour), LPA (light-intensity physical activity) and MVPA (moderate-to-vigorous-intensity physical activity) based on thigh data, high accuracy in classifying SB based on (non-dominant) wrist data, and low accuracy in classifying physical activities based on (dominant) wrist and hip data. Hence, they concluded that it is better to use thigh data or non-dominant wrist data in analysing different levels of physical activities. Cleland et al. [12] found that, of chest, wrist, lower back, hip, thigh and foot sensor data, hip data scored the highest accuracy in activity classification. However, they [12] also noted that further studies should be carried out in order to find the optimal sensor placement across multiple activities, since their study focused only on activities such as walking, lying and sitting. As both upper body and lower body movements contribute to locomotion [13], it is better to investigate movements from both sides of the body, rather than just one side.

Analysis of above mentioned sensor data related to activities may seek to find patterns of activities or movement quality. In most of the studies, pattern recognition algorithms were used in activity classification, such as decision trees ([10,14,15]), KNN (k-nearest neighbours algorithm) ([15–17]), SVM (Support Vector Machine) ([9,18,19]) and other algorithms (C4.5, RF (Random Forest), NB (Naive Bayes), Bayesian).

Even though there are numerous research studies on activity classification with sensor data, very few have been conducted on sensors attached to everyday clothes. One study highlighted that there was little to no research validating the measurements of IMUs (Inertial Measurement Unit) attached to loose clothes [20]. Their research aimed to validate the temporal motion from the sensors attached to the clothes. As the clothes, a tight fitting vest and a tight jacket were used. Their main intention was to validate the sensor readings by calculating four parameters, i.e., raw error, standardised error (Cohen scale), Pearson's correlation and mean difference. Five inertial sensor devices (weighing 23 g, with dimensions 55 mm × 30 mm × 13 mm) were used, where two were strapped onto the Cervical vertebrae segment(C7) and Thoracic vertebrae segment (T12), one was placed on a jacket at C7, and the other two sensors were sewn into two pockets of a tight fitting elastic heart rate monitor vest so that they were posterior to the C7 and T12 sensors. The study focused on only one activity, that is, dead-lifting. When comparing the raw error, Cohen scale, correlation and mean difference of the data sets, only the anterior-posterior acceleration was used. They were able to see a high similarity between the sensor values that were obtained from both mechanisms, owing to the single activity that they conducted with the tight clothes.

A second research study reported that sensors mounted onto clothes, instead of strapping them onto a structure with rigid bands, gives a better signal variation so that it may make the activity recognition procedure easier [21]. For their data collection, a pendulum and three different fabric materials (denim, jersey and roma) and three tri-axial accelerometers were used. The fabric was attached to the end of the pendulum and three accelerometers attached such that one was at the tip of the pendulum (fixed in place with a rigid band), a second one was in the middle of the fabric, and a third was at the edge of the fabric. After attaching the calibrated sensors, the pendulum was released from a horizontal position and data was collected for 10 seconds. The experiment was done with and without an additional weight at the end of the pendulum. The Euclidean distance and one-way analysis of variance were calculated when calculating the similarity of the signals (data from sensors attached with rigid bands as compared with sensors attached to different fabric materials). The objective was to predict whether the pendulum was swinging with or without a weight attached to the end. For this prediction, SVM and DRM (Discriminative Regression Machines) were used. The conclusion of their research work was that the fabric's nature of deforming movements in various directions makes it easier to predict the motion, compared with the sensor data obtained from the sensors attached with the rigid bands.

Hence it can be concluded that more information is needed to assess the true value of embedding sensors into clothing to allow better representation of human movement and activity classification.

3. Materials and Methodology

The aim of the present study is to compare and contrast how clothing sensor data patterns correlate/deviate from body worn sensor data, across three different types of clothing.

3.1. Data Collection Procedure

Data were collected from one participant (the first author) over three normal working days. On each day, the participant wore a different type of clothing (loose slacks, pencil skirt, and frock/knee-length dress), and multiple sensors were worn in pairs on the clothing and the body. The sensors and their placement are described further in the next section. An activity log was kept and used to annotate the data files. The main activities were walking, running, sitting as well as other daily activities including riding on a bus.

3.2. Sensor Placement

Actigraph tri-axial accelerometers (wGT3X-BT, weighing 19 g and measuring 4.6 cm × 3.3 cm × 1.5 cm, as shown in Figure 1) were worn in pairs, such that one sensor was strapped onto the body and the other was sewn to the clothes in a similar location to the body-worn sensor. As the optimal places to mount sensors are not yet well defined [12], we mounted one sensor pair on the waist to track upper body movements, and two other sensor pairs on the upper thigh and ankle to track lower body movements [13]. Hence, sensor pairs were placed at the participant's waist and upper-thigh for the pencil skirt (41 cm long, with a 38 cm inch perimeter at the thigh) and the frock (48 cm inch perimeter at the thigh). For loose slacks, a further pair of sensors was worn on the ankle and hem of the slacks. The body worn sensors were always placed just below the sensors on the clothes, as shown in Figure 2. The participant was 152 cm in height, and wore UK women's size 6 clothes. The orientation of the sensors was set such that the *y*-axis was aligned most closely to the axis of acceleration from gravity. Table 1 shows the duration of data collection, type of clothing and sensor placement.

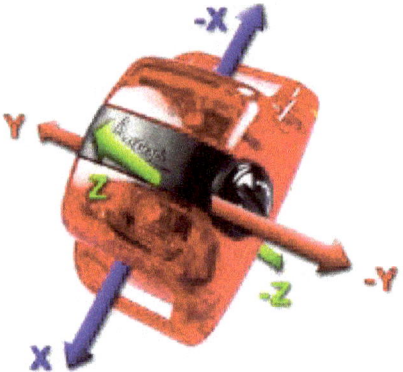

Figure 1. Coordinate frame of the Actigraph device. (Image from Actigraph website https://www.actigraphcorp.com).

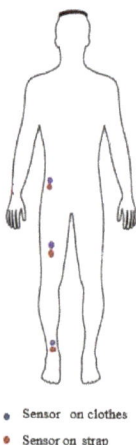

Figure 2. Sensor placement on subject and on subject's clothes.

The sensor devices were initialised with the Actilife (https://www.actigraphcorp.com/support/software/actilife/) software to synchronise their internal clocks. Additionally, at the start of each day of data collection, the participant performed a jump in order to create a distinctive marker in the accelerometry data that could be used to further check the synchronisation. Furthermore, each pair of sensors (one in clothes and one on the body) were tapped synchronously four times to ensure data from sensor pairs could be time-aligned. At the end of each data collection period, another jump was performed to identify the point where the data collection was completed, and provide an indication of any potential sensor time drift.

Table 1. Sensor placement over three days and three types of clothing.

		Day 1	Day 2	Day 3
	Clothes	Loose slacks	Pencil skirt	Frock (knee-length dress)
	Duration	5 hours	3 hours	3 hours
	Frequency	50 Hz	50 Hz	50 Hz
Sensor placement	on Body	Waist	Waist	Waist
		Right thigh	Right thigh	Right thigh
		Right ankle	n/a	n/a
	on Clothes	Waist band of slacks	Waist band of skirt	Waist band of frock
		On seam of slacks near thigh	On seam of skirt near thigh	On seam of frock near thigh
		Hem of slacks near ankle	n/a	n/a

3.3. Data Analysis

The data were analysed in terms of sensor pairs, in order to compare the body worn with the clothing worn data. Comparisons were also made across different activities and the different clothing types. The data were analysed in MATLAB.

3.3.1. Preprocessing the Data

The data from both sensors in a pair were first time-aligned, based on the "jump" and the "tap" markers. Next, the time lag between the two sets of sensor readings for each activity was estimated using a cross correlation, because there can be time lags between the body-worn and the clothing-mounted sensor readings owing to factors such as the stiffness of clothing material (which causes swing) and cloth dynamics for each activity. The maximum cross correlation value was then used to determine the lag between the two signals, and this lag was adjusted in order to bring the two signals into alignment.

Secondly, an orientation correction was applied to both sets of data. When attaching the sensors onto the body and to the clothes, there may be discrepancies in the orientations between the two sensors in a pair. Hence in order to maintain a reasonably similar orientation for each sensor pair, each data set was rotated along a common axis so as to align the principal direction of gravity with the y-axis of the sensor. This correction can be computed easily using Rodrigues' rotation formula [22] and identifying the axis of rotation as being perpendicular to both the gravity vector and the y-axis, and the rotation about this axis is therefore the angle between these two vectors. Data where this rotational correction has been applied is termed the 'rotated data set'.

These preprocessing techniques were carried out in order that the data from the two sensors in each pair could be meaningfully compared.

3.3.2. Activity Extraction

Using the activity log, data segments corresponding to four activities (walking, running, sitting, bus ride) were extracted for each day/clothing type. From these segments, three shorter instances (30–40 s/1500–2000 data points) of each activity were identified and extracted for further analysis.

3.3.3. Comparing the Similarity of the Body-Worn and Clothing-Mounted Sensors

After establishing the normality of the data [23], Pearson's correlation coefficient was calculated for each sensor pair to assess the strength of the linear relationship between the two signals [24].

3.3.4. Activity Classification

We also wished to investigate the possibility of using the clothing sensor data in activity classification as productively as the body worn sensors. For this purpose, the data were categorised into four classes: walking/running, transition of a movement, sitting and standing. The analysis examined only the 'thigh' sensor data. When a subject is sitting, the thigh is often in a perpendicular posture with respect to the standing posture, hence sitting and standing would be more easily distinguished with thigh sensor orientation data as compared with waist or ankle sensor data.

Furthermore, the y-axis accelerations (gravity axis) were used for the classification, because this axis exhibited the most noticeable differences across activities in acceleration values. When a subject is standing, the gravity axis acceleration is (following alignment) close to the y-axis value. When the subject is sitting, the y-axis is now perpendicular to the gravity vector so values are close to zero. When the subject is moving, the y-axis values are changing significantly based on the additional accelerations that result from these movements.

The features used for classification were chosen to emphasise information about posture and movement, including movement transitions. Transitions include sit-to-stand/stand-to-sit activities which would cause the y-axis acceleration to increase/decrease suddenly, sit-to-walk/run could again increase the acceleration suddenly, and walk/run-to-stand would cause a sudden reduction of the acceleration. Two features were used in this classification. To track postural changes, the y-axis acceleration values were used, while the moving variance of the y-axis acceleration values was calculated to track these transitions. A window size of 250 milliseconds was chosen to ensure that even the acceleration changes in short periods were captured.

A decision tree was implemented to classify the data into activities by defining threshold values, based on visual inspection, for the y-axis (gravity) acceleration and the y-axis moving variance values. Threshold values were estimated for both body-worn and clothing-mounted sensor data.

Both body worn and clothing data files were then classified into activities by using the decision tree. Finally, a confusion matrix was created to observe how the classification outputs differed from body worn data and clothing sensor data, by considering the classifications of body worn sensor data as the benchmark data set.

4. Results

4.1. Activity-Wise Time-Alignment

Figure 3 illustrates the cross correlation values plotted over time for one of the running data segments. The point at which the cross correlation reaches a maximum value indicates the lag between the two signals. The graph shows Day 3 (Frock) running data from the thigh sensor, and for this specific activity, the lag was 38 data points (approximately 0.76 s delay).

After adjusting for the delay based on the cross correlation maximum value, the time-aligned signals are as shown in the right-hand plots in Figure 3, with a maximum cross-correlation now appearing at 0 s, indicating that the delay between the two signals was minimised after applying this technique. When the correlation coefficient is calculated without considering this time lag, for this running instance, the value was 0.4136 and after the lag was corrected the correlation coefficient value was 0.6345. Likewise, the time lag between body worn and clothing worn data set for each activity segment was calculated and corrected before examining the correlation coefficient values for each activity.

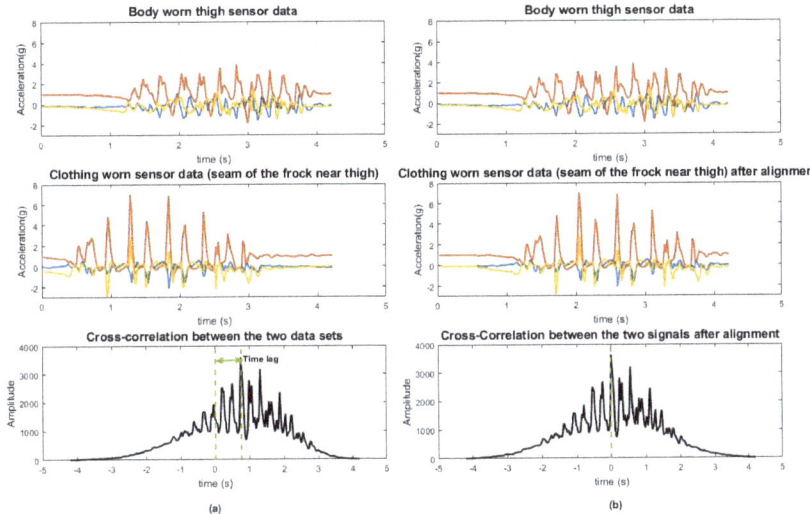

Figure 3. (**a**): Left side 3 plots: Tracked time lag between body worn and clothing sensor data for running when the subject was wearing a frock, (**b**) Right side 3 plots: Signals after the alignment using cross-correlation value. (**b**) After alignment, maximum cross correlation was observed at 0 s.

4.2. Descriptive Analysis of Acceleration Data

Figure 4 illustrates walking data extracted from thigh and ankle sensor pairs when the subject was wearing slacks. The sensors were on the right leg, thus two peaks can be interpreted as a single stride (2 steps) as indicated. According to the data it was calculated that typical stride (two steps) time here was approximately 0.7 s.

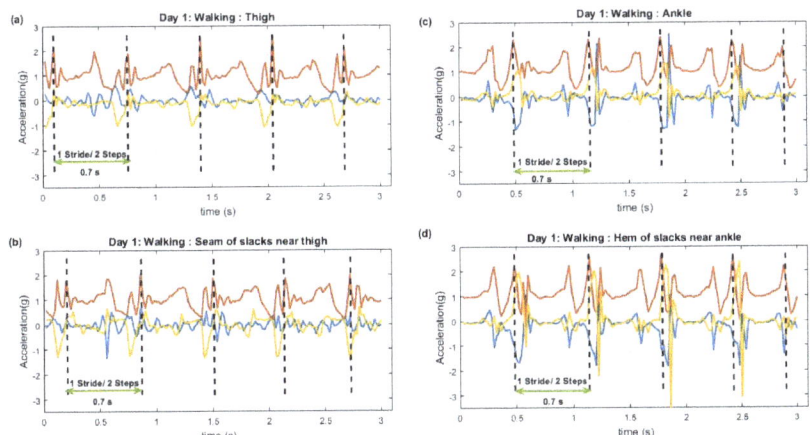

Figure 4. Walking from Day 1 (slacks). (**a**): Data from thigh worn sensor, (**b**): Data from seams of slacks near thigh, (**c**): Data from ankle worn sensor, (**d**): Data from hem of slacks near ankle. Red axis: vertical acceleration, Blue axis: anterior-posterior acceleration, yellow axis: mediolateral acceleration. Note the similarity of signals between clothing and body worn sensors for walking

Figure 5 shows running data from the sensor pairs that were on (and over) the thigh when the subject was wearing a pencil skirt (left graphs) and frock (right graphs) respectively. According to these data it can be seen that typical stride time (two steps) for running was approximately 0.3 s. Even though the acceleration values of pencil skirt data have relatively similar values with body worn sensor data, the frock data in contrast comprise higher acceleration values with sharp peaks when compared to body worn data.

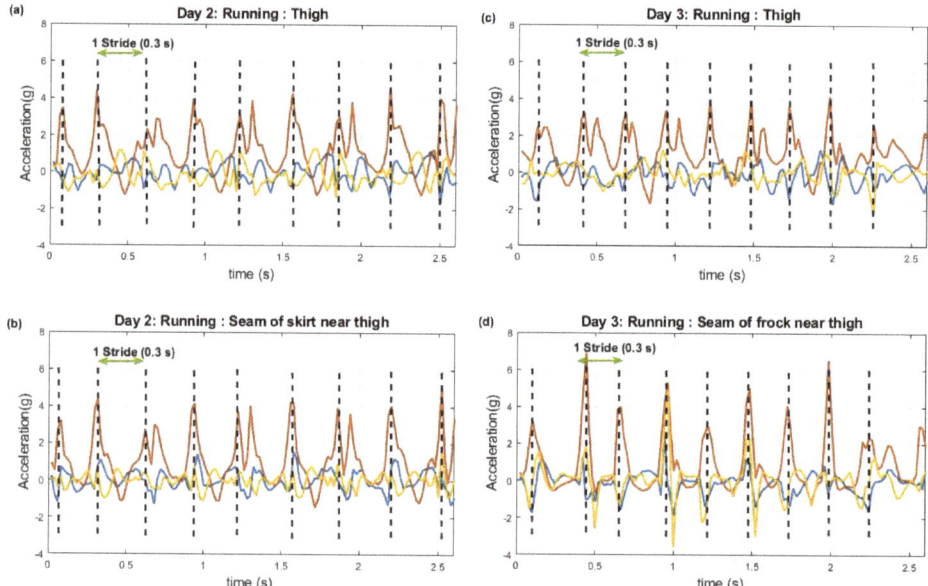

Figure 5. Running data from Day 2 (Skirt; left graphs) and Day 3 (Frock; right graphs). (**a**): Day 2 data from thigh, (**b**): Day 2 data from seams of skirt near thigh, (**c**): Day 3 data from thigh, (**d**): Day 3 data from seams of frock near thigh. Red axis: vertical acceleration, Blue axis: anterior-posterior acceleration, yellow axis: mediolateral acceleration. Note the similarity of signals between clothing and body worn sensors for skirt data verses the high accelerations present in frock data.

4.3. Correlation Coefficient Value Analysis

When examining the correlation coefficient values, five different sets of data were compared to determine from which data set the maximum correlation coefficient could be found. The five different data sets were the original data set, the time aligned data set, rotated data along the gravity axis, time-aligned and rotated data and finally the time-aligned, rotated and activity wise time-aligned data. After comparing all the values, it was noted that for activities like walking and running, maximum correlation coefficient values were found after applying a rotation matrix and activity-wise alignment.

Table 2 shows correlation coefficient values for each activity (multiple walking, running and sitting segments) after applying a rotation matrix and activity-wise alignment. They are listed by clothing type (slacks, skirt and frock) for both waist and thigh sensor data.

From Table 2, the waist sensor data had the highest correlation coefficients, irrespective of clothing type. However, thigh data also showed reasonable correlation values for each activity depending on the clothing type.

Table 2. Median correlation coefficient values for different activities for different clothes based on the 'Waist' and 'Thigh' sensors. Where there were multiple instances of the same activity in a day, the correlation coefficient was calculated for each instance, and the median and variance of the multiple instances is shown. There was a good correlation between body-worn and clothing sensors, apart from the sensor pair on the thigh and seam of the frock.

	Slacks		Skirt		Frock	
	Waist	Thigh	Waist	Thigh	Waist	Thigh
Walking	0.985± 0.022	0.945± 0.013	0.991± 0.006	0.973 ± 0.013	0.978 ± 0.018	0.921 ± 0.059
Running	0.811 ± 0.065	0.802 ± 0.067	0.926 ± 0.0007	0.835 ± 0.094	0.901 ± 0.008	0.642 ± 0.014
Sitting	0.993 ± 0.014	0.967 ± 0.001	0.999 ± 0.0002	0.995 ± 0.004	0.974	0.705
Bus Ride	0.988	0.987	-	-	-	-

4.4. Activity Classification

Figure 6 shows a segment of the output of the activity classifier, based on both body worn and clothing sensors (thigh data on the slacks). This classifier attempted to identify activities i.e., walking/running, transitions, sitting and standing, as denoted on Figure 6. In addition to the classification results, the activities performed by the participant as recorded in the diary are indicated on both graphs.

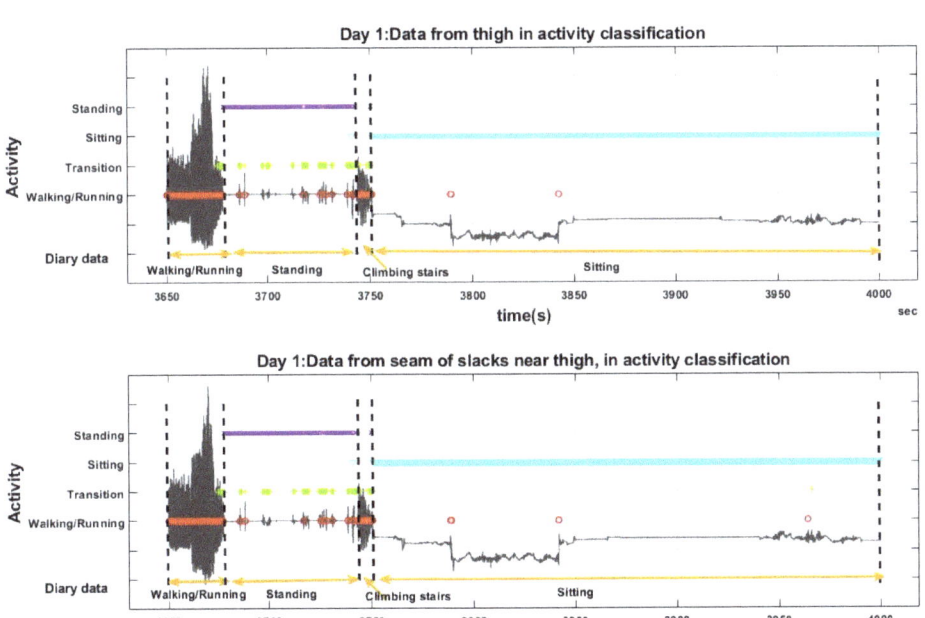

Figure 6. Activity recognition using a decision tree: Day 1 (slacks) data from body worn (top graph) and clothing sensors (bottom graph) were classified into one of four activities i.e., Walking/Running, Transitions of activities, Sitting and Standing. This figure shows a segment of the day's data. The gravity axis acceleration is plotted in grey, and the outputs of the classifier are denoted in different colours. Red: Walking/Running, Green: Transitions, Cyan: Sitting, Purple: Standing. The participant's activities according to the diary data are also shown in yellow. The outputs of the classifier are similar in both data files, with minor mismatches.

As the main intention of this research was to examine how the classifier outputs for the clothing sensor data compared with those from the body worn sensor data, and not to calculate the "true" activity classification accuracy, a confusion matrix (Table 3) was created considering the classifications from the body worn data set as the true class. For example, the first cell (row 1, column 1) of Table 3 indicates that 88.0% of the data that was classified as "walking" based on the body worn sensor are also classified as walking based on the clothing worn sensor. Similarly, 9.5% of the data classified as walking based on the body worn sensor are classified as transitions based on the clothing worn sensor.

Table 3. Confusion matrix showing the level to which activity classification based on the clothing sensor data was in agreement with classification based on the body worn sensor data (Day 1 data: when the subject was wearing slacks). Green boxes show when the highest value was expected and also achieved, Yellow boxes indicate where a high value was expected, but a lower value than expected was observed.

		Classification Data from Clothing Worn Sensor against Body Worn Data			
		Walking	Transitions	Sitting	Standing
Classification Data from the Body Worn Sensor as the "True" Class	Walking	88.00%	9.50%	0.70%	1.8%
	Transitions	16.10%	45.58%	11.42%	26.90%
	Sitting	0.32%	0.26%	88.37%	11.05%
	Standing	1.20%	9.58%	0.08%	89.14%

5. Discussion

When using correlation coefficients to compare the data sets, it was important to perform a data alignment for all the sensors, as the correlation was affected by time lags between the sensors' starting times. Orientation correction at this level is also important as the sensors can become misplaced while the subject is moving and it can mislead the comparisons of data sets. The long term goal is to eliminate the need for time lag and orientation correction by embedding the sensors more effectively in the clothes and engineering synchronous data readings.

The first analysis was done calculating correlation coefficient values for both data files. Table 2 was prepared with a summary of all data from the four common activities that were conducted on three days for waist and thigh sensors. It was clear that thigh data were less correlated than waist sensor data sets. Yet, these values were also significantly correlated with each other. The frock data indicate the possibility of considering clothing dynamics in the sensor data as the frock was a loose dress. Thus the frock could swing with the movements of the leg when the subject was running and walking. Further, when the subject was sitting on a chair, it was noted that the sensor on the clothes near the thigh tended to shift with respect to the sensor worn on the thigh itself. Typically the sensor on the frock would fall away from the leg and onto the chair thus losing a strong relationship to the underlying limb. In addition to the swinging attribute of the frock, the weight of the sensor device (Actigraph) emphasised the movement of the clothing rather than the body. Even though there are no established measures of the looseness of clothes relative to body size, clothing sensor readings would allow these concepts to be explored.

The final analysis was the comparison of the outputs of the activity classifiers. Based on the confusion matrix (Table 3), it was noted that all the activities except the transitions were identified in a high true positive rate, i.e., more than 80%, where the classifier output based on the body-worn sensor was considered as "true". Hence it can be taken as a positive indication that this would work more accurately when an advanced classifier would be used in activity classification. The findings of [21], mentioned that the accuracy of activity recognition was higher when the sensors were mounted onto clothes. However, they collected the data from a cloth attached to a pendulum. When it comes to data collection from a human with actual clothes, it could be said that our evidence demonstrates a more complex relationship. However, it should be noted that owing to the weight and the size of the

Actigraph devices, the correlation of data could have been decreased, and it is better to use smaller, lightweight sensors in a study like this.

When clothing worn sensor data is used for activity classification, it is reasonable to expect that the results will depend on factors that include subject characteristics (e.g., size, gender) as well as clothing styles (looseness, placement). However this study is intended to assess the viability of this approach and hence considers only a single subject across three different clothing types. In future studies, if the sensor positions may vary slightly from day to day due to different positioning of the clothes on the body, this issue can be minimised by rotating the three axis sensor readings along a common axis so as to align the principal direction of gravity with the y-axis of the sensor. Moreover, the data distribution for each activity is expected to be the same for x, y and z axis acceleration for sensor readings from different positions. Out of the three types of clothing, the pencil skirt data had the highest correlation as it was the tightest fitting of the clothing used in the study. Moreover, as the clothing waist sensors were more tightly attached to the waist with the clothes, waist sensor data were significantly correlated with each other irrespective of the clothing type.

6. Conclusions

This study aimed to assess the suitability of clothing sensor data for use in activity recognition when compared to similarly placed body worn sensors. In this study the clothing sensor data are shown to be well correlated with body worn sensor data as indicated by an analysis of correlation coefficient values. Furthermore the classification results from the clothing sensors are promising when compared to body worn sensors. This is a first study reporting data from sensors embedded into loose clothing in everyday activities. Results indicate that this approach has good potential for daily monitoring, for example in healthcare applications, and that this is an area worthy of further investigation.

This was a single person study intended to gain insight into how data might vary across three different clothing types across a range of likely daily activities. As such the study does not consider benefits of the wide range of different algorithms that could be used for classification. Rather the study checks whether it is possible to collect meaningful data from clothing worn sensors compared to body worn ones. Future studies are now encouraged to improve activity classifiers based on clothing types and supporting the use of multiple lightweight sensors that are networked and time synchronised.

All data used in the paper is available at 10.5281/zenodo.3597391.

Author Contributions: Conceptualisation, U.J., W.S.H. and F.H.; methodology, U.J.; software, U.J.; validation, U.J.; formal analysis, U.J., W.S.H. and F.H.; investigation, U.J., W.S.H. and F.H.; resources, U.J., W.S.H. and F.H.; data curation, U.J.; writing—original draft preparation, U.J.; writing—review and editing, ALL; visualization, U.J.; supervision, W.S.H. and F.H.; project administration, W.S.H.; funding acquisition, U.J., W.S.H. and F.H. All authors read and approved the final manuscript.

Funding: This research was partially funded by the UK Engineering and Physical Sciences Research Council(EPSRC, Grant number EP/K031910/1), an award from the Higher Education Funding Council for England to the University of Reading under the Global Challenges Research Fund, and University Grant Commission, Sri Lanka (UGC/VC/DRIC/PG2016(I)/UCSC/01).

Acknowledgments: We thank Giacomo Zanello for use of his Actigraph devices.

Conflicts of Interest: The authors declare no conflict of interest. The funders had no role in the design of the study; in the collection, analyses, or interpretation of data; in the writing of the manuscript, or in the decision to publish the results.

References

1. United Nations, N.Y. *World Population Ageing the 2015 Highlights*; Department of Economic and Social Affairs: New York City, NY, USA, 2015.
2. WHO. *Global Health and Aging*; World Health Organization: Geneva, Switzerland, 2010.
3. WHO. *World Report on Ageing and Health*; World Health Organization: Geneva, Switzerland, 2015.

4. Muro-De-La-Herran, A.; Garcia-Zapirain, B.; Mendez-Zorrilla, A. Gait analysis methods: An overview of wearable and non-wearable systems, highlighting clinical applications. *Sensors* **2014**, *14*, 3362–3394. [CrossRef] [PubMed]
5. Wang, Z.; Yang, Z.; Dong, T. A review of wearable technologies for elderly care that can accurately track indoor position, recognize physical activities and monitor vital signs in real time. *Sensors* **2017**, *17*, 341. [CrossRef] [PubMed]
6. Preece, S.J.; Goulermas, J.Y.; Kenney, L.P.; Howard, D.; Meijer, K.; Crompton, R. Activity identification using body-mounted sensors—A review of classification techniques. *Physiol. Meas.* **2009**, *30*, R1. [CrossRef] [PubMed]
7. Yang, J.Y.; Wang, J.S.; Chen, Y.P. Using acceleration measurements for activity recognition: An effective learning algorithm for constructing neural classifiers. *Pattern Recognit. Lett.* **2008**, *29*, 2213–2220. [CrossRef]
8. Kwapisz, J.R.; Weiss, G.M.; Moore, S.A. Activity recognition using cell phone accelerometers. *ACM SigKDD Explor. Newsl.* **2011**, *12*, 74–82. [CrossRef]
9. Ronao, C.A.; Cho, S.B. Deep convolutional neural networks for human activity recognition with smartphone sensors. In Proceedings of the 22nd International Conference on Neural Information Processing, ICONIP 2015, Istanbul, Turkey, 9–12 November 2015; Springer: Berlin/Heidelberg, Germany, 2015; pp. 46–53.
10. Bonomi, A.G.; Goris, A.H.; Yin, B.; Westerterp, K.R. Detection of type, duration, and intensity of physical activity using an accelerometer. *Med. Sci. Sport. Exerc.* **2009**, *41*, 1770–1777. [CrossRef] [PubMed]
11. Montoye, A.H.; Pivarnik, J.M.; Mudd, L.M.; Biswas, S.; Pfeiffer, K.A. Validation and comparison of accelerometers worn on the hip, thigh, and wrists for measuring physical activity and sedentary behavior. *AIMS Public Health* **2016**, *3*, 298. [CrossRef] [PubMed]
12. Cleland, I.; Kikhia, B.; Nugent, C.; Boytsov, A.; Hallberg, J.; Synnes, K.; McClean, S.; Finlay, D. Optimal placement of accelerometers for the detection of everyday activities. *Sensors* **2013**, *13*, 9183–9200. [CrossRef] [PubMed]
13. Boström, K.J.; Dirksen, T.; Zentgraf, K.; Wagner, H. The contribution of upper body movements to dynamic balance regulation during challenged locomotion. *Front. Hum. Neurosci.* **2018**, *12*, 8. [CrossRef] [PubMed]
14. Khan, A.M. Recognizing physical activities using Wii remote. *Int. J. Inf. Educ. Technol.* **2013**, *3*, 60. [CrossRef]
15. Ravi, N.; Dandekar, N.; Mysore, P.; Littman, M.L. Activity recognition from accelerometer data. *Aaai* **2005**, *5*, 1541–1546.
16. Wang, A.; Chen, G.; Yang, J.; Zhao, S.; Chang, C.Y. A comparative study on human activity recognition using inertial sensors in a smartphone. *IEEE Sens. J.* **2016**, *16*, 4566–4578. [CrossRef]
17. Wang, Z.; Wu, D.; Chen, J.; Ghoneim, A.; Hossain, M.A. A triaxial accelerometer-based human activity recognition via EEMD-based features and game-theory-based feature selection. *IEEE Sens. J.* **2016**, *16*, 3198–3207. [CrossRef]
18. Attal, F.; Mohammed, S.; Dedabrishvili, M.; Chamroukhi, F.; Oukhellou, L.; Amirat, Y. Physical human activity recognition using wearable sensors. *Sensors* **2015**, *15*, 31314–31338. [CrossRef] [PubMed]
19. Bedogni, L.; Di Felice, M.; Bononi, L. By train or by car? Detecting the user's motion type through smartphone sensors data. In Proceedings of the 2012 IFIP Wireless Days, Dublin, Ireland, 21–23 November 2012; pp. 1–6.
20. Gleadhill, S.; James, D.; Lee, J. Validating Temporal Motion Kinematics from Clothing Attached Inertial Sensors. In Proceedings of the 12th Conference of the International Sports Engineering Association, Brisbane, Australia, 26–29 March 2018; Volume 2, p. 304.
21. Michael, B.; Howard, M. Activity recognition with wearable sensors on loose clothing. *PLoS ONE* **2017**, *12*, e0184642. [CrossRef] [PubMed]
22. Rodrigues' Rotation Formula. MathWorld—A Wolfram Web Resource, created by Eric W. Weisstein. Available online: http://mathworld.wolfram.com/RodriguesRotationFormula.html (accessed on 19 December 2019).

23. Mukaka, M.M. Statistics corner: A guide to appropriate use of correlation coefficient in medical research. *Malawi Med. J.* **2012**, *24*, 69–71. [CrossRef] [PubMed]
24. Sarin, H.; Kokkolaras, M.; Hulbert, G.; Papalambros, P.; Barbat, S.; Yang, R.J. Comparing Time Histories for Validation of Simulation Models: Error Measures and Metrics. *J. Dyn. Syst. Meas. Control* **2010**, *132*, 061401. [CrossRef]

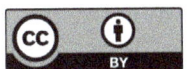

© 2019 by the authors. Licensee MDPI, Basel, Switzerland. This article is an open access article distributed under the terms and conditions of the Creative Commons Attribution (CC BY) license (http://creativecommons.org/licenses/by/4.0/).

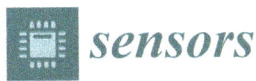

Article

Using Accelerometer and GPS Data for Real-Life Physical Activity Type Detection

Hoda Allahbakhshi [1],*, Lindsey Conrow [1,2], Babak Naimi [3] and Robert Weibel [1,2]

[1] Department of Geography, Geographic Information Systems Unit, University of Zurich (UZH), Winterthurerstrasse 190, 8057 Zurich, Switzerland; Lindsey.Conrow@geo.uzh.ch (L.C.); Robert.Weibel@geo.uzh.ch (R.W.)
[2] University Research Priority Program "Dynamics of Healthy Aging", University of Zurich, Andreasstrasse 15, 8050 Zurich, Switzerland
[3] Department of Geosciences and Geography, University of Helsinki, P.O. Box 64, 00014 Helsinki, Finland; Naimi.b@gmail.com
* Correspondence: Hoda.Allahbakhshi@geo.uzh.ch

Received: 14 December 2019; Accepted: 17 January 2020; Published: 21 January 2020

Abstract: This paper aims to examine the role of global positioning system (GPS) sensor data in real-life physical activity (PA) type detection. Thirty-three young participants wore devices including GPS and accelerometer sensors on five body positions and performed daily PAs in two protocols, namely semi-structured and real-life. One general random forest (RF) model integrating data from all sensors and five individual RF models using data from each sensor position were trained using semi-structured (Scenario 1) and combined (semi-structured + real-life) data (Scenario 2). The results showed that in general, adding GPS features (speed and elevation difference) to accelerometer data improves classification performance particularly for detecting non-level and level walking. Assessing the transferability of the models on real-life data showed that models from Scenario 2 are strongly transferable, particularly when adding GPS data to the training data. Comparing individual models indicated that knee-models provide comparable classification performance (above 80%) to general models in both scenarios. In conclusion, adding GPS data improves real-life PA type classification performance if combined data are used for training the model. Moreover, the knee-model provides the minimal device configuration with reliable accuracy for detecting real-life PA types.

Keywords: physical activity type; real-life; GPS; GIS

1. Introduction

In today's societies, the increase in sedentary lifestyles in people's homes and workplaces has caused severe health problems such as obesity and chronic diseases [1,2]. A physically active lifestyle can contribute to maintaining quality of life and preventing challenges related to people's health status, particularly for older adults. Many studies have been designed to objectively measure physical activity (PA) using wearable sensors; however, they have been conducted in controlled conditions. The data collected under controlled conditions are unable to reproduce PA behavior as it happens in real-life [3]. Studying such behaviors in natural daily settings is therefore important in order to discover how daily PA types can affect health status.

Accurate PA type detection is a prerequisite to recognize humans' daily activity behavior. Once we detect PA type, we can also estimate the other PA measures such as activity duration or level [4]. Detecting PA type helps to understand how much each activity type (e.g., walking or sitting) contributes to human physical and mental health. This also provides useful guidance regarding the amount of time that people should spend on a specific activity type to maintain their health. Moreover, PA type is a more understandable concept than PA level, particularly for laypersons [5]. Thus, it is imperative to improve daily PA type detection to identify humans' daily PA patterns and their association with health outcomes.

During the past decade, rapid progress in wearable sensor technologies has facilitated long-term PA behavior monitoring in real-life conditions. Among the existing wearable sensors, three-dimensional (3D) accelerometers have gained the most attention. A 3D accelerometer (ACC) measures acceleration forces in y, x and z dimensions, and therefore can sense the status of a body's motion or postures. Although the 3D accelerometer is the most common and informative sensor for PA type detection, it is challenging to accurately detect real-life activity types using only a single 3D accelerometer [5–7]. Researchers have extensively examined the usefulness of complementing accelerometer-based PA measures with additional sensors such as gyroscope, magnetometer, barometer and heart rate [8–11] or using multiple accelerometer devices on different body locations to improve the activity recognition [5,12]. However, these solutions entail mounting more devices on a person's body or rendering data analysis more complex due to dealing with different sensors featuring different data formats and sampling rates. Moreover, few studies have investigated the role of global positioning system (GPS) data in informing classifiers for detecting PA types [5,13], despite the great potential that a GPS sensor might have in contributing spatial context information that could further facilitate the PA type detection process.

Combining GPS and accelerometer sensors has been useful in improving movement monitoring of humans, particularly in daily life. In the transport mode detection domain, the combination of GPS and accelerometer sensors is more useful than using each sensor individually, specifically in differentiating transport-related activities such as walking, cycling and running. In the PA literature, we can categorize the use of GPS sensors into two broad applications. The first application mainly focuses on utilizing GPS spatial coordinates to link PA behavior derived from accelerometer data to the location and relevant spatial data such as land use, walkability, green spaces, neighborhood and exposure in a geographic information systems (GIS) environment [14–16]. These links enhance our contextual knowledge of the relationship between objectively measured PA and physical and social environments [17–21]. The second application uses features such as time, distance, altitude and speed derived from GPS data to inform classifiers in PA detection [5,22–25]. However, few studies in the PA domain attempted to assess the potential benefit of using GPS data as additional input to PA type detection.

Previous studies indicated that utilizing GPS devices is a practical method to accurately estimate humans' locomotion speed [26–30]. While adding GPS data (i.e., speed) to accelerometer data increases transport mode detection performance when differentiating between active and passive modes of transport [24,31–33], these studies rarely included different types of walking or cycling activities or different sub-types of the stationary class such as sitting, standing and lying. Although studies have included GPS speed to improve PA type detection for more fine-grained activities [5,13,34], they have a number of limitations that still have to be addressed.

Many of the models in the literature used data collected in controlled environments [5,13] to detect a limited number of activities from a small sample size [5,13,24,31,32,34]. Using GPS speed in combination with accelerometer data, models reliably detected activities that generate distinct accelerometer and GPS data profiles. However the models were unable to accurately detect activities with similar movement data profiles, such as non-level and level walking, which require different energy expenditure (EE) and have differing health impacts [6]. Exploiting GPS data to provide distinctive features would allow these similar types of activities to be distinguished. The previous studies have reported that the combination of GPS and accelerometer sensors generates better results for activity detection than using an accelerometer alone, but they did not fully discuss the role of the individual sensors in detail [5,24,32,34]. For example, it is unclear that to what extent adding GPS data improves activity recognition when using data collected in different environments (controlled and uncontrolled) or when using data from different sensor positions. It is also unknown whether adding GPS data addresses concerns about participant burden (e.g., wearing multiple sensors) during real-life data collection. To our knowledge, no study has explored the potential benefit of also using GPS spatial coordinates to classify PA type. The potential for combining GPS and accelerometer data to enhance real-life activity recognition is therefore a research area that is yet to be explored in detail.

This paper contributes to the body of literature on sensors and PA type detection first by calculating an informative elevation difference feature by linking the GPS spatial coordinates to GIS data, namely a digital elevation model (DEM), rather than using GPS speed alone. Second, we investigate the extent to which GPS sensors, in conjunction with accelerometer data, can enhance the prediction performance of detecting the major posture and transport-related motion activity types (sitting, standing, lying, walking, non-level walking, running and cycling). We then explore whether GPS data informs PA monitoring such that their inclusion minimizes the number of accelerometer devices that are required to reliably differentiate between the above posture and motion activity types under real-life conditions, with the aim of reducing participant burden. Finally, we advance research on real-life PA type detection through not only developing a single classification model, but also by assessing the contribution of GPS data in addressing the limitations of accelerometer sensor data and by studying the contribution of these sensors in detail within different realistic and stringent validation scenarios.

Our results provide insights that can assist future PA study design, especially when PA type detection is a focus. In particular, this research gives guidance regarding relevant data sources (accelerometer, GPS) and their usage, appropriate evaluation methods and optimal sensor positions for studies aiming to detect the major posture and transport-related motion activities.

2. Materials and Methods

2.1. Experimental Overview

The target PAs are lying, sitting, standing and walking on level ground at different speeds (slow, normal and fast), running, cycling, walking uphill, walking downhill, walking downstairs and walking upstairs. The rationale for selecting these target activities is to consider a subset of PAs from prior research including, (1) simple PAs classified by [35]. (2) Mobility-related activities of the International Classification of Functioning, Disability and Health (ICF) and (3) global body motion activities classified by [12]. (4) Activities that are commonly performed in everyday life and (5) activities that can cover different levels/intensities of PA and EE.

We used two study designs for data collection, semi-structured and real-life, to assess the transferability of the model trained with a semi-controlled data set on data collected in real-life conditions.

2.1.1. Semi-Structured Protocol

Participants reported to the sport center of the University. After completing a questionnaire regarding their socio-demographic information and typical PA based on the Global Physical Activity Questionnaire (GPAQ) [36], they put the six devices on in the following configuration: one smartphone (Motorola Moto E, 2nd gen) inside their right pocket and five wearable customized uTrail devices [37] on different body locations including left and right hips, inside their left pocket, chest and right knee (Figure 1). Two elastic straps, each holding the uTrail, were adjusted around their chest and below their right knee. For the hip positions, we fixed the uTrail devices to their waistband using the device clip.

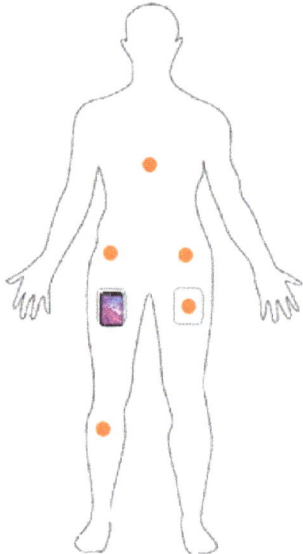

Figure 1. The location of smartphone and uTrail devices (orange circles) on the participants' body.

The uTrail device includes an audio sensor, a GPS sensor (uBlox UC530M) and an accelerometer that includes three magnetic field channels and three acceleration channels (ST Microelectronics LSM303D). The GPS recorded data at 1 Hz and has the ability of concurrent reception of up to three global navigation satellite systems (out of GPS (GPS = USA), Galileo (Galileo = European), GLONASS (GLONASS = Russia) and BeiDou (BeiDou = China)). The sampling rate for the accelerometer was 50 Hz. The uTrail device can be connected to a computer via a micro-USB port to download stored data; we were able to configure the device and retrieve the data via software developed for the uTrail. The smartphone and audio sensor data were not used in the present study. For all sensor positions except the right hip, the devices were oriented to have the y, x and z axes, recording acceleration data in the vertical, medio-lateral and antero-posterior direction of the body, respectively. For the right hip, the device was oriented to have the y, x and z axes, recording acceleration data in the vertical, antero-posterior and medio-lateral direction of the body, respectively.

Participants performed a number of activities, each completed twice in an outdoor area (see Appendix A, Table A1). They performed the motion activities at their own comfortable speed and were not restricted in this sense. We applied a direct observation approach for activity annotation using the "aTimeLogger" free app installed on a smartphone.

2.1.2. Real-Life Protocol

The real-life experiment was conducted a few days after the participants completed the semi-structured protocol. Participants wore the devices in the same configuration as the semi-structured protocol and they were instructed to use the "aTimeLogger" app to make their own data annotation during the real-life data collection. No instruction regarding how to perform the activities was given to the participants. They performed the target activities in an outdoor environment as part of their daily life spontaneously and in a random order. The only criteria were to meet the required minimum time duration for each activity task described in (see Appendix A, Table A2) and perform the transport-related activities such as walking, cycling and jogging in two different environments, namely an urban area and a leisure area; this data collection protocol took 3 h on average. The total amount of labeled data collected in both protocols (semi-structured + real-life) is about 161 h (29,017,465 data recordings), corresponding to an average of 4.8 h labeled data for each participant (Table 1). We anonymized all data (with the personal data stored separately from the ACC and GPS data) and instructed the participants to perform all PAs away from their home and workplace, such that their home and workplace location could not be inferred from the GPS data. This dataset is not yet publicly available as we intend to use it in a future publication [38].

Table 1. Labeled data collected for the study.

Dataset	Total Acc. Data	Total GPS Data	Acc. Data per Person	GPS Data per Person
Semi-structured	61.6 h (11,098,581)	59.6 h (214,628)	1.8 h (336,320.6)	1.8 h (6503.879)
Real-life	99.5 h (17,918,884)	101.5 h (365,631)	3 h (542,996.5)	3 h (11,079.73)
Total	161 h (29,017,465)	161 h (580,259)	4.8 h (879,317.1)	4.8 h (17,583.61)

2.1.3. Participants

A sample of 33 (20 male and 13 female) young participants ranging in age from 20 to 35 from 15 different countries (see Appendix A, Figure A1) participated in data collection (Table 2). As inclusion criteria, participants were required to be physically healthy and be able to walk and run without walking aids (self-report), and accept the instructions of the study protocol. The study was carried out following the rules of the Declaration of Helsinki of 1975. According to the rules of the University of Zurich (UZH) Ethics Policy, which are in accordance with the Swiss Human Research Act, it was not necessary to obtain separate ethics approval from the UZH Ethics Committee and our study was conducted in compliance with the ethical guidelines of the Philosophical Faculty of the University of Zurich. All participants provided written informed consent.

Table 2. Physical characteristics of the participants involved in the study.

Physical Characteristics	Mean (SD)
No. (F/M)	33 (13/20)
Age (year)	29 ± (5.6)
Height (cm)	173 ± (10.05)
Weight (kg)	67 ± (9.8)
BMI (kg·m^{-2})	22 ± (1.9)

2.2. Model Development

2.2.1. Accelerometer Preprocessing

After removing duplicates and missing values, we synchronized the data from five accelerometers. The synchronization was based on a sudden jump (i.e., "standing still-jump-standing still") as introduced in [7] and was performed by the participant before and after performing each activity task, as instructed. The jump activity generated a distinguishable acceleration profile (i.e., peaks) within the standing still segments. We detected the peak acceleration of the start and end jumps, and aligned the data recordings of the five sensors based on those peaks. We used the start and end timestamps recorded by the "aTimeLogger" app to annotate the data. For each activity task, we removed 10 s before and after the activity segment to exclude data recorded during the sudden jump period for each activity. We also removed long stops (more than 1 s) within the motion activities. To do this, we firstly developed a threshold-based stop-move detection algorithm based on accelerometer data, secondly we found the stop segments longer than 1 s, thirdly we removed them from each motion activity segment and finally, we assigned the corresponding label to the raw accelerometer data of that segment. Visual inspection helped to ensure signal alignment to the corresponding activities.

We used an overlapping fixed size windowing technique to segment the labeled data. We applied a sensitivity analysis (i.e., we altered and tested different segment sizes) using segments of 2, 5, 10, 20, 30 and 60 s to investigate how robust the model's classification performance was to the segment size.

After signal segmentation, we calculated time and frequency domain features from each segment to use as inputs to the classifier. Time domain features are typically mathematical or statistical measures derived directly from the sensor data. To derive frequency domain features, the segment of sensor data must first be transformed into the frequency domain, normally using a fast Fourier transform (FFT). In total, we extracted 85 features from each sensor's accelerometer data. The initial target features from accelerometer data include:

- Time domain features: mean, standard deviation and range of three axes and total acceleration, correlation among three axes, kurtosis, skewness and average absolute difference of three axes, number of observations falling within each of 10 bins of the three axes, time interval between local peaks and number of peaks of three axes.
- Frequency domain features using FFT: power spectral density, energy of the signal, mean of the first three dominant frequencies, amplitude of the first three dominant frequencies of three axes and total acceleration.

2.2.2. GPS Preprocessing

The GPS data include latitude, longitude, date, time, horizontal dilution of precision (HDOP), vertical dilution of precision (VDOP), number of satellites, altitude and instantaneous speed. To preprocess the GPS data, we firstly removed duplicates and missing values. We used linear interpolation based on latitude, longitude and timestamps to fill the data gaps greater than 1 s between consecutive GPS fixes. We extracted an elevation value for each interpolated GPS point from a DEM to fill in the altitude value for the interpolated GPS points. A DEM is a representation of the altitude of the earth's surface, today typically generated using remote sensing techniques such as stereo photogrammetry or laser scanning. We used the swissALTI3D DEM, which has a spatial resolution of 2 m and is provided by the Swiss national mapping agency swisstopo.

After filling gaps in the GPS data, it was important to keep the spatial error of GPS coordinates at a minimum. Map matching is a helpful solution to improve the spatial accuracy [39]. We used the point-to-curve geometric map-matching approach according to Quddus et al.'s (2007) categorization [39]. We applied an existing map matching algorithm on interpolated GPS data using road data obtained from OpenStreetMap (OSM) [40] and R software [41] (Figure 2).

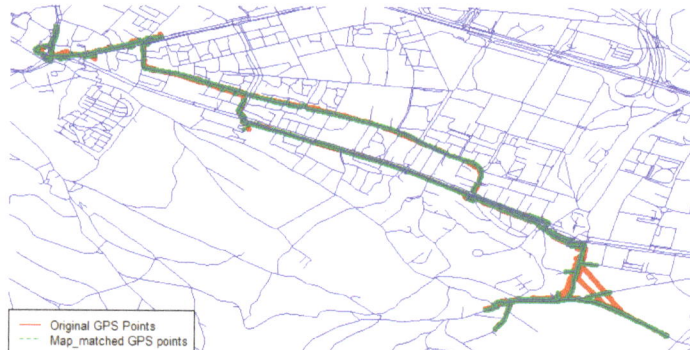

Figure 2. Map-matched global positioning system (GPS) points of data collected by a single participant in real-life using OpenStreetMap (OSM) data.

Afterward, we used the map-matched GPS coordinates to derive an elevation value from swissALTI3D for each GPS point. SwissALTI3D is an accurate DEM, which describes the surface of Switzerland without vegetation and development and is updated every six years. We used ArcGIS software v.10.6.1 and the tool "Extract value to points" to assign an elevation value to each GPS point. We then used a weighted average filter to remove noise and outliers and smooth the extracted elevation data from DEM. We matched the GPS timestamps with the start and end timestamps of accelerometer segments to combine the GPS data with the accelerometer data. Finally, we calculated the average speed and elevation difference for each segment and appended these two GPS features to the accelerometer feature space.

2.2.3. RF Model Development

We built two different training datasets, one using data from the semi-structured protocol only and another one using the combined dataset of both the semi-structured and real-life protocols, and used the random forest (RF) classifier to build the classification models in different scenarios (Table 3). For each scenario, we examined both single (accelerometer data only) and multi-sensor (accelerometer and GPS data) approaches to build the RF classification models. We built a general model that was trained with data obtained from all five sensor positions (chest, left hip, right hip, left pocket and right knee) and also five individual models, each trained with data from a single sensor position. Each accelerometer-based individual model used 85 features (see Section 2.2.1) for classification, and each accelerometer-based general model integrated features from all five sensors and used a total of 425 (85 × 5) features.

Table 3. Scenarios for separating data into a train and test data set and the corresponding validation method.

Scenario No.	Training Dataset	Validation Method and Test Data
Scenario 1	Semi-structured dataset	L1SO cross validation on semi-structured data L1SO cross validation on real-life data k-fold cross validation on semi-structured data
Scenario 2	Combined semi-structured and real-life dataset	L1SO cross validation on combined data L1SO cross validation on real-life data k-fold cross validation on combined data

We grouped the activities of each protocol and detected seven classes including walking, non-level walking, running, cycling, sitting, standing and lying. We also validated the results using three approaches: Leave-One-Subject-Out (L1SO), k-fold cross validation and L1SO validation with the real-life data set. We tested different segment sizes (2, 5, 10, 20, 30 and 60 s) for general models to assess the effect of segment size on classification performance. The data analysis tasks were implemented using the R statistical computing software [41].

To report the classification performance, we used four metrics including accuracy, recall, precision and F1 (Equations (1)–(4)).

$$\text{Accuracy} = (\text{True positive} + \text{True negative})/(\text{True positive} + \text{True negative} + \text{False positive} + \text{False negative}). \quad (1)$$

$$\text{Precision} = \text{True positive}/(\text{True positive} + \text{False positive}). \quad (2)$$

$$\text{Recall} = \text{True positive}/(\text{True positive} + \text{False negative}). \quad (3)$$

$$F1 = 2 \times \text{precision} \times \text{recall}/((\text{beta}^2 \times \text{precision}) + \text{recall}). \quad (4)$$

3. Results

We presented the overall accuracies of the RF models (general model and individual models) as evaluated using L1SO, 10-fold cross validation and validation with a real-life dataset in Figure 3 and Figure 5. Based on the results, we realized that the L1SO cross validation (with a training or real-life dataset) led to more realistic results compared to 10-fold cross validation. The 10-fold cross validation always had the best performance (above 95%) for all models regardless of the sensor positions, training or testing dataset and there was significant difference between the classification accuracy measured using L1SO (with training or real-life dataset) and 10-fold cross validation. In other words, 10-fold cross validation produced artificially high scores for all models, therefore we focus on the results obtained by L1SO cross validation only.

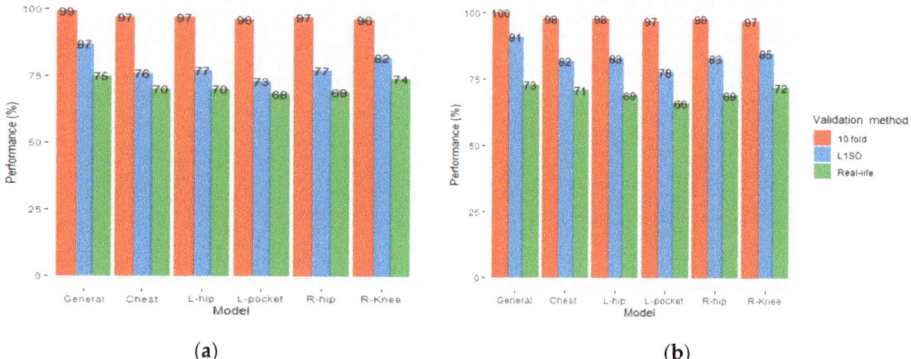

Figure 3. Overall accuracy of the RF classification models trained with semi-structured data, (**a**) accelerometer data only and (**b**) accelerometer and GPS data.

3.1. Results for Scenario 1

Using L1SO cross validation (with training data) and accelerometer data only, the general model with 87% accuracy performed better than individual models. Among individual models, the knee position scored highest with 82% accuracy followed by left/right hip (77%), chest (76%) and left pocket (73%). We observed a dramatic drop in accuracy under real-life dataset when using L1SO cross validation, indicating that the model trained with semi-structured data could weakly predict PA types in real-life (Figure 3a).

Adding GPS data to the accelerometer data improved the classification performance for all models validated by L1SO of the training dataset. The overall accuracy of hips and chest, pocket, general and knee positions increased by 6%, 5%, 4% and 3%, respectively. However, similar to accelerometer-based models, the classification performance decreased for all models when testing on real life data. General model performed the best with 73% accuracy followed by knee (72%), chest (71%), left/right hips (69%) and pocket (66%; Figure 3b).

Using L1SO of the training dataset, the overall accuracy for the general models ranged from 70% to 98% (using accelerometer data only) and from 81% to 99% (using accelerometer data combined with GPS data). Testing the general models with real-life data, the classification performance was between 56% and 95% and 56% and 95% using accelerometer data and ACC + GPS data, respectively. The interquartile range (IQR) of L1SO and the related real-life validation partially overlapped for all models excluding the general model when using accelerometer data only (Figure 4a). Conversely, there was no overlap between the IQR of L1SO and its related real-life validation when we added GPS data (Figure 4b). In addition, using multi-sensor data (Figure 4b) generated more outliers compared to using accelerometer data only (Figure 4a). The distribution range of the general and individual position models does not show a significant difference between Figure 4a,b. Results show that in an ideal situation (i.e., fewer GPS gaps and complete OSM data), adding GPS data could increase the overall classification accuracy for L1SO of training dataset by 15%.

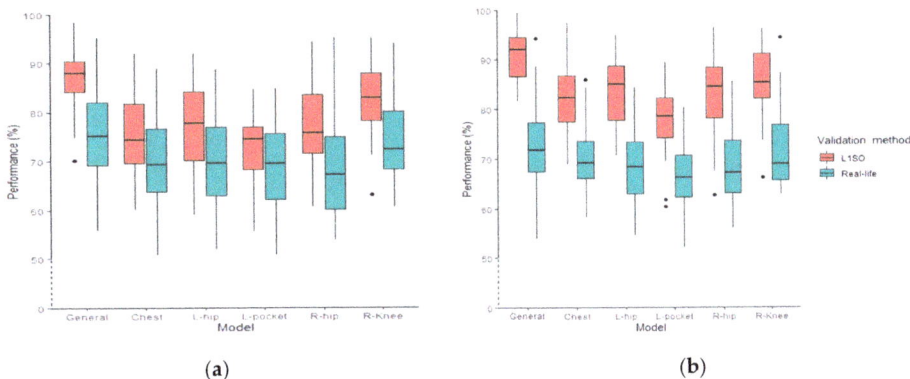

Figure 4. The distribution of overall accuracy among all participants for the RF classification models trained with semi-structured data, (**a**) accelerometer data only and (**b**) accelerometer and GPS data.

The general RF model using accelerometer data only detected lying, sitting, standing and running with high recall, precision and F1. However, the model obtained the lowest performance for non-level walking followed by walking and cycling (highlighted in bold in Table 4). Adding features derived from GPS data (speed and elevation differences) to the accelerometer feature space significantly improved the recall, precision and F1 for non-level walking, walking and cycling (highlighted in bold in Table 5).

Table 4. Confusion matrix of a participant (with the highest GPS contribution) when using accelerometer data only (Scenario 1).

Accelerometer Only	Cycle	Lie	N_Walk	Run	Sit	Stand	Walk	Recall	Precision	F1
Cycle	168	0	9	0	0	0	0	78	95	85
Lie	0	124	0	0	0	1	0	99	99	99
N_walk	0	0	209	0	0	0	163	42	56	48
Run	1	0	0	113	0	0	0	100	99	100
Sit	0	1	0	0	108	0	0	99	99	99
Stand	0	0	0	0	1	62	0	98	98	98
Walk	47	0	279	0	0	0	394	71	55	62

Table 5. Confusion matrix of a participant (with the highest GPS contribution) when using accelerometer and GPS data (Scenario 1).

Accelerometer & GPS	Cycle	Lie	N_Walk	Run	Sit	Stand	Walk	Recall	Precision	F1
Cycle	165	0	10	0	0	0	0	98	94	96
Lie	0	124	0	0	0	1	0	99	99	99
N_walk	0	0	278	0	0	0	89	58	76	66
Run	1	0	0	112	0	0	0	100	99	100
Sit	0	1	0	0	107	0	0	100	99	100
Stand	0	0	0	0	0	66	0	99	100	99
Walk	2	0	192	0	0	0	523	85	73	79

Feature Importance

Using accelerometer data only, the mean acceleration along the vertical and medio-lateral axes, standard deviation and energy of the signal of total acceleration and of the vertical axis, the number of observations falling within the fourth bin of the medio-lateral axis from the chest sensor's data; the mean acceleration along the medio-lateral axes of the left hip and pocket sensor's data and the number of observations falling within the fifth bin of the medio-lateral axis from the pocket's data were the top 10 best features for the general RF model (see Appendix B, Figure A2a).

Though the order of important features varied according to the different individual models, the mean acceleration along the vertical and medio-lateral axes, as well as power spectral density, and energy and amplitude of the first dominant frequency of total acceleration fell within the top 10 features for all individual models. We also observed that mean acceleration along the antero-posterior axis and total acceleration, average absolute difference of total acceleration, standard deviation of total acceleration, vertical and medio-lateral axes, energy of the signal along the vertical and medio-lateral axes, amplitude of the second dominant frequency of total acceleration, number of observations falling within the fourth, fifth and seventh bin of the medio-lateral axis and range of acceleration along the medio-lateral axis are among the top 10 features among different individual models.

Using the accelerometer and GPS data, excluding the features derived from GPS data, a similar feature importance pattern was seen for the general (see Appendix B, Figure A2b) and individual models.

3.2. Results for Scenario 2

In Scenario 2, for each participant, we combined all collected data in the semi-structured and real-life settings, and built the training data or "combined dataset" (Figure 5).

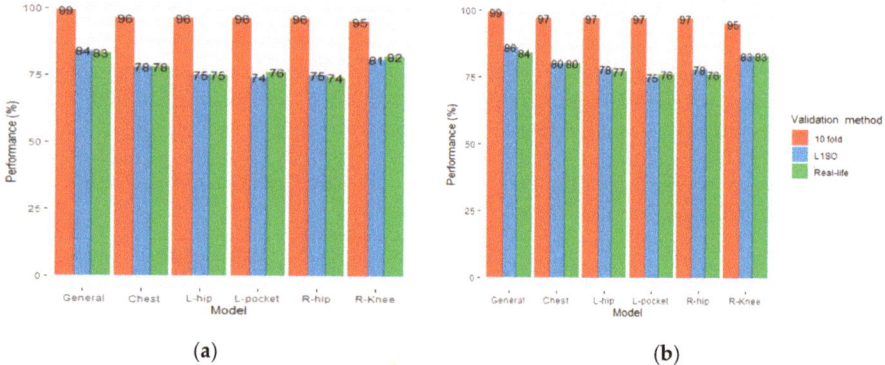

Figure 5. Overall accuracy of the RF classification models trained with combined dataset, (**a**) accelerometer data only and (**b**) accelerometer and GPS data.

Using L1SO cross validation (with training data) and accelerometer data only, the general model achieved 84% accuracy, a 3% decrease compared to the result obtained by using semi-structured data in training. Among individual models, the knee position again scored highest with 81% accuracy followed by chest (78%), hips (75%) and left pocket (74%). Using the combined data for training the RF, compared to Scenario 1, the model performance for chest and pocket positions slightly increased by 2% and 1%; whereas, it decreased by 3% and 1% for hips and knee position, respectively (Figure 5a).

Adding GPS data to the accelerometer data improved the classification performance for all models validated by L1SO of the training dataset by 2% with the exceptions of 1% for the pocket model and 3% for the hips position. This scenario also performed better with the real-life data, and ACC + GPS resulted in stable classification performance, unlike Scenario 1 where the performance dramatically dropped for all models. The general, knee, chest, pocket and right hip, and left hip models achieved 84%, 83%, 80%, 76% and 77% overall accuracy, respectively (Figure 5b).

The boxplots for the models' performance when using the combined dataset for training RF models shows that the overall accuracy ranges from 73% to 95% and from 74% to 95% when using accelerometer data only and when using data from both accelerometer and GPS sensors, respectively, and evaluated by L1SO (Figure 6). Testing the general models with real-life data, the overall accuracy ranges from 65% to 95% (Figure 6a) and 66% to 96% (Figure 6b). The IQR of L1SO and the related real-life validation overlapped for all models. The overall accuracies follow a similar distribution trend for both Figure 6a,b, regardless of sensor positions and validation methods. Both hip positions and the pocket models had the widest distribution followed by chest, knee and general models. Adding GPS data produced more outliers, as was the case in Scenario 1.

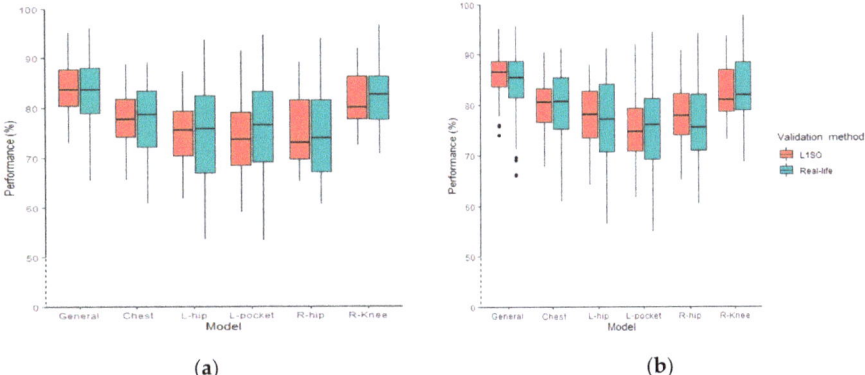

(a)   (b)

Figure 6. The distribution of overall accuracy among all participants for the RF classification models trained combined dataset, (**a**) accelerometer data only and (**b**) accelerometer and GPS data.

The confusion matrix for the participant with the highest GPS contribution (4%) shows that the most misclassification occurred for non-level walking and walking activities when using accelerometer data only and L1SO validation (highlighted in bold in Table 6). Similar to Scenario 1, adding GPS features improved the classification performance by reducing the misclassification errors for these two activities (highlighted in bold in Table 7).

Table 6. Confusion matrix of a participant (with the highest GPS contribution) when using accelerometer data only (Scenario 2).

Accelerometer only	Cycle	Lie	N_Walk	Run	Sit	Stand	Walk	Recall	Precision	F1
Cycle	743	0	2	0	0	0	0	100	100	100
Lie	0	185	1	0	1	0	0	99	99	99
N_walk	2	0	800	1	0	0	91	77	89	83
Run	0	0	0	320	0	0	0	99	100	100
Sit	0	1	0	0	170	1	0	99	99	99
Stand	0	1	0	0	0	157	0	99	99	99
Walk	0	0	233	2	0	1	885	91	79	84

Table 7. Confusion matrix of a participant (with the highest GPS contribution) when using accelerometer and GPS data (Scenario 2).

Accelerometer & GPS	Cycle	Lie	N_Walk	Run	Sit	Stand	Walk	Recall	Precision	F1
Cycle	738	0	0	0	0	0	0	100	100	100
Lie	0	186	1	0	0	0	0	99	99	99
N_walk	1	0	810	1	0	0	63	89	93	91
Run	0	0	0	318	0	0	1	99	100	99
Sit	0	1	0	0	166	1	0	98	99	99
Stand	0	1	0	0	3	158	0	99	98	98
Walk	1	0	97	2	0	1	1018	94	91	93

Feature Importance

As in Scenario 1, mean acceleration along the vertical and medio-lateral axes, standard deviation of acceleration along the vertical axis from the chest sensor's data, mean acceleration along the vertical axis and number of observations falling within the fifth bin of the medio-lateral axis from the pocket sensor's data fell within the top 10 features for the general model when using accelerometer data only (see Appendix B, Figure A3a). The average absolute difference of total acceleration and acceleration along the vertical axis, power spectral density of total acceleration from the chest's sensor data, number of observations falling within the fourth bin of the medio-lateral axis and amplitude of the third dominant frequency of acceleration along the medio-lateral axis from the pocket's sensor data were also among the top 10 important features for accelerometer data. The individual models' importance pattern for the top 10 features was similar to the individual models' feature importance in Scenario 1. There was again variation in the order of feature importance depending on the different individual models. The mean acceleration along the medio-lateral axis and power spectral density of total acceleration were among the top 10 features of all individual models.

Using accelerometer and GPS data, excluding the features derived from GPS data, we observed a similar feature importance pattern for the general (see Appendix B, Figure A3b) and individual models.

3.3. Sensitivity Analysis on Segment Size

We performed sensitivity analysis on different segment sizes using L1SO of training data to determine how sensitive the models are to the segment size. For both scenarios, we tested segment sizes of 2, 5, 10, 20, 30 and 60 s and performed L1SO cross validation on the general RF models. The results show that performance starts to converge with larger window size in (a) whereas (b) has the widest gap at 20 and 30s. Overall, there are slight changes ranging from 1% to 3% for the models' performance when using different segment sizes (Figure 7).

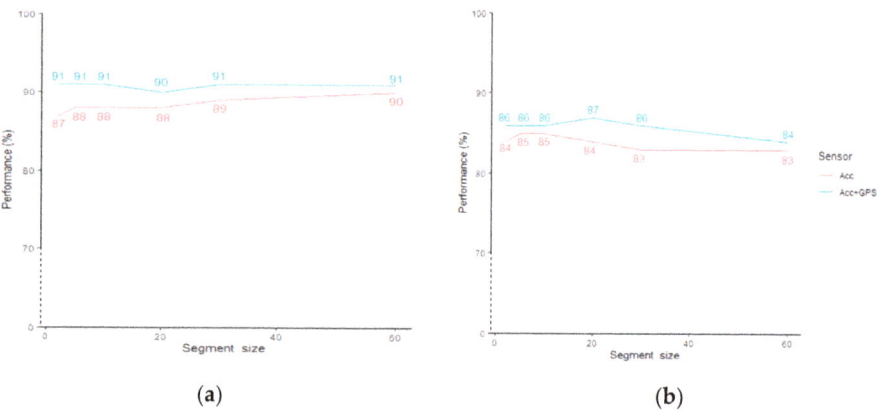

Figure 7. Sensitivity analysis on segment size, (**a**) general model trained with semi-structured dataset and (**b**) general model trained with combined dataset.

4. Discussion

4.1. Discussion of Results

The aim of this study was to investigate the extent to which using GPS sensor data, in conjunction with accelerometer data, enhances the prediction performance in detecting the major posture and transport-related motion activity types (sitting, standing, lying, level walking, non-level walking, running/jogging and cycling). Moreover, this study explored how adding GPS data allows the number of sensor devices to be minimized in PA monitoring.

The validation results show that using standard 10-fold cross validation, which allows data from the same participant in the test and training set produces artificially high accuracy scores. Though 10-fold cross validation is commonly used, it is a weak evaluation method, while L1SO cross validation corresponds to a more realistic setting in which the algorithm would be applied. In practical use, the data from a particular participant are never used as training data to classify another piece of data from that same participant, but will instead be used to classify data from another participant. Hence, it is likely that L1SO scored lower than 10-fold because different participants have different ways of performing individual activities. For these reasons, we recommend against using the 10-fold cross validation method in the PA type detection.

Adding GPS data to the general model improved the accuracy in Scenario 1, although the developed models showed a dramatic decrease when evaluated with L1SO applied on the real-life dataset. Performance decreased by 12% when using accelerometer only, and by 18% when using both accelerometer and GPS. This result indicates that adding GPS data to accelerometer data produces significant generalization error when tested with a real-life dataset. The generalization error may result from performing the activities in different real-life environments (leisure and urban), impacting the variable accuracy of GPS data. Urban areas in particular can affect GPS signal reception and therefore generate more GPS gaps and uncertainty in the data. Having more outliers in the boxplots when adding GPS data is also a manifestation of the increase in data uncertainty (Figure 4a). Moreover, incomplete OSM data is more often encountered in leisure (i.e., rural) environments, which influences the outcome of map matching GPS data collected in those areas. Thus, models developed using semi-structured data are weakly transferable to the data collected in real life, particularly when we add GPS data to the training data. The distribution of overall accuracy among all participants also shows the above-mentioned conclusion; by adding GPS data, there is a larger gap between IQR of L1SO and its related real-life validation for the general model (Figure 4b).

We used the combined dataset to train models in Scenario 2 to improve the transferability of our models for a real-life dataset and address the overfitting issue. In machine learning, overfitting refers to when a model learns the training data very well but performs weakly on a new dataset. Compared to the semi-structured dataset, there is more variation in the combined dataset, which explains the overall decrease in overall accuracy of the models between Scenarios 1 and 2. Using the combined data, the models showed comparable accuracy when evaluated by a L1SO of the training data and when evaluated with the real-life dataset. Testing the models on the real-life dataset of an unseen participant in the training data resulted in an overall accuracy of 83% for the accelerometer-based model (decreasing by only 1% compared to the result obtained by using L1SO validation of the training data) and 86% for the ACC + GPS based model. We therefore conclude that the new models trained with the combined dataset generate robust models with reproducible classification performance for real-life data from new subjects. The high degree of overlap between IQR of L1SO and the related real-life validation for all models in Scenario 2 also supports this conclusion. The advantage of using the combined dataset rather than the semi-structured dataset for training the model is that there is less generalization error in the classification performance when we use a real-life (i.e., a new) dataset for testing. This supports the results by Ermes et al. (2008) that in order to build a model that performs reliably on a real-life dataset, it is necessary to include labeled data collected in real-life in the training data [34]. It also explains why Scenario 2 performed better than Scenario 1 on the real-life data, with ACC + GPS increasing real-life performance.

Regarding the features, we did not apply any feature selection or dimensionality reduction algorithms as we used the random forest as a classifier, which performs feature selection throughout the classification process. Therefore, using the random forest classifier, the high number of features for general models does not lead to oscillations of the classification. We also used the R package ranger [42], which is a faster and more memory-efficient implementation of random forests, to improve the models' processing time. In general, when excluding GPS features, similar time and frequency domain features from accelerometer data appeared in all models, though the importance changes based on the sensor's position. The top 10 important features that gained the highest frequency among all models include the mean acceleration of the vertical, medio-lateral and antero-posterior axes; energy of acceleration along the vertical and medio-lateral axes; standard deviation of vertical axis and the average absolute difference, standard deviation, energy, power spectral density and amplitude of the first dominant frequency of total acceleration.

We performed a sensitivity analysis on six different segment sizes to assess the transferability of our models on data extracted from different time intervals. The highest GPS contribution to the classification performance was for the segment size of 2 s (4%) in Scenario 1 and for the segment sizes of 20 and 30 s (3%) in Scenario 2. Adding GPS data resulted in a high accuracy of 91% for all segment sizes except 20 s (90%) in Scenario 1. In Scenario 2, using multi-sensor data led to the highest accuracy of 87% when 20s segments were used. As there are only slight changes ranging from 1% to 3% for the models' performance when using different segment sizes, we could conclude that our models were stable and robust to the segment size. Using the longest, 60 s segment size, the ACC + GPS models in Scenario 1 and 2 reached 91% and 84% overall accuracy, respectively. This demonstrated that our models would be useful when collecting data with storage and battery limited devices (such as smartphones), which have limitations in recording sensor data at high sampling rates during long-term PA monitoring.

Comparing the five individual models, each trained on data from a single sensor position, showed that hips and chest models generate comparable accuracy with and without adding GPS data. For both hip positions, we usually gained similar classification performance, although we asked participants to wear the hip devices in different orientations. This shows that the orientation does not have a significant influence on the overall classification performance when using hip positions. However, looking more in detail, we found that the two hip models have distinguishable performance for different participants in detecting different activities. For example, the left hip model detects sitting activity better than the right hip model for some participants. The pocket position usually performed worse than other positions, possibly because the device in this position was not fixed as participants simply put the device in their pocket, which could cause flipping or rotating the device during activity performance. The knee model performed best both when using accelerometer only and when using multi-sensor data in both scenarios. In Scenario 2, the knee model showed comparable performance with the general model and achieved an accuracy above 80%. It also gained the most similar IQR compared to its related general model in this scenario. Moreover, in an ideal situation, the knee multi-sensor model obtained an overall accuracy of 94% for detecting the major posture and motion activities (see Appendix B, Table A4) when evaluated by L1SO on training data. This indicates that adding GPS data to knee-positioned accelerometer data provides classification performance with high accuracy, which further suggests that participant burden might be reduced as the number of sensor devices can be minimized for PA type detection.

4.2. Contributions and Limitations

This study has several strengths and limitations worth noting. A general strength of this study is that we comprehensively investigated the contribution of adding GPS data to enhance accelerometer-based PA type classification, as discussed above. We accurately detected activities that help to discover humans' daily activity behavior. For instance, Ermes et al., (2008) noted that the majority of data collected in the real-life environment by their participants (78%) include lying, sitting and standing, and emphasized the importance of detecting these three stationary activity types in real-life. However, they grouped sitting and standing to one group, as their model could not reliably distinguish these two activities [34]. There is a causal effect between spending too much time on these activities and the risk of negative health impacts such as diabetes or obesity. Detecting stationary activities, therefore, allows measurement of the amount of time people can spend on other more health-enhancing activities in their daily life. Related to this, Nguyen et al., (2013) were unable to accurately detect activities with similar GPS speed and accelerometer data profiles that require different EE and have a different health impact such as non-level and level walking [6]. In order to better detect these activities, in addition to GPS speed, we extracted another distinctive feature (elevation difference) by linking GPS spatial coordinates to DEM data.

Compared to most studies, which use a small sample size, we employed a large sample of thirty-three people that generated a comprehensive training dataset in terms of the diversity of the subjects' physical characteristics and also inspires confidence in our results. We used a customized light portable device with embedded accelerometer and GPS sensors for data collection, which overcomes the drawbacks of using smartphones or multiple devices. Using smartphones reduces the burden on the participant [24,31], as there is no need to carry extra devices; however, smartphones' limited battery and storage makes long-term activity monitoring problematic. Moreover, user interaction with the smartphone, such as making a phone call or sending a text message, can affect the sensor's data quality. Applying multi-devices [5,13,32,34] also entails carrying more devices and therefore a great burden on participants, particularly in real-life PA monitoring. In real-life experiments, well-designed data collection logistics are necessary to ensure that the process is minimally invasive for participants, while providing suitable data quality for researchers. Studies have addressed the question of how different body locations of accelerometers' can influence the performance of PA type detection [10,12,43]. However, it previously remained unknown how GPS sensor data can help in providing minimum a device configuration when used in combination with accelerometer data. Our examination of five device locations showed that the model developed using GPS and accelerometer data from a knee-worn device produces comparable high accuracy (above 80%) to the model developed by using data from multiple devices.

This study has some limitations that should be addressed in future research. The models that included GPS data are limited to detect outdoor activities because there are limitations regarding GPS signal reception in indoor environments and DEM data are only available for outdoor environments. We applied a high resolution DEM (2 m ground resolution) to extract elevation information for each GPS point; using a DEM with low resolution may not lead to similar results. We only used linear interpolation and point-to-curve geometric map matching to preprocess the GPS data. Other interpolation and map matching methods might help to advance the classification performance. The high performance of the developed models, however, can be achieved only when GPS data with few gaps and complete OSM data are available. Low data quality might lead to unreliable PA classification performance. Moreover, as in all such studies, the classification results depend on the target activities and study settings; selecting other activities and experimental conditions might lead to different outcomes. Though we accurately detected three major sub-types of postures (i.e., sitting, standing and lying), we did not aim to detect other sub-types of posture activity such as active standing (which occupies significant percentages of human daily activities) or complex activities [44]. In future studies, a wider range of activities should be included to provide more information about health-related daily PAs. Though we achieved a high classification performance using the RF classifier, applying other advanced machine learning models such as recurrent neural networks including long short-term memory (LSTM) networks [45,46] and comparing their performance may be considered as a future study. Finally, we trained the models using data collected by young healthy adults only. To what extent these models are transferable to older adults is a research question that we would like to answer in a future study.

Author Contributions: Conceptualization, H.A.; Data curation, H.A.; Formal analysis, H.A.; Investigation, H.A.; Methodology, H.A.; Project administration, H.A.; Resources, H.A. and R.W.; Software, H.A. in coordination with L.C. and B.N.; Supervision, R.W.; Validation, H.A.; Visualization, H.A.; Writing—original draft, H.A.; Writing—review and editing, H.A. in coordination with L.C., B.N. and R.W. All authors have read and agreed to the published version of the manuscript.

Funding: This research was in part supported by the University Research Priority Program, "Dynamics of Healthy Aging" of the University of Zurich and the Velux Stiftung (grant no. 917).

Acknowledgments: We would like to thank Alexander Sofios for his technical support. We would like to acknowledge the assistants for the data collection, and the participants who contributed their time for taking part in the study.

Conflicts of Interest: The authors declare no conflict of interest.

Appendix A

Table A1. Activity tasks for the semi-structured data collection.

Activity Task (I)	Activity Task (II)	Duration: 16.5 + 16.5 + 33 1.5 h
First step: Walking at different speed		
Jump and stand still for 5 s at starting point Walk at SLOW speed Turn left at turning point (sharp turn) Walk at SLOW speed Stop at the stop point for 5 s Walk at FAST speed Stop at the stop point for 5 s Walk at NORMAL speed turn left at point (smooth turn) Walk at NORMAL speed Stand still for 5 s at end point and jump	Jump and stand still for 5 s at starting point Walk at NORMAL speed Turn right at turning point (smooth turn) Walk at NORMAL speed Stop at the stop point for 5 s Walk at FAST speed Stop at the stop point for 5 s Walk at SLOW speed turn right at turning point (sharp turn) Walk at SLOW speed Stand still for 5 s at starting point and jump	3 + 3
Second step: Running		
Jump and stand still for 5 s at starting point Run at self-paced speed Turn left at turning point (sharp turn) Run at self-paced speed Stop at the stop point for 5 s Run at self-paced speed Turn left at turning point (smooth turn) Run at self-paced speed Stand still for 5 s at starting point and jump	Jump and stand still for 5 s at starting point Run at self-paced speed Turn right at turning point (smooth turn) Run at self-paced speed Stop at the stop point for 5 s Run at self-paced speed Turn right at turning point (sharp turn) Run at self-paced speed Stand still for 5 s at starting point and jump	1.5 + 1.5
Third step: Cycling		
Jump and stand still for 5 s at starting point Get on the cycle Cycle at self-paced speed Turn left at the turning point Cycle at self-paced speed Turn left at the turning point Stop at the ending point Get off the cycle Stand still for 5 s at starting point and jump	Jump and stand still for 5 s at starting point Get on the cycle Cycle at self-paced speed Turn right at the turning point Cycle at self-paced speed Turn right at the turning point Stop at the ending point Get off the cycle Stand still for 5 s at starting point and jump	1.5 + 1.5
Fourth step: Stairs walking		
Jump and stand still for 5 s at starting point Walk upstairs at normal speed Stand still for 5 s after first floor Walk upstairs at normal speed Stand still for 5 s at ending point and jump	Jump and stand still for 5 s at starting point Walk upstairs at normal speed Stand still for 5 s after first floor Walk upstairs at normal speed Stand still for 5 s at ending point and jump	1 + 1
Jump and stand still for 5 s at starting point Walk downstairs at normal speed Stand still for 5 s after first floor Walk downstairs at normal speed Stand still for 5 s at ending point and jump	Jump and stand still for 5 s at starting point Walk downstairs at normal speed Stand still for 5 s after first floor Walk downstairs at normal speed Stand still for 5 s at ending point and jump	1 + 1
Fifth step: Walking at different slopes		
Jump and stand still for 5 s at starting point Walk uphill at normal speed Stand still for 5 s at ending point and jump	Jump and stand still for 5 s at starting point Walk uphill at normal speed Stand still for 5 s at ending point and jump	2 + 2
Jump and stand still for 5 s at starting point Walk downhill at normal speed Stand still for 5 s at ending point and jump	Jump and stand still for 5 s at starting point Walk downhill at normal speed Stand still for 5 s at ending point and jump	2 + 2
Sixth step: Sedentary activities		

Table A1. Cont.

Activity Task (I)	Activity Task (II)	Duration: 16.5 + 16.5 + 33 1.5 h
Sit		
Jump	Jump	1 + 1
Go from standing position to sitting	Go from standing position to sitting	
Sit for 1 min	Sit for 1 min	
Go from sitting position to standing	Go from sitting position to standing	
Stand	Stand	
Jump	Jump	
Stand		
Jump	Jump	1 + 1
Stand for 1 min	Stand for 1 min	
Jump	Jump	
Lie		
Jump	Jump	1 + 1
Go from standing position to sitting	Go from standing position to sitting	
Sit	Sit	
Go from sitting position to lying on your back	Go from sitting position to lying on your back	
Lie on your back for 1 min	Lie on your back for 1 min	
Go from lying on your back to sitting position	Go from lying on your back to sitting position	
Sit	Sit	
Go from sitting position to standing	Go from sitting position to standing	
Stand	Stand	
Jump	Jump	

Table A2. Activity tasks for the real-life data collection.

Activity	Minimum Duration (Minute)	Location
Sedentary activities		
Lying	1	Outdoors (e.g., on a bench)
Sitting	1	Outdoors (not in a vehicle)
Standing	1	Outdoors (not in a vehicle)
Non-level walking		
Walking uphill	2	Outdoors
Walking downhill	2	Outdoors
Walking downstairs	2 floors (8 steps each)	Outdoors
Walking upstairs	2 floors (8 steps each)	Outdoors
Transport-related activities		
Walking, level ground	5	Leisure area (e.g., park)
	5	Urban area (e.g., street sidewalk)
Cycling, level ground	5	Leisure area (e.g., park)
	5	Urban area (e.g., street bike path)
Running, level ground	1	Leisure area (e.g., park)
	1	Urban area (e.g., street sidewalk)

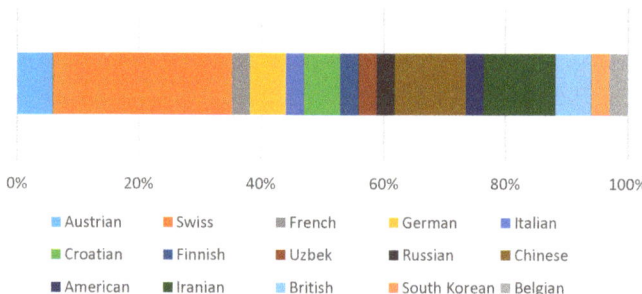

Figure A1. Nationality of the participants involved in the study.

Appendix B

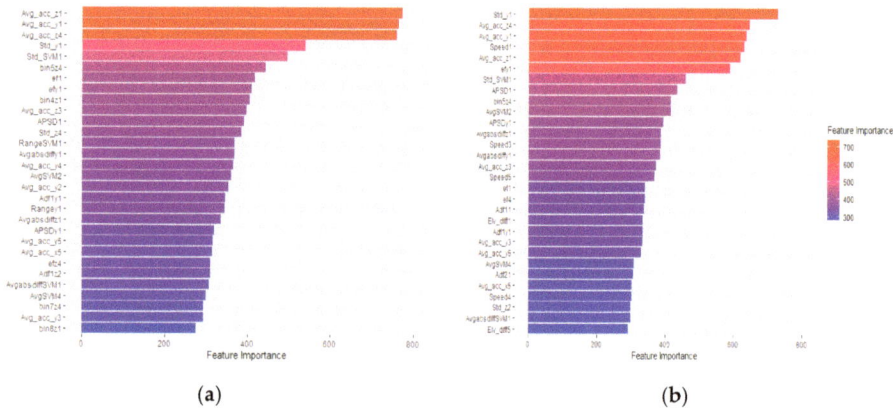

Figure A2. Top 30 important features of a participant's general RF model (with the highest GPS contribution) trained with semi-structured data (see the feature description in Table A3). (**a**) Accelerometer data only and (**b**) accelerometer and GPS data.

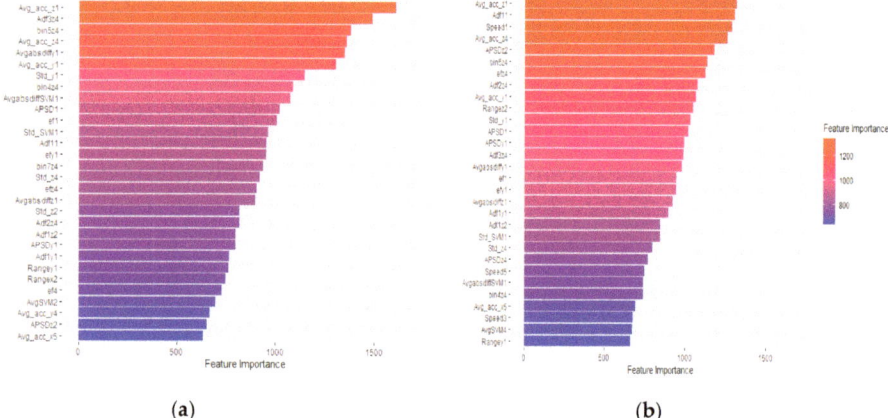

Figure A3. Top 30 important features of a participant's general RF model (with the highest GPS contribution) trained with combined data (see the feature description in Table A3). (**a**) Accelerometer data only and (**b**) accelerometer and GPS data.

Table A3. List of features appearing in Figures A2 and A3.

Feature Notation	Description
1, 2, 3, 4, 5	1 = Chest sensor's data 2 = Knee sensor's data 3 = left hip sensor's data 4 = left pocket sensor' data 5 = right hip sensors' data (e.g., ef1 = energy of total acceleration derived from chest sensor's data)
SVM	Total acceleration
Avg-SVM, Avg-acc-x, Avg-acc-y, Avg-acc-z	Mean of total acceleration and each axis
Std-SVM, Std-x, Std-y, Std-z	Standard deviation of total acceleration and each axis
BinN, BinNx, BinNy, BinNz	Number of observations falling within the Nth bin of total acceleration and each axis
Avgabsdiff, Avgabsdiffx, Avgabsdiffy, Avgabsdiffz	Average absolute difference of total acceleration and each axis
RangeSVM, Rangex, Rangey, Rangez	Range of total acceleration and each axis
APSD, APSDx, APSDy, APSDz	Power spectral density of total acceleration and each axis
ef, efx, efy, efz	Energy of total acceleration and each axis
ADF1, ADF1x, ADF1y, ADF1z	Amplitude of the first dominant frequency of total acceleration and each axis
ADF2, ADF2x, ADF2y, ADF2z	Amplitude of the second dominant frequency of total acceleration and each axis
ADF2, ADF2x, ADF2y, ADF2z	Amplitude of the third dominant frequency of total acceleration and each axis

Table A4. Confusion matrix of a participant when using accelerometer and GPS data for knee position. (Scenario 2).

Accelerometer & GPS	Cycle	Lie	N_Walk	Run	Sit	Stand	Walk	Recall	Precision	F1
Cycle	1245	0	8	1	0	0	11	98	98	98
Lie	0	196	0	0	0	0	0	100	100	100
N_walk	21	0	536	0	0	1	145	76	91	83
Run	0	0	3	254	0	0	3	98	99	98
Sit	1	0	1	0	195	2	0	98	93	95
Stand	0	0	0	0	15	259	0	95	99	97
Walk	0	0	43	1	0	0	1029	96	87	91

References

1. Lee, K.; Kwan, M.-P. Physical activity classification in free-living conditions using smartphone accelerometer data and exploration of predicted results. *Comput. Environ. Urban Syst.* **2018**, *67*, 124–131. [CrossRef]
2. Rippe, J.M.; Ward, A.; Porcari, J.P.; Freedson, P.S. Walking for Health and Fitness. *JAMA* **1988**, *259*, 2720. [CrossRef] [PubMed]
3. Van Hees, V.T.; Golubic, R.; Ekelund, U.; Brage, S. Impact of study design on development and evaluation of an activity-type classifier. *J. Appl. Physiol.* **2013**, *114*, 1042–1051. [CrossRef] [PubMed]
4. Lindemann, U.; Zijlstra, W.; Aminian, K.; Chastin, S.F.; De Bruin, E.D.; Helbostad, J.L.; Bussmann, J.B. Recommendations for Standardizing Validation Procedures Assessing Physical Activity of Older Persons by Monitoring Body Postures and Movements. *Sensors* **2014**, *14*, 1267–1277. [CrossRef]
5. Allahbakhshi, H.; Hinrichs, T.; Huang, H.; Weibel, R. The Key Factors in Physical Activity Type Detection Using Real-Life Data: A Systematic Review. *Front. Physiol.* **2019**, *10*, 75. [CrossRef]
6. Nguyen, D.M.T.; Lecoultre, V.; Sunami, Y.; Schutz, Y. Assessment of physical activity and energy expenditure by GPS combined with accelerometry in real-life conditions. *J. Phys. Act. Health* **2012**, *10*, 880–888. [CrossRef]

7. Gyllensten, I.C.; Bonomi, A.G. Identifying Types of Physical Activity with a Single Accelerometer: Evaluating Laboratory-trained Algorithms in Daily Life. *IEEE Trans. Biomed. Eng.* **2011**, *58*, 2656–2663. [CrossRef] [PubMed]
8. Adaškevičius, R. Method for Recognition of the Physical Activity of Human Being Using a Wearable Accelerometer. *Elektron. Elektrotechnika* **2014**, *20*, 127–131.
9. Barshan, B.; Yüksek, M.C. Recognizing Daily and Sports Activities in Two Open Source Machine Learning Environments Using Body-Worn Sensor Units. *Comput. J.* **2013**, *57*, 1649–1667. [CrossRef]
10. Skotte, J.; Korshøj, M.; Kristiansen, J.; Hanisch, C.; Holtermann, A. Detection of Physical Activity Types Using Triaxial Accelerometers. *J. Phys. Act. Health* **2014**, *11*, 76–84. [CrossRef]
11. El Achkar, C.M.; Lenoble-Hoskovec, C.; Paraschiv-Ionescu, A.; Major, K.; Büla, C.; Aminian, K.; Information, P.E.K.F.C. Instrumented shoes for activity classification in the elderly. *Gait Posture* **2016**, *44*, 12–17. [CrossRef] [PubMed]
12. Cornacchia, M.; Zheng, Y.; Velipasalar, S.; Ozcan, K. A Survey on Activity Detection and Classification Using Wearable Sensors. *IEEE Sens. J.* **2016**, *17*, 386–403. [CrossRef]
13. Troped, P.J.; Oliveira, M.S.; Matthews, C.E.; Cromley, E.K.; Melly, S.J.; Craig, B.A. Prediction of Activity Mode with Global Positioning System and Accelerometer Data. *Med. Sci. Sports Exerc.* **2008**, *40*, 972–978. [CrossRef] [PubMed]
14. Maddison, R.; Jiang, Y.; Hoorn, S.V.; Exeter, D.; Ni Mhurchu, C.; Dorey, E. Describing patterns of physical activity in adolescents using global positioning systems and accelerometry. *Pediatr. Exerc. Sci.* **2010**, *22*, 392–407. [CrossRef] [PubMed]
15. Quigg, R.; Gray, A.; Reeder, A.I.; Holt, A.; Waters, D.L. Using accelerometers and GPS units to identify the proportion of daily physical activity located in parks with playgrounds in New Zealand children. *Prev. Med.* **2010**, *50*, 235–240. [CrossRef] [PubMed]
16. Wheeler, B.W.; Cooper, A.R.; Page, A.S.; Jago, R. Greenspace and children's physical activity: A GPS/GIS analysis of the PEACH project. *Prev. Med.* **2010**, *51*, 148–152. [CrossRef]
17. Cebrecos, A.; Díez, J.; Gullón, P.; Bilal, U.; Franco, M.; Escobar, F. Characterizing physical activity and food urban environments: A GIS-based multicomponent proposal. *Int. J. Health Geogr.* **2016**, *15*, 35. [CrossRef]
18. Brown, G.; Schebella, M.F.; Weber, D. Using participatory GIS to measure physical activity and urban park benefits. *Landsc. Urban Plan.* **2014**, *121*, 34–44. [CrossRef]
19. E Thornton, L.; Pearce, J.R.; Kavanagh, A.M. Using Geographic Information Systems (GIS) to assess the role of the built environment in influencing obesity: A glossary. *Int. J. Behav. Nutr. Phys. Act.* **2011**, *8*, 71. [CrossRef]
20. Oakes, J.M.; Forsyth, A.; Schmitz, K.H. The effects of neighborhood density and street connectivity on walking behavior: The Twin Cities walking study. *Epidemiol. Perspect. Innov.* **2007**, *4*, 16. [CrossRef]
21. Saelens, B.E.; Sallis, J.F.; Black, J.B.; Chen, D. Neighborhood-Based Differences in Physical Activity: An Environment Scale Evaluation. *Am. J. Public Health* **2003**, *93*, 1552–1558. [CrossRef] [PubMed]
22. Almanza, E.; Jerrett, M.; Dunton, G.; Seto, E.; Pentz, M.A. A study of community design, greenness, and physical activity in children using satellite, GPS and accelerometer data. *Health Place* **2011**, *18*, 46–54. [CrossRef] [PubMed]
23. Troped, P.J.; Wilson, J.S.; Matthews, C.E.; Cromley, E.K.; Melly, S.J. The built environment and location-based physical activity. *Am. J. Prev. Med.* **2010**, *38*, 429–438. [CrossRef] [PubMed]
24. Lee, K.; Kwan, M.-P. Automatic physical activity and in-vehicle status classification based on GPS and accelerometer data: A hierarchical classification approach using machine learning techniques. *Trans. GIS* **2018**, *22*, 1522–1549. [CrossRef]
25. Miller, H.J.; Tribby, C.P.; Brown, B.B.; Smith, K.R.; Werner, C.M.; Wolf, J.; Wilson, L.; Oliveira, M.G.S. Public transit generates new physical activity: Evidence from individual GPS 583 and accelerometer data before and after light rail construction in a neighborhood of Salt Lake City, Utah, USA. *Health Place* **2015**, *36*, 8–17. [CrossRef]
26. Schutz, Y.; Chambaz, A. Could a satellite-based navigation system (GPS) be used to assess the physical activity of individuals on earth? *Eur. J. Clin. Nutr.* **1997**, *51*, 338–339. [CrossRef]
27. Townshend, A.D.; Worringham, C.J.; Stewart, I.B. Assessment of Speed and Position during Human Locomotion Using Nondifferential GPS. *Med. Sci. Sports Exerc.* **2008**, *40*, 124–132. [CrossRef]

28. Witte, T.; Wilson, A. Accuracy of non-differential GPS for the determination of speed over ground. *J. Biomech.* **2004**, *37*, 1891–1898. [CrossRef]
29. Larsson, P.; Henriksson-Larsén, K. The use of dGPS and simultaneous metabolic measurements during orienteering. *Med. Sci. Sports Exerc.* **2001**, *33*, 1919–1924. [CrossRef]
30. Perrin, O.; Terrier, P.; Ladetto, Q.; Merminod, B.; Schutz, Y. Improvement of walking speed prediction by accelerometry and altimetry, validated by satellite positioning. *Med. Biol. Eng.* **2000**, *38*, 164–168. [CrossRef]
31. Reddy, S.; Mun, M.; Burke, J.; Estrin, D.; Hansen, M.; Srivastava, M. Using mobile phones to determine transportation modes. *ACM Trans. Sens. Netw.* **2010**, *6*, 13. [CrossRef]
32. Ellis, K.; Godbole, S.; Marshall, S.; Lanckriet, G.; Staudenmayer, J.; Kerr, J. Identifying Active Travel Behaviors in Challenging Environments Using GPS, Accelerometers, and Machine Learning Algorithms. *Front. Public Health* **2014**, *2*, 2–36. [CrossRef]
33. Brondeel, R.; Pannier, B.; Chaix, B. Using GPS, GIS, and Accelerometer Data to Predict Transportation Modes. *Med. Sci. Sports Exerc.* **2015**, *47*, 2669–2675. [CrossRef] [PubMed]
34. Ermes, M.; Parkka, J.; Mantyjarvi, J.; Korhonen, I. Detection of Daily Activities and Sports with Wearable Sensors in Controlled and Uncontrolled Conditions. *IEEE Trans. Inf. Technol. Biomed.* **2008**, *12*, 20–26. [CrossRef] [PubMed]
35. Spinsante, S.; Angelici, A.; Lundström, J.; Espinilla, M.; Cleland, I.; Nugent, C. A Mobile Application for Easy Design and Testing of Algorithms to Monitor Physical Activity in the Workplace. *Mob. Inf. Syst.* **2016**, *2016*, 5126816. [CrossRef]
36. Armstrong, T.; Bull, F. Development of the World Health Organization Global Physical 609 Activity Questionnaire (GPAQ). *Public Health* **2016**, *14*, 66–70. [CrossRef]
37. Allahbakhshi, H.; Haosheng, H.; Weibel, R. A Study Design for Physical Activity 611 Reference Data Collection Using GPS and Accelerometer. In Proceedings of the 21th AGILE 612 Conference on Geographic Information Science, Lund, Sweden, 12–15 June 2018; pp. 1–6.
38. Allahbakhshi, H.; Weibel, R. Transferability of PA type detection models between different age cohorts. **2020**, in press.
39. Quddus, M.A.; Ochieng, W.Y.; Noland, R.B. Current map-616 matching algorithms for transport applications: State-of-the art and future research directions. *Transp. Res. Part C Emerg. Technol.* **2007**, *15*, 312–328. [CrossRef]
40. OpenStreetMap Contributors. "OpenStreetMap". Available online: www.openstreetmap.org (accessed on 15 August 2019).
41. R Core Team. *R: A Language and Environment for Statistical Computing*; R Foundation for Statistical Computing: Vienna, Austria, 2013. Available online: http://www.r-project.org/ (accessed on 13 February 2012).
42. Wright, M.N.; Ziegler, A. ranger: A Fast Implementation of Random Forests for High Dimensional Data in C++ and R. *J. Stat. Softw.* **2017**, *77*. [CrossRef]
43. De Vries, S.I.; Garre, F.G.; Engbers, L.H.; Hildebrandt, V.H.; Van Buuren, S. Evaluation of Neural Networks to Identify Types of Activity Using Accelerometers. *Med. Sci. Sports Exerc.* **2011**, *43*, 101–107. [CrossRef]
44. Liu, L.; Wang, S.; Hu, B.; Qiong, Q.; Wen, J.; Rosenblum, D.S. Learning structures of interval-based Bayesian networks in probabilistic generative model for human complex activity recognition. *Pattern Recognit.* **2018**, *81*, 545–561. [CrossRef]
45. Zhang, Y.; Wang, C.; Gong, L.; Lu, Y.; Sun, F.; Xu, C.; Li, X.; Zhou, X. A Power-Efficient Accelerator Based on FPGAs for LSTM Network. In Proceedings of the 2017 IEEE International Conference on Cluster Computing (CLUSTER), Honolulu, HI, USA, 5–8 September 2017; pp. 629–630.
46. Guan, Y.; Yuan, Z.; Sun, G.; Cong, J. FPGA-based accelerator for long short-term memory recurrent neural networks. In Proceedings of the 2017 22nd Asia and South Pacific Design Automation Conference (ASP-DAC), Chiba, Japan, 16–19 January 2017; pp. 629–634.

© 2020 by the authors. Licensee MDPI, Basel, Switzerland. This article is an open access article distributed under the terms and conditions of the Creative Commons Attribution (CC BY) license (http://creativecommons.org/licenses/by/4.0/).

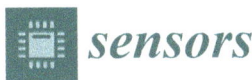

Article

Quantile Coarsening Analysis of High-Volume Wearable Activity Data in a Longitudinal Observational Study

Ying Kuen Cheung [1,*], Pei-Yun Sabrina Hsueh [2], Ipek Ensari [3], Joshua Z. Willey [4] and Keith M. Diaz [3]

1. Department of Biostatistics, Mailman School of Public Health, Columbia University, New York, NY 10032, USA
2. IBM Watson Research Center, Yorktown Heights, NY 10598, USA; phsueh@us.ibm.com
3. Center for Behavioral Cardiovascular Health, Department of Medicine, Columbia University Medical Center, New York, NY 10032, USA; ie2145@cumc.columbia.edu (I.E.); kd2442@cumc.columbia.edu (K.M.D.)
4. Department of Neurology, Columbia University Medical Center, New York, NY 10032, USA; jzw2@cumc.columbia.edu
* Correspondence: yc632@cumc.columbia.edu; Tel.: +1-212-305-3332

Received: 13 August 2018; Accepted: 6 September 2018; Published: 12 September 2018

Abstract: Owing to advances in sensor technologies on wearable devices, it is feasible to measure physical activity of an individual continuously over a long period. These devices afford opportunities to understand individual behaviors, which may then provide a basis for tailored behavior interventions. The large volume of data however poses challenges in data management and analysis. We propose a novel quantile coarsening analysis (QCA) of daily physical activity data, with a goal to reduce the volume of data while preserving key information. We applied QCA to a longitudinal study of 79 healthy participants whose step counts were monitored for up to 1 year by a Fitbit device, performed cluster analysis of daily activity, and identified individual activity signature or pattern in terms of the clusters identified. Using 21,393 time series of daily physical activity, we identified eight clusters. Employment and partner status were each associated with 5 of the 8 clusters. Using less than 2% of the original data, QCA provides accurate approximation of the mean physical activity, forms meaningful activity patterns associated with individual characteristics, and is a versatile tool for dimension reduction of densely sampled data.

Keywords: citizen science; cluster analysis; physical activity; sedentary behavior; walking

1. Introduction

Physical activity has been shown to improve cardiovascular health, reduce risk of mortality [1–4] and is an important component of primary prevention for many chronic diseases and conditions such as Type 2 diabetes and obesity [5,6]. Walking, in particular, is recognized as an easily accessible, convenient, and familiar mode of physical activity, and thus is an appealing strategy for the promotion of health and well-being. As such there is impetus for examining walking behaviors as a predictor of multiple health outcomes in ambulatory, community-dwelling adults.

Advances in sensor technologies on wearable devices have enabled the continuous and accurate collection of step counts and other walking parameters over an extended period of time, thus providing a voluminous stream of data. The large amount of data provides an opportunity to better understand the daily physical activity patterns across populations. However, conventional analytical approaches focus on measuring physical activity patterns by predefined summary statistics such as total step counts and average minutes with activity on a given day. By summarizing physical activity at the daily level, however, these methods ignore between-day heterogeneity within a person, as they fail to capture the within-day patterns of activity. An understanding of within-day patterns of physical activity is of importance to facilitate individualized mobile experience, such as when push notifications and activity updates are being sent [7,8], and identifying changes in an individual's daily routines, thereby facilitating tailored behavior intervention [9,10]. Given the broad use of step-counting trackers to monitor and improve physical activity [11–25], analyzing sensor data beyond predefined daily features thus can have significant public health impact.

Multivariate finite mixture modeling (MFMM) is a clustering method, whose purpose is to identify homogeneous subgroups wherein the number of subgroups is not assumed to be known in the analysis. The MFMM analysis is model-based, data-driven, and aims to produce subgroups with features arising from the same statistical distribution; dividing the data into an optimal number of subgroups based on specific criteria such as the Bayesian information criterion [26]. Clustering algorithms utilizing MFMM methods have been applied to identify dietary patterns [27,28] and physical activity patterns based on questionnaire data [29]. These algorithms often entail prespecifying only a small-to-moderate number of features as input variables, as the computational complexity grows exponentially with the addition of more features [30]. In the present context where the goal is to examine the within-day activity patterns, hundreds of physical activity inputs can be recorded from sensors throughout a day (e.g., minute-by-minute step counts), existing clustering algorithms may prove to be computationally infeasible without properly reducing the dimension of the data in a pre-processing step.

Dimension reduction of sensor data continuously collected can be achieved by time series modeling of the data [31–34]. Typically, a time series is first transformed to a domain relevant to the scientific interest, and is then summarized by a few parameters (e.g., autocorrelation). These parameters in turn serve as input features in a clustering algorithm. In this article, we take a similar approach and propose a two-step method for analyzing sensor data as time series: the proposed method first transforms the daily physical activity data into a coarsened probability density function of quantiles of activity time, and then applies the MFMM analysis using the quantiles as input features. The method is thus called quantile coarsening analysis (QCA). This approach is motivated by the consideration that time of activity, as well as the amount of activity, is of primary interest in our application. As will be shown in *Statistical Analyses* below, the resolution or coarseness of dimension reduction can be set by users in accordance with the needs in their application; such flexibility distinguishes the proposed method from the traditional parametric modeling of time series data [35]. The purposes of this article are to demonstrate the feasibility of QCA in a data set of 21,393 time series of daily physical activity, and to examine its estimation properties under various degrees of coarseness.

2. Materials and Methods

2.1. Study Cohort

A single cohort, 12-month, intensive observational study was conducted in healthy adults with an objective to collect their personal daily stress and physical activity for associative analysis. The study was approved by Columbia University Medical Center's (CUMC) institutional review board. All participants provided informed consent. Access to the study dataset and information about the study's execution and materials is publicly available [36].

Potentially eligible participants were identified and screened at CUMC. The inclusion criteria were (i) aged 18 years or older; (ii) self-reported intermittent exerciser (i.e., exercise 6–11 times per month but did not have a regular workout schedule); (iii) having access to a personal computer and a smartphone. Exclusion criteria included individuals who (i) were unavailable for 12 continuous months; (ii) had serious medical comorbidity that would compromise their ability to engage in usual physical activity; (iii) had occupational work demands that required rigorous activity; or (iv) were unable to read and speak English. From January 2014 to July 2015, a total of 79 participants were enrolled and followed for 12 months. For the purpose of this article, we considered the physical activity data (described below). Details of enrollment, participant characteristics, and other association studies of stress level were previously reported [37]. Briefly, the data set for the present analysis consisted of 45 females and 34 males, with an overall mean age of 31.9 years (±9.5 years). In addition, we considered the following variables for association with physical activity: race/ethnicity (27 non-Hispanic whites vs. 52 others), education as an ordinal variable (13 having less than college vs. 34 completing college vs. 32 attaining graduate or professional degrees), employment status (64 full-time employed vs. 8 part-time), and partner status (32 having a partner or spouse vs. 45 being single).

2.2. Physical Activity

Physical activity was monitored continuously for up to 12 months using a wrist-worn Fitbit activity monitor (Fitbit Flex) [38]. The Fitbit device, containing an accelerometer and an altimeter, tracks the wearer's daily physical activity including steps, distance walked, and stairs climbed, and has been previously validated for measuring physical activity [39]. While the Fitbit devices (including the Fitbit Flex) have been demonstrated to have good validity for the objective measurement of physical activity, their accuracy has largely been reported for stepping-related physical activities (e.g., walking and running) [40]. Similar to other research-grade accelerometers, the Fitbit devices have poor accuracy for the measurement of cycling [41,42]. Furthermore, Fitbit instructs users to not swim with the Fitbit Flex because it is not waterproof [43], thus rendering it unable to assess swimming-based exercise.

Data from the devices were automatically uploaded to the Fitbit website whenever the device was within 15 feet of the base station, which was plugged into the participant's own personal computer. Participants were instructed to sync and charge their device every 5–7 days to ensure no loss of activity data. The Fitbit accelerometer recorded data in one-minute epochs, starting at 12:00 a.m. and ending at 23:59 p.m. every day, yielding a time series of 1440 minute-epochs per day per individual. The raw minute-by-minute step count data were extracted from the manufacturer's website using Fitabase (Small Steps Labs, San Diego, CA, USA) and were reduced using a novel QCA, described in *Statistical Analyses* below. Specifically, the raw data that was relevant to the present article included the step counts over one-minute intervals with a timestamp; data for each participant was converted to an "RDATA" file each associated with a unique participant ID. Based on the raw data, we calculated other predefined physical activity measurements, including total daily step counts, the duration in minutes of physical activity (PA, defined as having at least 50 steps in a minute), and activity midday (defined as the time when 50% of daily step counts were achieved).

2.3. Statistical Analyses

2.3.1. Quantile Coarsening Analysis (QCA)

Let $Y(t)$ denote the step counts at time t and $S(t) = \int_0^t Y(u)du$ be the cumulative activity up to time $t \in (0, t_{max})$. Then

$$T(p) \inf\{t : S(t) \geq p\, S(t_{max})\} \tag{1}$$

denotes the time where $100p$ percent of the total activity has been achieved and will be referred to as the $100p$th quantile of the activity time [44]. Specifically, activity midday is defined by the 50th quantile, $T(0.5)$. The idea of QCA is to represent a time series $Y(t)$ using multiple quantiles $T(p_j)$ for a prespecified set of $p_1 < p_2 < \ldots < p_K$, together with the total daily counts $S(t_{max})$. The number K of quantiles determines the number of components used to represent $Y(t)$, and hence controls the resolution or coarseness of the approximation. Define the Kth order quantile-coarse function of $Y(t)$ as

$$C_K Y(t) = \frac{S(t_{max})}{(K+1)\{T(p_{j+1}) - T(p_j)\}} \text{ for } T(p_j) \leq t < T(p_{j+1}) \tag{2}$$

for $j = 0, \ldots, K$, with the convention that $T(0) = 0$ and $T(1) = t_{max}$. While p_j can be any values between 0 and 1, we consider an evenly spaced grid, i.e., setting $p_j = j/(K+1)$ for $j = 1, \ldots, K$. It can be easily shown that the quantile-coarse function is invariant under the quantile transformation. That is to say, applying the quantile transformation to $C_K Y(t)$ will result in the same quantile representation as applying the transformation to the original $Y(t)$, i.e., $C_K\{C_K Y(t)\} = C_K Y(t)$. As a result, there is no loss in information by converting between coarsened data and quantiles back and forth for any given K.

Our data set consisted of a total of 21,393 days of minute-by-minute step counts from 79 study participants. For each daily time series, we evaluated the quantile-coarse function. The mean time series $\overline{Y}(t)$ of each cluster was then approximated by the corresponding mean quantile-coarse function $\overline{C_K Y}(t)$. We calculated the integrated mean squared error:

$$\int_0^{t_{max}} \left\{\overline{C_K Y}(t) - \overline{Y}(t)\right\}^2 dt \tag{3}$$

to assess the accuracy of the quantile coarsening method under various coarseness values K.

2.3.2. Cluster Analysis

We performed cluster analysis using MFMM with the quantile-coarse function $C_K Y(t)$ as input. Specifically, we considered $K = 19$ so that each time series $Y(t)$ was represented by a total of 20 features, namely, $T(0.05)$, $T(0.10)$, $T(0.15)$, ..., $T(0.95)$, and $S(t_{max})$. Note that although we did not use common features such as PA minutes as direct inputs of the cluster analysis, these features were implicitly incorporated as they could be approximated from a quantile-coarse function. The number of clusters was determined based on the Bayesian information criterion [45]. After the MFMM analysis, physical activity features of each cluster were described using means and standard deviations, along with the mean time series $\overline{Y}(t)$ of each cluster.

2.3.3. Association Studies

In order to identify important factors affecting a participant's physical activity behaviors in terms of the identified clusters, association between the cluster membership and participant characteristics was assessed using generalized linear mixed model (GLMM) with a logit link in a univariate manner, with an adjustment for a weekend/weekday random effect nested within a subject random effect. For comparison purposes, we also examined the association of step-count based clusters with participant characteristics using the same GLMM approach.

3. Results

3.1. Physical Activity Clusters by Multivariate Finite Mixture Modeling

The MFMM analysis found an eight-cluster solution among the 21,393 series. Table 1 reports some summary physical activity measures in each cluster. The clusters were organized according to the average daily step counts, which were in concordance with PA duration. The least active cluster (Cluster 1) on average completed just below 1000 steps a day with 7.3 min in PA; this subgroup of activity either depicted a very sedentary pattern or effectively identified inactivity due to non-wear. The most active group (Cluster 8) had about 10,000 counts on average with 73 min in PA. The next two most active clusters (Clusters 6 and 7) had similar activity level to Cluster 8 and were within 1000 steps daily on average. However, activity midday in these clusters, ranging from noon to 3:00 p.m., occurred earlier than that of Cluster 8. While not as inactive as Cluster 1, Clusters 2 and 3 had low PA level when compared to the higher clusters, with different activity midday. Clusters 4 and 5 represented days of intermediate PA level.

Table 1. Physical activity clusters by multivariate finite mixture modeling.

Cluster ID	1	2	3	4	5	6	7	8
N	409	1302	2285	2751	7819	1678	2326	2823
Daily step counts	961	6227	6855	8037	8999	9379	9396	10,038
Activity midday [a]	11:30 a.m.	1:00 p.m.	2:00 p.m.	3:30 p.m.	2:00 p.m.	Noon	3:00 p.m.	5:00 p.m.
PA minutes [b]	7.3	42.3	45.6	52.8	59.9	65.9	65.1	72.7
Weekend [c]	37%	40%	39%	35%	16%	46%	30%	23%

[a] Time of day when 50% of daily counts were achieved; time was rounded to nearest half-hour. [b] Duration (in minutes) with ≥ 50 counts per minute. [c] Percent of time series in the cluster being on a weekend.

Figure 1 shows the mean activity curves of the clusters, and the superimposed cumulative activities of the clusters (lower right figure). These plots reveal additional cluster-defining features. Specifically, Cluster 2 was characterized by very early (i.e., late night) activity. Clusters 6 and 8 had peak activity averaged at around noon and 6:00 p.m. respectively, whereas Cluster 5 had multiple peaks throughout the day (at around 8:00 a.m., noon, and 5:00 p.m.).

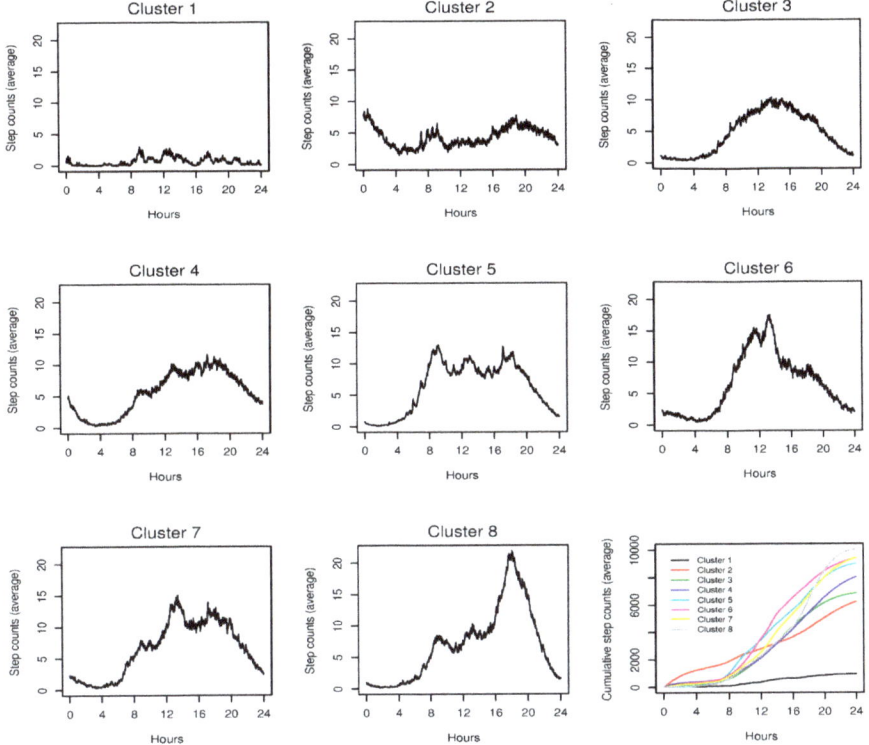

Figure 1. Mean activity of the 8 physical activity clusters by multivariate finite mixture modeling. Lower right: Superimposed cumulative step counts of the 8 clusters.

3.2. Activity Patterns and the Weekends

Table 1 also shows the proportion of daily activity falling on a weekend for each cluster, and demonstrates a range across the eight groups with $\geq 40\%$ of time series in Clusters 2 and 6 occurring on a weekend, and 16% in Cluster 5 being on a weekend. Generally, it is also noted that the time series in the inactive clusters (Clusters 1–3) tended to fall on weekends.

Figure 2 further shows the PA patterns of the 79 participants were very different on weekdays and on weekends, with Cluster 5 being clearly a weekday phenomenon in most participants. It was consistent with the fact that Cluster 5 was characterized by spikes in activity around morning commute, lunch, and evening commute (Figure 1). At the same time, the heatmaps showed variations among the participants and that some did not follow this weekday/weekend differential (e.g., Participants 11 and 16). In addition, the PA patterns on the weekends were more dispersed than those on the weekdays, suggesting weekend activities were less structured and more heterogenous across participants.

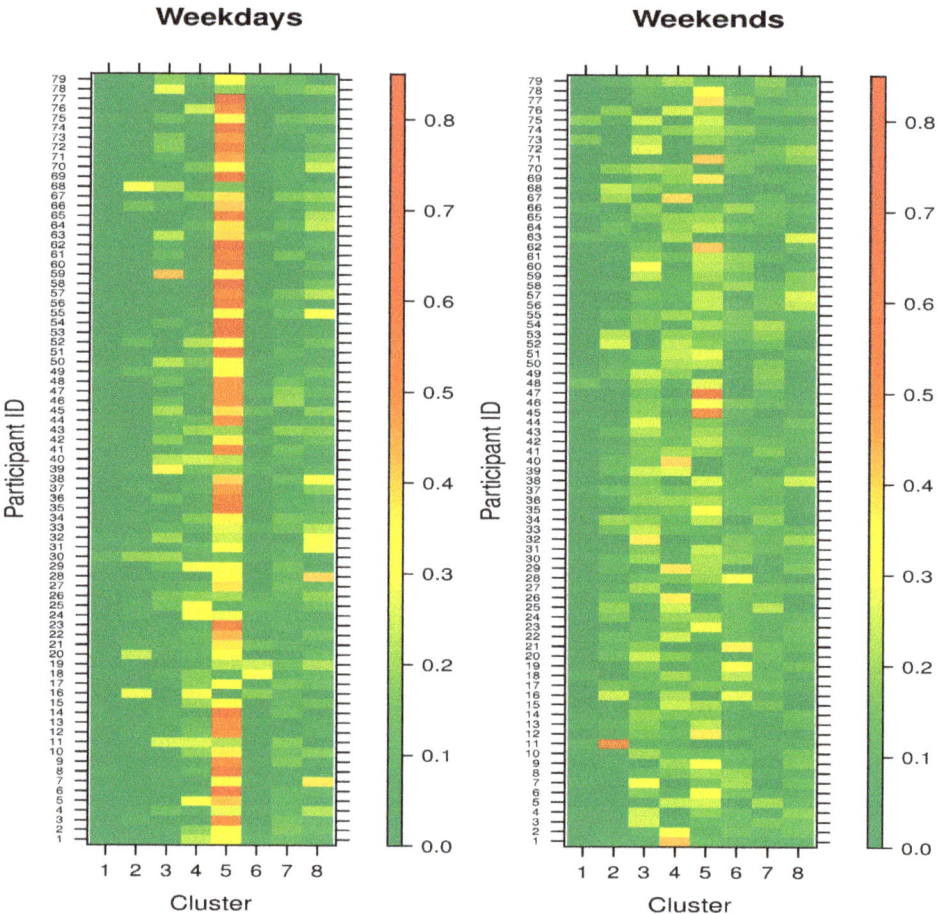

Figure 2. Heatmap of activity patterns of the 79 participants on weekdays and weekends. The color code indicates the proportion of days that a participant fell into each activity cluster.

3.3. Physical Activity Clusters and Participant Characteristics

Table 2 gives the association between each cluster and participant characteristics, in terms of odds ratio of falling into one activity cluster vs. the others using GLMM. In this cohort, employment and partner statuses were the most influential predictors of activity, each associated with 5 PA clusters. Specifically, Cluster 5 was highly significantly ($p < 0.01$) associated with being full-time employed and having a partner/spouse. Interestingly, the association between Cluster 5 and employment status was significant after adjusting for the weekend/weekday effect, suggesting that employment had a structural impact on an individual's behaviors and habits beyond the physical constraint it has during a workweek.

In contrast, Clusters 2 and 4, both having very early activity (Figure 1), were associated with singles with part-time jobs; having a younger age and receiving less education were also associated with these two clusters.

To a lesser extent, race/ethnicity was also predictive of an individual's activity behaviors. Specifically, non-Hispanic whites were more likely to engage in physical activities consistent with Clusters 5 and 8, and less with Cluster 2. Finally, it is interesting to note that the inactive cluster (Cluster 1) was not associated with any particular characteristics.

Table 2. Association (odds ratio) of physical activity clusters and participant characteristics.

Cluster ID	1	2	3	4	5	6	7	8
Age [a]	0.99	0.96 ***	0.99	0.98 *	1.02 *	1.01	1.00	1.01
Male (ref: Female)	0.77	0.94	0.80	1.37	0.86	1.04	1.02	0.95
NHW [b] (ref: others)	0.65	0.60 *	0.80	0.85	1.35 *	1.04	0.91	1.23 *
Education [c]	1.02	0.66 **	1.01	0.75 *	1.15	1.17	0.91	1.11
Full-time (FT) (ref: Part-time, PT)	1.17	0.44 *	0.93	0.42 ***	3.49 ***	0.57 **	1.01	1.41 *
Being single (ref: Partner/spouse)	0.74	2.37 ***	0.76*	1.72 ***	0.65 **	1.02	1.19 *	0.85

[a] Odds ratio per one-year increase in age. [b] NHW: Non-hispanic white. [c] Education as an ordinal variable: 0 = less than college; 1 = college graduate; 2 = above college. * ≤ 0.05, ** ≤ 0.01, *** ≤ 0.001.

3.4. Accuracy of Approximation

Table 3 gives the integrated mean squared errors of the quantile-coarse function using different values of K for estimating the mean activity of the 8 patterns. Accuracy improves as the original function $\overline{Y}(t)$ is represented with a larger number K of quantiles, with the initial improvement being most substantial. With K = 19, the mean squared error was about 3% on average of the error when daily activity was summarized using only the total daily counts (K = 0).

Table 3. Integrated mean squared errors in estimating the mean activity of the eight clusters.

K	1	2	3	4	5	6	7	8
0 [a]	563	3191	15,674	16,106	22,800	32,004	26,226	47,884
3	224	1690	5189	3926	13,473	8631	7356	15,360
9	59	609	880	908	2763	1519	2132	3084
19	29	255	253	342	676	506	626	826
39	19	131	98	135	181	188	211	237

[a] = 0 corresponds to approximation using daily step counts only; activity is assumed to be uniform throughout the day.

4. Discussion

We have proposed a novel QCA for reducing dimension of data collected from wearable devices, and for representing data in conjunction with downstream analyses such as MFMM and association studies. The proposed method contributes to the analysis and management of wearable data in two ways. First, quantile transformation lends itself to making inferences about the time of activity, which could be useful in distinguishing individuals and days from a single individual with differing patterns of PA accrual. Using data from an intensive, 12-month observational study, we were able to identify 8 unique clusters (or subgroups) that characterized the various types of PA accrual patterns observed at the day-level and were able to link these clusters with participant characteristics that provided important contextual information regarding the observed patterns. For example, we observed a "worker" cluster (Cluster 5) associated with employment status wherein spikes in activity were observed around times of day that typically coincide with morning commute, lunch, and evening commute. We also observed active clusters that accrued much of the activity earlier or later in the day (Clusters 6–8), possibly reflective of morning or evening exercise. On the other hand, it is interesting to note that the most active pattern (Cluster 8) accumulates steps late in the day and is associated with full-time employment, suggesting these are intentional leisure-time physical activities. This is consistent with the literature that individuals who meet physical activity guidelines are those who engage in leisure-time physical activity [46]. In contrast, when we performed cluster analysis using total step counts only (i.e., not including time of activity as inputs), all but one cluster had an activity midday at 2:30 p.m. (Table 1). And as a result, we identified fewer and weaker association between the step-count based clusters and participant characteristics (Table 2); this analysis did provide nuances about the nature of activity, which in turn could be useful for developing applications of individualized intervention.

Second, QCA facilitates large-scale data reduction, as quantile transformation requires only simple and scalable computations. We have demonstrated the method in a dataset of 21,393 time series (over 30 million minute-by-minute counts) from 79 participants for up to 1-year follow-up as a proof of concept. In real-life situations where deployment of mobile sensors such as Fitbit can occur at a much larger scale for a much longer duration, the large data volume will be a practical issue for storage and analyses and for the deployment of edge computing [47]. In a typical application, data are transmitted from the devices and stored externally on a server or in a cloud platform for specific analyses. Quantile coarsening in this context can be used as a data pre-processing step to minimize the volume of data transmission, storage, and persistence demand. As the size of the wearable devices tends to be small, their computational capacity is often limited. As such, continuous sensing may pose challenges to existing multi-modal analysis techniques using wearable devices. Since quantile transformation is easy to implement and can be computed independently of data from other individuals, simple scripts can be written to execute on the edge devices as well as on the server level. Depending on the purpose of the analysis, the end-user can specify the level of resolution in terms of the number K of quantiles needed. Our analyses show that the mean quantile-coarse function provides good approximation of the original mean function with only 20 data points per day per individual, representing less than 2% of the original amount of data (1440 data points). In addition, at the deployment time, QCA can also be applied on the incoming streams of data to compare to pre-stored cluster characteristics identified from the cluster analysis. This can lend support to the implementation of many other dynamic, just-in-time adaptive interventions that are key to persuasive reminder and sustainable behavioral changes [48].

The high volume of step count data offers the opportunities to tailor behavior intervention of each individual in a highly personalized manner. Specifically, we have created an activity behavior signature for each individual over time (Figure 2), which can serve as the basis of adaptive intervention. For instance, we could adapt the "dose" and time of push notifications if there are indications that an individual deviate from his/her own norm. The use of signature is broadly applicable to other behavioral intervention system such as centralized recommenders of health apps [49–51]. To allow for such tailored intervention, it is important to acknowledge individual behaviors are not monolithic, but heterogeneous. It is therefore important to note that our analysis goal was to identify clusters of daily activity as building blocks of each signature, as opposed to identify clusters of individuals. While within-day metrics (such as intensity and regularity [52]) have been examined to reflect enrich the heterogeneity in between-day activities of each individual, these approaches typically are semi-quantitative and are intended for visualization.

In the present article, we have shown the feasibility of QCA in a small cohort of relatively healthy individuals. The study design and analytical methods can be easily deployed to other populations. For example, the Northern Manhattan Study aims to assess risk factors for stroke and cardiovascular diseases, and has examined and analyzed the physical activity patterns of the cohort based on paper questionnaires [3,29]. It would be an interesting next step to follow up on these individuals to monitor and assess their mobility issues using wearables, and to provide additional information (signature) that contributes to cardiovascular risks.

We applied QCA to step count data. The method however is applicable to other data variety and supports monitoring of biometrics (e.g., heart rate, ambulatory blood pressure, etc.), location (e.g., indoor/outdoor), behaviors (e.g., medication adherence), exogenous factors such as weather, and user-input data via ecological momentary assessment. There is a growing trend towards self-monitoring on a daily basis with goals such as tracking health status, ameliorating exacerbations of chronic conditions, and avoiding episodic hospitalization; see [53–57] for example. As such, wearables devices are well-suited for this new approach to patient care, provided that they are capable of handling complex analysis efficiently (resulting in smaller and lighter devices with longer battery life). At the same time, we acknowledge that accelerometers are not capable of capturing some of the more common forms of aerobic exercise. Research- and commercial-grade accelerometers such as those made by Fitbit have poor accuracy for the measurement of cycling and cannot be worn while swimming due to not being waterproof [41,42]. However, given the versatility of the QCA, it shall provide useful unified analytical tools for the high data variety in multi-modal monitoring as sensing technologies advance.

Author Contributions: Conceptualization, Y.K.C. and K.M.D.; Methodology & Formal analysis, Y.K.C.; Resources, Y.K.C. and K.M.D.; Writing—Original Draft, Y.K.C.; Writing—Review & Editing, Y.K.C., P.-Y.S.H., I.E., J.Z.W. and K.M.D.

Funding: This work was partly supported by NIH grants R01HL111195 and R01MH109496.

Conflicts of Interest: The authors declare no conflict of interest.

References

1. World Health Organization. *Global Health Risks: Mortality and Burden of Disease Attributable to Selected Major Risks*; WHO Press: Geneva, Switzerland, 2009.
2. Garcia, M.C.; Bastian, B.; Rossen, L.M.; Anderson, R.; Minino, A.; Yoon, P.W.; Faul, M.; Massetti, G.; Thomas, C.C.; Hong, Y.; et al. *Potentially Preventable Deaths among the Five Leading Causes of Death—United States, 2010 and 2014*; Morbidity and Mortality Weekly Report (MMWR): Atlanta, GA, USA, 18 November 2016; Volume 65, pp. 1245–1255.
3. Cheung, Y.K.; Moon, Y.P.; Kulick, E.R.; Sacco, R.L.; Elkind, M.S.V.; Willey, J.Z. Leisure-time physical activity and cardiovascular mortality in an elderly population in northern Manhattan: A prospective cohort study. *J. Gen. Int. Med.* **2017**, *32*, 168–174. [CrossRef] [PubMed]
4. Diaz, K.M.; Howard, V.J.; Hutto, B.; Colabianchi, N.; Vena, J.E.; Safford, M.M.; Blair, S.N.; Hooker, S.P. Patterns of sedentary behavior and mortality in U.S. middle-aged and older adults. *Ann. Int. Med.* **2017**, *167*, 465–475. [CrossRef] [PubMed]
5. Motl, R.W. Theoretical models for understanding physical activity behavior among children and adolescents—Social cognitive theory and self-determination theory. *J. Teach. Phys. Edu.* **2007**, *26*, 350–357. [CrossRef]
6. Bravata, D.M.; Smith-Spangler, C.; Sundaram, V.; Gienger, A.L.; Lin, N.; Lewis, R.; Stave, C.D.; Olkin, I.; Sirard, J.R. Using pedometers to increase physical activity and improve health. *JAMA* **2007**, *298*, 2296–2304. [CrossRef] [PubMed]
7. Consolvo, S.; McDonald, D.W.; Toscos, T.; Chen, M.Y.; Froehlich, J.; Harrison, B.; Klasnja, P.; LaMarca, A.; LeGrand, L.; Libby, R.; et al. Activity sensing in the wild: A field trial of UbiFit Garden. In Proceedings of the SIGCHI Conference on Human Factors in Computing Systems, Florence, Italy, 5–10 April 2008; ACM Press: New York, NY, USA, 2008. [CrossRef]
8. Lin, J.J.; Mamykina, L.; Lindtner, S.; Delajoux, G.; Strub, H.B. Fish'n'Steps: Encouraging physical activity with an interactive computer game. In Proceedings of the 8th international conference on Ubiquitous Computing, Orange County, CA, USA, 17–19 September 2006; Dourish, P., Friday, A., Eds.; Springer: Berlin/Heidelberg, Germany, 2006; Volume 4206, pp. 261–278. [CrossRef]
9. Miller, A.D.; Mynatt, E.D. A School-based Pervasive Social Fitness System for Everyday Adolescent Health. In Proceedings of the SIGCHI Conference on Human Factors in Computing Systems, Toronto, ON, Canada, 26 April–1 May 2014; ACM Press: New York, NY, USA, 2014; pp. 823–2832. [CrossRef]

10. Munson, S.; Consolvo, S. Exploring goal-setting, rewards, self-monitoring, and sharing to motivate physical activity. In Proceedings of the 6th International. Conference on Pervasive Computing Technologies for Healthcare, San Diego, CA, USA, 21–24 May 2012; pp. 25–32. [CrossRef]
11. Pillay, J.D.; van der Ploeg, H.P.; Kolbe-Alexander, T.L.; Proper, K.I.; van Stralen, M.M.; Tomaz, S.A.; van Mechelen, W.; Lambert, E.V. The association between daily steps and health, and the mediating role of body composition: A pedometer-based, cross-sectional study in an employed South African population. *BMC Publ. Health* **2005**, *15*, 174. [CrossRef] [PubMed]
12. Evenson, K.R.; Wen, F.; Furberg, R.D. Assessing Validity of the Fitbit Indicators for U.S. Public Health Surveillance. *Am. J. Prev. Med.* **2017**, *53*, 931–932. [CrossRef] [PubMed]
13. Wang, J.B.; Cadmus-Bertram, L.A.; Natarajan, L.; White, M.M.; Madanat, H.; Nichols, J.F.; Ayala, G.X.; Pierce, J.P. Wearable Sensor/Device (Fitbit One) and SMS Text-Messaging Prompts to Increase Physical Activity in Overweight and Obese Adults: A Randomized Controlled Trial. *Telemed. E-Health* **2015**, *21*, 782–792. [CrossRef] [PubMed]
14. Bentley, F.; Tollmar, K.; Stephenson, P.; Levy, L.; Jones, B.; Robertson, S.; Price, E.; Catrambone, R.; Wilson, J. Health Mashups: Presenting Statistical Patterns between Wellbeing Data and Context in Natural Language to Promote Behavior Change. *ACM Trans. Comput. Hum. Interact.* **2013**, *20*, 1–27. [CrossRef]
15. Yoon, S.; Schwartz, J.E.; Burg, M.M.; Kronish, I.M.; Alcantara, C.; Julian, J.; Parsons, F.; Davidson, K.W.; Diaz, K.M. Using Behavioral Analytics to Increase Exercise: A Randomized N-of-1 Study. *Am. J. Prev. Med.* **2018**, *54*, 559–567. [CrossRef] [PubMed]
16. Cadmus-Bertram, L.A.; Marcus, B.H.; Patterson, R.E.; Parker, B.A.; Morey, B.L. Randomized Trial of a Fitbit-Based Physical Activity Intervention for Women. *Am. J. Prev. Med.* **2015**, *49*, 414–418. [CrossRef] [PubMed]
17. Auffray, C.; Balling, R.; Barroso, I.; Bencze, L.; Benson, M.; Bergeron, J.; Bernal-Delgado, E.; Blomberg, N.; Bock, C.; Conesa, A. Making sense of big data in health research: Towards an EU action plan. *Genome Med.* **2016**, *8*, 71. [CrossRef] [PubMed]
18. Cheung, Y.; Hsueh, P.; Qian, M.; Yoon, S.; Meli, L.; Diaz, K.M.; Schwartz, J.E.; Kronish, I.M.; Davidson, K.W. Are nomothetic or ideographic approaches superior in predicting daily exercise behaviors? Analyzing N-of-1 mHealth data. *Methods Inf. Med.* **2017**, *56*, 452–460. [CrossRef] [PubMed]
19. Hsiao, M.; Hsueh, P.; Ramakrishnan, S. Personalized adherence activity recognition via model-driven sensor data assessment. *Stud. Health Technol. Inf.* **2012**, *180*, 1050–1054.
20. Kim, Y.; Welk, G.J.; Braun, S.I.; Kang, M. Extracting Objective Estimates of Sedentary Behavior from Accelerometer Data: Measurement Considerations for Surveillance and Research Applications. *PLoS ONE* **2015**, *10*, e0118078. [CrossRef] [PubMed]
21. Swan, M. The Quantified Self: Fundamental Disruption in Big Data Science and Biological Discovery. *Big Data* **2013**, *1*, 85–99. [CrossRef] [PubMed]
22. Dijkhuis, T.B.; Blaauw, F.J.; van Ittersum, M.W.; Velthuijsen, H.; Aiello, M. Personalized Physical Activity Coaching: A Machine Learning Approach. *Sensors* **2018**, *18*, 623. [CrossRef] [PubMed]
23. Du, H.; Venkatakrishnan, A.; Youngblood, G.M.; Ram, A.; Pirolli, P. A Group-Based Mobile Application to Increase Adherence in Exercise and Nutrition Programs: A Factorial Design Feasibility Study. *JMIR MHealth UHealth* **2016**, *4*, e4. [CrossRef] [PubMed]
24. Burg, M.M.; Schwartz, J.E.; Kronish, I.M.; Diaz, K.M.; Alcantara, C.; Duer-Hefele, J.; Davidson, K.W. Does Stress Result in You Exercising Less? Or Does Exercising Result in You Being Less Stressed? Or Is It Both? Testing the Bi-directional Stress-Exercise Association at the Group and Person (N of 1) Level. *Ann. Behav. Med.* **2017**, *51*, 799–809. [CrossRef] [PubMed]
25. Hartman, S.J.; Nelson, S.H.; Weiner, L.S. Patterns of Fitbit Use and Activity Levels Throughout a Physical Activity Intervention: Exploratory Analysis from a Randomized Controlled Trial. *JMIR MHealth UHealth* **2018**, *6*, e29. [CrossRef] [PubMed]
26. McLachlan, G.; Peel, D. *Finite Mixture Models*; John Wiley & Sons, Inc.: Hoboken, NJ, USA, 2005.
27. Hu, F.B.; Rimm, E.; Smith-Warner, S.A.; Feskanich, D.; Stampfer, M.J.; Ascherio, A.; Sampson, L.; Willett, W.C. Reproducibility and validity of dietary patterns assessed with a food-frequency questionnaire. *Am. J. Clin. Nutr.* **1999**, *69*, 243–249. [CrossRef] [PubMed]
28. Hu, F.B. Dietary pattern analysis: A new direction in nutritional epidemiology. *Curr. Opin. Lipidol.* **2002**, *13*, 3–9. [CrossRef] [PubMed]

29. Cheung, Y.K.; Yu, G.; Wall, M.M.; Sacco, R.L.; Elkind, M.S.V.; Willey, J.Z. Patterns of leisure-time physical activity using multivariate finite mixture modeling and cardiovascular risk factors in the Northern Manhattan Study. *Ann. Epidemiol.* **2015**, *25*, 469–474. [CrossRef] [PubMed]
30. Inaba, M.; Katoh, N.; Imai, H. Applications of weighted Voronoi diagrams and randomization to variance-based k-clustering. In Proceedings of the 10th ACM Symposium on Computational Geometry, Stony Brook, NY, USA, 6–9 June 1994; pp. 332–339. [CrossRef]
31. Fan, J.; Yao, Q. *Nonlinear Time Series: Nonparametric and Parametric Methods*; Springer: Berlin, Germany, 2003.
32. Fryzlewicz, P.; Oh, H.S. Thick pen transformation for time series. *J. R. Stat. Soc. Ser. B* **2011**, *73*, 499–529. [CrossRef]
33. Tsay, R.S. Some methods for analyzing big dependent data. *J. Bus. Econ. Stat.* **2016**, *34*, 673–688. [CrossRef]
34. Lim, Y.; Oh, H.S.; Cheung, Y.K. Functional clustering of accelerometer data via transformed input variables. Unpublished manuscript.
35. Box, G.E.P.; Jenkins, G.M.; Reinsel, G.C. *Time Series Analysis*; John Wiley & Sons, Inc.: Hoboken, NJ, USA, 2008.
36. Diaz, K. Ecological Link of Psychosocial Stress to Exercise: Personalized Pathways. Available online: https://osf.io/kmszn/ (accessed on 11 September 2018).
37. Burg, M.M.; Schwartz, J.E.; Kronish, I.M.; Diaz, K.M.; Alcantara, C.; Duer-Hefele, J.; Davidson, K.W. Does stress result in you exercising less? Or does exercising result in you being less stressed? Or it is both? Testing the bi-directional stress-exercise association at the group and person (n of 1) level. *Ann. Behav. Med.* **2017**, *51*, 799–809. [CrossRef] [PubMed]
38. Fitbit Flex. Available online: http://www.fitbit.com (accessed on 11 September 2018).
39. Diaz, K.; Krupka, D.J.; Chang, M.J.; Peacock, J.; Ma, Y.; Goldsmith, J.; Schwartz, J.E.; Davidson, K.W. Fitbit: An accurate and reliable device for wireless physical activity tracking. *Int. J. Cardiol.* **2015**, *185*, 138–140. [CrossRef] [PubMed]
40. Evenson, K.R.; Goto, M.M.; Furberg, R.D. Systematic review of the validity and reliability of consumer-wearable activity trackers. *Int. J. Behav. Nutr. Phys. Act.* **2015**, *12*, 159. [CrossRef] [PubMed]
41. Sasaki, J.E.; Hickey, A.; Mavilia, M.; Tedesco, J.; John, D.; Kozey Keadle, S.; Freedson, P.S. Validation of the Fitbit wireless activity tracker for prediction of energy expenditure. *J. Phys. Act. Health* **2015**, *12*, 149–154. [CrossRef] [PubMed]
42. Wallen, M.P.; Gomersall, S.R.; Keating, S.E.; Wisloff, U.; Coombers, J.S. Accuracy of heart rate watches: Implications for weight management. *PLoS ONE* **2016**, *11*, e0154420. [CrossRef] [PubMed]
43. Fitbit Flex. Available online: https://staticcs.fitbit.com/content/assets/help/manuals/manual_flex_en_US.pdf (accessed on 11 September 2018).
44. Koenker, R. *Quantile Regression (Econometric Society Monographs)*; Cambridge University Press: Cambridge, UK, 2005.
45. Fraley, C.; Raftery, A.E. How many clusters? Which clustering method? Answers via model based cluster analysis. *Comput. J.* **1998**, *41*, 578–589. [CrossRef]
46. Nang, E.E.K.; Khoo, E.Y.; Salim, A.; Tai, E.S.; Lee, J.; Van Dam, R.M. Patterns of physical activity in different domains and implications for intervention in a multi-ethnic Asian population: A cross-sectional study. *BMC Public Health* **2010**, *10*, 644.
47. Garcia Lopez, P.; Montresor, A.; Epema, D.; Datta, A.; Higashino, T.; Iamnitchi, A.; Barcellos, M.; Felber, P.; Riviere, E. Edge-centric computing: Vision and challenges. *ACM SIGCOMM Comput. Commun. Rev.* **2015**, *45*, 37–42. [CrossRef]
48. Klasnja, P.; Hekler, E.B.; Shiffman, S.; Boruvka, A.; Almirall, D.; Tewari, A.; Murphy, S.A. Microrandomized trials: An experimental design for developing just-in-time adaptive interventions. *Health Psychol.* **2015**, *34*, 1220–1228. [CrossRef] [PubMed]
49. Mohr, D.C.; Cheung, K.; Schueller, S.M.; Brown, C.H.; Duan, N. Continuous evaluation of evolving behavioral intervention technologies. *Am. J. Prev. Med.* **2013**, *45*, 517–523. [CrossRef] [PubMed]
50. Cheung, K.; Ling, W.; Karr, C.J.; Weingardt, K.; Schueller, S.M.; Mohr, D.C. Evaluation of a recommender app for apps for the treatment of depression and anxiety: An analysis of longitudinal user engagement. *J. Am. Med. Inf. Assoc.* **2018**, *25*, 955–962. [CrossRef] [PubMed]
51. Hu, X.; Hsueh, P.S.; Qian, M.; Chen, C.-H.; Diaz, K.M.; Cheung, Y.K. A First Step Towards Behavioral Coaching for Managing Stress: A Case Study on Optimal Policy Estimation with Multi-stage Threshold Q-learning. *AMIA Annu. Symp. Proc.* **2017**, *2017*, 930–939.

52. Marschollek, M. A semi-quantitative method to denote generic physical activity phenotypes from long-term accelerometer data—The ATLAS index. *PLoS ONE* **2013**, *8*, e63522. [CrossRef] [PubMed]
53. Rodriguez-Paras, C.; Tippey, K.; Brown, E.; Sasangohar, F.; Creech, S.; Kum, H.-C.; Lawley, M.; Benzer, J.K. Posttraumatic Stress Disorder and Mobile Health: App Investigation and Scoping Literature Review. *JMIR MHealth UHealth* **2017**, *5*, e156. [CrossRef] [PubMed]
54. Kiral-Kornek, I.; Roy, S.; Nurse, E.; Mashford, B.; Karoly, P.; Carroll, T.; Payne, D.; Saha, S.; Baldassano, S.; O'Brien, T.; et al. Epileptic Seizure Prediction Using Big Data and Deep Learning: Toward a Mobile System. *EBioMedicine* **2018**, *27*, 103–111. [CrossRef] [PubMed]
55. Garcia-Alamino, J.M.; Ward, A.M.; Alonso-Coello, P.; Perera, R.; Bankhead, C.; Fitzmaurice, D.; Heneghan, C.J. Self-monitoring and self-management of oral anticoagulation. *Cochrane Database Syst. Rev.* **2010**, *7*, CD003839. [CrossRef]
56. Roditi, D.; Robinson, M.E. The role of psychological interventions in the management of patients with chronic pain. *Psy. Res. Behav. Manag.* **2011**, *4*, 41–49. [CrossRef] [PubMed]
57. Wells, N.; Pasero, C.; McCaffery, M. Improving the Quality of Care Through Pain Assessment and Management. In *Patient Safety and Quality: An Evidence-Based Handbook for Nurses*. Agency for Healthcare Research and Quality (US); NCBI: Bethesda, MD, USA, 2008. Available online: http://www.ncbi.nlm.nih.gov/pubmed/21328759 (accessed on 6 September 2018).

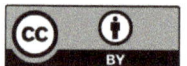

© 2018 by the authors. Licensee MDPI, Basel, Switzerland. This article is an open access article distributed under the terms and conditions of the Creative Commons Attribution (CC BY) license (http://creativecommons.org/licenses/by/4.0/).

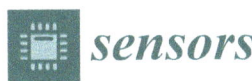

Article

A Device-Independent Efficient Actigraphy Signal-Encoding System for Applications in Monitoring Daily Human Activities and Health

Yashodhan Athavale * and Sridhar Krishnan

Department of Electrical, Computer and Biomedical Engineering, Ryerson University, Toronto, ON M5B 2K3, Canada; krishnan@ryerson.ca
* Correspondence: yashodhan.athavale@ryerson.ca; Tel.: +1-416-979-5000 (4931)

Received: 12 July 2018; Accepted: 28 August 2018; Published: 6 September 2018

Abstract: Actigraphs for personalized health and fitness monitoring is a trending niche market and fit aptly in the Internet of Medical Things (IoMT) paradigm. Conventionally, actigraphy is acquired and digitized using standard low pass filtering and quantization techniques. High sampling frequencies and quantization resolution of various actigraphs can lead to memory leakage and unwanted battery usage. Our systematic investigation on different types of actigraphy signals yields that lower levels of quantization are sufficient for acquiring and storing vital movement information while ensuring an increase in SNR, higher space savings, and in faster time. The objective of this study is to propose a low-level signal encoding method which could improve data acquisition and storage in actigraphs, as well as enhance signal clarity for pattern classification. To further verify this study, we have used a machine learning approach which suggests that signal encoding also improves pattern recognition accuracy. Our experiments indicate that signal encoding at the source results in an increase in SNR (signal-to-noise ratio) by at least 50–90%, coupled with a bit rate reduction by 50–80%, and an overall space savings in the range of 68–92%, depending on the type of actigraph and application used in our study. Consistent improvements by lowering the quantization factor also indicates that a 3-bit encoding of actigraphy data retains most prominent movement information, and also results in an increase of the pattern recognition accuracy by at least 10%.

Keywords: actigraphy; encoding; data compression; denoising; edge computing; signal processing; wearables; activity monitoring; machine learning

1. Introduction

The advent of smart devices and rapidly evolving communication technologies, has enabled the formation of the Internet of Things (IoT) environment. The IoT paradigm intends to connect and exchange information and user data between devices, physical environment and the individual. This translates into a smart, connected and interactive environment for an individual, thereby improving the quality of life. The devices could be computers, phones, wearables, home appliances, infrastructure and vehicles [1–3]. Therefore, any device which operates even with an ON/OFF switch can be integrated into an IoT environment. The IoT environment also allows for connecting devices with limited memory, power and CPU. Figure 1 shows how different components and users are interconnected in an IoT paradigm [1,4].

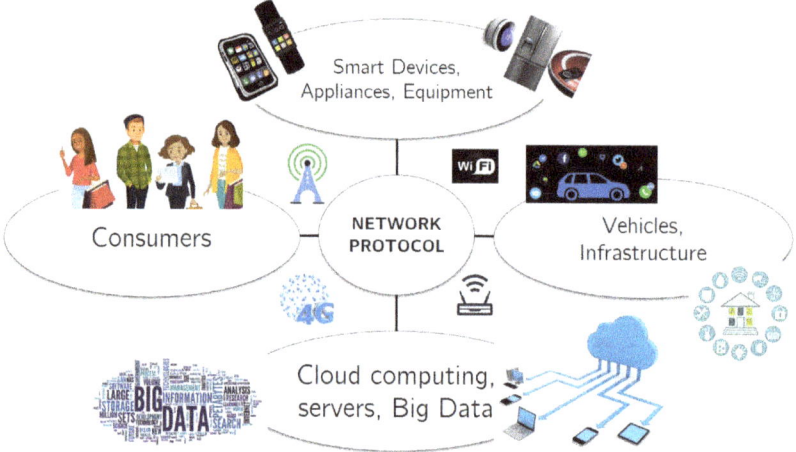

Figure 1. IoT Environment [4].

Advancements in sensor design have also enabled the rapid evolution of smart devices for personalized applications which include communication, health and fitness monitoring, virtual environments, autonomous transportation and smart homes. Considering the aspect of connected healthcare, the development of telehealth systems has resulted in coining of the term IoMT (Internet of Medical Things), which is a subset of IoT. The IoMT environment focuses on delivering clinical services to an individual via connected devices such as smart phones, wearables and infrastructure (see Figure 2). These services include [5]:

- Remote health monitoring via telecommunication network.
- Use of mobile health monitoring equipment and applications.
- Doctor-patient consultation via interactive technology.
- Continuous monitoring using smart devices for elderly and critical care individuals.

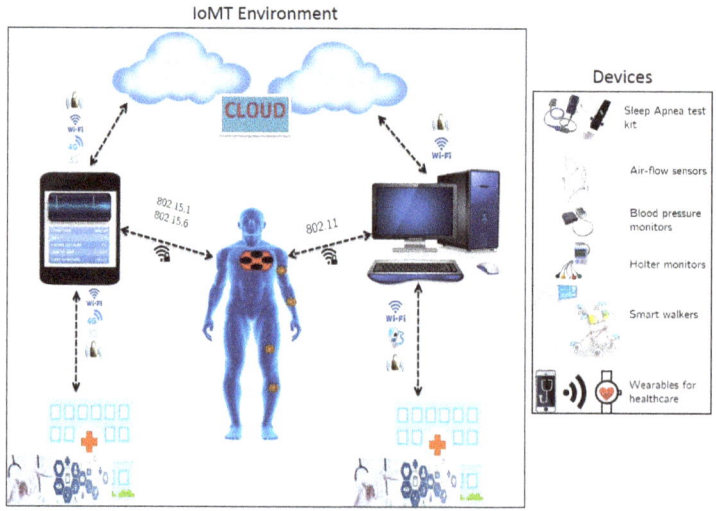

Figure 2. Connected Healthcare in an IoMT paradigm [5].

Our study is based on the use of wearables for home-based health monitoring in an IoMT environment. Wearables are devices embedded with accelerometers, gryoscopes, light and pressure sensors, for capturing and analyzing streaming physiological data from an individual during daily activity. Unlike smart phones or tablets, these devices can be comfortably worn on different body regions throughout the day, and can be used for various applications such as fitness monitoring, behavior tracking and vital signs analysis for critical disorders such as stroke, falls or seizures [6].

From our prior survey [6], we found that many currently available wearables such as Apple Watch^{TM} and FitBit^{TM} have embedded sensors for collecting and analyzing basic human activity parameters such as step counts, pulse rate, temperature and sleep times for fitness awareness. We also investigated into their respective SDKs (software development kits), which described how physiological data is collected, analyzed and shared with service providers for decision generation. In recent times, many clinical studies have been conducted to explore the validity of using wearables for physiological data analysis for disease or disorder detection. For example, accelerometer-based wearables have been used to study daily activity monitoring in individuals suffering from neuromuscular disorders, and validate their outputs with clinical standards [7].

As per a survey [8], considering that only about 90 out of 600 currently available wearables are being used for medical applications, we can see a clear potential for their usage in long-term, home-based health monitoring applications. Even though these numbers present a promising future for wearable-based health monitoring solutions, our review indicates that there still exist some crucial hurdles before implementing health monitoring devices and applications in real-time [6]. These include:

- Focusing on developing physiological signal analysis algorithms which promote edge computing approaches [4–6,9]. That is, the data acquisition, compression and analysis must be done at the device level without having the need to transmit long, streaming data to cloud services. This would lead to optimization of cloud resources by minimizing usage for data storage and analysis. The idea of edge computing is to help in optimizing on-device memory and power usage, thereby increasing operating efficiency and throughput [5,9].
- In addition to this, there is also a need for data acquisition standardization with respect to data formats and communication protocols [10,11].
- Ensuring seamless Internet connectivity across users, devices, infrastructure and services.
- Developing safe, non-invasive and comfortable wearables embedded with sensors for collecting and processing physiological data in a remote setting.

Meeting these challenges, could not only establish a set of standards with respect to device manufacturing and developing new communication protocols, but would also promote the development of novel data acquisition and storage algorithms in wearables. Since the most common sensor currently used in wearables is the accelerometer [6,8], we focus our study on activity monitoring applications. Note that wearables embedded exclusively with accelerometers are termed as actigraphs [12]. In the following section, we will discuss actigraphy applications, data acquisition and signal analysis.

2. Actigraphy

Actigraphs measure human body displacement in single or tri-axial directions, and have been used extensively in calculating gross motor activity for different applications. They are miniature devices which record and store motion data, which could then be further used for performing offline analysis. Actigraphs have been used by researchers in numerous clinical and consumer studies such as fitness monitoring, calorie consumption, sleep/wake activity analysis and for rehabilitation therapies in disabled individuals. To cite a few examples, actigraphy studies have been conducted in the following domains:

- Home-based sleep staging [13–15].
- Analyzing movements in individuals suffering from Parkinson's and Alzheimer's disease [16–18].
- Monitoring home activity of military personnel experiencing post-traumatic stress disorder (PTSD) [19].
- Routine of children diagnosed with autistic spectral disorder and ADHD (attention deficit hyperactivity disorder) [20,21].
- Estimating the severity of sleep related movement-disorders such as periodic limb movements (PLMs) [7,22,23].
- Therapeutic rehabilitation of joint disabilities in war veterans [24,25].
- Demographic studies for identifying differences in sleep patterns with respect to age, gender, ethnicity and sleep disorder prevalence [26].

A variety of actigraphs are currently available in the market (see Figure 3), and they are usually worn on wrist, waist or lower ankles for capturing human motor activity [27]. Typically, an actigraph is able to capture motion data with a sampling frequency in the range of 16–3200 Hz, coupled with an A-to-D quantization of 6–16 bits per sample, depending on the manufacturer [7,12,27,28].

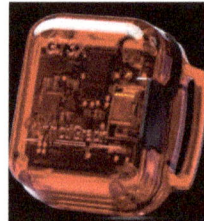
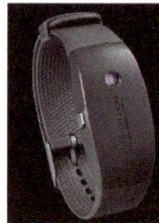
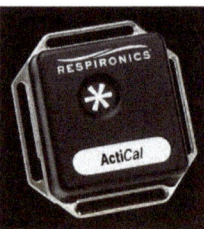

Figure 3. Example of actigraphs.

The reader must note that, due to device property variability from one manufacturer to another, data analysis of the same activity captured from two different actigraphs, might yield different results. This infers that actigraphy analysis algorithms must be designed to be device-independent and customizable as per application [6,29]. Typically, an actigraph consists of the following components [12,30]:

- Piezoelectric accelerometer for capturing motion/vibrations.
- Signal amplifier coupled with an A-to-D converter.
- low-pass filter to remove external vibrations.
- Flash-memory to store sampled and filtered amplitudes.
- Capacitive and rechargeable battery.
- A micro-USB^{TM}, serial or low power wireless interface to transfer data to a local computer.

The actigraph maintains a record of zero-crossings and minimal thresholds, and uses them to generate raw signal values from the motion. Most of the currently available actigraphy devices are able to record and store 24 h motion data for up to a week. Depending on the choice and application domain, actigraphs could be single axial or tri-axial. Note that, usually tri-axial devices are comparatively more sensitive than single axial ones, and may capture motion in scenarios which require real-time data analysis. Figure 4 illustrates single and tri-axial actigraphy signals captured from two different actigraphs.

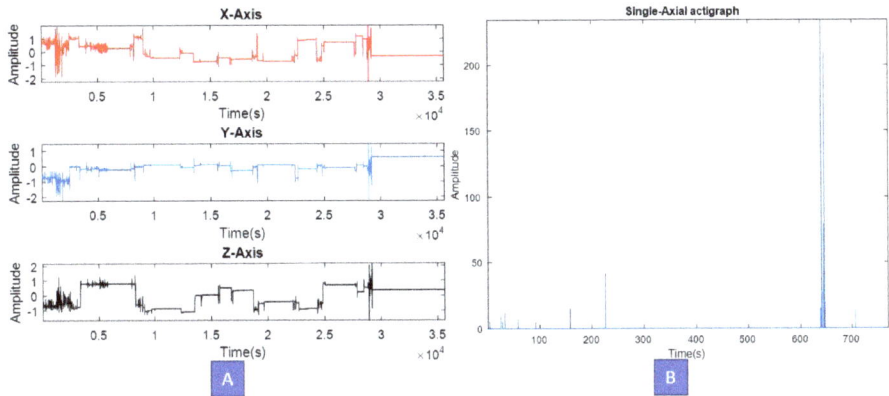

Figure 4. (**A**) Tri-axial, (**B**) Single axial actigraphy signal, captured from two different devices.

In case of tri-axial actigraphy data, our review of prior studies indicates that one must perform vector compounding of individual axial data before analysis, in order to simplify computations, and most importantly ensure that vibration information from all three directions is captured [14,31,32]. For example, given a tri-axial signal $S = <x, y, z>$, its vector magnitude would be computed as,

$$V = \sqrt{x^2 + y^2 + z^2} \tag{1}$$

In order to analyze an actigraphy signal, we must first run certain signal property tests to determine appropriate processing tools and techniques [29]. Following Table 1 highlights various tests and our observations on actigraphy data, computed in MATLAB^{TM}.

Table 1. Actigraphy signal tests.

Property Test	Observations
Visual inspection	Spiky data with a lot of transient information randomly distributed. Motion events seem uncorrelated when separated by significant time period.
Stationarity—KPSS test [33]	Non-stationary signals
Linearity— Augmented Dickey–Fuller test [34]	Non-linear data
Gaussianity—KS test [35]	Non-Gaussian distribution in most cases, since human motion is random.
Sparsity test—Gini Index [36]	Sparse in short windows. In case of tri-axial data, vector compounding and additional quantization may be needed.

Before an actigraphy signal is analyzed to detect specific movements or patterns, it must be pre-processed in order to remove noise and artifacts. Conventionally, actigraphy signals undergo the following operations before analysis:

(1) A-to-D conversion in order to assign discrete amplitudes to specific movements [29].
(2) As per our literature review, human activity is usually captured in the 0.3 to 6 Hz frequency range, and high frequency noise is captured around the sampling frequency. In order to remove the noise, a simple low-pass filter (Butterworth) is employed to capture movement data [12,14,31,32].

(3) Additional band-pass filters could be implemented in order to remove low frequency artifacts and noise.
(4) Depending on application, the actigraphy signal is annotated using time-stamps. For example, in many sleep studies, actigraphy data was clipped between "Lights-off" and "Lights-on" time periods, in order to ensure alignment with other clinical signals recorded in simultaneous PSG [7].

Although most actigraphs are designed for long-term recordings, there are certain shortcomings in their data acquisition and storage methods, which need to be met in order to optimize their usage and implementation as standalone devices, or in smart wearables. These limitations could be:

(1) Actigraphs that sample data at higher frequencies (typically 100 Hz and above) along with a high quantization rate (typically 12–16 bits per sample), often lead to memory leakage and underutilization of battery life during recording.
(2) Manufacturer-based variability in sampling and quantization. This limits algorithms from being designed as device-independent tools [27,37]. Some actigraphs tend to sample movement data too infrequently, thus leading to information loss in the output raw signal.
(3) Many prior studies have been conducted on short-duration actigraphy datasets and did not require extensive memory and computational resources for analysis [14,22]. Translating these studies into long-term activity monitoring solutions is not feasible unless the actigraphy data is subjected to significant compression and segmentation at the source.
(4) Increased use of computational resources (local or cloud) during offline processing of long-term recordings. Conventionally, actigraphy data is captured and entirely transferred to a local computer or cloud for analysis. Our review indicates that in most studies, no prior data processing is done at the source to retain only meaningful information and discard redundant values.

As stated in previous section, signal acquisition methods which promote an edge computing approach could overcome the afore-mentioned challenges in long-duration actigraphy data analysis and optimize device usage [5,6]. In the following section, we propose one such technique to pre-processing actigraphy data by performing data compression and denoising at the source. It should be noted that the proposed solution in this study is not an edge computing technique in itself, but rather focuses on optimizing data acquisition and storage which would then promote edge computing on the hardware.

Proposed Approach

In our review of actigraphy signals captured from different studies and applications, we found that employing a lower level of quantization to actigraphy data at the source, addresses a significant number of afore mentioned challenges. In this study, we propose a low-level encoding scheme which would improve actigraphy analysis in the following ways:

(1) Data compression at the source. The proposed encoding method intends to reduce the output actigraphy file size, thus enabling faster transfer and read time on a local computer.
(2) Signal normalization and denoising, which removes redundant and minute vibrations captured from highly sensitive accelerometers.
(3) SNR (signal-to-noise ratio) increase and enhancement of meaningful movement amplitudes in the signal.
(4) The proposed scheme also ensures operation across different types of actigraphs, thus promoting device-independency of this algorithm.

The reader must note that data compression might result an increase in energy consumption and latency at the source. But the proposed solution intends to reduce memory usage and optimize overall battery usage, which would balance-off these shortcomings. Figure 5 illustrates the methodology implemented in this study.

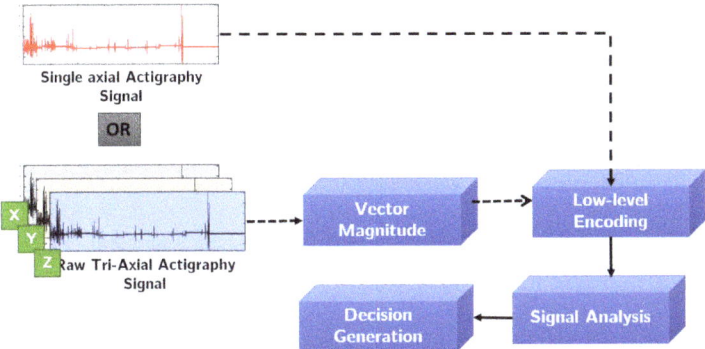

Figure 5. Flowchart of the proposed methodology.

In order to conduct a systematic investigation, we have conducted experiments on actigraphy data acquired from the following applications:

(1) Long-duration tri-axial actigraphy signals captured simultaneously with polysomnography in sleep studies [28].
(2) Activities of Daily Life (ADL) dataset obtained from Dua et al. [38].
(3) Vibroarthrographic signals captured from knee joints for osteoarthritis severity assessment [39].

The reader must note that in case of long-duration sleep actigraphy signals, the proposed encoding scheme's results have already been published in [28] by Athavale et al., and hence we've shown the same results in this paper, to augment our experiments with daily activity [38] and vibroarthrography datasets [39].

For the reader's reference, this paper has been further organized as follows: In Section 3.1 we will briefly explain the datasets used in our experiments, along with actigraph and signal properties used in each study. Next, in Section 3.2 we explain the proposed signal encoding scheme. Following this, we then proceed to check the validity of the proposed encoding scheme by performing simple machine learning and pattern classification of encoded signals, and comparing its results with those of raw actigraphy signals from each dataset, in Section 3.3 . In the next Sections 4.1 and 4.2 we present our experimental results from signal encoding and its validation. We finally conclude this paper with some critical discussions in Section 5.

3. Materials and Methods

3.1. Data Acquisition

In the proposed study, we have conducted experiments on three datasets:

- Long-duration, tri-axial,bi-lateral ankle actigraphy signals [28]
- Short-duration, tri-axial, wrist-actigraphy signals [38], and
- Short-duration, single-axial, vibroarthrographic actigraphy signals [39]

Following Table 2 highlights describes the datasets used in our study:

Table 2. Dataset Properties.

Application	Data-Type	No. of Signals	Length/Signal	Resolution	f_s
Sleep [28]	Tri-axial	50	6–8 h	16-bits/sample	25 Hz
ADL [38]	Tri-axial	274	5–60 s	6-bits/sample	32 Hz
VAG [39]	Single-axial	89	3–5 s	12-bits/sample	2 kHz

f_s is the sampling frequency.

In the next section, we will describe the proposed signal-encoding scheme applied to all the signals in the datasets described in Table 2.

3.2. Proposed Encoding Scheme

The proposed signal encoding scheme is then applied to afore mentioned actigraphy datasets as described in the following steps:

(1) The raw actigraphy signal is first normalized with respect to "g" factor using the device specifications. This operation removes signal components which have been amplified or caused due to earth's gravitational effect on the accelerometer sensor [31]. In this study, depending on the application and device used, one of the following normalization step has been applied. Given a raw actigraphy signal $S_r = <x_r, y_r, z_r>$, its corresponding normalized version can be computed as follows:

- For sleep, the normalized signal would be [28]

$$S = \frac{S_r}{2048 \; counts/g} \quad (2)$$

- For ADL, the normalized signal would be [38]

$$S = -1.5g + \frac{S_r}{63} \times 3g \quad (3)$$

- For VAG, the signal is normalized as [39],

$$S = \frac{(max_{S_{r_i}}(S_r) - S)}{(max_{S_{r_i}}(S_r) - min_{S_{r_i}}(S_r))} \quad (4)$$

Note that in case of Eqns.2 and 3, $g = 9.8 \; m/s^2$.

Note that the normalization operation is applied to each axis of the actigraphy signal.

(2) Next, depending on the signal type we perform vector compounding as shown in Equation (1). This operation is done only for tri-axial actigraphy data, and in case of single axial signals, we skip to normalization as shown in Equations (2)–(4).

(3) Assuming that b is the number of encoding bits, and $Q_f = \frac{2^b - 1}{2}$ is the quantization factor, we encode the signal S using the floor operation,

$$S_e = \lfloor (S \times Q_f + Q_f) \rfloor \quad (5)$$

The floor operation in Equation (5) digitally approximates each value generated from $(S \times Q_f + Q_f)$ to the greatest integer less than or equal to it. For example, a value of 3.4 would be mapped to 3. Note that in this study, we have experimented with different levels of encoding depending on the dataset. From our experiments, we have observed that a 3-bit encoding provides highest signal clarity.

(4) The SNR of the encoded actigraphy signal is then calculated as,

$$SNR_{S_e} = 20 \log \left(\frac{RMS_S}{RMS_{Q_e}} \right) \; dB \quad (6)$$

where, RMS_S and RMS_{Q_e} are the root mean square values of the input normalized signal and the quantization error respectively. The quantization error can be computed as $Q_e = (S - S_e)$.

The encoding scheme proposed in this section aims to perform on-the-fly denoising, SNR enhancement and compression of actigraphy data at the source. Our experimental results with different levels of encoding have been highlighted in Section 4.1. In the next section, we describe a validation process using a machine learning approach.

3.3. Validation Using Machine Learning

In order to ensure that no vital information is lost in the encoding process, we perform a machine learning validation in our study. This is done because unlike physiological data with characteristic patterns such as ECG, actigraphy signals do not show any specific structure or morphology, and hence obtaining a ground truth from experts proves to be trivial [29]. For example, in prior studies pertaining to actigraphy validation with PSG (polysomnography), clinical feedback was given only on PSG readings, and the actigraphy data was used only for comparing certain statistical parameters [7,23,40,41].

As shown in Table 1, the actigraphy data looks transient in nature, and requires ground truth information such as activity labels for further analysis. In order to validate the encoding scheme, we perform a simple feature extraction and pattern classification of raw and encoded actigraphy signals from each dataset used in this study, using the following steps:

(1) For each dataset, we create two distinct groups, namely:

- Group 1: Raw actigraphy signals, and;
- Group 2: Encoded actigraphy signals

(2) From each signal in Groups 1 and 2, we extract 13 time, frequency [7] and signal-specific features, defined in Table 3 as shown. For the reader's reference, in this research study we propose two new signal specific features, namely—rapid change factor and spiky index. The remaining 11 features have been used in prior works pertaining to actigraphy and other physiological signal analysis applications [29].

Table 3. Features and their description

Domain	Feature	Description
Time	RMS	Root mean square value of the signal
	Maxima	Maximum Peak value in the signal
	Peak-to-Peak	Difference between maximum and minimum peak
	Peak-to-RMS	Maximum peak to RMS ratio
	Peak-to-Avg.Power	Maximum peak to avg. power ratio
	SNDR	Signal to noise & distortion ratio
	Hjorth's Parameters [42]	First order mobility, $M_f = \sqrt{\frac{\sigma_f}{\sigma_x}}$ Second order mobility, $M_s = \sqrt{\frac{\sigma_s}{\sigma_x}}$ Complexity, $C_x = \frac{M_{fs}}{M_f}$
Frequency	Median Frequency	Median normalized frequency of power spectrum
	Band power	Average signal power
Signal-Specific	Spiky Index	$SI = \frac{\# \, of \, Prominent \, Peaks \, or \, events}{Total \, Activity \, Time(s)}$
	Rapid Change Factor	$RCF = \frac{Step \, Size}{b \times T_s}$

(3) Next, depending on the dataset and its corresponding application, we apply pre-defined labels to Group 1 and 2 feature sets as follows:

- **Sleep Data:** As the application is focused on distinguishing between mild and severe PLM (periodic limb movement) index, using the pre-defined labels in Athavale et al. [7,28], we divide the feature set into "Mild" and "Severe".
- **ADL Data:** Since this dataset contains signals of 14 multiple activities, we divide the feature set based on 14 labels [38].
- **VAG Data:** As per Krishnan et al., the feature set has been divided into "Normal" and "Abnormal" depending on the severity of knee-joint degeneration [39].

(4) Finally, using a 70–30 ratio of training and testing feature data, we use an LDA (linear discriminant analysis) tool to classify actigraphy feature data within Groups 1 and 2 of each dataset. Further to this, we also cross-validate our results with a support vector machine (SVM).

It should be noted that in this study, machine learning of actigraphy data is not the main objective but has been used to validate the effect of signal encoding at source. Hence, the choice of using a LDA classifier has been done only to observe the linear classification performance on the encoded data. The results from this machine learning based validation for each dataset have been presented in Section 4.2.

4. Results

4.1. Signal-Encoding Results

As evident from Equation (5), the encoding floor operation digitally approximates an actigraphy signal S by performing a non-linear mapping of each sample S_i to an integer less than or equal to S_i after multiplication with the quantization factor. Figure 6 illustrates a sample actigraphy signal from each dataset and its corresponding encoded version.

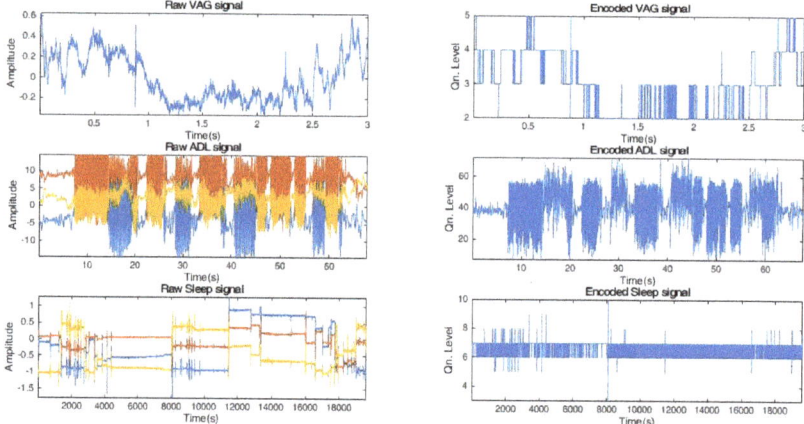

Figure 6. Sample Raw and Encoded signals from each dataset.

Additionally, we also perform a parameter-wise comparison, and observe that signal encoding not only inherently denoises and enhances SNR, but also performs significant data compression at the source. Following Table 4 highlights these results for a sample actigraphy signal obtained from each dataset.

Table 4. Parametric Encoding Results.

Signal Type	Parameter	Sleep	ADL	VAG
Raw	SNR (dB)	−18.9	−48.4	−0.1
	Bit Rate (bits/s)	400	192	20×10^3
Encoded	SNR (dB)	38.8	28.2	19.9
	Bit Rate (bits/s)	75	96	6×10^3
Overall	% Space Savings	92%	68%	88%

These results have also been illustrated in following Figures 7–9.

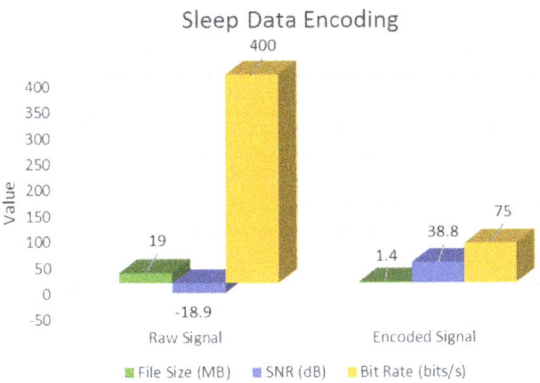

Figure 7. Encoding Sleep actigraphy signals.

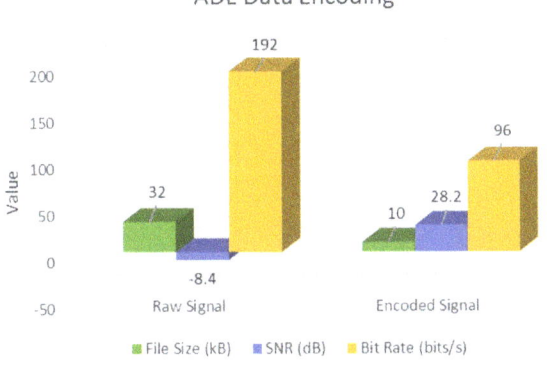

Figure 8. Encoding ADL actigraphy signals.

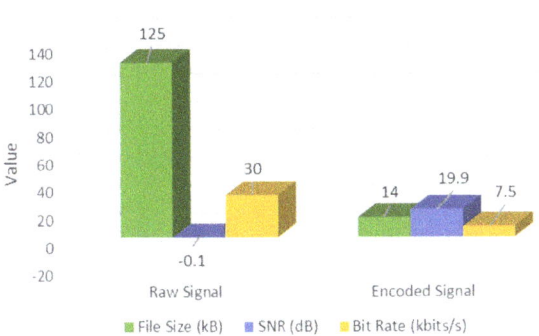

Figure 9. Encoding VAG actigraphy signals.

As evident from Table 4 and Figures 7–9, signal encoding not only enhances actigraphy data by retaining vital movement information and discarding redundant values, but also helps in signal compression at the source. Further to this, in Section 4.2, we highlight the machine learning validation results in order to show the encoding procedure's efficiency in improving actigraphy signal recognition.

4.2. Encoding Validation Results

As described in Section 3.3, we performed a machine learning based validation of the proposed encoding scheme, and find that for each dataset, the classification rate within Group 2 (encoded) features is higher than that of Group 1 (raw) feature set. Table 5 highlights the classification results for LDA and SVM. In addition to computing the classification accuracies between raw and 3-bit encoded feature sets, we also calculate the F1-score metric for each data-set's classification rate using the expression,

$$F1 = 2 \times \frac{Precision \times Recall}{Precision + Recall} \tag{7}$$

Table 5. Machine Learning Results along F1-Scores for each actigraphy dataset.

Data	Raw Features				Encoded Features			
	LDA		SVM		LDA		SVM	
	Accuracy (%)	F1-Score	Accuracy (%)	F1-Score	Accuracy (%)	F1-Score	Accuracy (%)	F1-Score
Sleep	87.1	0.78	83.3	0.71	93.3	0.90	93.3	0.91
ADL	88.3	0.82	82.8	0.73	89.1	0.85	84.9	0.76
VAG	57.7	0.45	65.4	0.59	76.0	0.70	84.6	0.81

As evident from Table 5, the classification accuracies for ADL data [38] does not increase significantly even after encoding. We investigated this further and found that the classification rates varied drastically within the 14 classes of the ADL data due to lack of sufficient number of signals for certain activities. Nevertheless, we have still included the encoding results in this study, in order show the applicability of the proposed technique to any type of actigraphy.

Further to this, we also compare the LDA classification accuracies of signals encoded using different bit-factors for each dataset. Through this, we find that a 3-bit encoding of actigraphy data ensures highest performance in data acquisition, storage and analysis. Following Figures 10–12 illustrates this trend on how the classification rate for each dataset decreases with increase in bit resolution of the signal.

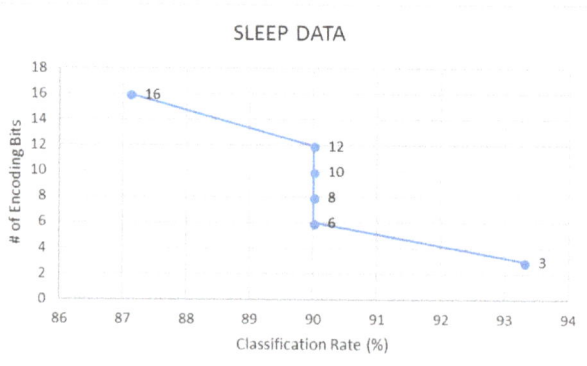

Figure 10. Classification rate vs. encoding - sleep data.

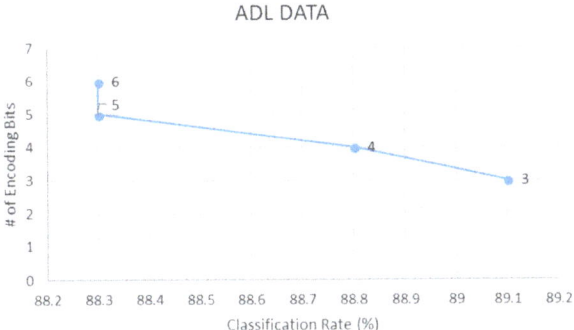

Figure 11. Classification rate vs. encoding - ADL data.

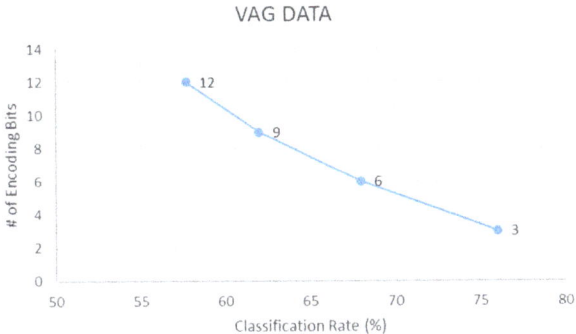

Figure 12. Classification rate vs. encoding - VAG data.

5. Discussions and Future Works

As evident from our investigation and experimental results, employing a very low-factor signal quantization greatly improves the device's data handling capacity by ensuring enhanced SNR, high compression ratio and removal of redundant movement information from the actigraphy signal. The 3-bit encoding proposed in this study, works best in compressing actigraphy data at the edge of an IoT-type setup. Considering the nature of actigraphy signals as highlighted in Table 1, the proposed encoding scheme addresses the transient, spiky information by retaining only significant movement amplitudes or true acceleration values. Movements which are very small are floored to zero in the encoding operation. Thus, redundant values and high frequency noise are removed in the encoded signal, which now contains only relevant movement information.

Although in this study we have used offline datasets, it must be noted that the objective of the proposed encoding scheme is to be applied at the recording source (i.e., on the device) in real-time. This supports an edge computing approach when coupled with activity-based adaptive segmentation techniques to extract regions of peak movements. The machine learning validation approach used in this study aptly supports the proposed encoding scheme as shown by the classification results in Table 5. Further to this, we observe that the 3-bit encoding provides the highest activity recognition rate. From our study on different actigraphy datasets, it should be noted that the proposed encoding algorithm is device-independent and signal-independent, and could easily be ported onto any accelerometer-based wearable.

Current trends in IoMT and related device developments highly promote the edge computing structure in smart devices, as it would significantly reduce cloud burden, and ensure data privacy and security at the consumer end. Home-based health monitoring using an IoMT framework is a burgeoning market and would help in significant reduction of patient-doctor visits and associated healthcare costs. One way to encourage this trend is to use wearables and sensors, embedded with edge computing friendly algorithms, such as the one proposed in this study. This would also promote the clinical validation and development of tools for long-term monitoring of vital physiological parameters in not just chronically ill or elderly patients, but for the betterment of all individuals [6,43].

As part of our future work, we would like to test the proposed algorithm's efficiency on commercially available wearables such as FitBit^{TM}, Apple Watch^{TM} as well as other generic actigraphs used in activity monitoring studies.

Author Contributions: Conceptualization, S.K.; Methodology, S.K.; Software, Y.A.; Validation, Y.A.; Formal Analysis, Y.A.; Investigation, Y.A.; Resources, S.K.; Data Curation, Y.A.; Writing—Original Draft Preparation, Y.A.; Writing—Review & Editing, S.K.; Visualization, Y.A.; Supervision, S.K.; Project Administration, S.K.; Funding Acquisition, Y.A., S.K.

Funding: This research was supported by Ryerson University. The funding was provided by NSERC DG (1-51-53712) and NSERC PGS-D (504725 - 2017).

Acknowledgments: We would like to thank Ryerson University and NSERC for supporting our ongoing research in physiological signal analysis using wearables. We would also like to thank Sunnybrook Health Sciences Centre for providing us the Sleep Actigraphy dataset, and University of Calgary for giving us access to the vibroarthrography dataset.

Conflicts of Interest: The authors declare no conflict of interest.The founding sponsors had no role in the design of the study; in the collection, analyses, or interpretation of data; in the writing of the manuscript, and in the decision to publish the results.

Abbreviations

The following abbreviations are used in this manuscript:

IoT	Internet of Things
IoMT	Internet of Medical Things
VAG	Vibroarthrography
ADL	Activities of Daily Life
SNR	signal-to-noise ratio
LDA	linear discriminant analysis
SVM	support vector machine

References

1. Miorandi, D.; Sicari, S.; De Pellegrini, F.; Chlamtac, I. Internet of things: Vision, applications and research challenges. *Ad Hoc Netw.* **2012**, *10*, 1497–1516. [CrossRef]
2. Wortmann, F.; Flüchter, K. Internet of things. *Bus. Inf. Syst. Eng.* **2015**, *57*, 221–224. [CrossRef]
3. Atzori, L.; Iera, A.; Morabito, G. Understanding the Internet of Things: definition, potentials, and societal role of a fast evolving paradigm. *Ad Hoc Netw.* **2017**, *56*, 122–140. [CrossRef]
4. Sethi, P.; Sarangi, S.R. Internet of things: Architectures, protocols, and applications. *J. Electr. Comput. Eng.* **2017**, *2007*, 9324035. [CrossRef]
5. Rodrigues, J.J.; Segundo, D.B.; Junqueira, H.A.; Sabino, M.H.; Prince, R.M.; Al-Muhtadi, J.; de Albuquerque, V.H.C. Enabling Technologies for the Internet of Health Things. *IEEE Access* **2018**, *6*, 13129–13141. [CrossRef]
6. Athavale, Y.; Krishnan, S. Biosignal monitoring using wearables: Observations and opportunities. *Biomed. Signal Process. Control* **2017**, *38*, 22–33. [CrossRef]
7. Athavale, Y.; Krishnan, S.; Dopsa, D.D.; Berneshawi, A.G.; Nouraei, H.; Raissi, A.; Murray, B.J.; Boulos, M.I. Advanced signal analysis for the detection of periodic limb movements from bilateral ankle actigraphy. *J. Sleep Res.* **2017**, *26*, 14–20. [CrossRef] [PubMed]

8. Vandrico—Wearable Technology Database. Available online: http://vandrico.com/wearables/ (accessed on 16 June 2016).
9. McMahon, E.; Williams, R.; El, M.; Samtani, S.; Patton, M.; Chen, H. Assessing medical device vulnerabilities on the Internet of Things. In Proceedings of the 2017 IEEE International Conference on Intelligence and Security Informatics (ISI), Beijing, China, 22–24 July 2017; pp. 176–178.
10. Before Wearables Can Be Used for Health Care Monitoring, These Issues Must Be Addressed-IEEE-The Institute. Available online: http://theinstitute.ieee.org/technology-topics/life-sciences/before-wearables-can-be-used-for-health-care-monitoring-these-issues-must-be-addressed/ (accessed on 7 October 2018).
11. Gazis, V. A Survey of Standards for Machine-to-Machine and the Internet of Things. *IEEE Commun. Surv. Tutor.* **2017**, *19*, 482–511. [CrossRef]
12. Acebo, C. Actigraphy. In *Sleep: A Comprehensive Handbook*; Wiley: Hoboken, NJ, USA, 2005; pp. 1035–1038.
13. Domingues, A.; Paiva, T.; Sanches, J.M. Sleep and wakefulness state detection in nocturnal actigraphy based on movement information. *IEEE Trans. Biomed. Eng.* **2014**, *61*, 426–434. [CrossRef] [PubMed]
14. Muns, I.W.; Lad, Y.; Guardiola, I.G.; Thimgan, M. Classification of Rest and Active Periods in Actigraphy Data Using PCA. *Procedia Comput. Sci.* **2017**, *114*, 275–280. [CrossRef]
15. El-Manzalawy, Y.; Buxton, O.; Honavar, V. Sleep/wake state prediction and sleep parameter estimation using unsupervised classification via clustering. In Proceedings of the 2017 IEEE International Conference on Bioinformatics and Biomedicine (BIBM), Kansas City, MO, USA, 13–16 November 2017; pp. 718–723.
16. Camargos, E.F.; Louzada, F.M.; Nóbrega, O.T. Wrist actigraphy for measuring sleep in intervention studies with Alzheimer's disease patients: Application, usefulness, and challenges. *Sleep Med. Rev.* **2013**, *17*, 475–488. [CrossRef] [PubMed]
17. Maglione, J.E.; Liu, L.; Neikrug, A.B.; Poon, T.; Natarajan, L.; Calderon, J.; Avanzino, J.A.; Corey-Bloom, J.; Palmer, B.W.; Loredo, J.S.; et al. Actigraphy for the assessment of sleep measures in Parkinson's disease. *Sleep* **2013**, *36*, 1209–1217. [CrossRef] [PubMed]
18. Barth, J.; Klucken, J.; Kugler, P.; Kammerer, T.; Steidl, R.; Winkler, J.; Hornegger, J.; Eskofier, B. Biometric and mobile gait analysis for early diagnosis and therapy monitoring in Parkinson's disease. In Proceedings of the 2011 Annual International Conference of the IEEE Engineering in Medicine and Biology Society, Boston, MA, USA, 30 August–3 September 2011; pp. 868–871.
19. Miller, N.L.; Shattuck, L.G.; Matsangas, P. Longitudinal study of sleep patterns of United States Military Academy cadets. *Sleep* **2010**, *33*, 1623–1631. [CrossRef] [PubMed]
20. De Crescenzo, F.; Licchelli, S.; Ciabattini, M.; Menghini, D.; Armando, M.; Alfieri, P.; Mazzone, L.; Pontrelli, G.; Livadiotti, S.; Foti, F.; et al. The use of actigraphy in the monitoring of sleep and activity in ADHD: A meta-analysis. *Sleep Med. Rev.* **2016**, *26*, 9–20. [CrossRef] [PubMed]
21. Wiggs, L.; Stores, G. Sleep patterns and sleep disorders in children with autistic spectrum disorders: Insights using parent report and actigraphy. *Dev. Med. Child Neurol.* **2004**, *46*, 372–380. [CrossRef] [PubMed]
22. Kye, S.; Moon, J.; Lee, T.; Lee, S.; Lee, K.; Shin, S.C.; Lee, Y.S. Detecting periodic limb movements in sleep using motion sensor embedded wearable band. In Proceedings of the IEEE International Conference on Systems, Man, and Cybernetics (SMC), Banff, AB, Canada, 5–8 October 2017; pp. 1087–1092.
23. Plante, D.T. Leg actigraphy to quantify periodic limb movements of sleep: A systematic review and meta-analysis. *Sleep Med. Rev.* **2014**, *18*, 425–434. [CrossRef] [PubMed]
24. Töreyin, H.; Hersek, S.; Teague, C.N.; Inan, O.T. A Proof-of-Concept System to Analyze Joint Sounds in Real Time for Knee Health Assessment in Uncontrolled Settings. *IEEE Sens. J.* **2016**, *16*, 2892–2893. [CrossRef]
25. Töreyin, H.; Jeong, H.K.; Hersek, S.; Teague, C.N.; Inan, O.T. Quantifying the Consistency of Wearable Knee Acoustical Emission Measurements During Complex Motions. *IEEE J. Biomed. Health Inf.* **2016**, *20*, 1265–1272. [CrossRef] [PubMed]
26. Morrish, E.; King, M.A.; Pilsworth, S.N.; Shneerson, J.M.; Smith, I.E. Periodic limb movement in a community population detected by a new actigraphy technique. *Sleep Med.* **2002**, *3*, 489–495. [CrossRef]
27. Khabou, M.A.; Parlato, M.V. Classification and feature analysis of actigraphy signals. In Proceedings of the 2013 Proceedings of IEEE Southeastcon, Jacksonville, FL, USA, 4–7 April 2013; pp. 1–5.
28. Athavale, Y.; Krishnan, S.; Raissiz, A.; Kirolos, N.; Murray, B.J.; Boulos, M.I. Integrated Signal Encoding and Analysis System for Actigraphy-based Long-term Monitoring of Periodic Limb Movements in Sleep. Presented at the 2018 IEEE EMBC International Conference, Honolulu, HI, USA, 17–21 July 2018. In Press, Engineering in Medicine and Biology Society.

29. Krishnan, S.; Athavale, Y. Trends in biomedical signal feature extraction. *Biomed. Signal Process. Control* **2018**, *43*, 41–63. [CrossRef]
30. Marcio de Almeida Mendes, M.; da Silva, I.C.; Ramires, V.V.; Reichert, F.F.; Martins, R.C.; Tomasi, E. Calibration of raw accelerometer data to measure physical activity: A systematic review. *Gait Posture* **2018**, *61*, 98–110. [CrossRef] [PubMed]
31. Gyllensten, I.C. *Physical Activity Recognition in Daily Life Using a Traxial Accelerometer*; Skolan för Datavetenskap och Kommunikation, Kungliga Tekniska högskolan: Stockholm, Sweden, 2010.
32. Zhang, S.; Rowlands, A.V.; Murray, P.; Hurst, T.L. Physical activity classification using the GENEA wrist-worn accelerometer. *Med. Sci. Sports Exerc.* **2012**, *44*, 742–748. [CrossRef] [PubMed]
33. Kwiatkowski, D.; Phillips, P.C.; Schmidt, P.; Shin, Y. Testing the null hypothesis of stationarity against the alternative of a unit root: How sure are we that economic time series have a unit root? *J. Econometr.* **1992**, *54*, 159–178. [CrossRef]
34. Fuller, W.A. *Introduction to Statistical Time Series*; John Wiley & Sons: New York, NY, USA, 1976.
35. Ghasemi, A.; Zahediasl, S. Normality tests for statistical analysis: A guide for non-statisticians. *Int. J. Endocrinol. Metab.* **2012**, *10*, 486. [CrossRef] [PubMed]
36. Zonoobi, D.; Kassim, A.A.; Venkatesh, Y.V. Gini index as sparsity measure for signal reconstruction from compressive samples. *IEEE J. Sel. Top. Signal Process.* **2011**, *5*, 927–932. [CrossRef]
37. Athavale, Y.; Boulos, M.; Murray, B.J.; Krishnan, S. Classification of periodic leg movements through actigraphy signal analysis. In Proceedings of the 2016 CMBES39 Conference, Calgary, AB, Canada, 24–27 May 2016.
38. Dheeru, D.; Karra Taniskidou, E. UCI Machine Learning Repository. 2017. Available online: https://archive.ics.uci.edu/ml/index.php (access on 23 July 2018).
39. Krishnan, S.; Rangayyan, R.M.; Bell, G.D.; Frank, C.B. Adaptive time-frequency analysis of knee joint vibroarthrographic signals for noninvasive screening of articular cartilage pathology. *IEEE Trans. Biomed. Eng.* **2000**, *47*, 773–783. [CrossRef] [PubMed]
40. Ferri, R. The time structure of leg movement activity during sleep: the theory behind the practice. *Sleep Med.* **2012**, *13*, 433–441. [CrossRef] [PubMed]
41. Gschliesser, V.; Frauscher, B.; Brandauer, E.; Kohnen, R.; Ulmer, H.; Poewe, W.; Högl, B. PLM detection by actigraphy compared to polysomnography: A validation and comparison of two actigraphs. *Sleep Med.* **2009**, *10*, 306–311. [CrossRef] [PubMed]
42. Hjorth, B. EEG analysis based on time domain properties. *Electroencephalogr. Clin. Neurophysiol.* **1970**, *29*, 306–310. [CrossRef]
43. Celler, B.G.; Sparks, R.S. Home Telemonitoring of Vital Signs Technical Challenges and Future Directions. *IEEE J. Biomed. Health Inform.* **2015**, *19*, 82–91. [CrossRef] [PubMed]

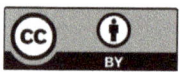 © 2018 by the authors. Licensee MDPI, Basel, Switzerland. This article is an open access article distributed under the terms and conditions of the Creative Commons Attribution (CC BY) license (http://creativecommons.org/licenses/by/4.0/).

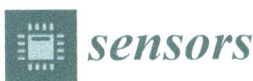

Article

Towards an Efficient One-Class Classifier for Mobile Devices and Wearable Sensors on the Context of Personal Risk Detection

Luis A. Trejo * and Ari Yair Barrera-Animas

Tecnologico de Monterrey, Escuela de Ingeniería y Ciencias, Carretera al Lago de Guadalupe Km. 3.5, Atizapán, Edo. de México C.P. 52926, Mexico; ybarrera@itesm.mx
* Correspondence: ltrejo@itesm.mx; Tel.: +52-55-5864-5647

Received: 27 June 2018; Accepted: 23 August 2018; Published: 30 August 2018

Abstract: In this work, we present a first step towards an efficient one-class classifier well suited for mobile devices to be implemented as part of a user application coupled with wearable sensors in the context of personal risk detection. We compared one-class Support Vector Machine (ocSVM) and OCKRA (One-Class K-means with Randomly-projected features Algorithm). Both classifiers were tested using four versions of the publicly available PRIDE (Personal RIsk DEtection) dataset. The first version is the original PRIDE dataset, which is based only on time-domain features. We created a second version that is simply an extension of the original dataset with new attributes in the frequency domain. The other two datasets are a subset of these two versions, after a feature selection procedure based on a correlation matrix analysis followed by a Principal Component Analysis. All experiments were focused on the performance of the classifiers as well as on the execution time during the training and classification processes. Therefore, our goal in this work is twofold: we aim at reducing execution time but at the same time maintaining a good classification performance. Our results show that OCKRA achieved on average, 89.1% of Area Under the Curve (AUC) using the full set of features and 83.7% when trained using a subset of them. Furthermore, regarding execution time, OCKRA reports in the best case a 33.1% gain when using a subset of the feature vector, instead of the full set of features. These results are better than those reported by ocSVM, in which case, even though the AUCs are very close to each other, execution times are significantly higher in all cases, for example, more than 20 h versus less than an hour in the worst-case scenario. Having in mind the trade-off between classification performance and efficiency, our results support the choice of OCKRA as our best candidate so far for a mobile implementation where less processing and memory resources are at hand. OCKRA reports a very encouraging speed-up without sacrificing the classifier performance when using the PRIDE dataset based only on time-domain attributes after a feature selection procedure.

Keywords: time-domain features; frequency-domain features; principal component analysis; behaviour analysis; classifier efficiency; personal risk detection; one-class classification; wearable sensors

1. Introduction

It is highly desirable to recognise as soon as possible whenever a person faces a risk-prone situation that could threaten that person's physical integrity. Barrera-Animas et al. in [1] introduce the term *Personal Risk Detection* as an attractive line of research focused on this timely detection. Their hypothesis is based on the observation that people express regular patterns, with small variations, regarding their normal physical and behavioural activities. These patterns would change, even drastically, whenever the person is facing a hazardous situation. A wearable device with a set of simple and common sensors, such as heart rate, accelerometer, gyroscope, and skin temperature, just to mention a few, is sufficient to capture deviations from normal behaviour. Personal risk detection can be tackled as an anomaly detection problem that aims at differentiating a normal condition from unusual behaviour. In this context, the use of one-class classification algorithms has shown very good results. Actually, Barrera-Animas et al. reported in [1] that one-class Support Vector Machine (ocSVM) achieved the best performance among the classifiers used in their experiments. Later on, a new one-class classifier named One-Class K-means with Randomly-projected features Algorithm (OCKRA) proposed by Rodríguez et al. in [2] was introduced for the personal risk detection problem. In their research, they showed that OCKRA achieved the best results in the classification task, leaving ocSVM in second place.

As stated in [1], Vital Signs Monitoring (VSM) and Human Activity Recognition (HAR) fields are closely related to the personal risk detection problem. From research works presented in both fields, a trend to use features in frequency and time domains can be noticed [3–6]. The rationale behind this approach lies in the nature of recorded sensors measurements and that their treatment in frequency-domain reveals several features that can not be appreciated in the time-domain. Thus, the inclusion of features in both domains generally gives a more complex and complete view of the observed scenario. Furthermore, in HAR and VSM research fields, several works pursue the use of distinct specialised sensors to gather the most possible information about individuals and their environment. For instance, an interesting review work on this subject is that of Rucco et al. [7], which describes the state-of-the-art research on fall risk assessment, fall prevention and detection. Their review surveys the most adopted sensor technologies used in this field and their position on the human body, with special interest in healthy elderly people. With this approach, it is also intended to increase the number of features obtained that characterise the study case.

Advantages such as to gain a better understanding of the physiological and behavioural patterns of an individual, and to avoid lack of information and data concurrency, result from increasing the number of used sensors and features. However, despite the fact that using several sensors and deriving diverse features in time/frequency-domain has some advantages, an important issue could arise from this approach: a high dimensionality problem. Reducing dimensionality comprises the process of project high-dimensional data into a low-dimensional space while retaining its variability [8]—that is, to reveal a relevant low-dimensional space embraced in the high-dimensional one [9]. Principal Component Analysis (PCA) is one of the classic techniques used in the literature to reduce the dimensionality of a dataset due to its capability to reveal the hidden structure of data, even on high-dimensional space, and to its low computational consumption requirements [9]. Regarding the personal risk detection problem, to the authors' knowledge, there is no research work based on this approach. However, several research studies across multiple disciplines integrate frequency-/time-domain features and deal with the dimensionality reduction problem, as we briefly describe in Section 2.

The aim of the present research is twofold. Firstly, we are interested in exploring the impact of using dimension reduction techniques and frequency domain features in the context of the personal risk detection problem. We use a correlation matrix and Principal Component Analysis for the dimension reduction task as they are well studied and implemented in related research concerning classification problems. The second aim is to speed-up the training and classification process of a given classifier, without sacrificing its performance. This is a very important requirement since our final classifier is meant to be implemented on mobile devices; thus, efficiency is paramount due to a limitation on memory and CPU resources.

The rest of the document is organised as follows: in Section 2, we briefly review recent work that is closely related to ours; in Section 3, we present the PRIDE dataset used in our experiments, the pre-processing of PRIDE and feature selection methodology in the time and frequency domains. Additionally, the one-class classifiers used in our experiments are introduced. Next, in Section 4, we present our experimental results and, to reinforce their validity, we discuss the outcome of statistical tests run over our algorithms. Finally, in Section 5, we give our conclusions about the outcomes of this work and ideas for current and future work.

2. Related Work

Pei et al. [3] work focused on three main topics: context sensing, modelling human behaviour, and the development of a new architecture intended for a cognitive phone platform. Time and frequency domain features were comprised in their study. Furthermore, a sequential forward selection algorithm was used during the feature selection process carried out before training any classifier. Test results showed an accuracy rate up to 92.9%.

Özdemir and Barshan [4] used an accelerometer, gyroscope, and magnetometer/compass tri-axial sensors to detect people's falls by means of six wearable sensors. They set up a controlled environment to capture data when falling occurs. In their work, they derived a 1404-dimensional feature vector, using variables in the time and frequency domains; later, they employed a Discrete Fourier Transform. Afterwards, PCA was used to reduce the feature vector high dimensionality and complexity in training and testing the classifiers, obtaining a 30-dimensional feature vector. As classifiers, they used Least Squared Method, k-Nearest Neighbour, Support Vector Machines, Bayesian Decision Making, Dynamic Time Warping, and Artificial Neural Networks. Furthermore, they computed the computational cost for training and testing of each classifier for a single fold. Results showed an accuracy over 95% for the six tested classifiers. The authors conclude that k-Nearest Neighbour and Least Squared Method are suitable for real-time applications since their computational requirements are acceptable in the training and testing phase.

Wundersitz et al. [5] research was centred on the classification of team sport-related activities using data obtained from accelerometers and gyroscopes. In their study, frequency and time domain features were calculated and used to train different classifiers. Frequency-domain features were calculated via the fast Fourier transformation. Moreover, ANOVA (Analysis of variance) and LASSO (Least absolute shrinkage and selection operator) regression analysis were used as feature selection methods to reduce the processing time and to make the model easier to interpret. As part of their conclusions, they stated that it is possible to reduce the processing time through feature selection, but decreasing the classification accuracy. However, they also concluded that further exploration of features and feature selection is needed.

Lian [10] showed that PCA can be used as a dimension reduction tool for an ocSVM classifier with good results. His research takes as a baseline one of the most popular dimension reduction tools used in unsupervised and supervised problems, PCA. However, instead of extracting eigenvectors associated with top eigenvalues, he extracts the eigenvectors associated with small eigenvalues. In this approach, the null of the eigenspace is of interest since common features contained in the training samples are described by the null space.

Su et al. [11] work explores the dimension reduction of a hyperspectral images (HSI) dataset through feature selection and feature extraction techniques. Their goal was to augment the classification accuracy obtained by SVM. To reduce the size of the training dataset, they tested the following algorithms: mutual information, minimal redundancy maximal relevance, PCA, and Kernel PCA. Their experiments were centred on the performance achieved by SVM using the number of features selected by each technique. Results showed that PCA was the most effective technique to reduce data dimensionality in terms of computational load, implementation complexity, and classification performance. Furthermore, they showed that using SVM in combination with PCA obtains better prediction performance in terms of accuracy than using SVM with the full dataset. The authors concluded that using SVM with PCA is suitable for real-time applications since there is a significant reduction in computational time.

As we have seen in the reviewed work, a common approach is to work with attributes in both domains, time and frequency, and then apply feature selection techniques before training any classifier. Following this approach, it is possible to minimise the number of computed features and thus reduce the processing time required to train the classifiers, but, at the same time, trying to keep a good classification performance.

3. Methods

In this section, we describe in detail the datasets used in our experiments as well as the feature selection procedures performed on the datasets. In addition, we describe the classifiers used to compare the efficiency of the feature selection process.

3.1. PRIDE Dataset

Barrera-Animas et al. [1] built a new dataset specifically oriented to the personal risk detection problem, so that the research community could use it for a fair comparison of algorithms. The dataset is known as PRIDE and contains sensor data from 23 subjects wearing a Microsoft Band v1$^{©}$ (Microsoft Corporation, Washington, DC, USA), and by means of a mobile application developed by the authors, they collected sensor data from the band, and uploaded it to an FTP (File Transfer Protocol) server. This procedure was done during one week, 24 h a day, to create the normal conditions dataset (NCDS), which is part of PRIDE. During this period, subjects made sure that their week was an ordinary one. PRIDE includes subjects with diverse individualities regarding gender, age, height and lifestyle. The dataset comprises 15 male and eight female volunteers aged in the range 21 to 52 years, statures from 1.56 to 1.86 m, weights in the range 42 to 101 kg, exercising practice of 0 to 10 h per week, and sedentary hours or leisure ranging from 20 to 84 h per week. Afterwards, to build the PRIDE's anomaly conditions dataset (ACDS), the same 23 subjects participated in another process to obtain data under specific conditions, for which five scenarios to simulate hazardous or abnormal conditions were designed. These scenarios involved the following activities: running 100 m as fast as possible, climbing the stairs in a multi-floor building as quick as possible, a two-minute boxing episode, falling back and forth, and holding one's breath for as long as possible. Each activity intended to simulate anomalous conditions, comprising possibly risk-prone situations from real world, e.g., running away from an unsafe situation, clearing a building due to an emergency alert, defending against an aggressor during a dispute, swooning and suffering from breathing problems. The session to perform all five scenarios by each subject lasted for about two hours, and it demanded major physical effort. They were realised indoors and outdoors with different weather conditions and levels of UV exposure, depending on the day the subject was able to present them. The elderly, and other groups such as people suffering a chronicle disease, comprise very important groups in our society; however, they were not included in the data collection process, due to the demanding nature of the method just described.

As mentioned previously, personal risk detection can be approached as an anomaly detection problem, to differentiate a normal condition from uncommon behaviour. The anomaly detector can be a one-class classifier, trained only with a user's normal conditions dataset. The stress scenarios serve to verify if the classifier is able to distinguish them as an anomaly, and not to recognise which scenario or activity is being observed. The stress scenarios are intended to simulate certain danger or abnormal behaviour; however, we acknowledge that they are only an estimate to real-life situations. Our goal is to detect anomalies that can be the result of, for example, a car accident, a health crisis, or a physical aggression. We decided to undertake this approach since we do not have the means to obtain data in the course of a real-life crisis. It is worth remarking that anomalous situations in some cases may be related to a personal risk-prone situation. However, labelling a behaviour as abnormal does not always imply risk; moreover, not all risk-prone situations will always turn into anomalous behaviour. In other words, we are able to differentiate abnormal behaviour from ordinary one, thereby spotting some (but not all) possible risk-prone circumstances.

Next, we briefly describe the sensors embedded in the wearable device. Table 1 lists the sensors in the band and their operating frequencies; using these values, a user gathered on average 1.6 millions of records per day. A readout from the accelerometer and gyroscope was obtained every 125 ms, using an operating frequency of 8 Hz. Ultraviolet exposure values are gathered every 1 min and skin temperature values every half a minute. The measurements of the rest of the band's sensors, distance, pedometer, heart rate, and calories are logged every 1 s.

Table 1. Description of sensors in the band.

Sensor	Description	Operation Frequency
Accelerometer	Provides x, y, and z acceleration in g units. 1 g = 9.81 m/s^2.	8 Hz
Gyroscope	Provides x, y, and z angular velocity in $°$/s units.	8 Hz
Distance	Gives the total distance in cm, current speed in cm/s, current pace in ms/m.	1 Hz
Heart Rate	Gives the number of beats per minute.	1 Hz
Pedometer	Delivers the total number of steps the user has accomplished.	1 Hz
Skin Temperature	Gives the current skin temperature of the user in Celsius.	33 mHz
Ultraviolet exposure	Delivers the current ultraviolet radiation exposure intensity.	16 mHz
Calories	Provides total calories burned by the user.	1 Hz

In the following sections, we present our methodology for feature selection in time and frequency domains, respectively. By running the Kruskal–Wallis test, we proved that all users' datasets are statistically different, that is, they are not drawn from the same population. Hence, we decided to use a subject-dependent approach during the feature selection process, i.e., on a user-by-user basis. It is important to notice that the feature selection process is performed only on the user's training dataset, that is, the Normal Conditions Dataset (NCDS).

3.2. PRIDE Pre-Processing and Feature Selection in the Time-Domain

During the pre-processing step, a feature vector is computed using windows of one second of sensor data; this process is done for every user in the PRIDE dataset. Depending on the readout interval of a sensor, three rules apply in order to assign a value to the feature vector:

$$\text{Feature vector} = \begin{cases} \text{Average and sample standard deviation} \\ \text{of all sensor measurements in a second,} & \text{if readout interval} < 1\text{ s,} \\ \text{Assign the sensor value,} & \text{if readout interval} = 1\text{ s,} \\ \text{Assign the last sensor value,} & \text{if readout interval} > 1\text{ s.} \end{cases}$$

Thus, a feature vector from a given window contains the following sensor values:

- Means and standard deviations of the gyroscope and accelerometer readouts.
- Absolute values from the heart rate, skin temperature, pace, speed, and ultraviolet exposure sensors.
- A Δ-value, computed as the difference between the current and previous values of the following measurements: total steps, total distance, and calories burned.

Using this procedure, a 26-dimensional feature vector is derived; its final structure is shown in Table 2. This feature vector in the time-domain was used to obtain all results reported in [1,2,12]. The subsets NCDS and ACDS of PRIDE are pre-processed using this procedure.

Table 2. Feature vector structure.

Feature Number	Feature Name	Feature Number	Feature Name
1	$\bar{x}$ Gyroscope Accelerometer x-axis	14	s Accelerometer x-axis
2	s Gyroscope Accelerometer x-axis	15	$\bar{x}$ Accelerometer y-axis
3	$\bar{x}$ Gyroscope Accelerometer y-axis	16	s Accelerometer y-axis
4	s Gyroscope Accelerometer y-axis	17	$\bar{x}$ Accelerometer z-axis
5	$\bar{x}$ Gyroscope Accelerometer z-axis	18	s Accelerometer z-axis
6	s Gyroscope Accelerometer z-axis	19	Heart Rate
7	$\bar{x}$ Gyroscope Angular Velocity x-axis	20	Skin Temperature
8	s Gyroscope Angular Velocity x-axis	21	Pace
9	$\bar{x}$ Gyroscope Angular Velocity y-axis	22	Speed
10	s Gyroscope Angular Velocity y-axis	23	Ultraviolet
11	$\bar{x}$ Gyroscope Angular Velocity z-axis	24	Δ Pedometer
12	s Gyroscope Angular Velocity z-axis	25	Δ Distance
13	$\bar{x}$ Accelerometer x-axis	26	Δ Calories

Finally, each of the user logs was divided into five folds to use them in a five-fold cross-validation. In the cross-validation, four folds of the normal behaviour of a user were used for training and one fold was joined with the anomaly dataset log to test the classifiers. This procedure was repeated five times alternating the user's fold that was retained for testing. Hence, five training datasets and five testing datasets were set.

After this pre-processing step, we have conducted a Principal Component and a Correlation Matrix (CM) analysis on the PRIDE time-domain dataset with the aim of reducing its dimensionality. PCA allows identifying those features that best describe the variability of the points in the dataset, whereas the correlation matrix performs a statistical correlation analysis that is often used to remove redundant (highly-correlated) features [6,13–16].

The experiments were conducted in R language, in the RStudio software (version:1.0.153 , RStudio Inc., Boston, MA, USA) [17]. The correlation matrix was computed using the well-known caret package [18]. Firstly, we performed the CM process to remove redundant features and then we applied PCA to remove features that do not contribute sufficiently to the principal components but at the same time retaining at least 60% of data variability [13,14,19]. This process is illustrated in Figure 1.

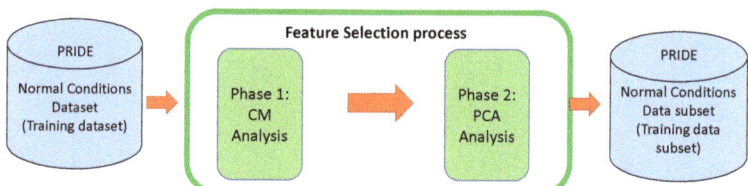

Figure 1. Feature selection process performed over every user of the PRIDE training dataset.

3.2.1. Correlation Matrix Analysis on the Time-Domain Attributes

We computed the correlation matrix for the 23 users in PRIDE. As a sample, the result for user 1 is shown in Figure 2. For each user, features with a correlation value equal to or greater than 0.75 are saved into a vector [20]. Next, we computed the frequency of occurrence of each feature along the 23 vectors. If a feature is reported as highly-correlated by at least 22 of the 23 vectors, then that feature is removed from the dataset.

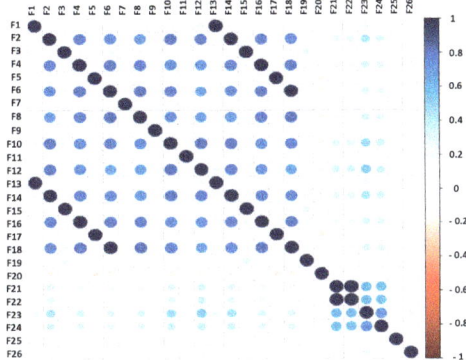

Figure 2. Correlation matrix of user 1.

The results in Table 3 show that features F2, F6, F10, F14, and F18 are highly-correlated consistently in at least 22 users, thus they were removed from the PRIDE dataset. Using the correlation matrix analysis for feature selection, the PRIDE dataset was downsized from 26 to 21 features.

Table 3. Results of the correlation matrix analysis for feature selection in the PRIDE dataset.

Feature Number	Frequency	Feature Name	Feature Number	Frequency	Feature Name
F1	9	$\bar{x}$ Gyro Accel x	F14	22	s Accel x
F2	23	s Gyro Accel x	F15	15	$\bar{x}$ Accel y
F3	8	$\bar{x}$ Gyro Accel y	F16	21	s Accel y
F4	19	s Gyro Accel y	F17	8	$\bar{x}$ Accel z
F5	15	$\bar{x}$ Gyro Accel z	F18	23	s Accel z
F6	23	s Gyro Accel z	F19	0	Heart Rate
F7	0	$\bar{x}$ Gyro Ang Vel x	F20	0	Skin Temperature
F8	2	s Gyro Ang Vel x	F21	3	Δ Pedometer
F9	0	$\bar{x}$ Gyro Ang Vel y	F22	13	Δ Distance
F10	22	s Gyro Ang Vel y	F23	2	Speed
F11	0	$\bar{x}$ Gyro Ang Vel z	F24	0	Pace
F12	10	s Gyro Ang Vel z	F25	1	Δ Calories
F13	14	$\bar{x}$ Accel x	F26	0	Ultraviolet

3.2.2. Principal Component Analysis on the Time-Domain Attributes

We run a Principal Component Analysis over every user of the PRIDE dataset in order to identify those features that best describe the variability of the data in the dataset; in this way, we are able to remove those features that do not contribute sufficiently to data variability.

Figure 3 shows the results of PCA computed over the PRIDE user with more data, user 1. It shows the percentage of the explained variances across ten dimensions. It can be observed, by aggregating the contribution of each dimension, that the first five dimensions explain approximately 60% of data variability [13,14,19]. Figure 4a–e depict a plot for each of the first five dimensions, with contribution percentage per variable in such dimension. Additionally, Figure 4f shows the contribution percentage of each variable to the aggregated first five dimensions. All plots are related to user 1.

After we computed PCA over the 23 users, we totalled the frequency of occurrence of each feature along the first five dimensions of all users. A feature is included in this count if it had a contribution value over the expected average contribution of all features. The red line in each plot of Figure 4 represents the expected average contribution of all features if their contributions were uniform. This means that the highest possible value of a feature is 115, i.e., it is above a threshold in all five dimensions for every user (5 × 23). From this sum, we removed from the dataset those features that never contributed (or contributed insufficiently) to any of the first five dimensions, i.e., the dimensions necessary to preserve at least 60% of data variability.

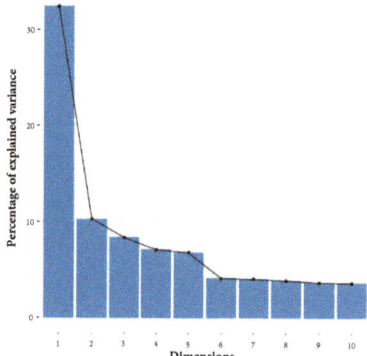

Figure 3. PCA results for user 1 from PRIDE that shows the percentage of explained variance of the first 10 dimensions.

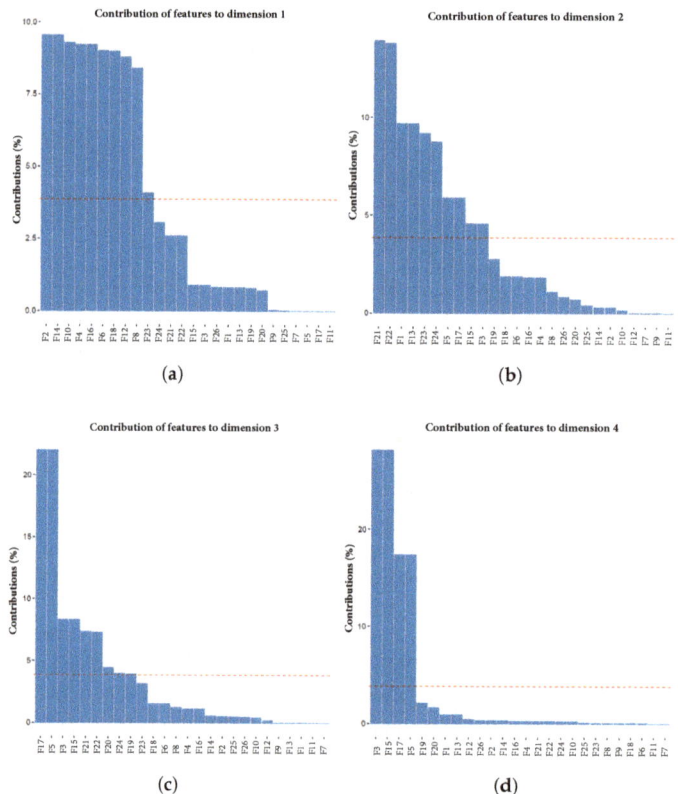

Figure 4. *Cont.*

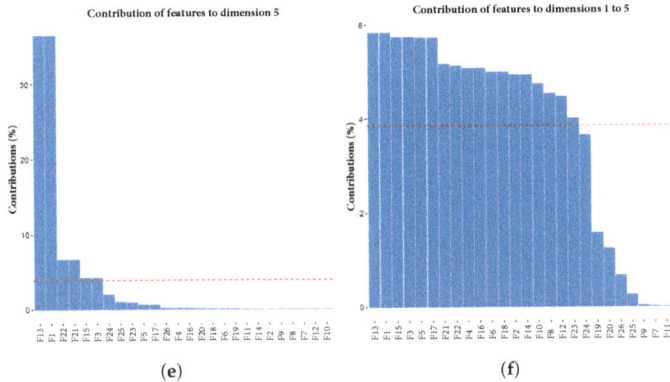

(e) (f)

Figure 4. PCA results for user 1. Each graph represents the contribution of every feature to data variability in (**a**) dimension 1; (**b**) dimension 2; (**c**) dimension 3; (**d**) dimension 4; and (**e**) dimension 5; (**f**) contribution of every feature in the aggregated five dimensions.

The results in Table 4 show that features F7, F9, and F11 are never used in the PCA analysis; that is, these features do not contribute to explaining the data variability. Furthermore, feature F26 is used only once across the first five dimensions, making its contribution negligible. Hence, it is feasible to remove these features from the PRIDE dataset without losing data representativeness.

Table 4. Principal Component Analysis results for feature selection in the PRIDE dataset.

Feature Number	Frequency	Feature Name	Feature Number	Frequency	Feature Name
F1	52	$\bar{x}$ Gyro Accel x	F16	37	s Accel y
F3	31	$\bar{x}$ Gyro Accel y	F17	53	$\bar{x}$ Accel z
F4	37	s Gyro Accel y	F19	18	Heart Rate
F5	53	$\bar{x}$ Gyro Accel z	F20	16	Skin Temperature
F7	**0**	**$\bar{x}$ Gyro Ang Vel x**	F21	29	Δ Pedometer
F8	28	s Gyro Ang Vel x	F22	29	Δ Distance
F9	**0**	**$\bar{x}$ Gyro Ang Vel y**	F23	31	Speed
F11	**0**	**$\bar{x}$ Gyro Ang Vel z**	F24	29	Pace
F12	26	s Gyro Ang Vel z	F25	15	Δ Calories
F13	52	$\bar{x}$ Accel x	**F26**	**1**	**Ultraviolet**
F15	58	$\bar{x}$ Accel y			

At this point, we have performed a feature selection procedure based on a correlation matrix and Principal Component Analysis in order to reduce the dimension of the PRIDE dataset and thus reduce execution time by keeping a comparable performance of the classifiers. After this procedure, nine attributes in the time-domain were removed without losing data representativeness: five attributes by means of the correlation matrix analysis (F2, F6, F10, F14, and F18) and four attributes by applying Principal Component Analysis (F7, F9, F11, and F26). The complete feature selection process just described is summarised and shown in Figures 5 and 6.

In the next section, we describe the pre-processing of the PRIDE dataset using attributes in the time and frequency domains. Then, a similar procedure for feature selection as the one just described is also presented.

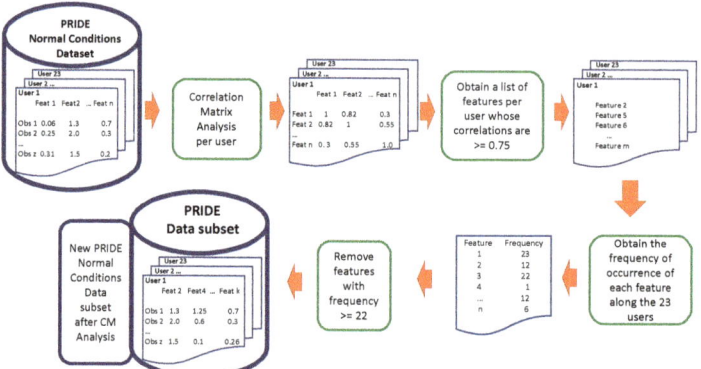

Figure 5. Feature selection process. Phase 1: CM Analysis.

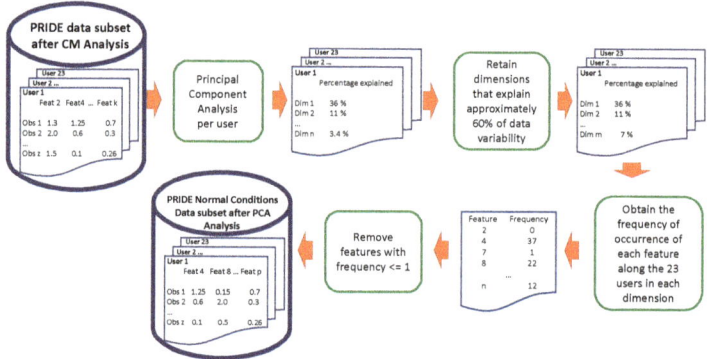

Figure 6. Feature selection process. Phase 2: PCA analysis.

3.3. PRIDE Pre-Processing and Feature Selection in the Time/Frequency-Domain

Inspired by [21] and following the aim to obtain features that could describe the behavioural and physiological patterns of a person, several features were calculated in the frequency-domain. Hence, we extended the feature vector presented in Section 3.2 by calculating new frequency-domain attributes; as a result, ten new features in the frequency-domain were derived for each axis of the accelerometer and gyroscope sensors. These features are computed using a non-overlapping one-second time sliding window, similar to the process described in Section 3.2. The accelerometer and gyroscope provide eight data samples every window, since the operation frequency of these sensors is set up at 8 Hz, as recalled from Table 1.

Table 5 shows the new frequency-domain features, computed according to [21–24]. These attributes come from the signal analysis area and have been widely used to reveal more properties normally not appreciated in the domain of time, to attain a richer view of the observed scenario; the interested reader is referred to these works, for a complete description of the signal processing methods. In total, 90 features in the frequency-domain were obtained. Furthermore, the eight features of non-motion sensors from Table 2 were preserved. Thus, we end up with a 98-dimensional feature vector that combines attributes from both dimensions. For the sake of simplicity to the reader, the final vector is listed in the Appendix. The feature selection process described next is performed over this new feature vector, containing both time and frequency domain features.

Table 5. New frequency-domain attributes.

Feature Name	Feature Formula
FFT energy	$\sum_{i=1}^{(\frac{n}{2})+1} x[i]^2$
FFT mean energy	$\frac{1}{n} \times \sum_{i=1}^{n} x_i$
FFT STD energy	$(\frac{1}{n} \times \sum_{i=1}^{n} x_i((|x_i - \frac{1}{n} \times \sum_{i=1}^{n} x_i|)^2))^2$
Peak power	$\max \frac{P(w_i)}{\sum_i P(w_i)}$
Peak DFT bin	$\max_{ith} (n \times Fs/N)$
Peak magnitude	$\max |fft(x)|$
Entropy	$\sum_{j=1}^{(\frac{n}{2})+1} \frac{|x_i|}{\sum_{i=1}^{(\frac{n}{2})+1} x[i]^2} \times \log(\frac{|x_i|}{\sum_{i=1}^{(\frac{n}{2})+1} x[i]^2})$
Spectral Entropy	$-\sum_{i=1}^{n} \frac{P(w_i)}{\sum_i P(w_i)} \times \ln(\frac{P(w_i)}{\sum_i P(w_i)})$
Peak Frequency	$\max (n \times Fs/N)$
Peak energy	$\max \sum_{i=1}^{(\frac{n}{2})+1} x[i]^2$

Note: FFT stands for Fast Fourier Transform; STD stands for Standard Deviation; DFT stands for Discrete Fourier Transform.

In this case, we have also conducted a Principal Component Analysis and a Correlation Matrix analysis on the extended PRIDE dataset with attributes in the time and frequency domains, with the aim of reducing its dimensionality. As in the time-domain case, we first performed the CM process to remove redundant features and then we applied PCA to remove features that do not contribute sufficiently to the principal components, retaining at least 60% of data variability.

We used the same criteria to remove attributes to the dataset as described in Section 3.2; thus, for the sake of simplicity, we only present in the following sections the outcome of the correlation matrix and the Principal Component Analysis.

3.3.1. Correlation Matrix Analysis on the Time/Frequency-Domain Attributes

After performing a correlation matrix analysis on the new feature vector, we were able to remove 11 features from the PRIDE dataset, since their correlation values were consistently above 0.75 in all 23 users. Table 6 shows the features that appeared at least 22 times, thus removed. Since the new vector contains 98 attributes, we only show in the table those attributes removed by the CM analysis, downsizing the vector to 87 attributes.

Table 6. Results of the correlation matrix analysis for feature selection in the extended PRIDE dataset. Only removed features are shown.

Feature Number	Frequency	Feature Name
F1	23	Energy GyroSensor xAccel
F3	23	Standard Deviation Energy GyroSensor xAccel
F5	23	Peak DFT Bin GyroSensor xAccel
F7	23	Peak Magnitude GyroSensor xAccel
F10	23	Peak Energy GyroSensor xAccel
F11	22	Energy GyroSensor yAccel
F15	23	Peak DFT Bin GyroSensor yAccel
F17	23	Peak Magnitude GyroSensor yAccel
F18	22	Entropy GyroSensor yAccel
F20	23	Peak Energy GyroSensor yAccel
F21	23	Energy GyroSensor zAccel

3.3.2. Principal Component Analysis on the Time/Frequency-Domain Attributes

We run a Principal Component Analysis over every user of the extended PRIDE dataset in order to get rid of those features that do not contribute sufficiently to data variability. After running PCA, we found out that, in this case, the first eight dimensions explain at least 60% of data variability. Then, we added up the frequency of occurrence of each feature along the first eight dimensions of all users. A feature is included in this count if it had a contribution value over the expected average contribution of all features. In this case, the highest possible value of a feature is 184, i.e., it is above a threshold in all eight dimensions for every user (8×23). From this sum, we removed from the dataset those features that never contributed to any of the eight dimensions, i.e., the dimensions necessary to retain at least 60% of data variability.

Results in Table 7 show that features F38, F48, F58 and F98 are never used in the PCA analysis; that is, these features do not contribute to explaining the data variability. Hence, it is feasible to get rid of these features from the PRIDE dataset without losing data representativeness.

Table 7. Principal Component Analysis results for feature selection in the extended PRIDE dataset. Only removed features are shown.

Feature Number	Frequency	Feature Name
F38	0	Entropy GyroSensor xAngVel
F48	0	Entropy GyroSensor yAngVel
F58	0	Entropy GyroSensor zAngVel
F98	0	Ultraviolet

In summary, we performed a feature selection procedure based on a correlation matrix and Principal Component Analysis in order to reduce the dimension of the new PRIDE dataset and thus reduce execution time by keeping a comparable performance of the classifiers. After this procedure, fifteen attributes in the time/frequency-domain were removed without losing data representativeness: eleven attributes based on the correlation matrix analysis (F1, F3, F5, F7, F10, F11, F15, F17, F18, F20, and F21) and four attributes after applying a Principal Component Analysis (F38, F48, F58, and F98), resulting in an 83-dimension feature vector.

3.4. The Classifiers

We decided to use in our experiments two classifiers, ocSVM and OCKRA. ocSVM is well known in the literature [25] and it was reported by Barrera-Animas et al. in [1] as the best classifier for the personal risk detection problem. On the other hand, OCKRA is a new algorithm proposed in [2] specially designed to improve previous results in the same context and particularly having in mind its implementation in a mobile device. OCKRA is an ensemble of one-class classifiers, based on multiple projections of the dataset according to random subsets of features. Refer to [2] for a detailed description of this new algorithm. For our experiments, we used four different versions of PRIDE, which are:

- Dataset 1. Original dataset as described in [1] based on 26 time-domain features.
- Dataset 2. A subset of Dataset 1, after a feature selection procedure, as described in Section 3.2. Each vector holds 19 attributes.
- Dataset 3. An extended feature vector based on Dataset 1, with new frequency-domain attributes. Each vector comprises 98 attributes.
- Dataset 4. A subset of Dataset 3, after a feature selection procedure, as described in Section 3.3. Each vector holds 83 attributes.

We used the implementation of ocSVM [25] built-in in LibSVM [26] using the radial basis function kernel with default parameter values ($\gamma = 0.038$ and $\nu = 0.5$). Both classifiers, ocSVM and OCKRA, were tested using a five-fold cross-validation, as described in Section 3.2.

In the context of personal risk detection, our intention is to find a classifier that is able to distinguish every possible abnormal behaviour from those that are normal. For that reason, the goal is to build a classifier that maximises true positive classifications (i.e., true abnormal conditions) while minimising false positive ones (i.e., false abnormal or hazardous situations). To evaluate the performance of our classifiers, we compute the Area Under the Curve (AUC) of the true positive detection rate (TPR) versus the false positive detection rate (FPR). This indicator describes the general performance of the classifier for all false positive detection rates.

We only use AUC as the metric to evaluate and compare the classifiers performance since our focus in this work is mainly on the feature selection procedure and the speed-up achieved during training, without sacrificing the classifier performance. We consider AUC a very valuable and robust metric to monitor the overall performance of the classifiers when trained over the four datasets, which all come from the same problem domain, that is, the publicly available PRIDE dataset. For the interested reader, an exhaustive performance comparison between ocSVM and OCKRA over the PRIDE dataset (Dataset 1) is presented in [2]. Therein, in addition to AUC values, Precision–Recall curves and ROC curves (Receiver Operating Characteristic) per user and for the total population are presented, along with several statistical tests.

4. Results

Table 8 shows our results regarding the performance of the classifiers based on the AUC metric, where DS-i refers to Dataset i. In this particular case, averages are acceptable as a quick reference, since the multiple datasets are related to the same problem domain [27]. In general, both classifiers perform better when using datasets DS-1 and DS-2 (i.e., based on time-domain attributes and a subset of it, respectively) than when they are trained using datasets DS-3 and DS-4 (i.e., the extended vector with new attributes in the time/frequency domains and a subset of it, respectively). Based on the performance of both classifiers, we discarded DS-3 and DS-4 for further analysis.

Table 8. ocSVM and OCKRA performance based on the AUC with different datasets.

User	ocSVM				OCKRA			
	DS-1	DS-2	DS-3	DS-4	DS-1	DS-2	DS-3	DS-4
User 1	97.3	97.3	79.1	78.5	98.8	95.5	78.0	81.0
User 2	94.5	94.3	82.2	81.6	95.7	92.0	85.5	82.9
User 3	87.4	87.2	74.5	73.9	91.2	84.1	82.4	81.9
User 4	83.9	82.1	57.7	57.1	88.2	83.6	61.4	61.0
User 5	80.8	80.8	65.7	65.8	90.2	71.5	68.8	61.9
User 6	96.1	96.1	81.8	81.8	98.2	97.4	87.9	82.3
User 7	69.4	68.1	64.9	64.1	79.2	76.9	65.6	59.5
User 8	93.8	94.0	73.2	71.6	92.4	86.8	77.6	72.8
User 9	95.3	95.5	76.4	75.6	92.7	89.3	81.5	77.8
User 10	94.0	94.3	70.0	69.8	93.7	91.5	69.3	71.9
User 11	93.4	93.8	66.5	66.1	90.9	79.4	69.9	66.8
User 12	74.6	73.4	73.2	73.3	80.3	77.6	71.4	69.4
User 13	75.8	73.4	74.1	73.4	80.5	76.0	70.7	69.2
User 14	78.0	78.2	63.0	62.9	81.9	79.0	66.8	65.1
User 15	93.8	94.4	71.5	70.8	94.5	89.9	77.4	69.3
User 16	83.2	83.0	73.6	73.2	87.9	84.3	73.0	73.8
User 17	98.1	99.0	82.5	82.1	98.0	84.1	81.6	81.9
User 18	89.1	89.0	77.0	77.0	86.9	75.9	70.6	72.5
User 19	89.4	90.0	64.7	64.2	89.6	86.3	64.5	61.8
User 20	90.5	90.2	78.0	77.8	92.2	88.2	79.8	73.6
User 21	98.4	98.4	89.5	89.4	97.9	94.2	87.2	88.3
User 22	78.3	77.8	70.8	70.1	79.2	77.4	70.2	71.5
User 23	53.0	52.6	63.3	62.9	68.9	64.2	72.3	60.9
Average	86.44	86.2	72.8	72.3	89.1	83.7	74.5	72.0

We run a set of Wilcoxon signed-ranks tests to verify whether the two classifiers are statically significantly different or the differences between their performance are random. The first test compares OCKRA against ocSVM run over DS-1, and the second test run over DS-2. According to the results shown in Table 9, we reject the null-hypothesis and decide that OCKRA improves ocSVM with a level of significance $\alpha = 0.95$ and a p-value of 0.01. For the second test, Wilcoxon test result is shown in Table 10. We can appreciate that there is also a significant difference between the two classifiers, ocSVM performing better than OCKRA when running over DS-2, this time at a level of significance $\alpha = 0.90$ and a p value of 0.049. Although this significant difference is weak ($p \approx 0.05$), at this point, we cannot conclude that either classifier improves the other in all cases; hence, further analysis is needed.

Table 9. Wilcoxon signed-ranks test comparison between AUC obtained respectively by ocSVM and OCKRA classifiers when using the DS-1 dataset.

Comparison	R^+	R^-	Hypothesis ($\alpha = 0.05$)	p-Value
OCKRA vs. ocSVM	221.0	55.0	Rejected	0.010793

Table 10. Wilcoxon signed-ranks test comparison between AUC obtained respectively by ocSVM and OCKRA classifiers when using the DS-2 dataset.

Comparison	R^+	R^-	Hypothesis ($\alpha = 0.10$)	p-Value
ocSVM vs. OCKRA	202.0	74.0	Rejected	0.04979

Regarding execution time, Table 11 shows our results in hh:mm:ss format. We chose the datasets from two users, the ones with more and less number of observations in the PRIDE dataset; that is, users 1 and 17, respectively.

Table 11. Execution time required by the classifier training phase using different datasets. The $\mathcal{G}$ column indicates the gain in percentage when using a subset against the full feature vector. Experiments were performed using an Intel core i7-6600U (Mountain View, CA, USA) at 2.60–2.81 GHz and 16 GB RAM.

Domain	Dataset	Dimension	ocSVM				OCKRA			
			User 1	$\mathcal{G}$	User 17	$\mathcal{G}$	User 1	$\mathcal{G}$	User 17	$\mathcal{G}$
Time	DS-1	full	21:14:59		02:39:36		00:55:23		00:04:52	
	DS-2	subset	21:07:07	0.6%	02:38:28	0.7%	00:37:01	33.1%	00:03:55	19.5%
Time+Freq	DS-3	full	19:31:21		01:56:13		03:37:53		00:20:52	
	DS-4	subset	19:05:31	2.2%	01:55:05	0.9%	03:11:17	12.2%	00:17:37	15.5%

In the case of OCKRA, there is in all instances a reduction in the execution time when training with a subset of the attributes instead of using the full feature vector. The best speed-up is obtained when training user 1 with a subset of attributes in the time-domain (DS-2). In this case, the execution time was approximately 37 min compared to approximately 55.4 min when trained using the full set of attributes (DS-1), which corresponds to a speed-up of 33.1%. For user 17, the attained acceleration is 19.5%. The achieved acceleration is smaller when working with a subset of attributes in the time/frequency domain (DS-3, DS-4); for user 1, 12.2% and for user 17, 15.5%. However, the execution time is much higher, above three hours in the worst case (user 1) compared to 37 min in the previous case. In the case of ocSVM, there is a minimum gain in the execution time when using a subset of attributes against the full feature vector ($\leq 2.2\%$); however, execution times are much higher in all cases than those reported by OCKRA.

Concerning execution time, it is clear that our best candidate to be implemented on a mobile device is OCKRA using a subset of the time-domain dataset (DS-2). However, as for the performance of the classifiers when using DS-2, we recall from Table 10 that the Wilcoxon test reports a very weak statistical difference, which allows us to take a safe decision when choosing OCKRA as our best candidate without sacrificing performance. Additionally, the gain in speed-up is considerably higher when compared to the execution time reported by ocSVM.

Besides training times, testing and classification times are also important in several real-world applications; however, in our case, these times are very short. We registered the time required for testing by the same users, both classifiers, and the four datasets. We observed seven seconds in the worst case (user 1, OCKRA, DS-3, that is, the extended dataset in the time and frequency domains before feature selection), and less than one second in 25% of the cases. Taking into account that a testing fold contains approximately 94,000 observations for user 1, and 27,000 observations for user 17, the time needed to classify a new object by either OCKRA or ocSVM is negligible.

We can note that, when using the PRIDE dataset based only on time-domain attributes and a subset of it, both classifiers guarantee a good classification performance, which is not the case when using the extended feature vector and a subset of it, as classification performance is notably degraded; however, in the case of OCKRA, the time needed for training can be reduced considerably using the dataset after feature selection. This is a very important fact to consider during the design process, in order to select the more efficient classifier that is to be implemented in a mobile device, assuming less processing and memory resources.

5. Discussion

In this work, we built upon previous results reported by Barrera-Animas et al. in [1], in which the authors claimed that it is likely to use PRIDE, a dataset with information drawn from a number of users wearing a device with built-in sensors, to develop a personal risk detection mechanism, and showed that abnormal behaviour could be automatically detected by a one-class classifier. In addition, they showed that OCKRA stands so far as the state-of-the-art classifier in the context of personal risk detection, followed by ocSVM [2]. Our current goal is to derive an efficient classifier to be implemented on mobile devices, as part of a user application for automatic personal risk detection, thus low-consumption of physical resources, such as CPU time and memory, must be taken into account.

First, we decided to extend the PRIDE dataset by adding features in the frequency-domain by transforming current time-domain features on the search to attain a better classification accuracy. Concerning CPU time, we decided to apply feature selection techniques on the PRIDE dataset; in our case, we used correlation matrix and Principal Component Analysis.

We conclude that, in the context of personal risk detection, using the PRIDE dataset based on time-domain attributes and a subset of it should be enough to guarantee a good classification performance. Additionally, OCKRA showed a very important speed-up during the training process when using the dataset after feature selection. Considering the trade-off between classification performance and efficiency, our results support the choice of OCKRA as our best candidate so far for a mobile implementation, using a reduced dataset on the time-domain after a feature selection procedure. By using this subset, OCKRA reported a very important gain on execution time without sacrificing the classifier performance. This result is promising since it can translate into a better user experience, thus reducing the chance to stop using the wearable and its application in the short and mid-term.

Our results are encouraging since they represent the first step towards an efficient classifier well suited for mobile devices and to be implemented as part of a user application coupled with wearable sensors, in order to deal with the problem of timely detecting risk-prone situations experienced by a person.

However, by using our methodology, we acknowledge the possibility that the feature selection process performed on the training dataset could result in removing features that may contribute to the detection of abnormal situations. For example, concerning the UV attribute, the CM analysis kept this feature and the PCA analysis left this variable out, meaning that even though it is not highly correlated to other variables, it does not contribute enough to explain the dataset variability, thus it was removed without losing data representativeness. Therefore, even if we initially thought that UV was a very important feature, PCA tells us that, at least in this dataset, we can safely get rid of it, for the purpose of dimension reduction. The performance of the classifiers was maintained, meaning that the selection process was satisfactory. Nevertheless, it is of great interest to perform the feature selection process on the complete dataset, that is, using the training and testing datasets. Although we believe this can result in overfitting of the dataset, we might be reducing the possibility of leaving out an important feature capable of detecting unseen abnormal behaviours. Therefore, it is clearly a trade-off issue inherent in the feature selection problem for one-class datasets, which is worth further exploring. Indeed, we are currently reviewing other feature selection techniques that allow for a similar reduction on the execution time, but at the same time could achieve a statistically equivalent or better classification performance.

According to Yousef et al. [16,28], feature selection is well studied for two-class classification problems while few methods are proposed for one-class classification ones. Furthermore, two-class feature selection methods may not apply to one-class classification problems because of the use of the two classes during the feature ranking procedure. Thus, this further step becomes challenging, since feature selection is NP-hard according to Yousef et al. Recall from computational complexity theory that a problem is NP-hard if there is an algorithm to solve it that can be transformed into one for solving any NP (non-deterministic polynomial-time) problem. NP-hard is then "at least as hard as any NP-problem", or even harder. Therefore, additional work must be performed to determine an appropriate feature selection method for the personal risk detection problem.

Author Contributions: Conceptualization, L.A.T. and A.Y.B.-A.; Data curation, A.Y.B.-A.; Formal analysis, A.Y.B.-A.; Investigation, A.Y.B.-A.; Methodology, L.A.T. and A.Y.B.-A.; Project administration, L.A.T.; Resources, L.A.T.; Software, A.Y.B.-A.; Supervision, L.A.T.; Validation, L.A.T. and A.Y.B.-A.; Visualization, L.A.T. and A.Y.B.-A.; Writing—Original draft, L.A.T.; Writing—Review and editing, L.A.T. and A.Y.B.-A.

Funding: This research received no external funding.

Acknowledgments: We thank the GIEE-ML group (Grupo de Investigación con Enfoque Estratégico-Machine Learning) at Tecnológico de Monterrey for providing useful observations and advice during the preparation of this work; in particular, we would like to give special thanks to Octavio Loyola, for his precious help regarding the statistical tests. We also thank the Hasso Plattner Institut Future SOC (Service-Oriented Computing) Lab for providing the computing infrastructure, which comprises a VM with 64 cores, to perform part of the experiments.

Conflicts of Interest: The authors declare no conflicts of interest.

Abbreviations

The following abbreviations are used in this manuscript:

ACDS	Anomaly conditions dataset
AUC	Area under the curve
CM	Correlation matrix
FPR	False positive detection rate
LibSVM	Support vector machine library
NCDS	Normal conditions dataset
OCKRA	One-class K-means with randomly projected features algorithm
ocSVM	One-class support vector machine
PCA	Principal component analysis
PRIDE	Personal risk detection
ROC	Receiver operating characteristic
TPR	True positive detection rate
NP-hard	Non-deterministic polynomial-time hard

Appendix A

Table A1. Time/frequency-domain feature vector part 1.

Feature Number	Feature Name
1	Energy Gyroscope x-Axis
2	Mean Energy Gyroscope x-Axis
3	Standard Deviation of Energy Gyroscope x-Axis
4	Peak Power Gyroscope x-Axis
5	Peak DFT Bin Gyroscope x-Axis
6	Spectral Entropy Gyroscope x-Axis
7	Peak Magnitude Gyroscope x-Axis
8	Entropy Gyroscope x-Axis
9	Peak Frequency Gyroscope x-Axis
10	Peak Energy Gyroscope x-Axis
11	Energy Gyroscope y-Axis
12	Mean Energy Gyroscope y-Axis
13	Standard Deviation of Energy Gyroscope y-Axis
14	Peak Power Gyroscope y-Axis
15	Peak DFT Bin Gyroscope y-Axis
16	Spectral Entropy Gyroscope y-Axis
17	Peak Magnitude Gyroscope y-Axis
18	Entropy Gyroscope y-Axis
19	Peak Frequency Gyroscope y-Axis
20	Peak Energy Gyroscope y-Axis
21	Energy Gyroscope z-Axis
22	Mean Energy Gyroscope z-Axis
23	Standard Deviation of Energy Gyroscope z-Axis
24	Peak Power Gyroscope z-Axis
25	Peak DFT Bin Gyroscope z-Axis
26	Spectral Entropy Gyroscope z-Axis
27	Peak Magnitude Gyroscope z-Axis
28	Entropy Gyroscope z-Axis
29	Peak Frequency Gyroscope z-Axis
30	Peak Energy Gyroscope z-Axis
31	Energy Gyroscope Angular Velocity x-Axis
32	Mean Energy Gyroscope Angular Velocity x-Axis
33	Standard Deviation of Energy Gyroscope Angular Velocity x-Axis
34	Peak Power Gyroscope Angular Velocity x-Axis
35	Peak DFT Bin Gyroscope Angular Velocity x-Axis
36	Spectral Entropy Gyroscope Angular Velocity x-Axis
37	Peak Magnitude Gyroscope Angular Velocity x-Axis
38	Entropy Gyroscope Angular Velocity x-Axis
39	Peak Frequency Gyroscope Angular Velocity x-Axis
40	Peak Energy Gyroscope Angular Velocity x-Axis
41	Energy Gyroscope Angular Velocity y-Axis
42	Mean Energy Gyroscope Angular Velocity y-Axis
43	Standard Deviation of Energy Gyroscope Angular Velocity y-Axis
44	Peak Power Gyroscope Angular Velocity y-Axis
45	Peak DFT Bin Gyroscope Angular Velocity y-Axis
46	Spectral Entropy Gyroscope Angular Velocity y-Axis
47	Peak Magnitude Gyroscope Angular Velocity y-Axis
48	Entropy Gyroscope Angular Velocity y-Axis
49	Peak Frequency Gyroscope Angular Velocity y-Axis
50	Peak Energy Gyroscope Angular Velocity y-Axis

Table A2. Time-/Frequency-domain feature vector part 2.

Feature Number	Feature Name
51	Energy Gyroscope Angular Velocity z-Axis
52	Mean Energy Gyroscope Angular Velocity z-Axis
53	Standard Deviation of Energy Gyroscope Angular Velocity z-Axis
54	Peak Power Gyroscope Angular Velocity z-Axis
55	Peak DFT Bin Gyroscope Angular Velocity z-Axis
56	Spectral Entropy Gyroscope Angular Velocity z-Axis
57	Peak Magnitude Gyroscope Angular Velocity z-Axis
58	Entropy Gyroscope Angular Velocity z-Axis
59	Peak Frequency Gyroscope Angular Velocity z-Axis
60	Peak Energy Gyroscope Angular Velocity z-Axis
61	Energy Accelerometer x-Axis
62	Mean Energy Accelerometer x-Axis
63	Standard Deviation of Energy Accelerometer x-Axis
64	Peak Power Accelerometer x-Axis
65	Peak DFT Bin Accelerometer x-Axis
66	Spectral Entropy Accelerometer x-Axis
67	Peak Magnitude Accelerometer x-Axis
68	Entropy Accelerometer x-Axis
69	Peak Frequency Accelerometer x-Axis
70	Peak Energy Accelerometer x-Axis
71	Energy Accelerometer y-Axis
72	Mean Energy Accelerometer y-Axis
73	Standard Deviation of Energy Accelerometer y-Axis
74	Peak Power Accelerometer y-Axis
75	Peak DFT Bin Accelerometer y-Axis
76	Spectral Entropy Accelerometer y-Axis
77	Peak Magnitude Accelerometer y-Axis
78	Entropy Accelerometer y-Axis
79	Peak Frequency Accelerometer y-Axis
80	Peak Energy Accelerometer y-Axis
81	Energy Accelerometer z-Axis
82	Mean Energy Accelerometer z-Axis
83	Standard Deviation of Energy Accelerometer z-Axis
84	Peak Power Accelerometer z-Axis
85	Peak DFT Bin Accelerometer z-Axis
86	Spectral Entropy Accelerometer z-Axis
87	Peak Magnitude Accelerometer z-Axis
88	Entropy Accelerometer z-Axis
89	Peak Frequency Accelerometer z-Axis
90	Peak Energy Accelerometer z-Axis
91	Heart Rate
92	Skin Temperature
93	Δ Pedometer
94	Δ Distance
95	Speed
96	Pace
97	Δ Calories
98	Ultraviolet

References

1. Barrera-Animas, A.Y.; Trejo, L.A.; Medina-Pérez, M.A.; Monroy, R.; Camiña, J.B.; Godínez, F. Online Personal Risk Detection Based on Behavioural and Physiological Patterns. *Inf. Sci.* **2017**, *384*, 281–297. [CrossRef]
2. Rodríguez, J.; Barrera-Animas, A.Y.; Trejo, L.A.; Medina-Pérez, M.A.; Monroy, R. Ensemble of One-Class Classifiers for Personal Risk Detection Based on Wearable Sensor Data. *Sensors* **2016**, *16*, 1619. [CrossRef] [PubMed]

3. Pei, L.; Guinness, R.; Chen, R.; Liu, J.; Kuusniemi, H.; Chen, Y.; Chen, L.; Kaistinen, J. Human behavior cognition using smartphone sensors. *Sensors* **2013**, *13*, 1402–1424. [CrossRef] [PubMed]
4. Özdemir, A.T.; Barshan, B. Detecting falls with wearable sensors using machine learning techniques. *Sensors* **2014**, *14*, 10691–10708. [CrossRef] [PubMed]
5. Wundersitz, D.W.; Josman, C.; Gupta, R.; Netto, K.J.; Gastin, P.B.; Robertson, S. Classification of team sport activities using a single wearable tracking device. *J. Biomech.* **2015**, *48*, 3975–3981. [CrossRef] [PubMed]
6. Del Rosario, M.B.; Redmond, S.J.; Lovell, N.H. Tracking the evolution of smartphone sensing for monitoring human movement. *Sensors* **2015**, *15*, 18901–18933. [CrossRef] [PubMed]
7. Rucco, R.; Sorriso, A.; Liparoti, M.; Ferraioli, G.; Sorrentino, P.; Ambrosanio, M.; Baselice, F. Type and Location of Wearable Sensors for Monitoring Falls during Static and Dynamic Tasks in Healthy Elderly: A Review. *Sensors* **2018**, *18*, 1613. [CrossRef] [PubMed]
8. Roweis, S.T.; Saul, L.K. Nonlinear dimensionality reduction by locally linear embedding. *Science* **2000**, *290*, 2323–2326. [CrossRef] [PubMed]
9. Tenenbaum, J.B.; De Silva, V.; Langford, J.C. A global geometric framework for nonlinear dimensionality reduction. *Science* **2000**, *290*, 2319–2323. [CrossRef] [PubMed]
10. Lian, H. On feature selection with principal component analysis for one-class SVM. *Pattern Recognit. Lett.* **2012**, *33*, 1027–1031. [CrossRef]
11. Su, J.; Yi, D.; Liu, C.; Guo, L.; Chen, W.H. Dimension reduction aided hyperspectral image classification with a small-sized training dataset: Experimental comparisons. *Sensors* **2017**, *17*, 2726. [CrossRef] [PubMed]
12. López-Cuevas, A.; Medina-Pérez, M.A.; Monroy, R.; Márquez, J.R.; Trejo, L.A. FiToViz: A Visualisation Approach for Real-time Risk Situation Awareness. *IEEE Trans. Affect. Comput.* **2017**. [CrossRef]
13. Jolliffe, I. *Principal Component Analysis*, 2nd ed.; Wiley Online Library: New York, NY, USA, 2002.
14. Jolliffe, I. Principal Component Analysis. In *Encyclopedia of Statistics in Behavioral Science*; John Wiley & Sons, Ltd.: Hoboken, NJ, USA, 2005. [CrossRef]
15. Wan, C.; Mita, A. An automatic pipeline monitoring system based on PCA and SVM. *World Acad. Sci. Eng. Technol.* **2008**, *47*, 90–96.
16. Yousef, M.; Allmer, J.; Khalifa, W. Feature selection for microRNA target prediction comparison of one-class feature selection methodologies. In Proceedings of the 9th International Joint Conference on Biomedical Engineering Systems and Technologies (BIOSTEC 2016), Rome, Italy, 21–23 February 2016; Volume 3, pp. 216–225.
17. RStudio. Available online: https://www.rstudio.com/ (accessed on 5 January 2018).
18. Max Kuhn. The Caret Package. Available online: http://topepo.github.io/caret/index.html (accessed on 5 January 2018).
19. Statistical tools for High-Throughput Data Analysis (STHDA). Principal Component Methods in R: Practical Guide, 2017. Available online: http://www.sthda.com/english/articles/31-principal-component-methods-in-r-practical-guide/ (accessed on 23 August 2018).
20. Cohen, J. *Statistical Power Analysis for the Behavioral Sciences*, 1st ed.; Academic Press: New York, NY, USA 1977.
21. Maxhuni, A.; Muñoz-Meléndez, A.; Osmani, V.; Perez, H.; Mayora, O.; Morales, E.F. Classification of bipolar disorder episodes based on analysis of voice and motor activity of patients. *Pervasive Mob. Comput.* **2016**, *31*, 50–66. [CrossRef]
22. Randall, R.B.; Tech, B. *Frequency Analysis*; Brüel & Kjær: Nærum, Denmark, 1987.
23. Proakis, J.G.; Manolakis, D.G. *Digital Signal Processing: Principles, Algorithms, and Applications*, 3rd ed.; Prentice Hall: Upper Saddle River, NJ, USA, 1996.
24. Harris, F.J. On the use of windows for harmonic analysis with the discrete Fourier transform. *Proc. IEEE* **1978**, *66*, 51–83. [CrossRef]
25. Vapnik, V.N. *Statistical Learning Theory*, 1st ed.; Wiley-Interscience: Hoboken, NJ, USA, 1998; Volume 1.
26. Chang, C.C.; Lin, C.J. LIBSVM: A Library for Support Vector Machines. *ACM Trans. Intell. Syst. Technol.* **2011**, *2*, 1–27. [CrossRef]

27. Demšar, J. Statistical Comparisons of Classifiers over Multiple Data Sets. *J. Mach. Learn. Res.* **2006**, *7*, 1–30.
28. Yousef, M.; Saçar Demirci, M.D.; Khalifa, W.; Allmer, J. Feature selection has a large impact on one-class classification accuracy for MicroRNAs in plants. *Adv. Bioinf.* **2016**, *2016*, 5670851. [CrossRef] [PubMed]

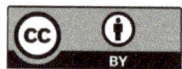

© 2018 by the authors. Licensee MDPI, Basel, Switzerland. This article is an open access article distributed under the terms and conditions of the Creative Commons Attribution (CC BY) license (http://creativecommons.org/licenses/by/4.0/).

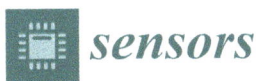

Article

Activity Recognition Invariant to Wearable Sensor Unit Orientation Using Differential Rotational Transformations Represented by Quaternions

Aras Yurtman [1], Billur Barshan [1,*] and Barış Fidan [2]

[1] Department of Electrical and Electronics Engineering, Bilkent University, Bilkent, Ankara 06800, Turkey; yurtman@ee.bilkent.edu.tr
[2] Department of Mechanical and Mechatronics Engineering, University of Waterloo, 200 University Ave W, Waterloo, ON N2L 3G1, Canada; fidan@uwaterloo.ca
* Correspondence: billur@ee.bilkent.edu.tr; Tel.: +90-312-290-2161

Received: 5 July 2018; Accepted: 15 August 2018; Published: 19 August 2018

Abstract: Wearable motion sensors are assumed to be correctly positioned and oriented in most of the existing studies. However, generic wireless sensor units, patient health and state monitoring sensors, and smart phones and watches that contain sensors can be differently oriented on the body. The vast majority of the existing algorithms are not robust against placing the sensor units at variable orientations. We propose a method that transforms the recorded motion sensor sequences invariantly to sensor unit orientation. The method is based on estimating the sensor unit orientation and representing the sensor data with respect to the Earth frame. We also calculate the sensor rotations between consecutive time samples and represent them by quaternions in the Earth frame. We incorporate our method in the pre-processing stage of the standard activity recognition scheme and provide a comparative evaluation with the existing methods based on seven state-of-the-art classifiers and a publicly available dataset. The standard system with fixed sensor unit orientations cannot handle incorrectly oriented sensors, resulting in an average accuracy reduction of 31.8%. Our method results in an accuracy drop of only 4.7% on average compared to the standard system, outperforming the existing approaches that cause an accuracy degradation between 8.4 and 18.8%. We also consider stationary and non-stationary activities separately and evaluate the performance of each method for these two groups of activities. All of the methods perform significantly better in distinguishing non-stationary activities, our method resulting in an accuracy drop of 2.1% in this case. Our method clearly surpasses the remaining methods in classifying stationary activities where some of the methods noticeably fail. The proposed method is applicable to a wide range of wearable systems to make them robust against variable sensor unit orientations by transforming the sensor data at the pre-processing stage.

Keywords: activity recognition and monitoring; patient health and state monitoring; wearable sensing; orientation-invariant sensing; motion sensors; accelerometer; gyroscope; magnetometer; pattern classification

1. Introduction

As a consequence of the development and pervasiveness of sensor technology and wireless communications, wearable sensors have been reduced in size, weight, and cost, gained wireless transmission capabilities, and been integrated into mobile devices such as smart phones, watches, and bracelets [1]. Such smart devices, however, have limited resources. Their effectiveness is determined by the screen size, sensor, computing processor, battery and storage capacities, as well as the wireless data transmission capability [2,3]. Activity recognition with wearables has various potential applications in the healthcare domain in the form of medical state monitoring, memory enhancement, medical data access, and emergency communications [4,5]. Health state monitoring and activity recognition using wearable sensors is advantageous compared to approaches based on computer vision and radio frequency identification that rely on external sensors such as cameras or antennas [6].

With the advancements mentioned above, placing wearable devices on the body properly has become a challenging and intrusive task for the user, making wearable devices prone to be fixed to the body at incorrect orientations. For instance, disabled, injured, elderly people or children whose health, state, or activities can be monitored using wearables [7] tend to place the sensor units at incorrect or variable orientations. Mobile phones can be carried in pockets at different orientations. However, the majority of existing wearable activity recognition studies neglect this issue and assume that the sensor units are properly oriented or, alternatively, use simple features (such as the vector norms) that are invariant to sensor unit orientation. In this study, we focus on orientation invariance in a generic activity recognition framework. Our aim is to develop a methodology that can be applied at the pre-processing stage of activity recognition to make this process robust to variable sensor unit orientation, as depicted in Figure 1.

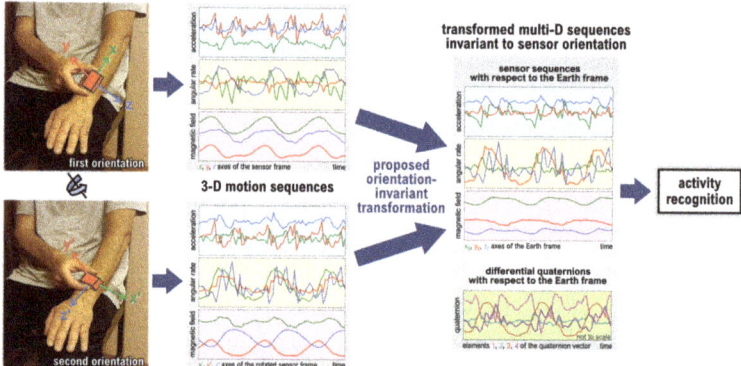

Figure 1. An overview of the proposed method for sensor unit orientation invariance.

We utilize tri-axial wearable motion sensors (accelerometer, gyroscope, and magnetometers) to capture the body motions. Data acquired by these sensors not only contain information about the body movements but also about the orientation of the sensor unit. However, these two types of information are coupled in the sensory data and it is not straightforward to decouple them. More specifically, a tri-axial accelerometer captures the vector sum of the gravity vector and the acceleration resulting from the motion. A tri-axial gyroscope detects the angular rate about each axis of sensitivity and can provide the angular velocity vector. A tri-axial magnetometer captures the vector sum of the magnetic field of the Earth and external magnetic sources, if any.

The acceleration vector acquired by an accelerometer approximately points in the down direction of the Earth frame, provided that the gravitational component of the total acceleration is dominant over the acceleration components resulting from the motion of the sensor unit. However, even if the acceleration vector consists of mainly the gravitational component, by itself it is not sufficient to estimate the sensor unit orientation because there exist infinitely many solutions to the sensor unit orientation, obtained by rotating the correct solution about the direction of the acquired acceleration vector (Figure 2a). Hence, we need to incorporate the magnetometer into the orientation estimation as well. The magnetic field vector acquired by a magnetometer points in a fixed direction in the Earth frame (the magnetic North) (Figure 2b), provided that there are no external magnetic sources or distortion and the variation of the Earth's magnetic field is neglected.

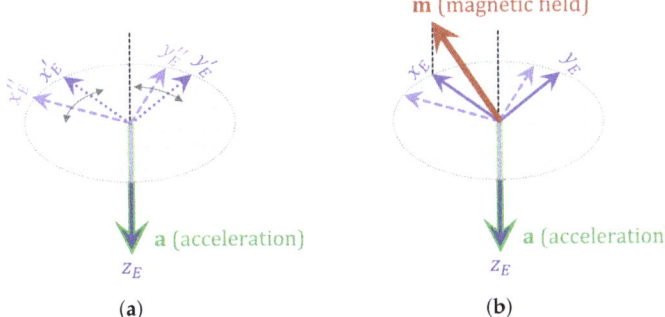

Figure 2. (**a**) With only the acquired acceleration field vector **a**, there exist infinitely many solutions to the sensor unit orientation (two are shown); (**b**) the acquired magnetic field vector **m** uniquely identifies the sensor unit orientation.

By taking the reference directions obtained from the accelerometer and the magnetometer as the vertical axis and the (magnetic) North axis of the Earth frame, respectively, we can calculate the orientation of the sensor unit with respect to the Earth frame. However, this estimation is reliable only in the long term because the gravity component is superposed with the acceleration caused by the motion of the unit and the Earth's magnetic field is superposed with the external magnetic sources (if any). Hence, we also estimate the sensor unit orientation by integrating the gyroscope angular rate output, which is reliable only in the short term because of the drift error [8]. To obtain an accurate orientation estimate both in the short and long term, we merge these two sources of information. Thus, we exploit the information provided by the three types of sensors to determine the sensor unit orientation with respect to the Earth frame as a function of time.

Once we estimate the sensor unit orientation with respect to the Earth frame, we can transform the acquired data from the sensor frame to the Earth frame such that they become invariant to sensor unit orientation. In addition, to include the information about the rotational motion of the sensor unit, we represent the sensor unit rotation between consecutive time samples in the Earth frame by using a similarity transformation. We show that appending this rotational motion data to the sensor data and representing both in the Earth frame improves the activity recognition accuracy. Figure 1 provides an overview of the proposed method with experimentally acquired sensor sequences during a walking activity.

We utilize widely available sensor types and do not make any assumptions about the sensor configuration, data acquisition, activities, and activity recognition procedure. Our proposed method can be integrated into existing activity recognition systems by applying a transformation to the time-domain data in the pre-processing stage without modifying the rest of the system or the methodology. We outperform the existing methods for orientation invariance and achieve an accuracy close to the fixed orientation case.

The rest of the article is organized as follows: In Section 2, we summarize the related work on wearable sensing that allows versatility in sensor placement. Section 3 presents the transformations applied to the sensor data to achieve orientation invariance. In Section 4, we describe the dataset together with the proposed and existing methodology on orientation invariance, explain the activity recognition procedure, and present the data analysis results including accuracies and run times of the data transformation techniques and the classifiers. In Section 5, we provide a discussion of the results. Section 6 summarizes our contributions, draws conclusions, and indicates some directions for future research.

2. Related Work

Although most of the existing activity recognition studies assume fixed sensor unit orientations [9,10], a number of methods have been proposed to achieve orientation invariance with wearable sensors. These methods can be grouped as transformation-based geometric methods, learning-based methods, and other approaches.

2.1. Transformation-Based Geometric Methods

A straightforward method for achieving orientation invariance is to calculate the magnitudes (the Euclidean norms) of the 3D vectors acquired by tri-axial sensors and to use these magnitudes as features in the classification process instead of individual vector components. When the sensor unit is placed at a different orientation, the magnitude of the sensor readings remains the same, making this method invariant to sensor unit orientation [10–12]. Reference [10] states that a significant amount of information is lost with this approach and the accuracy drops off even for classifying simple daily activities. Instead of using only the magnitude, references [13–15] append the magnitude of the tri-axial acceleration vector as a fourth axis to the tri-axial data. Reference [13] shows that this modification slightly increases the accuracy compared to using only the tri-axial acceleration components. Even if the magnitude of the acceleration is not appended to the data, the limited number of sensor unit orientations considered (only four) allows accurate classification to be achieved with Support Vector Machine (SVM) classifiers [13]. Reference [16] uses the magnitude, the y-axis data, and the squared sum of x and y axes of the tri-axial acceleration sequences acquired by a mobile phone, assuming that the orientation of the phone carried in a pocket has natural limitations: the screen of the phone either faces inward or outward.

In a number of studies [17–19], the direction of the gravity vector is estimated by averaging the acceleration vectors in the long term. This is based on the assumption that the acceleration component associated with daily activities averages out to zero, causing the gravity component to remain dominant. Then, the amplitude of the acceleration along the gravity vector direction and the magnitude of the acceleration perpendicular to that direction are used for activity recognition [17–19], which is equivalent to transforming tri-axial sensor sequences into bi-axial ones. In terms of activity recognition accuracy, in reference [17], this method is shown to perform slightly better and in reference [19], significantly worse than using only the magnitude of the acceleration vector.

In addition to the direction of the gravity vector, reference [20] also estimates the direction of the forward-backward (saggital) axis of the human body based on the assumption that most of the body movements as well as the variance of the acceleration sequences are in this direction. The sensor data are transformed into the body frame whose axes point in the direction of the gravity vector, the forward-backward direction of the body that is perpendicular to that, and a third direction perpendicular to both, forming a right-handed coordinate frame. The method in [20] does not distinguish between the forward and backward directions of the body, whereas reference [10] determines the forward direction from the sign of the integral of the acceleration as the subject walks.

Reference [21] assumes that incorrect placement of a sensor unit causes only shifts in the class means in the feature space. The class means of a Bayesian classifier are adapted to the data by using the expectation-maximization algorithm, and it is shown that the accuracy improves for one dataset and diminishes for another. To test for orientation invariance, sensor data are artificially rotated either about the x or z axis of the sensor unit. In this study, sensor unit rotation about an arbitrary axis is not considered and the assumption regarding the shifts in the class means is a strong one since such shifts may not always be significant.

Reference [22] proposes a coordinate transformation from the sensor frame to the Earth frame to achieve orientation invariance. To transform the data, the orientation of a mobile phone is estimated based on the data acquired from the accelerometer, gyroscope, and magnetometer of the sensor unit embedded in the device. An accuracy level close to the fixed orientation case is obtained by representing the sensor data with respect to the Earth frame. However, only two different orientations of the phone are considered, which is a major limitation of the study in [22]. Reference [23] calculates three principal axes based on acceleration and angular rate sequences by using principal component analysis (PCA) and represents the sensor data with respect to these axes.

2.2. Learning-Based Methods

Reference [24] proposes a high-level machine-learning approach for activity recognition that can tolerate incorrect placement (both position and orientation) of *some of* multiple wearable sensor units. In the standard approach, features extracted from all the sensor units are aggregated and the activity is classified at once. In reference [24], the performed activity is classified by processing the data acquired from each sensor unit separately and the decisions are fused by using the confidence values. The proposed method is compared with the standard approach for different sets of activities, features, and different numbers of incorrectly placed sensor units by using three types of classifiers. When the subjects are requested to place the sensor units at any position and orientation on the appropriate body parts, incorrect placement of some of the units can be tolerated when all nine units are employed, but not with only a single unit.

Among the references [25–27] that employ deep learning for activity recognition, reference [27] increases robustness to variable sensor unit orientations by summing the features extracted from the x, y, z axes.

2.3. Other Approaches

Reference [28] proposes to classify the sensor unit orientation to compensate for variations in orientation. Dynamic portions of the sensor sequences are extracted by thresholding the standard deviation of the acceleration sequence and four pre-determined sensor unit orientations are perfectly recognized by a one-nearest-neighbor (1-NN) classifier. Then, the sensory data are rotated accordingly prior to activity recognition. However, the number of sensor unit orientations considered is again very limited and the direction of one of the sensor axes is common to all four orientations.

Reference [29] proposes an activity recognition scheme invariant to sensor orientation and position, based on tri-axial accelerometers. Orientation invariance is achieved by calibration movements to estimate the sensor orientation. With sensor units fixed to the body, the subject performs two static postures for a few seconds. Then, the axes of a new coordinate frame are determined by using Gram-Schmidt ortho-normalization applied to the average acceleration vectors corresponding to the calibration postures.

In some studies [30,31], the sensor unit is allowed to be placed at an incorrect position on the same body part but its orientation is assumed to remain fixed throughout the activity, which is not realistic. Reference [30] claims that the sensor unit orientation can be estimated without much effort in most cases, which is not always true according to the results obtained in the literature [32,33].

In our earlier work [34–36], we have proposed two different approaches to transform and make time-domain sensor data invariant to the orientations at which the sensor units are fixed to the body. The first approach is a heuristic transformation where geometrical features invariant to the sensor unit orientation are extracted from the sensor data and used in the classification process [34,35], analogous to a method proposed by [37] for gait analysis. In the second approach, sensor sequences are represented with respect to three principal axes that are calculated using singular value decomposition (SVD) [34,36]. In both approaches, the transformed sequences are mathematically proven to be invariant to sensor unit orientations. Unlike most of the other studies that investigate orientation invariance, the proposed heuristic and SVD-based methods are compared with the fixed orientation case and shown to decrease the accuracy by 15.5% and 7.6%, respectively, on average, over five publicly available datasets, four state-of-the-art classifiers, and two cross-validation techniques. It is also shown in [34] that randomly oriented sensor units degrade the accuracy by 21.2% when the untransformed sensor data are used for classification. In this article, as explained in Section 4.3, we use a wider set of classifiers and leave-one-subject-out (L1O) cross-validation technique for better generalizability [38], in which case our newly proposed method achieves a noticeably higher accuracy than our previously proposed methods [34–36].

2.4. Discussion

The activity recognition methods in most of the existing studies are not generic and the results are neither consistent nor comparable because they use different datasets and sensor configurations. Furthermore, in most studies, the proposed orientation-invariant methods are not evaluated comparatively including the case with fixed sensor unit orientations. These methods either impose a major restriction on the possible sensor unit orientations or the types of body movements, which prevents them from being used in a wide range of applications such as health, state, and activity monitoring of elderly or disabled people. The aim of our study is to propose a novel orientation-invariant transformation and to comparatively and fairly observe its impact on the activity recognition accuracy based on the same dataset. To this end, we execute the activity recognition scheme with and without applying our transformation in the pre-processing stage for comparison between fixed and variable sensor unit orientations. We also implement the existing orientation invariance methods to compare them with ours. Furthermore, we artificially rotate the sensor data to observe the effects of incorrectly oriented sensor units on the standard activity recognition system that is originally designed for fixed sensor unit orientations.

3. Proposed Methodology to Achieve Invariance to Sensor Unit Orientation

To achieve orientation invariance with wearable motion sensor units in activity recognition, we propose to transform the acquired sensor data such that they become invariant to the orientations at which the sensor units are worn on the body. To transform the data, we first estimate the orientation of each sensor unit with respect to the Earth frame as a function of time. Unlike most existing studies, we consider a continuum of sensor orientations.

3.1. Estimation of Sensor Orientation

We define the Earth's coordinate frame E such that the Earth's z axis, z_E, points downwards and the Earth's x axis, x_E, points in the direction of the component of the Earth's magnetic field that is perpendicular to the z axis, which is roughly the North direction, as illustrated in Figure 3. The Earth frame is also called the North-East-Down frame [39].

Let S_n be the rotating sensor frame at time sample n. Estimating the sensor unit orientation involves calculating a 3×3 rotational transformation matrix $\mathbf{R}_{S_n}^{E}$ that describes the sensor frame S_n with respect to the Earth frame E at each time sample n. The Earth frame and the sensor frame at consecutive time samples n and $n+1$ are depicted in Figure 4 together with the rotation matrices relating these coordinate frames. We adopt the orientation estimation method in [40], which is explained in the Appendix A. The short-term orientation estimate is calculated by integrating the angular rate acquired by the gyroscope. For the long-term orientation estimation, Gauss-Newton method is used to minimize a cost function which decreases as the acceleration vector points downwards in the Earth frame and as the horizontal component of the magnetic field vector is aligned with the North direction of the Earth frame. Then, the short- and long-term orientation estimates are combined through weighted averaging [40].

3.2. Sensor Signals with Respect to the Earth Frame

The tri-axial data acquired on the x, y, and z axes of each sensor in the sensor coordinate frame S_n naturally depend on the orientations of the sensor units. Our approach is based on transforming the acquired data from the sensor frame to the Earth frame.

Let $\mathbf{v}^S[n] = \left(v_x^S[n], v_y^S[n], v_z^S[n]\right)^T$ be the data vector in $\mathbb{R}^3$ acquired from the x, y, z axes of a tri-axial sensor at time sample n. To represent $\mathbf{v}^S[n]$ with respect to the Earth frame, we pre-multiply it by the estimated sensor unit orientation at that time sample, which is the rotation matrix relating the S_n frame to the E frame:

$$\mathbf{v}^E[n] = \mathbf{R}_{S_n}^E \, \mathbf{v}^S[n] \qquad (1)$$

The components of the vector $\mathbf{v}^E[n] = \left(v_x^E[n], v_y^E[n], v_z^E[n] \right)^T$ are represented with respect to the x_E, y_E, z_E axes of the Earth frame and are invariant to the sensor orientation.

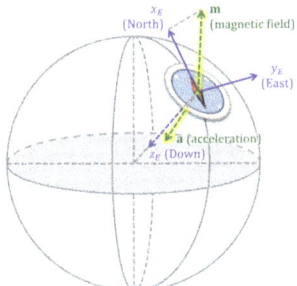

Figure 3. The Earth frame illustrated on an Earth model with the acquired reference vectors.

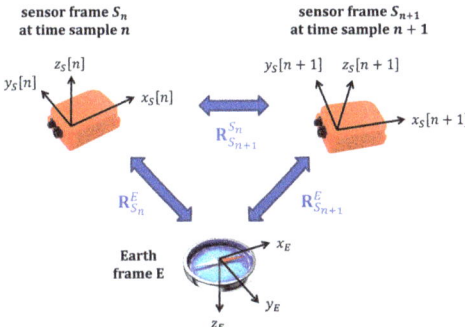

Figure 4. The Earth and the sensor coordinate frames at two consecutive time samples with the rotational transformations relating them.

3.3. Differential Sensor Rotations with Respect to the Earth Frame

In addition to the data transformed to the Earth frame, we propose to incorporate the information contained in the change in the sensor unit orientation over time. While the sensor units can be placed at arbitrary orientations, we require that during data acquisition their orientations remain fixed with respect to the body part they are placed on. In other words, the sensor units need to be firmly attached to the body and are not allowed to rotate freely during the motion. However, this restriction is only necessary in the short term over one time segment (5 s in this study). Under this restriction, the rotational motion of the body parts on which the sensor units are worn can be extracted from the acquired data correctly regardless of the initial orientations of the units.

Note that we can easily calculate the sensor unit orientation $\mathbf{R}_{S_{n+1}}^{S_n}$ at time sample $n+1$ relative to the sensor orientation at time sample n as

$$\mathbf{C}_n \triangleq \mathbf{R}_{S_{n+1}}^{S_n} = \mathbf{R}_E^{S_n} \, \mathbf{R}_{S_{n+1}}^E = \left(\mathbf{R}_{S_n}^E \right)^{-1} \mathbf{R}_{S_{n+1}}^E \qquad (2)$$

for each n as shown in Figure 4. The matrix $\mathbf{C}_n$ is not invariant to sensor orientation because it represents the orientation of frame S_{n+1} with respect to S_n and depends on the orientation at which the sensor unit is fixed to the body. To observe this, let us assume that the sensor unit is placed at a different arbitrary orientation; that is, the sensor unit is rotated by an arbitrary rotation matrix $\mathbf{P}$ that is constant over time. Then, the acquired data are $\tilde{\mathbf{v}}^S[n] = \mathbf{P}^{-1}\mathbf{v}^S[n]$ for all n, represented with respect to the new sensor orientation $\tilde{S}_n$, and the sensor unit orientation with respect to the Earth is estimated as $\tilde{\mathbf{R}}^E_{\tilde{S}_n} = \mathbf{R}^E_{S_n}\mathbf{P}$ for all n. Note that the original rotation matrix is post-multiplied by $\mathbf{P}$ because $\mathbf{P}$ describes a rotational transformation with respect to the sensor frame, not the Earth frame [41]. For the new sensor unit orientation, the rotation of the sensor unit between time samples n and $n+1$ can be calculated as

$$\begin{aligned}
\tilde{\mathbf{C}}_n &= \tilde{\mathbf{R}}^{S_n}_{S_{n+1}} \\
&= \tilde{\mathbf{R}}^{S_n}_E \tilde{\mathbf{R}}^E_{S_{n+1}} \\
&= \left(\tilde{\mathbf{R}}^E_{S_n}\right)^{-1} \tilde{\mathbf{R}}^E_{S_{n+1}} \\
&= \left(\mathbf{R}^E_{S_n}\mathbf{P}\right)^{-1} \left(\mathbf{R}^E_{S_{n+1}}\mathbf{P}\right) \\
&= \mathbf{P}^{-1}\left(\mathbf{R}^E_{S_n}\right)^{-1}\mathbf{R}^E_{S_{n+1}}\mathbf{P} \\
&= \mathbf{P}^{-1}\mathbf{R}^{S_n}_E \mathbf{R}^E_{S_{n+1}}\mathbf{P} \\
&= \mathbf{P}^{-1}\mathbf{R}^{S_n}_{S_{n+1}}\mathbf{P} \\
&= \mathbf{P}^{-1}\mathbf{C}_n\mathbf{P}
\end{aligned} \quad (3)$$

Since $\tilde{\mathbf{C}}_n \neq \mathbf{C}_n$ in general, $\mathbf{C}_n$ is *not* invariant to sensor orientation.

We can make the rotational transformation $\mathbf{C}_n$ invariant to sensor unit orientation by representing it in the Earth frame. Hence, we transform $\mathbf{C}_n$ from the sensor frame S_n to the Earth frame E by using a similarity transformation [42]:

$$\mathbf{D}_n = \left(\mathbf{R}^{S_n}_E\right)^{-1}\mathbf{C}_n\left(\mathbf{R}^{S_n}_E\right) = \mathbf{R}^E_{S_n}\mathbf{R}^{S_n}_{S_{n+1}}\mathbf{R}^{S_n}_E = \mathbf{R}^E_{S_{n+1}}\mathbf{R}^{S_n}_E \quad (4)$$

We call this transformation $\mathbf{D}_n$ *differential sensor rotation with respect to the Earth frame*.

It is straightforward to show that $\mathbf{D}_n$ is invariant to sensor orientation. Using a constant arbitrary rotation matrix $\mathbf{P}$ that relates the original and modified sensor orientations as before, we have:

$$\begin{aligned}
\tilde{\mathbf{D}}_n &= \tilde{\mathbf{R}}^E_{S_{n+1}} \tilde{\mathbf{R}}^{S_n}_E \\
&= \tilde{\mathbf{R}}^E_{S_{n+1}} \left(\tilde{\mathbf{R}}^E_{S_n}\right)^{-1} \\
&= \left(\mathbf{R}^E_{S_{n+1}}\mathbf{P}\right)\left(\mathbf{R}^E_{S_n}\mathbf{P}\right)^{-1} \\
&= \mathbf{R}^E_{S_{n+1}}\underbrace{\mathbf{P}\mathbf{P}^{-1}}_{\mathbf{I}_{3\times 3}}\left(\mathbf{R}^E_{S_n}\right)^{-1} \\
&= \mathbf{R}^E_{S_{n+1}}\mathbf{R}^{S_n}_E \\
&= \mathbf{D}_n
\end{aligned} \quad (5)$$

Thus, we observe that the differential rotation $\tilde{\mathbf{D}}_n$ with respect to the Earth frame, calculated based on the rotated data, is the same as the one calculated based on the original data ($\mathbf{D}_n$).

4. Comparative Evaluation of Proposed and Existing Methodology on Orientation Invariance for Activity Recognition

4.1. Dataset

To demonstrate our methodology, we use the publicly available daily and sports activities dataset acquired by our research group earlier [43]. To acquire the dataset, each subject wore five Xsens MTx sensor units [44] (see Figure 5), each unit containing three tri-axial devices: an accelerometer, a gyroscope, and a magnetometer. The sensor units are placed on the chest, on both wrists, and on the outer sides of both knees, as shown in Figure 6. Nineteen activities are performed by eight subjects. For each activity performed by each subject, there are 45 ($= 5$ units $\times$ 9 sensors) time-domain sequences of 5 min duration, sampled at 25 Hz, and consisting of 7500 time samples each. The dataset comprises the following activities:

Sitting (A_1), standing (A_2), lying on back and on right side (A_3 and A_4), ascending and descending stairs (A_5 and A_6), standing still in an elevator (A_7), moving around in an elevator (A_8), walking in a parking lot (A_9), walking on a treadmill in flat and 15° inclined positions at a speed of 4 km/h (A_{10} and A_{11}), running on a treadmill at a speed of 8 km/h (A_{12}), exercising on a stepper (A_{13}), exercising on a cross trainer (A_{14}), cycling on an exercise bike in horizontal and vertical positions (A_{15} and A_{16}), rowing (A_{17}), jumping (A_{18}), and playing basketball (A_{19}).

The activities can be broadly grouped into two: In stationary activities (A_1–A_4), the subject stays still without moving significantly, whereas non-stationary activities (A_5–A_{19}) are associated with some kind of motion.

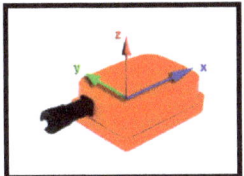

Figure 5. The Xsens MTx unit [44].

4.2. Description of the Proposed and Existing Methodology on Orientation Invariance

In the pre-processing stage, seven data transformation techniques are considered to observe the effects of different sensor orientations on the accuracy and the improvement obtained with the existing and the proposed orientation-invariant transformations:

- **Reference:** Data are not transformed and the sensor units are assumed to maintain their fixed positions and orientations during the whole motion. This corresponds to the standard activity recognition scheme, as in [45–47].
- **Random rotation:** This case is considered to assess the accuracy of the standard activity recognition scheme (without any orientation-invariant transformation) when the sensor units are oriented randomly at their fixed positions. Instead of recording a new dataset with random sensor orientations, we randomly rotate the original data to make a fair comparison with the reference case. For this purpose, we randomly generate a rotational transformation:

$$\mathbf{P} = \begin{bmatrix} 1 & 0 & 0 \\ 0 & \cos\theta & -\sin\theta \\ 0 & \sin\theta & \cos\theta \end{bmatrix} \begin{bmatrix} \cos\phi & 0 & \sin\phi \\ 0 & 1 & 0 \\ -\sin\phi & 0 & \cos\phi \end{bmatrix} \begin{bmatrix} \cos\psi & -\sin\psi & 0 \\ \sin\psi & \cos\psi & 0 \\ 0 & 0 & 1 \end{bmatrix} \quad (6)$$

where yaw, pitch, roll angles θ, ϕ, ψ are independent and uniformly distributed in the interval $[-\pi, \pi)$ radians. For each time segment of each sensor unit (see Section 4.3 for segmentation), we generate a different $\mathbf{P}$ matrix and pre-multiply each of the three tri-axial sequences of that unit by the random rotation matrix corresponding to that segment of the unit: $\tilde{\mathbf{v}}[n] = \mathbf{P}\mathbf{v}^S[n]$. In this way, we simulate the situation where each sensor unit is placed at a possibly different random orientation in each time segment.

- **Euclidean norm method:** The Euclidean norm of the x, y, z components of the sensor sequences are taken at each time sample and used instead of using the original tri-axial sequences. As reviewed in Section 2, this technique has been used in activity recognition to achieve sensor orientation invariance [10–12] or as an additional feature as in [13–16,48,49].
- **Sequences along and perpendicular to the gravity vector:** In this method, the acceleration sequence in each time segment is averaged over time to approximately calculate the direction of the gravity vector. Then, for each sensor type, the sensor sequence's amplitude in this direction and the magnitude that is perpendicular to this direction are taken. This method has been used in [17–19] to achieve orientation invariance.
- **SVD-based transformation:** Sensory data are represented with respect to three principal axes that are calculated by SVD [34,36]. The transformation is applied to each time segment of each sensor unit separately so that sensor units are allowed to be placed at different orientations in each segment.

To calculate the orientation-invariant transformations in the remaining two methods, we estimate the orientation $\mathbf{R}_{S_n}^E$ of each of the five sensor units as a function of time sample n as explained in the Appendix A. For the algorithm to reach steady state rapidly, we append to the acquired signal a prefix signal of duration 1 s that consists of zero angular rate, a constant acceleration, and a constant magnetic field that are the same as the measurements at the first time sample.

- **Sensor sequences with respect to the Earth frame:** We transform the sensor sequences into the Earth frame using the estimated sensor orientations, as described by Equation (1). This method has been used in [22] to achieve invariance to sensor orientation in activity recognition.
  As an example, Figure 7a shows the accelerometer, gyroscope, and magnetometer data ($\mathbf{v}^S[n]$) acquired during activity A_{10} and Figure 7b shows the same sequences transformed into the Earth frame. We observe that the magnetic field with respect to the Earth frame does not significantly vary over time because the Earth's magnetic field is nearly constant in the Earth frame provided that there are no external magnetic sources in the vicinity of the sensor unit.
- **Proposed method: sensor sequences and differential quaternions, both with respect to the Earth frame:** We calculate the differential rotation matrix $\mathbf{D}_n$ with respect to the Earth frame for each sensor unit at each time sample n, as explained in Section 3.3. This rotation matrix representation is quite redundant because it has nine elements while any 3D rotation can be represented by only three angles. Since the representation by three angles has a singularity problem, we represent the differential rotation $\mathbf{D}_n$ compactly by a four-element quaternion $\mathbf{q}_n^{\text{diff}}$ as

$$\mathbf{q}_n^{\text{diff}} = \begin{bmatrix} q_1^{\text{diff}} \\ q_2^{\text{diff}} \\ q_3^{\text{diff}} \\ q_4^{\text{diff}} \end{bmatrix} = \begin{bmatrix} \frac{\sqrt{1+d_{11}+d_{22}+d_{33}}}{2} \\ \frac{d_{32}-d_{23}}{4\sqrt{1+d_{11}+d_{22}+d_{33}}} \\ \frac{d_{13}-d_{31}}{4\sqrt{1+d_{11}+d_{22}+d_{33}}} \\ \frac{d_{21}-d_{12}}{4\sqrt{1+d_{11}+d_{22}+d_{33}}} \end{bmatrix} \quad (7)$$

where d_{ij} ($i, j = 1, 2, 3$) are the elements of $\mathbf{D}_n$ [50]. The vector $\mathbf{q}_n^{\text{diff}}$ is called *differential quaternion with respect to the Earth frame* (the dependence of the elements of $\mathbf{q}_n^{\text{diff}}$ and $\mathbf{D}_n$ on n has been dropped from the notation for simplicity). In the classification process, we use each element of $\mathbf{q}_n^{\text{diff}}$ as a function of n, as well as the sensor sequences with respect to the Earth frame. Hence, there are four time sequences for the differential quaternion in addition to the three axes each of accelerometer, gyroscope, and magnetometer data for each of the five sensor units. Therefore, the transformed data comprises $(4+3+3+3)$ sequences $\times$ 5 sensor units $= 65$ sequences in total. We have observed that the joint use of the sensor sequences and differential quaternions, both with respect to the Earth frame, achieves the highest activity recognition accuracy compared to the other combinations. Representing rotational transformations by rotation matrices instead of quaternions degrades the accuracy. Omitting magnetometer sequences with respect to the Earth frame causes a slight reduction in the accuracy. Activity recognition results of the various different approaches that we have implemented are not presented in this article for brevity, and can be found in [51].

Figure 7c shows the nine elements of the differential rotation matrix $\mathbf{D}_n$ with respect to the Earth frame over time, which are calculated based on the sensor data shown in Figure 7a. Figure 7d shows the elements of the differential quaternion $\mathbf{q}_n^{\text{diff}}$ as a function of n. The almost periodic nature of the sensor sequences (Figure 7a) is preserved in $\mathbf{D}_n$ and $\mathbf{q}_n^{\text{diff}}$ (Figure 7c,d). The differential rotation is calculated between two consecutive time samples that are only a fraction of a second apart, hence the amplitudes of the elements of $\mathbf{D}_n$ and $\mathbf{q}_n^{\text{diff}}$ do not vary much. Since differential rotations involve small rotation angles (close to $0°$), the $\mathbf{D}_n$ matrices are close to the 3×3 identity matrix ($\mathbf{I}_{3\times3}$) because they can be expressed as the product of three rotation matrices as in Equation (6) where each of the basic rotation matrices (as well as their product) is close to $\mathbf{I}_{3\times3}$ because of the small angles. Hence, the diagonal elements which are close to one and the upper- and lower-diagonal elements which are close to zero are plotted separately in Figure 7c for better visualization. When $\mathbf{D}_n$ is close to $\mathbf{I}_{3\times3}$, the $\mathbf{q}_n^{\text{diff}}$ vectors calculated by using Equation (7) are close to $(1,0,0,0)^T$, as observed in Figure 7d.

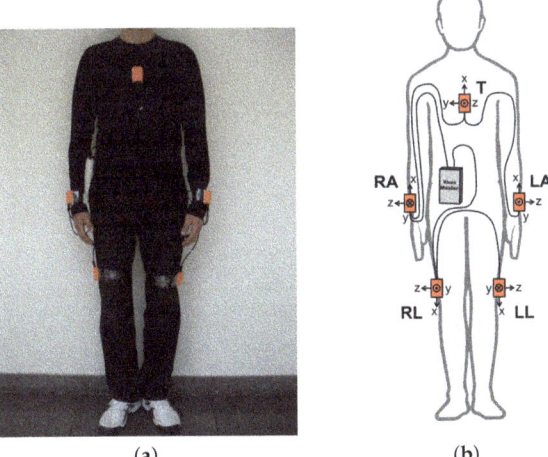

Figure 6. (a) Positioning of the MTx units on the body; (b) connection diagram of the units (the body drawing in the figure is from http://www.clker.com/clipart-male-figure-outline.html; the cables, Xbus Master, and sensor units were added by the authors).

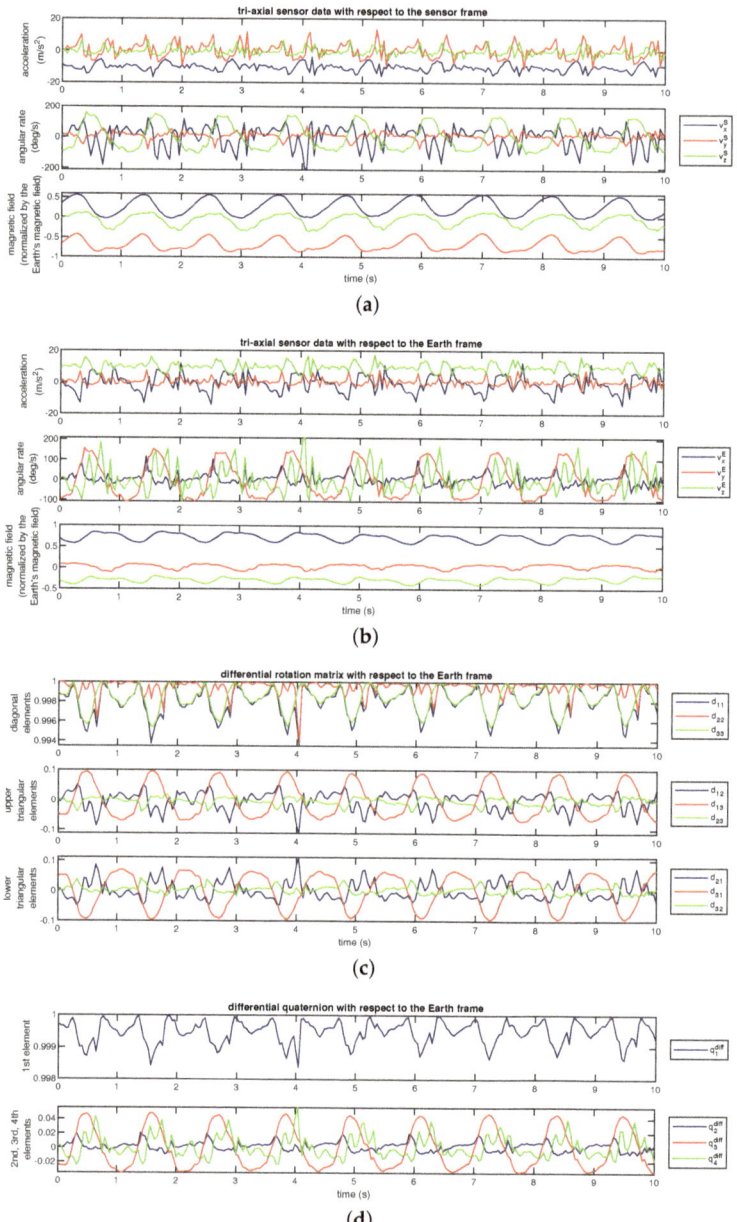

Figure 7. Original and orientation-invariant sequences from a walking activity plotted over time. (**a**) Original sensor sequences; (**b**) sensor sequences; elements of (**c**) the differential rotation matrix and (**d**) the differential quaternion. Sequences in (**b**–**d**) are represented in the Earth frame and are invariant to sensor orientation.

4.3. Activity Recognition and Classifiers

A procedure similar to that in [34,45] is followed for activity recognition. The sensor sequences are divided into 9120 (= 60 feature vectors × 19 activities × 8 subjects) non-overlapping segments of 5 s duration each and transformed according to one of the seven approaches described in Section 4.2.

Then, statistical features are extracted for each segment of each axis of each sensor type. The following features are calculated: minimum, maximum, mean, variance, skewness, kurtosis, 10 coefficients of the autocorrelation sequence (autocorrelation sequence for the lag values of $5, 10, \ldots, 45, 50$ samples is used), and the five largest discrete Fourier transform (DFT) peaks with the corresponding frequencies (the separation between any two peaks in the DFT sequence is taken to be at least 11 samples), resulting in a total of 26 features per segment of each axis. For the reference approach that does not involve any transformation, there are 5 sensor units $\times$ 9 axes $\times$ 26 features per axis $= 1170$ features that are stacked to form a 1170-element feature vector for each segment. The number of axes as well as the number of features vary depending on the transformation technique; however, the total number of feature vectors is fixed (9120). For instance, in the Euclidean norm, there is a three-fold decrease in the number of axes and hence in the number of features. The features are normalized to the interval $[0, 1]$ over all the feature vectors for each subject.

The number of features is reduced through PCA, which is a linear and orthogonal transformation where the transformed features are sorted to have variances in descending order [52]. This allows one to consider only a certain number of features that exhibit the largest variances to reduce the dimensionality. Thus, for each approach, the eigenvalues of the covariance matrix of the feature vectors are calculated, sorted in descending order, and plotted in Figure 8. Using the first 30 eigenvalues appears to be suitable for most of the approaches; hence, we reduce the dimensionality down to $F = 30$.

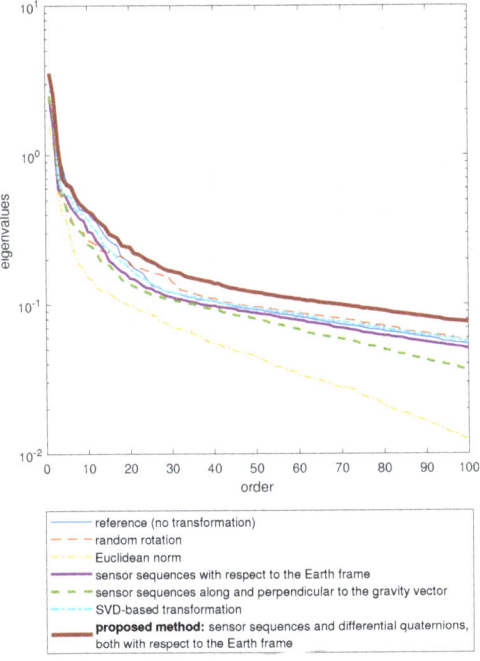

Figure 8. The first 100 eigenvalues of the covariance matrix of the feature vectors sorted in descending order, calculated based on the features extracted from the data transformed according to the seven approaches.

We perform activity classification with seven state-of-the-art classifiers that are briefly described below.

- **Support Vector Machines (SVM):** The feature space is nonlinearly mapped to a higher-dimensional space by using a kernel function and divided into regions by hyperplanes. In this study, the kernel is selected to be a Gaussian radial basis function $f_{\text{RBF}}(\mathbf{x}, \mathbf{y}) = e^{-\gamma \|\mathbf{x}-\mathbf{y}\|^2}$ with parameter γ because it can perform at least as accurately as the linear kernel if the parameters of the SVM are optimized [53]. To extend the binary SVM to more than two classes, a binary SVM classifier is trained for each class pair, and the decision is made according to the classifier with the highest confidence level [54]. The penalty parameter C (see Equation (1) in [55]) and the kernel parameter γ are jointly optimized over all the data transformation techniques by performing a two-level grid search. The optimal parameter values in the coarse grid $(C, \gamma) \in \{10^{-5}, 10^{-3}, 10^{-1}, \ldots, 10^{15}\} \times \{10^{-15}, 10^{-13}, 10^{-11}, \ldots, 10^3\}$ are obtained as $(C^*, \gamma^*) = (10^1, 10^{-1})$. Then, a finer grid is constructed around (C^*, γ^*) as $(C, \gamma) \in 100\,\mathcal{P} \times \mathcal{P}$ with $\mathcal{P} = \{0.01, 0.05, 0.1, 0.2, 0.3, 0.4, 0.5, 0.7, 1, 3, 5\}$ and the optimal parameter values found by searching the fine grid, $(C^{**}, \gamma^{**}) = (5, 0.1)$, are used in SVM throughout this study. The SVM classifier is implemented by using the MATLAB toolbox LibSVM [56].
- **Artificial Neural Networks (ANN):** We use three layers of neurons, where each neuron has a sigmoid output function [57]. The number of neurons in the first (input) and the third (output) layers are as many as the reduced number of features, F, and the number of classes, K, respectively. The number of neurons in the second (or hidden) layer is selected as the integer nearest to the average of $\frac{\log(2K)}{\log 2}$ and $2K - 1$, with the former expression corresponding to the optimistic case where the hyperplanes intersect at different positions and the latter corresponding to the pessimistic case where the hyperplanes are parallel to each other. The weights of the linear combination in each neuron are initialized randomly in the interval $[0, 0.2]$ and during the training phase, they are updated by the back-propagation algorithm [58]. The learning rate is selected as 0.3. The algorithm is terminated when the amount of error reduction (if any) compared to the average of the last 10 epochs is less than 0.01. The ANN has a scalar output for each class. A given test feature vector is fed to the input and the class corresponding to the largest output is selected.
- **Bayesian Decision Making (BDM):** In the training phase, a multi-variate Gaussian distribution with an arbitrary covariance matrix is fitted to the training feature vectors of each class. Based on maximum likelihood estimation, the mean vector is estimated as the arithmetic mean of the feature vectors and the covariance matrix is estimated as the sample covariance matrix for each class. In the test phase, for each class, the test vector's conditional probability given that it is associated with that class is calculated. The class that has the maximum conditional probability is selected according to the maximum a posteriori decision rule [52,57].
- **Linear Discriminant Classifier (LDC):** This classifier is the same as BDM except that the average of the covariance matrices individually calculated for each class is used for all of the classes. Since the Gaussian distributions fitted to the different classes have different mean vectors but the same covariance matrix in this case, the classes have identical probability density functions centered at different points in the feature space. Hence, the classes are linearly separated from each other, and the decision boundaries in the feature space are hyperplanes [57].
- **k-Nearest Neighbor (k-NN):** The training phase consists only of storing the training vectors with their class labels. In the classification phase, the class corresponding to the majority of the k training vectors that are closest to the test vector in terms of the Euclidean distance is selected [57]. The parameter k is chosen as $k = 7$ because it is suitable among the k values ranging from 1 to 30.
- **Random Forest (RF):** A random forest classifier is a combination of multiple decision trees [59]. In the training phase, each decision tree is trained by randomly and independently sampling the training data. Normalized information gain is used as the splitting criterion at each node. In the classification phase, the decisions of the trees are combined by using majority voting. The number of decision trees is selected as 100 because we have observed that using a larger number of trees does not significantly improve the accuracy while increasing the computational cost considerably.

- **Orthogonal Matching Pursuit (OMP):** The training phase consists of only storing the training vectors with their class labels. In the classification phase, each test vector is represented as a linear combination of a very small portion of the training vectors with a bounded error, which is called the sparse representation. The vectors in the representation are selected iteratively by using the OMP algorithm [60] where an additional training vector is selected at each iteration. The algorithm terminates when the desired representation error level is reached, which is selected to be 10^{-3}. Then, a residual for each class is calculated as the representation error when the test vector is represented as a linear combination of the training vectors of only that class, and the class with the minimum residual error is selected.

To determine the accuracies of the classifiers, L1O cross-validation technique is used [57]. In this type of cross validation, feature vectors of a given subject are left out while training the classifier with the remaining subjects' feature vectors. The left out subject's feature vectors are then used for testing (classification). This process is repeated for each subject. Thus, in our implementation, the dataset is partitioned into eight and there are 1140 feature vectors in each partition. L1O is highly affected by the variation in the data across the subjects, and hence, is more challenging than subject-unaware cross-validation techniques such as repeated random sub-sampling or multi-fold cross validation [61].

4.4. Comparative Evaluation Results

The activity recognition performance of the different data transformation techniques and classifiers is shown in Figure 9. In the figure, the lengths of the bars correspond to the classification accuracies and the thin horizontal sticks indicate plus/minus one standard deviation about the accuracies averaged over the cross-validation iterations.

In the lower part of Figure 9, the accuracy values averaged over the seven classifiers are also provided for each approach and compared with the reference case, as well as with the proposed method. Referring to this part of the figure, the standard system that we take as reference, with fixed sensor orientations, provides an average accuracy of 87.2%. When the sensor units are randomly oriented, the accuracy drops by 31.8% on average with respect to the standard reference case. This shows that the standard system is not robust to incorrectly or differently oriented sensors. The existing methods for orientation invariance result in a more acceptable accuracy reduction compared to the reference case: The accuracy drop is 18.8% when the Euclidean norms of the tri-axial sensor sequences are taken, 12.5% when the sensor sequences are transformed to the Earth frame, 12.2% when the sensor sequences are represented along and perpendicular to the gravity vector, and 8.4% when the SVD-based transformation is applied.

Our approach that uses the sensor sequences together with differential quaternions, both with respect to the Earth frame, achieves an average accuracy of 82.5% over all activities with an average accuracy drop of only 4.7% compared to the reference case. Such a decrease in the accuracy is expected when the sensor units are allowed to be placed freely at arbitrary orientations because this flexibility entails the removal of fundamental information such as the direction of the gravity vector measured by the accelerometers and the direction of the Earth's magnetic field detected by the magnetometers. Hence, the average accuracy drop of 4.7% is considered to be acceptable when such information related to the sensor unit orientations is removed inevitably.

In the lower part of Figure 9, we also provide the improvement achieved by each method compared to the random rotation case which corresponds to the standard system using random sensor orientations. The method that we newly propose in this article performs the best among all the methods considered in this study when the sensor units are allowed to be placed at arbitrary orientations.

The activity recognition accuracy highly depends on the classifier. According to Figure 9, in almost all cases, the SVM classifier performs the best among the seven classifiers compared. SVM outperforms the other classifiers especially in approaches targeted to achieve orientation invariance where the classification problem is more challenging. The robustness of SVM in such non-ideal conditions is consistent with other studies [13,46]. Besides the SVM classifier, ANN and LDC also obtain high classification accuracy. Although reference [22] states that k-NN has been shown to perform remarkably well in activity recognition, it is not the most accurate classifier that we have identified.

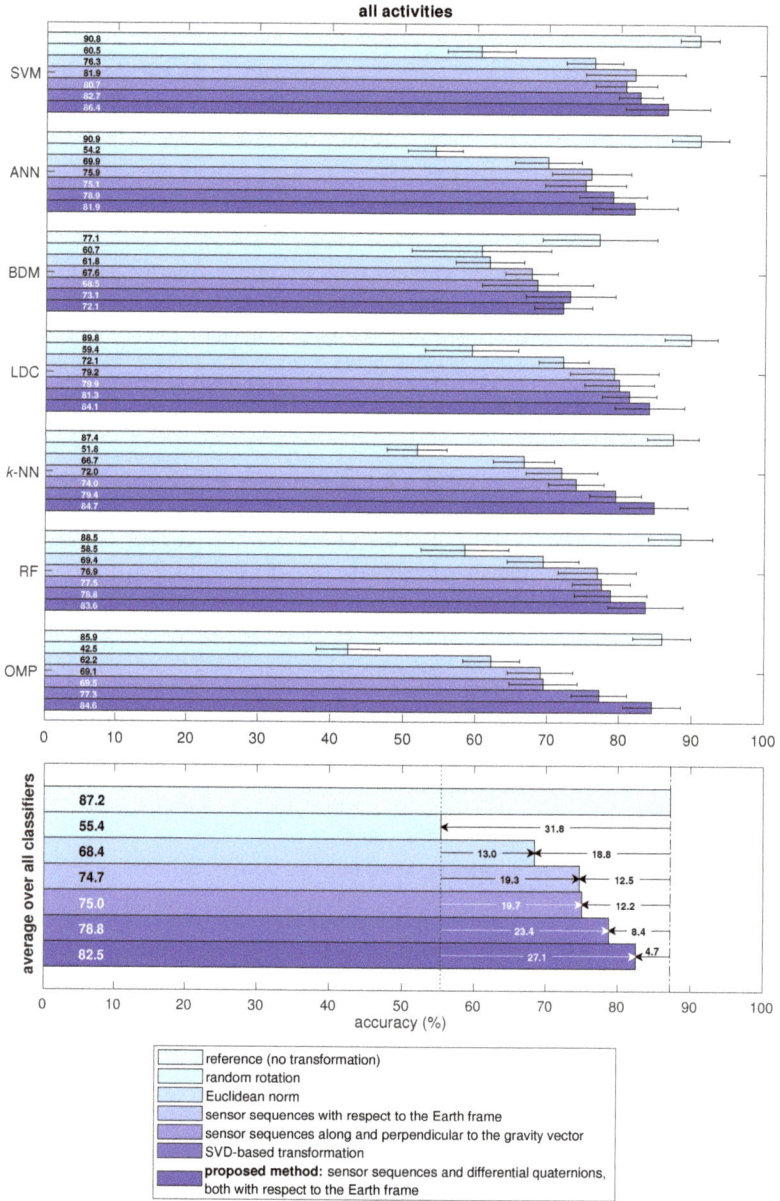

Figure 9. Activity recognition performance for all the data transformation techniques and classifiers over all activities. The lengths of the bars represent the accuracies and the thin horizontal sticks indicate plus/minus one standard deviation over the cross-validation iterations.

To observe the recognition rates of the individual activities, a confusion matrix associated with the SVM classifier is provided in Table 1 for the proposed method. It is apparent that the proposed transformation highly misclassifies the stationary activities A_1–A_4. These activities contain stationary postures, namely, sitting, standing, and two types of lying, which are misclassified probably because we remove the information about sensor orientation from the data. In particular, activity A_1 (sitting) is mostly misclassified and confused with activities A_3 (lying on back side) and A_7 (standing still in an elevator). The remaining stationary activities are also misclassified as A_7. Among the 15 non-stationary activities, activities A_{10} and A_{11} (walking on a treadmill in flat and 15° inclined position, respectively) are confused with each other because of the similarity between the body movements in the two activities. Other misclassifications occur between activity pairs that have similarities such as A_7/A_8, A_8/A_7, A_2/A_8, A_{18}/A_6, and A_{13}/A_9, although rarely. Activities A_{12} (running on a treadmill at a speed of 8 km/h) and A_{17} (rowing) are perfectly classified by SVM for the proposed method, probably because they are associated with unique body movements and do not resemble any of the other activities.

We present the classification performance separately for stationary and non-stationary activities in Figure 10. For each classifier and each approach, we calculate the accuracy values by averaging out the accuracies of the stationary activities (A_1–A_4) and non-stationary activities (A_5–A_{19}).

For stationary activities (see Figure 10a), an average accuracy of 81.2% is obtained for fixed sensor orientations. When the sensor units are oriented randomly, the average accuracy drops to 42.6%. The existing orientation-invariant methods exhibit accuracies between 31.7% and 62.2%, some of them being higher and some being lower than the accuracy for random rotation. The Euclidean norm method performs particularly poorly in this case. The proposed method achieves an average accuracy of 66.8%, which is considerably higher than random rotation and all the existing orientation-invariant transformations. Although two of the existing transformations provide some improvement compared to the random rotation case, their accuracies are much lower than the standard reference system. Hence, removing the orientation information from the data makes it particularly difficult to classify stationary activities.

For non-stationary activities (see Figure 10b), the accuracy decreases from 88.8% to 58.8% on average when the sensor units are placed randomly and no transformation is applied. The existing orientation-invariant methods obtain accuracies ranging from 78.2% to 83.2%, which are comparable to the reference case with fixed sensor orientations. The method we propose obtains an average accuracy of 86.7%, which is higher than all the existing methods and only 2.1% lower than the reference case. This shows that when the sensor units are fixed to the body at arbitrary orientations, the proposed method can classify non-stationary activities with a performance similar to that of fixed sensor unit orientations. In the last two rows of the confusion matrix provided in Table 1, the average accuracy of the stationary activities (A_1–A_4) and non-stationary activities (A_5–A_{19}) are provided separately for the proposed method, again using the SVM classifier.

Referring to Figure 10a, we observe that the recognition rate of stationary activities highly depends on the classifier. On average, the best classifier is LDC, probably because the recognition of stationary activities is quite challenging and the LDC classifier separates the classes from each other linearly and smoothly in the feature space. For the proposed method, the OMP classifier performs much better than the remaining six classifiers. On the other hand, for non-stationary activities (see Figure 10b), the classifiers obtain comparable accuracy values, unlike the case for stationary activities. In this case, SVM is the most accurate classifier, both on average and for the proposed method.

Table 1. Confusion matrix of the SVM classifier for the proposed method over all activities.

Estimated Labels	A_1	A_2	A_3	A_4	A_5	A_6	A_7	A_8	A_9	A_{10}	A_{11}	A_{12}	A_{13}	A_{14}	A_{15}	A_{16}	A_{17}	A_{18}	A_{19}	Total
A_1	286	1	68	20	0	0	8	0	0	0	0	0	0	0	0	0	0	0	0	383
A_2	0	330	0	0	0	0	26	1	0	0	0	0	0	0	0	0	0	0	0	357
A_3	81	0	372	0	0	0	0	0	0	0	0	0	0	0	0	0	0	0	0	453
A_4	1	0	0	367	0	0	0	0	0	0	0	0	0	0	0	0	0	0	0	368
A_5	0	0	0	0	477	0	0	2	11	0	12	0	0	0	0	0	0	0	1	503
A_6	0	0	0	0	0	453	2	5	0	0	0	0	6	0	0	0	0	42	0	508
A_7	97	102	33	83	0	0	354	61	0	0	0	0	0	0	0	0	0	0	0	730
A_8	15	47	6	10	1	27	90	409	1	0	1	0	9	2	2	1	0	0	8	628
A_9	0	0	0	0	2	0	0	1	416	19	4	0	36	0	0	0	0	0	0	479
A_{10}	0	0	0	0	0	0	0	0	13	354	84	0	0	0	0	0	0	0	0	451
A_{11}	0	0	0	0	0	0	0	0	38	105	374	0	11	0	0	0	0	0	0	528
A_{12}	0	0	0	0	0	0	0	0	0	0	0	480	0	0	0	0	0	0	0	480
A_{13}	0	0	0	0	0	0	0	1	1	2	5	0	399	7	0	0	0	0	1	416
A_{14}	0	0	0	0	0	0	0	0	0	0	0	0	19	471	0	0	0	0	0	490
A_{15}	0	0	0	0	0	0	0	0	0	0	0	0	0	0	478	1	0	0	0	479
A_{16}	0	0	0	0	0	0	0	0	0	0	0	0	0	0	0	477	0	0	0	477
A_{17}	0	0	1	0	0	0	0	0	0	0	0	0	0	0	0	1	480	0	0	482
A_{18}	0	0	0	0	0	0	0	0	0	0	0	0	0	0	0	1	0	438	0	439
A_{19}	0	0	0	0	0	0	0	0	0	0	0	0	0	0	0	0	0	0	469	469
total	480	480	480	480	480	480	480	480	480	480	480	480	480	480	480	480	480	480	480	9120
accuracy (%)	59.6	68.8	77.5	76.5	99.4	94.4	73.8	85.2	86.7	73.8	77.9	100.0	83.1	98.1	99.6	99.4	100.0	91.3	97.7	86.5 (overall)
	(for stationary activities) 70.6								(for non-stationary activities) 90.7											

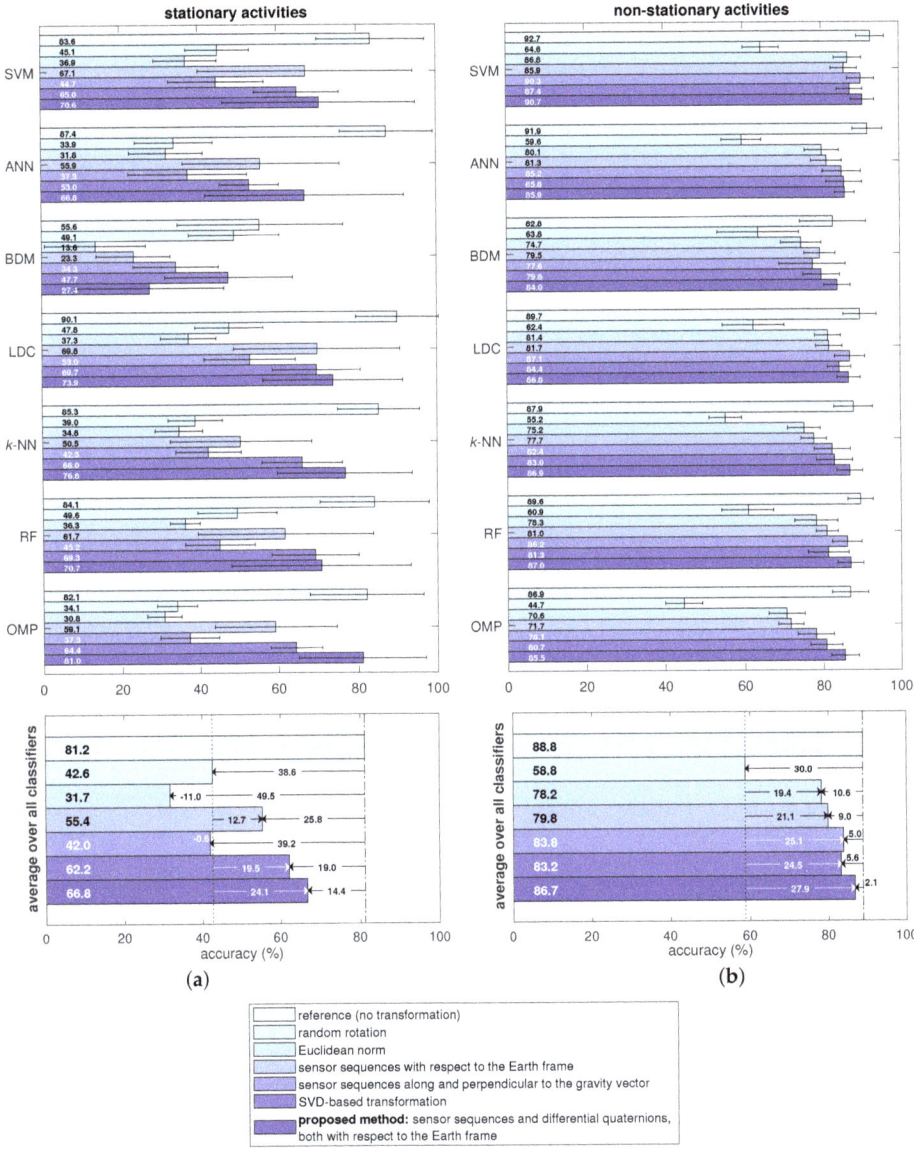

Figure 10. Activity recognition performance for all the data transformation techniques and classifiers for (**a**) stationary and (**b**) non-stationary activities. The lengths of the bars represent the accuracies and the thin horizontal sticks indicate plus/minus one standard deviation over the cross-validation iterations.

4.5. Run Time Analysis

The average run times of the data transformation techniques per one 5-s time segment are provided in Table 2. All the processing in this work was performed on a laptop with a quad-core Intel® Core™ i7-4720HQ processor at 2.6–3.6 GHz and 16 GB of RAM running 64-bit

MATLAB® R2017b. The proposed method has an average run time of about 61 ms per 5-s time segment and can be executed in near real time since the run time is much shorter than the duration of the time segment.

Table 2. Average run times of the data transformation techniques per 5-s time segment.

Data Transformation Technique	Run Time (ms)
Euclidean norm	0.69
sensor sequences with respect to the Earth frame	56.25
sensor sequences along and perpendicular to the gravity vector	1.09
SVD-based transformation	8.94
proposed method: sensor sequences and differential quaternions, both with respect to the Earth frame	61.08

The run times of the classifiers are presented in Table 3 for each of the seven data transformation techniques. Table 3a contains the total run times of the classifiers for an average cross-validation iteration, including the training phase and classification of all the test feature vectors. We observe that k-NN, LDC, and BDM are much faster than the other classifiers for all of the data transformation techniques. Table 3b contains the average training times of the classifiers for a single cross-validation iteration. The k-NN and OMP classifiers only store the training feature vectors in the training phase; therefore, their training time is negligible. Among the remaining classifiers, training of BDM is the fastest. Table 3c contains the average classification time of a single test feature vector, extracted from a segment of 5 s duration. ANN and LDC are about an order of magnitude faster than the others in classification. The classification time of OMP is the largest. Note that, because of programming overheads, the total classification times provided in Table 3a are greater than the sum of the training and classification times (Table 3b,c, respectively) multiplied by 1140 (the number of feature vectors per L1O iteration).

This study is a proof-of-concept for a comparative analysis of the accuracies and run times of the proposed and existing methods as well as state-of-the-art classifiers. Therefore, we have implemented them as well as the remaining parts of the activity recognition framework on a laptop computer rather than on a mobile platform.

Given that the data transformation techniques and most of the classifiers have been implemented in MATLAB in this study, it is possible to further improve the efficiency of the algorithms by programming them in other languages such as C++, by implementing them on an FPGA platform, or by embedding the algorithms in wearable hardware. As such, our methodology can be handled by the limited resources of wearable systems. Alternatively, transmitting the data acquired from wearable devices wirelessly to a cloud server would allow performing the activity recognition in the cloud [14,62]. Despite the latency issues that will arise in this case, this approach would provide additional flexibility and enable the applications of wearables to further benefit from the proposed methodology and the advantages of cloud computing.

Table 3. (a) Total run time (including training and classification of all test feature vectors) and (b) training time in an average L1O iteration; (c) average classification time of a single test feature vector.

	Classifier	Reference (No Transformation)	Random Rotation	Euclidean Norm	Sensor Sequences with Respect to the Earth Frame	Sensor Sequences Along and Perpendicular to the Gravity Vector	SVD-Based Transformation	Proposed Method: Sensor Sequences and Differential Quaternions, Both with Respect to the Earth Frame
(a) total run time (s)	SVM	6.42	14.20	7.22	11.71	8.19	6.24	10.05
	ANN	7.37	8.49	8.54	6.58	12.04	7.91	6.14
	BDM	1.67	1.61	1.59	1.55	2.12	1.48	1.69
	LDC	1.10	0.87	0.84	1.52	0.84	0.93	1.51
	k-NN	0.24	0.12	0.12	0.21	0.19	0.12	0.22
	RF	16.81	22.51	26.40	24.34	19.05	19.71	23.98
	OMP	1018.27	798.90	92.32	99.41	96.48	75.18	114.68
(b) training time (s)	SVM	6.01	13.39	6.61	10.31	7.58	5.36	8.60
	ANN	7.35	8.47	8.52	6.57	12.01	7.89	6.12
	BDM	0.01	0.01	0.01	0.01	0.01	0.01	0.01
	LDC	0.33	0.23	0.22	0.38	0.22	0.26	0.33
	k-NN	–	–	–	–	–	–	–
	RF	15.20	20.90	24.11	21.75	17.45	17.87	21.25
	OMP	–	–	–	–	–	–	–
(c) classification time (ms)	SVM	0.26	0.60	0.42	0.39	0.40	0.24	0.31
	ANN	0.02	0.02	0.01	0.01	0.02	0.01	0.01
	BDM	1.46	1.41	1.39	1.35	1.85	1.29	1.47
	LDC	0.04	0.03	0.03	0.05	0.03	0.03	0.04
	k-NN	0.21	0.11	0.11	0.19	0.16	0.11	0.19
	RF	0.71	0.73	0.99	0.83	0.72	0.74	0.87
	OMP	892.55	700.17	80.55	86.38	84.20	65.43	99.69

5. Discussion

Overall, the recognition rates of non-stationary activities are considerably better than those of stationary ones for all the approaches considered in this study. This is because in non-stationary activities, the activity type is encoded in the body motion whereas in stationary activities, since there is no significant body motion, the removal of sensor orientation information to achieve orientation invariance has a major impact on the accuracy. The classification of stationary activities is a more challenging problem and it is clear that sensor unit orientations provide essential information for this purpose.

The direction of the gravity vector measured by the accelerometer and the direction of the magnetic field vector determined by the magnetometer provide essential information about the orientation of the sensor unit. When the sensor sequences are represented with respect to the Earth frame to achieve orientation invariance, this information is lost because the gravity and the magnetic field of the Earth are roughly in the fixed z_E and x_E directions of the Earth frame, respectively. Hence, in our proposed method, we incorporate the change in the sensor unit orientation over time by calculating differential quaternions with respect to the Earth, which represent the rotation between consecutive time samples invariantly to the sensor unit orientation. The use of differential quaternions increases the accuracy considerably because they effectively represent the rotational motion of the sensor unit related to the activities. When the rotational transformation is represented with respect to the Earth frame, it is invariant to sensor unit orientation, as desired.

For all the methods compared in this study, we use the same dataset which was acquired by placing the sensor units on the body at fixed orientations. This enables us to make a fair comparison between all of the seven approaches considered in this work. In the random rotation case, we rotate the data arbitrarily for each time segment and each sensor unit; hence, we obtain new data that simulate random sensor orientations and match exactly the same level of difficulty of the original data except for the rotational difference. In the last five approaches that correspond to orientation-invariant methods, it is mathematically guaranteed that the transformed data are exactly invariant to sensor orientations; hence, they can be directly compared with the reference and random rotation cases. Had we recorded an additional dataset with different sensor unit orientations, we would not be able to fairly compare the accuracies obtained with the two datasets because it is not possible to guarantee the same level of difficulty in activity recognition in different experiments. This fact can be observed even within the current dataset from the non-negligible standard deviations in the activity recognition accuracy over the cross-validation iterations (see Figures 9 and 10). This shows that the variation among the subjects is significant, as also observed in [38].

6. Conclusions and Future Work

We have demonstrated that the standard activity recognition paradigm cannot handle incorrectly or differently oriented sensors when the position remains fixed. To overcome this problem, we have proposed a transformation that we apply on the sensor data at the pre-processing stage to increase the robustness of the system to errors in the orientations at which the sensor units are worn on the body. The method we have proposed extracts the activity-related information from the sensor sequences while removing the information associated with the absolute sensor unit orientations. This way, we ensure that the transformed sequences do not depend on the absolute sensor unit orientations. The transformed sequences have the same form as the original sequences except the number of axes, which enables us to apply this method in the pre-processing stage of any system that can handle multi-axial data, including systems that directly use time-domain data in its raw form as well as those that use extracted features. We have shown that our method significantly reduces the accuracy degradation caused by incorrect/different sensor unit orientations. The proposed method performs substantially better than the existing methods developed specifically for this problem and achieves nearly the same accuracy level as the fixed orientation case for non-stationary activities. The transformation we propose can be computed in a time much shorter than the duration of one segment of the data, therefore, it can be efficiently implemented and used in near real time.

The next step of this research may involve calculating the differential quaternions with respect to the Earth over a wider time window rather than over only two consecutive time samples, which may improve robustness against high-frequency noise. The transformation proposed here can be used in other wearable sensing applications such as detecting and classifying falls and automated evaluation of physical therapy exercises. By transforming the sensor data at the pre-processing stage, orientation invariance can be achieved without the need to modify the rest of the system. Position invariance can also be investigated to allow the sensor units to be interchanged and/or placed at different positions on the body. The two can be combined to develop activity recognition systems that are invariant to both the position and orientation of the sensor units.

Author Contributions: A.Y. developed and implemented the algorithms and applied them to the dataset; B.B. supervised the research; B.F. reviewed the study with his corrections, suggestions, and critical feedback; all three authors contributed to the writing of the article.

Funding: This research received no external funding.

Conflicts of Interest: The authors declare no conflict of interest.

Abbreviations

The following abbreviations are used in this manuscript:

SVM	Support Vector Machines
PCA	Principal Component Analysis
1-NN	One-Nearest-Neighbor
SVD	Singular Value Decomposition
DFT	Discrete Fourier Transformation
ANN	Artificial Neural Networks
BDM	Bayesian Decision Making
LDC	Linear Discriminant Classifier
k-NN	k-Nearest Neighbor
RF	Random Forest
OMP	Orthogonal Matching Pursuit
L1O	Leave-One-Subject-Out

Appendix A. Sensor Unit Orientation Estimation

The orientation estimation method in [40] combines orientation estimates based on two sources of information. The first estimate is obtained simply by integrating the gyroscope angular rate measurements. This estimate is accurate in the short term but drifts in the long term. The second relies on the direction of the gravity vector measured by the accelerometer and the magnetic field of the Earth detected by the magnetometer in the long term. For the long-term estimation, the Gauss-Newton method [40] is used to solve a minimization problem where the cost function decreases as the acquired acceleration vector is aligned with the gravity vector and as the acquired magnetic field vector is aligned with the magnetic North of the Earth. The short- and long-term estimates are combined through weighted averaging [40].

In the orientation estimation algorithm, we relate the sensor and the Earth frames by a quaternion $\hat{\mathbf{q}}_n = (q_1, q_2, q_3, q_4)^T$ corresponding to the rotation matrix $\hat{\mathbf{R}}_E^{S_n} = \left(\hat{\mathbf{R}}_{S_n}^E\right)^{-1}$ for all n as follows [50]:

$$\hat{\mathbf{R}}_E^{S_n} = \begin{bmatrix} q_1^2 + q_2^2 - q_3^2 - q_4^2 & 2(q_2 q_3 - q_1 q_4) & 2(q_1 q_2 + q_2 q_4) \\ 2(q_2 q_3 + q_1 q_4) & q_1^2 - q_2^2 + q_3^2 - q_4^2 & 2(q_3 q_4 - q_1 q_2) \\ 2(q_2 q_4 - q_1 q_3) & 2(q_1 q_2 + q_3 q_4) & q_1^2 - q_2^2 - q_3^2 + q_4^2 \end{bmatrix} \quad (A1)$$

The short- and long-term orientation estimates are denoted by $\hat{\mathbf{q}}_{n,\text{ST}}$ and $\hat{\mathbf{q}}_{n,\text{LT}}$ and the overall estimate is denoted by $\hat{\mathbf{q}}_n$.

The short-term estimate of the sensor quaternion $\hat{\mathbf{q}}_{n,\text{ST}}$ at time sample n based on the overall estimate $\hat{\mathbf{q}}_{n-1}$ at the previous time sample is given by:

$$\hat{\mathbf{q}}_{n,\text{ST}} = \hat{\mathbf{q}}_{n-1} + \Delta t \left(\frac{1}{2}\hat{\mathbf{q}}_{n-1} \otimes \boldsymbol{\omega}^S[n]\right) \quad (A2)$$

where $\boldsymbol{\omega}^S[n] = \left(0, \omega_x^S[n], \omega_y^S[n], \omega_z^S[n]\right)^T$ is an augmented vector consisting of zero and the angular rate vector acquired by the gyroscope at time sample n [40] and Δt is the sampling interval. Note that the equation involves feedback because $\hat{\mathbf{q}}_{n,\,\text{ST}}$ is calculated based on $\hat{\mathbf{q}}_{n-1}$.

For the long-term estimation, let $\mathbf{a}^S[n]$ and $\mathbf{m}^S[n]$ be the acceleration and the magnetic field vectors, respectively, represented in the sensor frame and normalized by their magnitudes. To align $\mathbf{a}^S[n]$ with the z_E axis of the Earth frame, we represent it in the Earth frame as $\mathbf{a}^E[n] = \mathbf{q}_n \otimes \mathbf{a}^S[n] \otimes \mathbf{q}_n^*$, and solve the following minimization problem [40]:

$$\hat{\mathbf{q}}_{n,\,\text{LT-1}} = \arg\min_{\mathbf{q}_n} f_1\left(\mathbf{q}_n, \mathbf{a}^S[n]\right) \quad \text{where} \quad f_1\left(\mathbf{q}_n, \mathbf{a}^S[n]\right) = \left\|(0,\,0,\,1)^T - \mathbf{q}_n \otimes \mathbf{a}^S[n] \otimes \mathbf{q}_n^*\right\| \quad (A3)$$

where $\|\cdot\|$ denotes the Euclidean norm and $\otimes$ denotes the quaternion product operator.

We represent the magnetic field vector $\mathbf{m}^S[n]$ as $\mathbf{m}^E[n] = \mathbf{q}_n \otimes \mathbf{m}^S[n] \otimes \mathbf{q}_n^*$ in the Earth frame and allow it to have only a vertical component along the z_E direction and a horizontal component along the x_E direction. Hence, we align $\mathbf{m}^E[n]$ with the magnetic reference vector defined as $\mathbf{m}_0[n] \triangleq \left(\sqrt{(m_x^E[n])^2 + (m_y^E[n])^2},\, 0,\, m_z^E[n]\right)^T$ in the Earth frame by solving the following minimization problem [40]:

$$\hat{\mathbf{q}}_{n,\,\text{LT-2}} = \arg\min_{\mathbf{q}_n} f_2\left(\mathbf{q}_n, \mathbf{m}^S[n]\right) \quad \text{where} \quad f_2\left(\mathbf{q}_n, \mathbf{m}^S[n]\right) = \left\|\mathbf{m}_0[n] - \mathbf{q}_n \otimes \mathbf{m}^S[n] \otimes \mathbf{q}_n^*\right\| \quad (A4)$$

To simultaneously align the acceleration and magnetic field vectors, we combine the minimization problems defined in Equations (A3) and (A4) into one and solve the following joint minimization problem:

$$\hat{\mathbf{q}}_{n,\,\text{LT}} = \arg\min_{\mathbf{q}_n} f\left(\mathbf{q}_n, \mathbf{a}^S[n], \mathbf{m}^S[n]\right) \quad (A5)$$

where the combined objective function is

$$f\left(\mathbf{q}_n, \mathbf{a}^S[n], \mathbf{m}^S[n]\right) = f_1^2\left(\mathbf{q}_n, \mathbf{a}^S[n]\right) + f_2^2\left(\mathbf{q}_n, \mathbf{m}^S[n]\right) \quad (A6)$$

We use the Gauss-Newton method to solve the problem defined in Equation (A5) iteratively [40]. The quaternion at iteration $i+1$ can be calculated based on the estimate at the ith iteration as follows:

$$\mathbf{q}_{n,\,\text{LT}}^{(i+1)} = \mathbf{q}_{n,\,\text{LT}}^{(i)} - \left(\mathbf{J}^T\mathbf{J}\right)^{-1}\mathbf{J}^T\,f\left(\mathbf{q}_{n,\,\text{LT}}^{(i)}, \mathbf{a}^S[n], \mathbf{m}^S[n]\right) \quad (A7)$$

where $\mathbf{J}$ is the 6×4 Jacobian matrix of $\mathbf{f}$ with respect to the elements of $\mathbf{q}_n^{(i)}$. This matrix is provided in closed form in [40].

Finally, the short- and long-term estimates are merged by using weighted averaging [40]:

$$\hat{\mathbf{q}}_n = \mathcal{K}\hat{\mathbf{q}}_{n,\,\text{ST}} + (1-\mathcal{K})\hat{\mathbf{q}}_{n,\,\text{LT}} \quad (A8)$$

where the parameter $\mathcal{K}$ is selected as 0.98 as in [40]. The estimated quaternion $\hat{\mathbf{q}}_n$ represents the rotation matrix $\hat{\mathbf{R}}_E^{S_n}$ compactly, where we drop the hat notation ($\hat{}$) in the main text for simplicity.

References

1. Lara, O.D.; Labrador, M.A. A survey on human activity recognition using wearable sensors. *IEEE Commun. Surv. Tutor.* **2013**, *15*, 1192–1209. [CrossRef]
2. Rawassizadeh, R.; Price, B.A.; Marian, P. Wearables: Has the age of smartwatches finally arrived? *Commun. ACM* **2015**, *58*, 45–47. [CrossRef]

3. Mortazavi, B.; Nemati, E.; VanderWall, K.; Flores-Rodriguez, H.G.; Cai, J.Y.J.; Lucier, J.; Arash, N.; Sarrafzadeh, M. Can smartwatches replace smartphones for posture tracking? *Sensors* **2015**, *15*, 26783–26800. [CrossRef] [PubMed]
4. Darwish, A.; Hassanien, A.E. Wearable and implantable wireless sensor network solutions for healthcare monitoring. *Sensors* **2011**, *11*, 5561–5595. [CrossRef] [PubMed]
5. Pantelopoulos, A.; Bourbakis, N.G. A survey on wearable sensor-based systems for health monitoring and prognosis. *IEEE Trans. Syst. Man Cybern. Part C* **2010**, *40*, 1–12. [CrossRef]
6. Yurtman, A.; Barshan, B. Human activity recognition using tag-based radio frequency localization. *Appl. Artif. Intell.* **2016**, *30*, 153–179. [CrossRef]
7. Yurtman, A.; Barshan, B. Automated evaluation of physical therapy exercises using multi-template dynamic time warping on wearable sensor signals. *Comput. Methods Progr. Biomed.* **2014**, *117*, 189–207. [CrossRef] [PubMed]
8. Seçer, G.; Barshan, B. Improvements in deterministic error modeling and calibration of inertial sensors and magnetometers. *Sens. Actuators A Phys.* **2016**, *247*, 522–538. [CrossRef]
9. Morales, J.; Akopian, D. Physical activity recognition by smartphones, a survey. *Biocybern. Biomed. Eng.* **2017**, *37*, 388–400. [CrossRef]
10. Kunze, K.; Lukowicz, P. Sensor placement variations in wearable activity recognition. *IEEE Pervasive Comput.* **2014**, *13*, 32–41. [CrossRef]
11. Reddy, S.; Mun, M.; Burke, J.; Estrin, D.; Hansen, M.; Srivastava, M. Using mobile phones to determine transportation modes. *ACM Trans. Sens. Netw.* **2010**, *6*, 13. [CrossRef]
12. Bhattacharya, S.; Nurmi, P.; Hammerla, N.; Plötz, T. Using unlabeled data in a sparse-coding framework for human activity recognition. *Pervasive Mob. Comput.* **2014**, *15*, 242–262. [CrossRef]
13. Sun, L.; Zhang, D.; Li, B.; Guo, B.; Li, S. Activity recognition on an accelerometer embedded mobile phone with varying positions and orientations. In *Lecture Notes in Computer Science, Proceedings of the 7th International Conference on Ubiquitous Intelligence and Computing, Xi'an, China, 26–29 October 2010*; Yu, Z., Liscano, R., Chen, G., Zhang, D., Zhou, X., Eds.; Springer: Berlin/Heidelberg, Germany, 2010; Volume 6406, pp. 548–562.
14. Shoaib, M.; Bosch, S.; İncel, Ö.D.; Scholten, H.; Havinga, J.M. Fusion of smartphone motion sensors for physical activity recognition. *Sensors* **2014**, *14*, 10146–10176. [CrossRef] [PubMed]
15. Janidarmian, M.; Fekr, A.R.; Radecka, K.; Zilic, Z. A comprehensive analysis on wearable acceleration sensors in human activity recognition. *Sensors* **2017**, *17*, 529. [CrossRef] [PubMed]
16. Siirtola, P.; Röning, J. Recognizing human activities user-independently on smartphones based on accelerometer data. *Int. J. Interact. Multimed. Artif. Intell.* **2012**, *1*, 38–45. [CrossRef]
17. Yang, Y. Toward physical activity diary: Motion recognition using simple acceleration features with mobile phones. In Proceedings of the 1st International Workshop on Interactive Multimedia for Consumer Electronics, Beijing, China, 23 October 2009; pp. 1–10.
18. Lu, H.; Yang, J.; Liu, Z.; Lane, N.D.; Choudhury, T.; Campbell, A.T. The Jigsaw continuous sensing engine for mobile phone applications. In Proceedings of the 8th ACM Conference on Embedded Networked Sensor Systems, Zürich, Switzerland, 3–5 November 2010; pp. 71–84.
19. Wang, N.; Redmond, S.J.; Ambikairajah, E.; Celler, B.G.; Lovell, N.H. Can triaxial accelerometry accurately recognize inclined walking terrains? *IEEE Trans. Biomed. Eng.* **2010**, *57*, 2506–2516. [CrossRef] [PubMed]
20. Henpraserttae, A.; Thiemjarus, S.; Marukatat, S. Accurate activity recognition using a mobile phone regardless of device orientation and location. In Proceedings of the International Conference on Body Sensor Networks, Dallas, TX, USA, 23–25 May 2011; pp. 41–46.
21. Chavarriaga, R.; Bayati, H.; Millán, J.D. Unsupervised adaptation for acceleration-based activity recognition: Robustness to sensor displacement and rotation. *Pers. Ubiquitous Comput.* **2011**, *17*, 479–490. [CrossRef]
22. Ustev, Y.E.; İncel, Ö.D.; Ersoy, C. User, device and orientation independent human activity recognition on mobile phones: Challenges and a proposal. In Proceedings of the ACM Conference on Pervasive and Ubiquitous Computing, Zürich, Switzerland, 8–12 September 2013; pp. 1427–1436.
23. Morales, J.; Akopian, D.; Agaian, S. Human activity recognition by smartphones regardless of device orientation. In Proceedings of the SPIE-IS&T Electronic Imaging: Mobile Devices and Multimedia: Enabling Technologies, Algorithms, and Applications, San Francisco, CA, USA, 18 February 2014; Creutzburg, R., Akopian, D., Eds.; SPIE: Bellingham, WA, USA; IS&T: Springfield, VA, USA, 2014; Volume 9030, pp. 90300I-1–90300I-12.

24. Banos, O.; Toth, M.A.; Damas, M.; Pomares, H.; Rojas, I. Dealing with the effects of sensor displacement in wearable activity recognition. *Sensors* **2014**, *14*, 9995–10023. [CrossRef] [PubMed]
25. Yang, J.B.; Nguyen, M.N.; San, P.P.; Li, X.L.; Krishnaswamy, S. Deep convolutional neural networks on multichannel time series for human activity recognition. In Proceedings of the 24th International Conference on Artificial Intelligence (IJCAI'15), Buenos Aires, Argentina, 25–31 July 2015; pp. 3995–4001.
26. Alsheikh, M.A.; Selim, A.; Niyato, D.; Doyle, L.; Lin, S.; Tan, H.-P. Deep activity recognition models with triaxial accelerometers. In Proceedings of the Workshop at the Thirtieth AAAI Conference on Artificial Intelligence: Artificial Intelligence Applied to Assistive Technologies and Smart Environments, Phoenix, AZ, USA, 12–17 February 2016.
27. Ravi, D.; Wong, C.; Lo, B.; Yang, G. A deep learning approach to on-node sensor data analytics for mobile or wearable devices. *IEEE J. Biomed. Health* **2017**, *21*, 56–64. [CrossRef] [PubMed]
28. Thiemjarus, S. A device-orientation independent method for activity recognition. In Proceedings of the International Conference on Body Sensor Networks, Biopolis, Singapore, 7–9 June 2010; pp. 19–23.
29. Jiang, M.; Shang, H.; Wang, Z.; Li, H.; Wang, Y. A method to deal with installation errors of wearable accelerometers for human activity recognition. *Physiol. Meas.* **2011**, *32*, 347–358. [CrossRef] [PubMed]
30. Kunze, K.; Lukowicz, P. Dealing with sensor displacement in motion-based onbody activity recognition systems. In Proceedings of the 10th International Conference on Ubiquitous Computing, Seoul, Korea, 21–24 September 2008; pp. 20–29.
31. Förster, K.; Roggen, D.; Troster, G. Unsupervised classifier self-calibration through repeated context occurrences: Is there robustness against sensor displacement to gain? In Proceedings of the International Symposium on Wearable Computers, Linz, Austria, 4–7 September 2009; pp. 77–84.
32. Bachmann, E.R.; Yun, X.; Brumfield, A. Limitations of attitude estimation algorithms for inertial/magnetic sensor modules. *IEEE Robot. Autom. Mag.* **2007**, *14*, 76–87. [CrossRef]
33. Ghasemi-Moghadam, S.; Homaeinezhad, M.R. Attitude determination by combining arrays of MEMS accelerometers, gyros, and magnetometers via quaternion-based complementary filter. *Int. J. Numer. Model. Electron. Netw. Devices Fields* **2018**, *31*, 1–24. [CrossRef]
34. Yurtman, A.; Barshan, B. Activity recognition invariant to sensor orientation with wearable motion sensors. *Sensors* **2017**, *17*, 1838. [CrossRef] [PubMed]
35. Yurtman, A.; Barshan, B. Recognizing activities of daily living regardless of wearable device orientation. In Proceedings of the Fifth International Symposium on Engineering, Artificial Intelligence, and Applications, Book of Abstracts, Kyrenia, Turkish Republic of Northern Cyprus, 1–3 November 2017; pp. 22–23.
36. Yurtman, A.; Barshan, B. Classifying daily activities regardless of wearable motion sensor orientation. In Proceedings of the Eleventh International Conference on Advances in Computer-Human Interactions (ACHI), Rome, Italy, 25–29 March 2018.
37. Zhong, Y.; Deng, Y. Sensor orientation invariant mobile gait biometrics. In Proceedings of the IEEE International Joint Conference on Biometrics, Clearwater, FL, USA, 29 September–2 October 2014; pp. 1–8.
38. Barshan B.; Yurtman, A. Investigating inter-subject and inter-activity variations in activity recognition using wearable motion sensors. *Comput. J.* **2016**, *59*, 1345–1362. [CrossRef]
39. Cai, G.; Chen, B.M.; Lee, T.H. Chapter 2: On Coordinate Systems and Transformations. In *Unmanned Rotorcraft Systems*; Springer: London, UK, 2011; pp. 23–34.
40. Comotti, D. *Orientation Estimation Based on Gauss-Newton Method and Implementation of a Quaternion Complementary Filter*; Technical Report; Department of Computer Science and Engineering, University of Bergamo: Bergamo, Italy, 2011. Available online: https://storage.googleapis.com/google-code-archive-downloads/v2/code.google.com/9dof-orientation-estimation/GaussNewton_QuaternionComplemFilter_V13.pdf (accessed on 16 August 2018).
41. Spong, M.W.; Hutchinson, S.; Vidyasagar, M. Section 2.3: On Rotational Transformations. In *Robot Modeling and Control*; John Wiley & Sons: New York, NY, USA, 2006; pp. 4–48.
42. Chen, C.-T. Section 3.4: On Similarity Transformation. In *Linear System Theory and Design*; Oxford University Press: New York, NY, USA, 1999; pp. 53–55.
43. Altun, K.; Barshan, B. Daily and Sports Activities Dataset. In *UCI Machine Learning Repository*; School of Information and Computer Sciences, University of California, Irvine: Irvine, CA, USA, 2013. Available online: http://archive.ics.uci.edu/ml/datasets/Daily+and+Sports+Activities (accessed on 16 August 2018).

44. Xsens Technologies B.V. *MTi, MTx, and XM-B User Manual and Technical Documentation*; Xsens: Enschede, The Netherlands, 2018. Available online: http://www.xsens.com (accessed on 16 August 2018).
45. Altun, K.; Barshan, B.; Tunçel, O. Comparative study on classifying human activities with miniature inertial and magnetic sensors. *Pattern Recognit.* **2010**, *43*, 3605–3620. [CrossRef]
46. Barshan, B.; Yüksek, M.C. Recognizing daily and sports activities in two open source machine learning environments using body-worn sensor units. *Comput. J.* **2014**, *57*, 1649–1667. [CrossRef]
47. Altun, K.; Barshan, B. Human activity recognition using inertial/magnetic sensor units. In *Lecture Notes in Computer Science, Proceedings of the International Workshop on Human Behaviour Understanding, Istanbul, Turkey, 22 August 2010*; Salah, A.A., Gevers, T., Sebe, N., Vinciarelli, A., Eds.; Springer: Berlin/Heidelberg, Germany, 2010; Volume 6219, pp. 38–51.
48. Rulsch, M.; Busse, J.; Struck, M.; Weigand, C. Method for daily-life movement classification of elderly people. *Biomed. Eng.* **2012**, *57*, 1071–1074. [CrossRef] [PubMed]
49. Özdemir, A.T.; Barshan, B. Detecting falls with wearable sensors using machine learning techniques. *Sensors* **2014**, *14*, 10691–10708. [CrossRef] [PubMed]
50. Diebel, J. *Representing Attitude: Euler Angles, Unit Quaternions, and Rotation Vectors*; Technical Report; Department of Aeronautics and Astronautics, Stanford University: Stanford, CA, USA, 2006. Available online: http://www.swarthmore.edu/NatSci/mzucker1/papers/diebel2006attitude.pdf (accessed on 16 August 2018).
51. Yurtman, A.; Barshan, B. *Choosing Sensory Data Type and Rotational Representation for Activity Recognition Invariant to Wearable Sensor Orientation Using Differential Rotational Transformations*; Technical Report; Department of Electrical and Electronics Engineering, Bilkent University: Ankara, Turkey, 2018.
52. Webb, A. *Statistical Pattern Recognition*; John Wiley & Sons: New York, NY, USA, 2002.
53. Keerthi, S.S.; Lin, C.-J. Asymptotic behaviors of support vector machines with Gaussian kernel. *Neural Comput.* **2003**, *15*, 1667–1689. [CrossRef] [PubMed]
54. Duan, K.-B.; Keerthi, S.S. Which is the best multiclass SVM method? An empirical study. In *Lecture Notes in Computer Science, Proceedings of the 6th International Workshop on Multiple Classifier Systems, Seaside, CA, USA, 13–15 June 2005*; Nikunj, C.O., Polikar, R., Kittler, J., Roli, F., Eds.; Springer: Berlin/Heidelberg, Germany, 2005; Volume 3541, pp. 278–285.
55. Hsu, C.W.; Chang, C.C.; Lin, C.J. *A Practical Guide to Support Vector Classification*; Technical Report; Department of Computer Science, National Taiwan University: Taipei, Taiwan, 2003.
56. Chang, C.C.; Lin, C.J. LIBSVM: A library for support vector machines. *ACM Trans. Intell. Syst. Technol.* **2011**, *2*, 27. [CrossRef]
57. Duda, R.O.; Hart, P.E.; Stork, D.G. *Pattern Classification*; John Wiley & Sons: New York, NY, USA, 2000.
58. Haykin, S. *Neural Networks: A Comprehensive Foundation*, 2nd ed.; Prentice Hall: Upper Saddle River, NJ, USA, 1998.
59. Witten, I.H.; Frank, E.; Hall, M.A.; Pal, C.J. *Data Mining: Practical Machine Learning Tools and Techniques*, 4th ed.; Elsevier: Cambridge, MA, USA, 2016.
60. Pati, Y.C.; Rezaiifar, R.; Krishnaprasad, P.S. Orthogonal matching pursuit: Recursive function approximation with applications to wavelet decomposition. In Proceedings of the 27th Asilomar Conference on Signals, Systems and Computers, Pacific Grove, CA, USA, 1–3 November 1993; pp. 40–44.
61. Wang, L.; Cheng, L.; Zhao, G. *Machine Learning for Human Motion Analysis: Theory and Practice*; IGI Global: Hershey, PA, USA, 2000.
62. Rawassizadeh, R.; Pierson, T.J.; Peterson, R.; Kotz, D. NoCloud: Exploring network disconnection through on-device data analysis. *IEEE Pervasive Comput.* **2018**, *17*, 64–74. [CrossRef]

© 2018 by the authors. Licensee MDPI, Basel, Switzerland. This article is an open access article distributed under the terms and conditions of the Creative Commons Attribution (CC BY) license (http://creativecommons.org/licenses/by/4.0/).

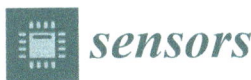

Article

Identifying Free-Living Physical Activities Using Lab-Based Models with Wearable Accelerometers

Arindam Dutta [1,*], Owen Ma [1], Meynard Toledo [2], Alberto Florez Pregonero [3], Barbara E. Ainsworth [2], Matthew P. Buman [2] and Daniel W. Bliss [1]

1. School of Electrical, Computer and Energy Engineering, Arizona State University, Tempe, AZ 85281, USA; owenma@asu.edu (O.M.); d.w.bliss@asu.edu (D.W.B.)
2. College of Health Solutions, Arizona State University, Phoenix, AZ 85281, USA; mltoledo@asu.edu (M.T.); bainswor@asu.edu (B.E.A.); mbuman@asu.edu (M.P.B.)
3. Departamento de Formación, Pontificia Universidad Javeriana, Bogotá D.C. 110231, Colombia; floreza@javeriana.edu.co
* Correspondence: adutta7@asu.edu

Received: 11 October 2018; Accepted: 6 November 2018; Published: 12 November 2018

Abstract: The purpose of this study was to classify, and model various physical activities performed by a diverse group of participants in a supervised lab-based protocol and utilize the model to identify physical activity in a free-living setting. Wrist-worn accelerometer data were collected from ($N = 152$) adult participants; age 18–64 years, and processed the data to identify and model unique physical activities performed by the participants in controlled settings. The Gaussian mixture model (GMM) and the hidden Markov model (HMM) algorithms were used to model the physical activities with time and frequency-based accelerometer features. An overall model accuracy of 92.7% and 94.7% were achieved to classify 24 physical activities using GMM and HMM, respectively. The most accurate model was then used to identify physical activities performed by 20 participants, each recorded for two free-living sessions of approximately six hours each. The free-living activity intensities were estimated with 80% accuracy and showed the dominance of stationary and light intensity activities in 36 out of 40 recorded sessions. This work proposes a novel activity recognition process to identify unsupervised free-living activities using lab-based classification models. In summary, this study contributes to the use of wearable sensors to identify physical activities and estimate energy expenditure in free-living settings.

Keywords: physical activity classification; free-living; GENEactiv accelerometer; machine learning; Gaussian mixture model; hidden Markov model; wavelets

1. Introduction

Engaging in sufficient amounts of physical activity (PA) is associated with decreased risk of premature mortality from cardiovascular diseases [1–3]. The 2008 physical activity guidelines recommend engaging in at least 150 minutes per week of moderate-vigorous physical activity [4]. Without an accurate PA measurement tool, our ability to determine the relationship between physical activity and health, develop effective interventions to promote these healthy behaviors, and evaluate the effectiveness of these interventions, is severely limited. Human beings perform a wide range of complex activities, varying based on age, profession, time of the day and other demographics. Physical activities of many forms including daily household activities, walking, aerobics, and strength training are performed at various intensities (i.e., light, moderate or vigorous), based on the individual. Hence, we need measurement tools to quantify complex human activities accurately, and make necessary interventions to maintain healthy behaviors.

With the advent of wearable and remote sensors, it has become easier to monitor PA due to their objectivity, minimal participant burden and rich data that can be collected for a long period. Human activity recognition using video processing has become a widely studied area of research. Video analysis approaches based on template-based methods [5,6], generative models [7–9], and discriminative models [10] have been used to classify complex human activities and gait patterns. However, in this paper we focused on wearable accelerometers, which have become inexpensive, small and lightweight, can gather high-frequency data and can be used by the population across all demographics. Accelerometer-based systems have been used to gain insights about physical activity of all age groups, adolescents [11,12], young adults [13–16], old adults [17–22] and seniors [17,23–25]. There are two major research foci in PA monitoring studies: (a) energy expenditure (EE) estimation and (b) activity classification. The traditional approach to EE estimation using accelerometer data is to estimate the intensity (MET value) of an activity through simple linear regression modeling [26]. Another approach attempts to identify the type of activity performed, and calculate EE using knowledge of the activity's intensity. Current methodological development, especially in signal processing and machine learning techniques, have led researchers to implement alternative frameworks for estimating EE. Of which, methods such as artificial neural network [27], novel estimation framework based on statistical estimation theory [28] and piecewise linear regression model [29], deserve special mention due to their high prediction accuracy. Activity classification studies have been performed with both supervised laboratory and free-living protocols. Most PA classification approaches involve extracting features from raw or processed accelerometer data and using them to identify unique physical activities using machine learning or deep learning based classifiers. Various studies have investigated different types of features and classifiers to identify a wide range of PA, reporting efficiency ranging between 68 and 99% [11,18,19,22,30–34]. All these studies have proposed methods to identify various PA performed by study participants ($N \leq 130$) using single [11,18,22,32] or multiple accelerometer units [30,31,35], but strictly in supervised, controlled settings and lack free-living applications. The studies [11,30] that have analyzed a large database of PA (≥ 20) lack in diversity and total number of study participants ($N \leq 53$). Simultaneously, studies [18,32] that dealt with a large number of study participants ($N \geq 100$) analyzed less PA (≤ 12). In this study, however, we have used a larger dataset of ($N = 152$) participants to model 24 PA in a lab-based study using just a single wrist-worn accelerometer. Previous work has generally relied on lab-based activity trials to train and test classification models. However, validity of these previously studied methodologies applied toward free-living contexts is starting to emerge. One such study [36] cross-validated four PA classification models ($N = 21$) and classified four activities in free-living setting from ($N = 16$) participants wearing a wrist-worn accelerometer. Supervised classification was performed with reference to recorded labels using another thigh worn accelerometer. In this study, we use a novel unsupervised framework to identify PA performed by 20 participants in a free -living setting. In the first part of this paper, we train and test classifiers to model physical activities using accelerometer data from lab-based settings. In the second part of the paper, we use the lab-based classification model to identify free -living activities in an unsupervised framework.

The data used in this analysis were gathered through two separate studies conducted in a southwestern university in the USA. The first study provided accelerometer data on structured, lab-based activities that were used to train and validate the proposed machine learning method. The data from the free-living protocol were used to evaluate the developed algorithm in its capacity to estimate activity intensities in a free -living setting. The details of each study (recruitment, participant characteristics, and data collection methods) are described in the following sections.

2. Lab-Based Study Protocol

2.1. Data Collection

A total of 152 adult participants (48% male, age 18–64 years old) were recruited in the lab-based protocol. The recruitment method and participant eligibility criteria were similar in both lab-based and free-living protocol and accomplished via fliers, emails, and social networks (e.g., Twitter, Facebook). Interested participants completed an online screener and scheduled a lab visit to determine eligibility by performing a wide array of physical activities. Participants were screened for conditions that could limit their physical activity (e.g., cardiovascular disease, high blood pressure) as well as completed a physical activity readiness questionnaire. For both studies, informed consent was obtained from each participant prior to enrollment. The university's institutional review board approved all study materials and procedures.

After obtaining consent, each participant was scheduled for a two-hour laboratory visit. They were instructed to wear comfortable clothing and were fitted with a GENEActiv accelerometer (Activinsights Ltd., Kimbolton, Huntingdon, UK) on their non-dominant wrist along with other activity monitors. The GENEActiv is a lightweight, waterproof, wrist-worn sensor that collects raw acceleration data. Adult participants performed a set of ambulatory and lifestyle activities randomly selected from a predetermined pool of activities (see Table 1). Participants were video-recorded completing each of the activities using a custom-designed Android app developed by our research team. This application provided automated start and stop times for each activity and an electronic video file of each activity performed. Table 1 shows the major groups of PA, the metabolic equivalent (MET) values (defined as the ratio between energy expenditure during an activity and energy expenditure at rest) associated to each PA, according to the 2011 Adult Compendium of PA [37], and their corresponding intensity levels.

Table 1. Laboratory dataset and physical activity details, showing the unique physical activities performed by the participants, with the associated metabolic equivalent (MET) values and intensities.

Dataset (Adults)	PA No	PA Class	MET Value [a]	Intensity Label [b]
Stationary	1	Seated, folding/stacking laundry	2.0	L
	2	Standing/fidgeting with hands while talking	1.8	L
	3	1 minute brushing teeth + 1 minute brushing hair	2.0	L
	4	Driving a car	2.5	L
Walking	5	Treadmill at 1 mph	2.0	L
	6	Treadmill at 2 mph	2.8	L
	7	Treadmill at 3 mph	3.5	M
	8	Treadmill at 3 mph, 5% grade	5.3	M
	9	Treadmill at 4 mph	4.9	M
	10	Hard surface walking	2.8	L
	11	Hard surface, hand in pocket	3.5	M
	12	Hard surface, while carrying 8 lb. object	5.0	M
	13	Hard surface, holding cell phone	4.5	M
	14	Hard surface, holding filled coffee cup	3.5	M
	15	Carpet with high heels or dress shoes	2.8	L
	16	Grass barefoot	4.8	M
	17	Uneven dirt	4.5	M
	18	Uphill with high heels or dress shoes, 5% grade	5.3	M
	19	Downhill with high heels or dress shoes, 5% grade	3.3	M
Running	20	Treadmill at 5 mph	8.3	V
	21	Treadmill at 6 mph	9.8	V
	22	Treadmill at 6 mph, 5% grade	12.3	V
Stair climbing	23	Walking upstairs (5 floors)	4.0	M
	24	Walking down stairs (5 floors)	3.5	M

[a] MET values obtained from the Adults Compendium of PA, Ainsworth et al. 2011;
[b] L = light intensity, M = moderate intensity, V = vigorous intensity.

2.2. Data Processing

Tri-axial accelerometer data (X, Y and Z axes) were collected at a sampling rate of 100 Hz, during which the participants had to stay still for the first 5 seconds, and then perform a specific PA for a fixed period of time. As a part of pre-processing, the resultant acceleration, $R = \sqrt{X^2 + Y^2 + Z^2}$, was calculated and used as a fourth signal along with the X, Y and Z direction acceleration signals. After the activity transitions were identified from observed labels, the four acceleration signals were divided into windows of 10 seconds (1000 samples) without overlap, which is enough to capture both stationary and properties of the signal. To find descriptors of unique PA, various features were extracted from windowed accelerometer signals, followed by a feature selection method. Supervised classification was performed using the Gaussian mixture model (GMM) and the hidden Markov model (HMM), and their performances were compared. The entire lab-based process chain is shown in Figure 1.

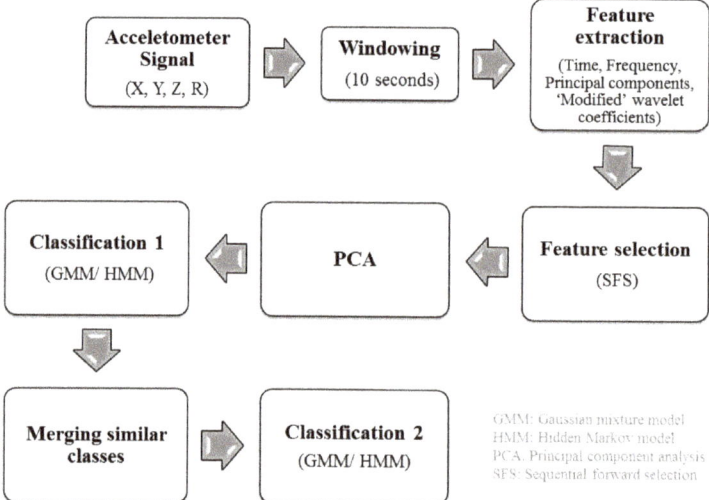

Figure 1. Lab-based activity classification process chain.

2.2.1. Feature Extraction

In this study, we have investigated some state-of-the-art features and introduced some novel ones as descriptors of PA for each window of accelerometer signals. 130 such features were extracted from every 10 second window (1000 samples) from different combinations of the four acceleration signals. We have briefly explained some essential backgrounds of the features investigated in this study.

- *Time-Domain Features*: Mean, standard deviation, skewness, kurtosis, energy and the squared sum of the Y and Z acceleration signals under the 25th and 5th percentile.
- *Frequency-Domain Features*: Maximum magnitude between 1 → 5 Hz, sum of frequency component heights below 5 Hz and number of peaks in spectrum below 5 Hz.
- *Principal Component Features*: First four principal components of X, Y, Z and R.
- *'Modified' Wavelet Coefficient Features*: The wavelet transform provides a time-frequency representation of a signal, as it gives an optimal resolution in both time and frequency domains [38]. In our case we used a three level Haar wavelet decomposition to extract wavelet coefficients from each 10 seconds window. We used the Kolmogorov-Smirnov (KS) test, to automatically

select 20 coefficients out of 1000 (10 secs window). Given a wavelet coefficient x, across all the windows of a specific PA, the test compares the cumulative distribution function $F(x)$ with that of a Gaussian distribution with the same mean and variance $G(x)$, and hence it finds the coefficients that show maximum deviation as a sign of multi-modal distribution.

2.2.2. Feature Selection

Machine learning algorithms always present problems when dealing with high dimensional inputs, so we selected the most 'efficient' features out of 130 features. For this purpose, we used the sequential forward selection (SFS) method. The SFS is a greedy search algorithm that works in tandem with classifiers and compares classification accuracy at each step. We used the SFS algorithm for training on a random subset of 40 adult participants' laboratory accelerometer data, using a GMM classifier. Results showed that the 'modified' wavelet coefficients extracted from the resultant acceleration signal (R) were the most 'efficient' or highest ranked features. This suggests that the 'modified' wavelet coefficients of R can be used as a descriptor of unique PA. To make use of all the 20 wavelet coefficients we computed the principal components of these coefficients, and used the first 10 components as the feature space for PA classification.

2.2.3. Classification

For classification of physical activities, we explored two classification algorithms, GMM and HMM, with the first 10 principal components of the 'modified' wavelet features, used as the input feature vector. We assume that wavelet features of each PA follows a Gaussian distribution. Based on this assumption, the principal components which are orthogonal vectors also follow Gaussian distributions. Thus, the choice of GMM and HMM with Gaussian distribution as their output distribution is justified. To measure the specificity of classification, we executed two levels of classification. The first level was used to combine similar activities and reduce the number of activity classes and the second level was used to extract the models for each activity (unique or combined).

- *Gaussian Mixture Model*: GMM is one of the most commonly used classifiers, which models the probability distribution of data as a linear combination of multiple Gaussian distributions. To create a model, the optimal values of each Gaussian distribution in the mixture must be estimated, using the Expectation-Maximization (EM) procedure [39]. GMMs have been extensively used for supervised classification problems, in which a GMM can model a single class, but can also be used for unsupervised clustering problems [40]. Before estimating the Gaussian distribution, we initialized the GMM using the Linde-Buzo-Gray (LBG) k-means algorithm [41].
- *Hidden Markov Model*: We used the GMM as the probability distribution function of the HMM output, otherwise known as the emission probability parameter. The Viterbi approximation path algorithm [42] was used to estimate the new labels for which the joint distribution of X (feature vector) and Z (observed PA labels) is maximized. The algorithm considers the most likely path instead of summing over all possible state sequences, which saves computation time.
- *Merging Similar Classes*: One shortcoming of using a single accelerometer is that there is a high possibility that similar activities (e.g., 'Hard surface walking, while carrying 8 lb. object' and 'Hard surface walking, while holding filled coffee cup') might be hard to classify. Consequently, we executed a simple method to measure the specificity of classification and find out which classes are more likely to get merged. The confusion matrix was constructed after first level of classification using the predicted and actual classes as its rows and columns, respectively. We employed a thresholding technique to combine similar classes into one larger class. For any class, if more than 50% of the class was predicted as another class, we combined them into a single class. This method helped us to find similar PAs in an unsupervised manner. After combining the similar classes, we performed a second level of classification to construct the final confusion matrix. We have shown the final number of combined classes as the measure of specificity.

2.3. Results

We trained the classification process with a random subset of 40 adult participants using SFS and GMM. The rest (112 adults) were used as the test data. The classification results for the adult samples are shown below.

2.3.1. Lab-Based PA Classification Results

We have shown classification results for the four major classes of activities; stationary, walking, running and stair climbing in Table 2. The table shows the number of initial activity classes, the number of combined classes after merging and the final classification accuracy using GMM and HMM. Out of 15 walking activities, 5 classes (PA classes 5, 10, 12, 14 and 16 from Table 1) and two classes (PA classes 15 and 19 from Table 1) were merged into two single PA classes using GMM. With HMM, two classes (PA classes 6 and 9), four classes (PA classes 10, 12, 14 and 16) and two classes (PA class 15 and 19) were merged into three single PA classes. Similar groups of classes were merged with both classifiers. In all other activities, the classes mostly remained unmerged. Observing the PAs that were merged, we can see that most of the walking activities were merged. PA classes 5, 10, 12, 14 and 16 were walking activities with or without carrying something with their dominant hand, and 15 and 19 were both activities wearing dress shoes. Some of these merges were similar activities of different intensity. In this study, we were limited to a single accelerometer on the non-dominant wrist, which might be the reason why both the classifiers were not able to distinguish between these classes. This suggests that the features from just the non-dominant wrist accelerometer are not able to capture unique descriptors of these PAs. This limitation might be because of less variability in the intensity of movement of the non-dominant arm. However, despite such limitations, the classifiers could identify various complex activities. This suggests that the 'modified' wavelet features can be an accurate descriptor of physical activities. Comparing the two classifiers, the final classification accuracies for all the major classes were 99.91% (GMM) for stationary, 84.87% (HMM) for walking, 99.86% (HMM) for running and 100% (GMM) for stair climbing activities.

Table 2. Classification accuracy for various lab-based physical activities using Gaussian mixture model (GMM) and hidden Markov model (HMM) (showing the initial and the final number of PA classes after merging).

Activities	Original PA Classes	PA Classes after Merging (GMM)	PA Classes after Merging (HMM)	Classification Accuracy% (GMM)	Classification Accuracy% (HMM)
Stationary	4	4	4	99.91	89.32
Walking	15	10	10	79.57	84.87
Running	3	2	3	91.4	99.86
Stair-climbing	2	2	2	100	99.8
All activities	24	21	17	78.54	90.2

2.3.2. Best Classification Model Selection

The best classification model was estimated by comparing the two classification algorithms. Three parameters were used to compare the performances of the classifiers: trace of the confusion matrix after the two levels of classification, final classification accuracy (mean of the trace of the final confusion matrix) and total number of classes identified after merging (specificity). Given the input feature vector of 10 principal components (of 'modified' wavelet features), we tested the classifiers in multiple feature spaces (2-D to 10-D, each dimension representing a principal component) to find the best classification model and feature space. The GMM gave the best classification performance in 10-D feature space with an accuracy of 78.5% (21 final classes), and HMM gave the best performance in 6-D feature space with accuracy 90.5% (17 final classes). Upon comparing both classifiers, the GMM achieved higher average trace with fewer classes combined, while the HMM achieved higher classification accuracy with more classes combined. To decide on the better classifier, we made a comparison between the two best cases of GMM and HMM by combining one class at a time and comparing the accuracy after each step, until all classes were merged to one whole class (Figure 2). It can be seen in Figure 2, as we kept combining PA classes, HMM showed a better convergence than GMM. Thus, the classification model of the HMM in 6-D feature space was selected as the best classification model. We used the models of all the 24 classes to identify PA in the free-living setting.

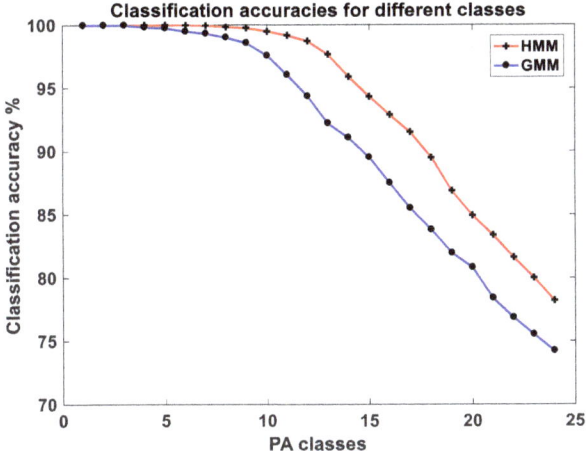

Figure 2. Convergence characteristics of each classifier (GMM and HMM), comparing the classification accuracies, as a PA class is merged at every step.

3. Free-Living Study Protocol

3.1. Data Collection

The 20 participants (50% male, age 21–46 years old) who participated in the free-living protocol were instructed to indicate two typical days (one weekday and one weekend day) for data collection. The participants included students, office workers, professors and home-makers. On those selected days, they were instructed to maintain their usual daily activity pattern while two researchers were independently classifying their activities through direct observation [43]. The researchers continuously classified a participant's activity over a 6–8 hour period using a researcher-developed mobile app that allowed for continuous activity classification. Activities were labeled based on the type and context of activities. The six physical activity type labels were walking, sitting, jogging, reclining, standing and squatting whereas the context labels were sports/exercise, household chores, transportation, occupation and leisure. Approximately 8% of the data were classified as unobserved, when participants required private time (e.g., restroom use) or were out of sight of the researchers. On both days, participants were asked to wear the GENEActiv continuously along with other activity monitors.

3.2. Data Processing

In the lab-based settings, we modeled unique PA by distribution of Gaussian mixtures in a 6-D space. From the lab-based results, it was shown that the best supervised classification model was accomplished using HMM with the first six principal components of the 'modified' wavelet features. We used all the 24 PA models to identify PA in the free-living settings in an unsupervised classification framework. The primary goal of the free-living data analysis was to identify PA and the PA intensity associated to the identified activity types. The entire process was divided into the following sub-sections based on the order they were performed: pre-processing, feature extraction, unsupervised classification and Gaussian model matching (see Figure 3).

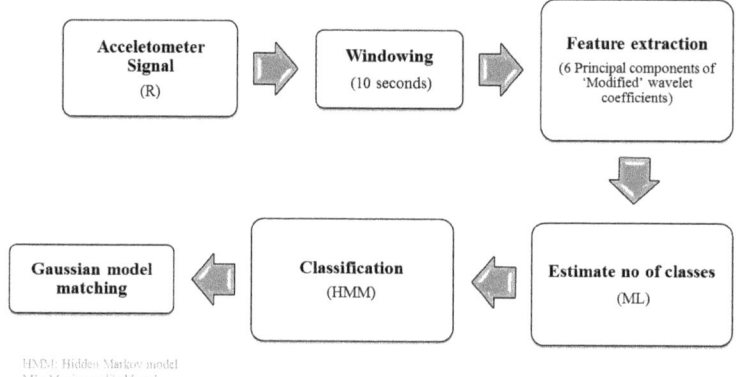

Figure 3. Free-living activity identification process chain.

3.2.1. Pre-Processing

The resultant acceleration, R, was calculated from the tri-axial acceleration signals and was used as the main signal from which features (PA descriptors) were extracted from 10 second windows of the signal.

3.2.2. Feature Extraction

The 'modified' wavelet coefficients proved to be the most efficient feature choice for the lab-based settings study. The first six principal components of 20 'modified' wavelet coefficients were used as feature vector.

3.2.3. Unsupervised Classification

Since the number of activities performed during a session was unknown, we first estimated the total number of activities performed using Gaussian mixture maximum likelihood estimation. The maximum log likelihood is calculated using the following equation,

$$M_l = \arg\max_{K} \sum_{n=1}^{N} \{ \sum_{k=1}^{K} \pi_k N(x_n | \mu_k, \Sigma_k) \}$$

where, x_n are the data points, N is total number of data points from a session and K is the total number of PA classes for each session. μ_k and Σ_k are the mean and standard deviation of the Gaussian distributions corresponding to each PA class. After estimating the total number of classes, we performed classification using HMM with output distribution of Gaussian mixtures to find the Gaussian distribution corresponding to each activity.

3.2.4. Gaussian Model Matching

Using unsupervised classification, we managed to estimate the total number of activities and modeled them by a mixture of Gaussians in the 6-D feature space. However, we still needed to identify the activities. We identified an unsupervised activity as the lab-based PA that had the 'minimum distance' in the feature space. We defined this 'distance' as the distance between the means of the

Gaussians of the unsupervised model and the best supervised model. The predicted unsupervised PA is given by L_c and computed as follows,

$$k_c = \underset{L_c, c=1,\ldots,24}{\arg\min} |\mu_k - \mu_{L_c}|$$

μ_x and μ_{L_c} are the means of the kth free-living PA class from the unsupervised model and cth lab-based PA class from the best supervised model Gaussian distributions.

3.3. Results

We first estimated the total number of activities performed by a participant in each session using Gaussian mixture maximum likelihood. HMM and Gaussian model matching were used to identify the estimated activities among the pool of lab-based activities. In Figure 4, we have shown the proportion of the identified PA performed by the participants in each free-living session. It can be seen that 'Standing/fidgeting with hands while talking' was the most commonly performed PA. Most of the study participants spent the majority of their sessions performing stationary activities, and at most 10% of the time performing ambulatory activities. Result shows that participants 3, 5, 6 and 16 mostly performed ambulatory activities during their second sessions. We also estimated the intensity levels of the activities using the corresponding MET values of the estimated classes. A correlation coefficient of 0.80 was achieved between the estimated and the actual intensity level, which was approximately calculated from direct observations. Figure 5 shows the estimated number of activities performed by a participant (total 20) in each session (total 2) and the estimated intensity levels along with the recorded activity and context labels. Results are shown in terms of percentage of time spent on different activities (estimated and observed).

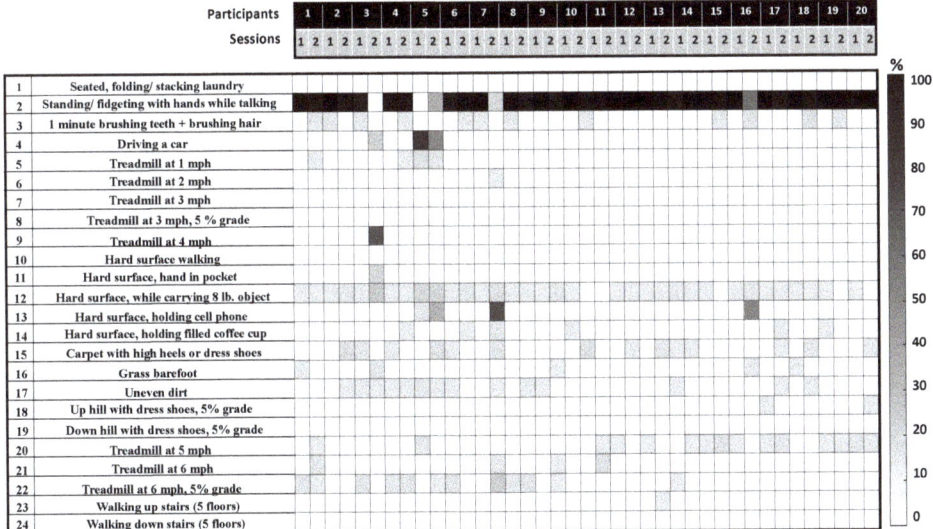

Figure 4. Free-living analysis results, showing the proportion of identified PA for each participant in each session; each column represents a session, showing the percentage of time spent on unique activities (out of 24 lab-based PA) by a participant in that session.

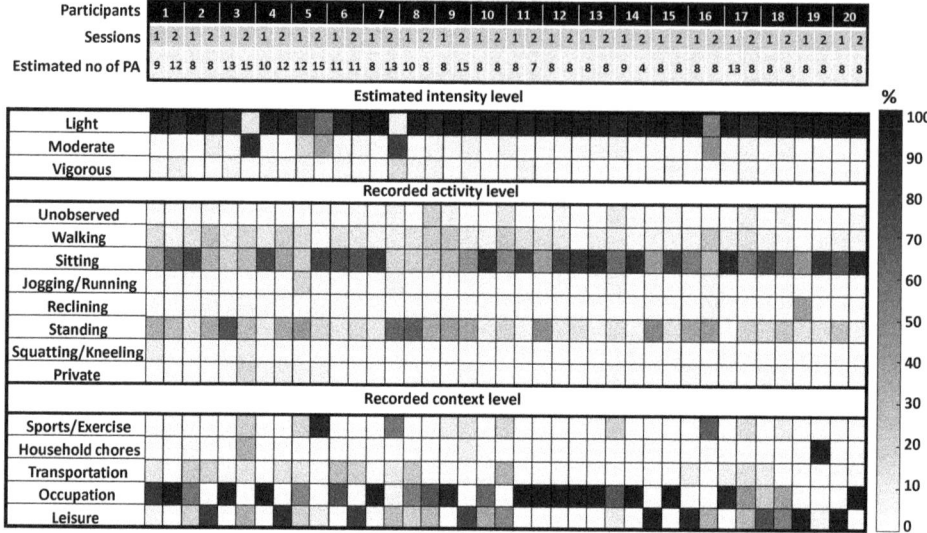

Figure 5. Free-living analysis results, showing the estimated number of PA and intensity levels (estimated), the observed activity types and contexts for every participant in each session. Results are shown in the form of percentage of time spent on each type of activity in a session. For example, participant 1 performed more that 90% of his 1st session performing sedentary or light intensity physical activities (estimated), and from the observed labels, it can be seen that he performed sitting and standing activities for more than 90% of the time, which was mostly during his workday.

4. Discussion

This study systematically classified 24 lab-based supervised PAs and used the best classification model to identify activities in free-living settings. The lab-based participants ($N = 152$) performed activities from a pool of four stationary, 15 walking, three running and two stair climbing activities. We achieved fairly high accuracy, identifying classes from each activity group with both GMM (79–100%) and HMM (85–99%), with some limitations in specificity regarding a few walking activities. We then tested both the classifiers with the entire dataset in different feature spaces to find out the best classification space. The HMM in a 6-D feature space proved to be the best classification model and this model was used to identify unsupervised activities in the free-living settings. We estimated the total number of activities and identified them for 20 participants in each session. We further estimated the PA intensity levels with high accuracy (approximately 80%) and found that nearly all participants spent most of their time doing stationary and light intensity activities. The recorded activity levels showed that participants spent most of their time performing stationary (i.e., sitting and standing) activities.

In the last decade, GMMs and HMMs have been successfully applied in classification problems for their low computational complexity and robustness. HMMs make use of both the similarity of shapes between test and reference signals and the probabilities of shapes appearing and succeeding in time series signals, which makes it a dynamic modeling scheme. The GMM, on the other hand, is a static modeling scheme and it can be thought of as a single state HMM. In this study, the GMM does a better job classifying stationary activities, but overall the HMM outperforms GMM. This suggests that dynamic models are more suitable to recognize complex PA, especially non-stationary activities. On the other hand, a static model like GMM is more likely to classify stationary activities with better precision.

This study is unique because both lab-based and free-living dataset were investigated, with one dataset co-dependent on the other. We identified novel descriptors of PA from accelerometer signals ('modified' wavelet coefficients) that can be used to classify PA and produce near-accurate models. In our previous paper [34], we already showed that these features were efficient descriptors of gait patterns in 99 older adults with disabilities. With the use of a novel unsupervised classification technique we identified free-living PA and estimated energy expenditure. Generally, activities performed on a daily basis are more complex than the 24 activities investigated in this study. This study suggests that although the identified activities might not be exactly the same as the real activity, it can be a close approximation. Of note, our results suggest less degradation in activity classification accuracy from laboratory to free-living settings than previous studies. We posit that this may be because of the robust activity classifier that was developed given the large sample size and diverse set of laboratory-based activities.

This study has important implications for physical activity researchers. First, because these data were collected using a raw waveform accelerometry on the wrist, these computations can be replicated across a large range of wearable sensors that capture and make available to the researcher raw accelerations, and are not limited to the GENEactiv sensors used here. Accelerometers that can record the magnitude and intensity of movement by measuring acceleration between the magnitudes of $\pm 8g$ (where g is equal to 9.825 ms^{-2}, the acceleration of gravity), within a frequency range of 0 to 1 kHz, produce good spatiotemporal resolution. A good spatiotemporal resolution of the accelerometer waveform is sufficient to extract the 'modified' wavelet coefficients as descriptors of PA. Second, the study posits limitations regarding identification of some walking activities, which is due to the use of only one accelerometer on the non-dominant wrist. Although wrist-worn accelerometers are most convenient to wear and associated with greater wear-time compliance, we might be able to improve our results with the use of multiple accelerometers at various other locations of the body. Third, although ample details are provided here for data scientists to replicate this approach, the methods are not computationally intensive and more user-friendly tools are currently being prepared to make this approach available for physical activity researchers. The manufacturers of wearable sensors that are commonly used by physical activity researchers are encouraged to include this algorithm in data analysis packages they are made available to their customers.

In summary, this study contributes to the use of wearable sensors to identify physical activities and estimate energy expenditure in free-living settings by applying state-of-the-art machine learning approaches to a diverse set of laboratory-based, supervised activities. This study has demonstrated success in transferring lab-based validation techniques to the estimation of free-living activities that can be applied to future studies that wish to estimate physical activity in cohort or intervention studies.

Supplementary Materials: The following are available online at http://www.mdpi.com/1424-8220/18/11/3893/s1, Section 1: Summary of features extracted for lab-based activity classification, Section 2: Sequential Forward Selection Algorithm, Section 3: Gaussian mixture model, Section 4: Hidden Markov model, Section 5: Class merging using confusion matrix, Section 6: Lab-based classifier comparisons.

Author Contributions: Each author made substantial contributions to the conception or design of the work and has approved the submitted version (and version substantially edited by journal staff that involves the authors' contribution to the study) and agrees to be personally accountable for the authors' own contributions and for ensuring that questions related to the accuracy or integrity of any part of the work, even ones in which the author was not personally involved, are appropriately investigated, resolved, and documented in the literature. Their individual contributions in specific areas of this paper are provided below.

Conceptualization, A.D. and D.W.B.; Methodology, A.D.; Validation, O.M., M.T. and A.F.P.; Formal Analysis, A.D.; Investigation, A.D.; Resources, M.T., A.F.P., B.E.A., M.P.B. and D.W.B.; Data Curation, M.T., A.D., O.M. and A.F.B.; Writing—Original Draft Preparation, A.D.; Writing—Review & Editing, A.D., O.M., M.T., A.F.P., B.E.A. and M.P.B.; Supervision, D.W.B. and M.P.B.; Project Administration, M.P.B.

Funding: This research received no external funding.

Acknowledgments: The authors would like to thank Pavan Turaga and his students, Suhas Lohit and Qiao Wang of the Arizona State University for their help and suggestions.

Conflicts of Interest: The authors declare no conflict of interest.

References

1. Choo, J.; Elci, O.U.; Yang, K.; Turk, M.W.; Styn, M.A.; Sereika, S.M.; Music, E.; Burke, L.E. Longitudinal relationship between physical activity and cardiometabolic factors in overweight and obese adults. *Eur. J. Appl. Physiol.* **2010**, *108*, 329–336. [CrossRef] [PubMed]
2. Craig, S.B.; Bandini, L.G.; Lichtenstein, A.H.; Schaefer, E.J.; Dietz, W.H. The impact of physical activity on lipids, lipoproteins, and blood pressure in preadolescent girls. *Pediatrics* **1996**, *98*, 389–395. [PubMed]
3. Ekelund, U.; Franks, P.W.; Sharp, S.; Brage, S.; Wareham, N.J. Increase in physical activity energy expenditure is associated with reduced metabolic risk independent of change in fatness and fitness. *Diabetes Care* **2007**, *30*, 2101–2106. [CrossRef] [PubMed]
4. U.S. Department of Health and Human Services. *2008 Physical Activity Guidelines for Americans*; President's Council on Physical Fitness & Sports Research Digest: Washington, DC, USA, 2008; Volume 9, pp. 1–8. [CrossRef]
5. Bobick, A.F.; Davis, J.W. The recognition of human movement using temporal templates. *IEEE Trans. Pattern Anal. Mach. Intell.* **2001**. [CrossRef]
6. Veeraraghavan, A.; Roy-Chowdhury, A.K.; Chellappa, R. Matching shape sequences in video with applications in human movement analysis. *IEEE Trans. Pattern Anal. Mach. Intell.* **2005**. [CrossRef] [PubMed]
7. Duong, T.V.; Bui, H.H.; Phung, D.Q.; Venkatesh, S. Activity recognition and abnormality detection with the switching hidden semi-Markov model. In Proceedings of the 2005 IEEE Computer Society Conference on Computer Vision and Pattern Recognition (CVPR 2005), San Diego, CA, USA, 20–25 June 2005. [CrossRef]
8. Liu, L.; Wang, S.; Su, G.; Huang, Z.G.; Liu, M. Towards complex activity recognition using a Bayesian network-based probabilistic generative framework. *Pattern Recognit.* **2017**, *68*, 295–309. [CrossRef]
9. Liu, L.; Wang, S.; Hu, B.; Qiong, Q.; Wen, J.; Rosenblum, D.S. Learning structures of interval-based Bayesian networks in probabilistic generative model for human complex activity recognition. *Pattern Recognit.* **2018**, *81*, 545–561. [CrossRef]
10. Schüldt, C.; Laptev, I.; Caputo, B. Recognizing human actions: A local SVM approach. In Proceedings of the 17th International Conference on Pattern Recognition, Cambridge, UK, 23–26 August 2004. [CrossRef]
11. Mannini, A.; Rosenberger, M.; Haskell, W.L.; Sabatini, A.M.; Intille, S.S. Activity recognition in youth using single accelerometer placed at wrist or ankle. *Med. Sci. Sports Exerc.* **2017**, *49*, 801–812. [CrossRef] [PubMed]
12. Chowdhury, A.K.; Tjondronegoro, D.; Chandran, V.; Trost, S.G. Ensemble Methods for Classification of Physical Activities from Wrist Accelerometry. *Med. Sci. Sports Exerc.* **2017**. [CrossRef] [PubMed]
13. Dinger, M.K.; Behrens, T.K. Accelerometer-determined physical activity of free-living college students. *Med. Sci. Sports Exerc.* **2006**, *38*, 774–779. [CrossRef] [PubMed]
14. De Vries, S.I.; Engels, M.; Garre, F.G. Identification of children's activity type with accelerometer-based neural networks. *Med. Sci. Sports Exerc.* **2011**, *43*, 1994–1999. [CrossRef] [PubMed]
15. Hikihara, Y.; Tanaka, C.; Oshima, Y.; Ohkawara, K.; Ishikawa-Takata, K.; Tanaka, S. Prediction models discriminating between nonlocomotive and locomotive activities in children using a triaxial accelerometer with a gravity-removal physical activity classification algorithm. *PLoS ONE* **2014**, *9*. [CrossRef] [PubMed]
16. Del Rosario, M.B.; Wang, K.; Wang, J.; Liu, Y.; Brodie, M.; Delbaere, K.; Lovell, N.H.; Lord, S.R.; Redmond, S.J. A comparison of activity classification in younger and older cohorts using a smartphone. *Physiol. Meas.* **2014**, *35*, 2269–2286. [CrossRef] [PubMed]
17. Hansen, B.H.; Kolle, E.; Dyrstad, S.M.; Holme, I.; Anderssen, S.A. Accelerometer-Determined Physical Activity in Adults and Older People. *Med. Sci. Sports Exerc.* **2012**, *44*, 266–272. [CrossRef] [PubMed]
18. Welch, W.A.; Bassett, D.R.; Thompson, D.L.; Freedson, P.S.; Staudenmayer, J.W.; John, D.; Steeves, J.A.; Conger, S.A.; Ceaser, T.; Howe, C.A.; et al. Classification accuracy of the wrist-worn gravity estimator of normal everyday activity accelerometer. *Med. Sci. Sports Exerc.* **2013**, *45*, 2012–2019. [CrossRef] [PubMed]
19. Dong, B.; Montoye, A.H.K.; Pfeiffer, K.A.; Biswas, S. Energy-aware activity classification using wearable sensor networks. In *Sensing Technologies for Global Health, Military Medicine, and Environmental Monitoring*; The International Society for Optical Engineering: Baltimore, MD, USA, 2013; Volume 8723, p. 87230Y. [CrossRef]
20. Mannini, A.; Intille, S.S.; Rosenberger, M.; Sabatini, A.M. Activity Recognition Using a Single Accelerometer Placed at the Wrist or Ankle. *Med. Sci. Sports Exerc.* **2014**, *45*, 2193–2203. [CrossRef] [PubMed]

21. Skotte, J.; Korshøj, M.; Kristiansen, J.; Hanisch, C.; Holtermann, A. Detection of Physical Activity Types Using Triaxial Accelerometers. *J. Phys. Act. Health* **2014**, *11*, 76–84. [CrossRef] [PubMed]
22. Zhang, S.; Rowlands, A.V.; Murray, P.; Hurst, T.L. Physical activity classification using the GENEA wrist-worn accelerometer. *Med. Sci. Sports Exerc.* **2012**, *44*, 742–748. [CrossRef] [PubMed]
23. Rosenberg, D.; Godbole, S.; Ellis, K.; Di, C.; Lacroix, A.; Natarajan, L.; Kerr, J. Classifiers for Accelerometer-Measured Behaviors in Older Women. *Med. Sci. Sports Exerc.* **2017**, *49*, 610–616. [CrossRef] [PubMed]
24. Sasaki, J.E.; Hickey, A.M.; Staudenmayer, J.W.; John, D.; Kent, J.A.; Freedson, P.S. Performance of activity classification algorithms in free-living older adults. *Med. Sci. Sports Exerc.* **2016**, *48*, 941–949. [CrossRef] [PubMed]
25. Tedesco, S.; Barton, J.; O'Flynn, B. A review of activity trackers for senior citizens: Research perspectives, commercial landscape and the role of the insurance industry. *Sensors* **2017**, *17*, 1277. [CrossRef]
26. Freedson, P.S.; Melanson, E.; Sirard, J. Calibration of the Computer Science and Applications, Inc. accelerometer. *Med. Sci. Sports Exerc.* **1998**, *30*, 777–781. [CrossRef] [PubMed]
27. Montoye, A.H.; Mudd, L.M.; Biswas, S.; Pfeiffer, K.A. Energy Expenditure Prediction Using Raw Accelerometer Data in Simulated Free Living. *Med. Sci. Sports Exerc.* **2015**, *47*, 1735–1746. [CrossRef] [PubMed]
28. Wang, Q.; Lohit, S.; Toledo, M.J.; Buman, M.P.; Turaga, P. A statistical estimation framework for energy expenditure of physical activities from a wrist-worn accelerometer. In Proceedings of the Annual International Conference of the IEEE Engineering in Medicine and Biology Society (EMBS), Orlando, FL, USA, 16–20 August 2016; pp. 2631–2635. [CrossRef]
29. Sirichana, W.; Dolezal, B.A.; Neufeld, E.V.; Wang, X.; Cooper, C.B. Wrist-worn triaxial accelerometry predicts the energy expenditure of non-vigorous daily physical activities. *J. Sci. Med. Sport* **2017**, *20*, 761–765. [CrossRef] [PubMed]
30. Tapia, E.M.; Intille, S.S.; Haskell, W.; Larson, K.W.J.; King, A.; Friedman, R. Real-Time Recognition of Physical Activities and their Intensitiies Using Wireless Accelerometers and a Heart Monitor. In Proceedings of the International Symposium on Wearable Computers, Boston, MA, USA, 11–13 October 2007; pp. 37–40. [CrossRef]
31. Ellis, K.; Kerr, J.; Godbole, S.; Staudenmayer, J.; Lanckriet, G. Hip and wrist accelerometer algorithms for free-living behavior classification. *Med. Sci. Sports Exerc.* **2016**, *48*, 933–940. [CrossRef] [PubMed]
32. Trost, S.G.; Wong, W.K.; Pfeiffer, K.A.; Zheng, Y. Artificial Neural Networks to Predict Activity Type and Energy Expenditure in Youth. *Med. Sci. Sports Exerc.* **2012**, *44*, 1801–1809. [CrossRef] [PubMed]
33. Dutta, A.; Ma, O.; Buman, M.P.; Bliss, D.W. Learning approach for classification of GENEActiv accelerometer data for unique activity identification. In Proceedings of the 13th Annual Body Sensor Networks Conference (BSN 2016), San Francisco, CA, USA, 14–17 June 2016; pp. 359–364. [CrossRef]
34. Dutta, A.; Ma, O.; Toledo, M.; Buman, M.P.; Bliss, D.W. Comparing Gaussian mixture model and hidden Markov model to classify unique physical activities from accelerometer sensor data. In Proceedings of the 2016 15th IEEE International Conference on Machine Learning and Applications (ICMLA 2016), Anaheim, CA, USA, 18–20 December 2016; pp. 339–344. [CrossRef]
35. Semwal, V.B.; Singha, J.; Sharma, P.K.; Chauhan, A.; Behera, B. An optimized feature selection technique based on incremental feature analysis for bio-metric gait data classification. *Multimed. Tools Appl.* **2017**. [CrossRef]
36. Pavey, T.G.; Gilson, N.D.; Gomersall, S.R.; Clark, B.; Trost, S.G. Field evaluation of a random forest activity classifier for wrist-worn accelerometer data. *J. Sci. Med. Sport* **2017**, *20*, 75–80. [CrossRef] [PubMed]
37. Ainsworth, B.E.; Haskell, W.L.; Herrmann, S.D.; Meckes, N.; Bassett, D.R.; Tudor-Locke, C.; Greer, J.L.; Vezina, J.; Whitt-Glover, M.C.; Leon, A.S. 2011 compendium of physical activities: A second update of codes and MET values. *Med. Sci. Sports Exerc.* **2011**, *43*, 1575–1581. [CrossRef] [PubMed]
38. Barford, L.A.; Fazzio, R.S.; Smith, D.R. *An Introduction to Wavelets*; Tech. Rep. HPL-92-124; Hewlett-Packard Labs: Bristol, UK, 1992; Volume 2, pp. 1–29. [CrossRef]
39. Moon, T. The expectation-maximization algorithm. *IEEE Signal Process. Mag.* **1996**, *13*, 47–60. [CrossRef]
40. Reynolds, D.A.; Rose, R.C. Robust Text-Independent Speaker Identification Using Gaussian Mixture Speaker Models. *IEEE Trans. Speech Audio Process.* **1995**, *3*, 72–83. [CrossRef]

41. Ortega, J.P.; del Rocio Boone Rojas, M.; Somodevilla Garcia, M.J. Research issues on K-means Algorithm: An Experimental Trial Using Matlab. In Proceedings of the 2nd Workshop on Semantic Web and New Technologies, Puebla, Mexico, 23–24 March 2009; pp. 83–96.
42. Forney, G.D., Jr. The viterbi algorithm. *Proc. IEEE* **1973**, *61*, 302–309 [CrossRef]
43. Florez Pregonero, A.A. Monitors-Based Measurement of Sedentary Behaviors and Light Physical Activity in Adults. Ph.D. Thesis, Arizona State University, Tempe, AZ, USA, 2017.

© 2018 by the authors. Licensee MDPI, Basel, Switzerland. This article is an open access article distributed under the terms and conditions of the Creative Commons Attribution (CC BY) license (http://creativecommons.org/licenses/by/4.0/).

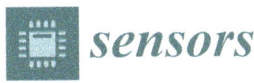

Article

Comparison of Different Sets of Features for Human Activity Recognition by Wearable Sensors

Samanta Rosati *, Gabriella Balestra and Marco Knaflitz

Department of Electronics and Telecommunications, Politecnico di Torino, 10129 Torino, Italy; gabriella.balestra@polito.it (G.B.); marco.knaflitz@polito.it (M.K.)
* Correspondence: samanta.rosati@polito.it; Tel.: +39-011-090-4136

Received: 29 October 2018; Accepted: 27 November 2018; Published: 29 November 2018

Abstract: Human Activity Recognition (HAR) refers to an emerging area of interest for medical, military, and security applications. However, the identification of the features to be used for activity classification and recognition is still an open point. The aim of this study was to compare two different feature sets for HAR. Particularly, we compared a set including time, frequency, and time-frequency domain features widely used in literature (*FeatSet_A*) with a set of time-domain features derived by considering the physical meaning of the acquired signals (*FeatSet_B*). The comparison of the two sets were based on the performances obtained using four machine learning classifiers. Sixty-one healthy subjects were asked to perform seven different daily activities wearing a MIMU-based device. Each signal was segmented using a 5-s window and for each window, 222 and 221 variables were extracted for the *FeatSet_A* and *FeatSet_B* respectively. Each set was reduced using a Genetic Algorithm (GA) simultaneously performing feature selection and classifier optimization. Our results showed that Support Vector Machine achieved the highest performances using both sets (97.1% and 96.7% for *FeatSet_A* and *FeatSet_B* respectively). However, *FeatSet_B* allows to better understand alterations of the biomechanical behavior in more complex situations, such as when applied to pathological subjects.

Keywords: human activity recognition; wearable sensors; MIMU; genetic algorithm; feature selection; classifier optimization; machine learning

1. Introduction

Human Activity Recognition (HAR) is a growing research field of great interest for medical, military, and security applications. Focusing on the healthcare domain, HAR was successfully applied for monitoring and observation of the elderly [1], remote detection and classification of falls [2], medical diagnosis [3], rehabilitation and physical therapy [4].

A HAR system is usually made up of two components: (1) a wearable device, equipped with a set of sensors (i.e., accelerometers, gyroscopes, magnetometers, ...) suitable for capturing human movements during daily life, and (2) a processing tool that recognizes the activity performed in a given instant by the subject. The most common systems employed for HAR are miniature magnetic and inertial measurement units (MIMUs) that work only as a data logger, performing the signal acquisition and storage, while an external system (pc, tablet, smartphone) is needed to process signals and recognize the activities. However, for all those applications in which a real-time feedback is required, it is important to create a stand-alone device able both to acquire several magnetic-inertial signals for long periods of time and to identify the performed activities as fast as possible. From this perspective, the desired device should be lightweight, small and easy to be worn from the subject, provided with a long-lasting battery, and equipped with a microcontroller having enough internal memory for signals and activities storage and able to support the implementation of a classifier for activity recognition. From the classifier point of view, it should be as fast as possible, in order to return a real-time feedback, with low storage requirements and easy to be realized on a microcontroller. In a previous work, we showed that a suitable machine learning classifier is Decision Tree (DT), that is also able to reduce the number of input variables, decreasing the computational time, even if its accuracy was lower than other methods [5].

Another challenging and still open aspect when dealing with HAR is the identification of the correct set of input variables (or features) for the classifier. Analyzing the literature, different approaches can be found. The most popular approach is based on time-domain features [6–8], that are usually of a statistical nature: mean value, median, variance, skewness, kurtosis, percentiles and interquartile range. Some studies use cross-correlation coefficients to quantify the similarity between signals coming from different axes [9,10], but other studies demonstrated the inefficiency of these features [11]. To give an idea of the energy and power contained in signals, frequency-domain features, such as signal power, root mean square value, auto-correlation coefficients, mean and median frequency, and spectral entropy, are commonly extracted [8,12]. Finally, some approaches based on the time-frequency domain can be found in the literature, in particular using the Discrete Wavelet Transform (DWT), that allows a decomposition of signals into several coefficients, each containing frequency data across temporal changes [13]. A detailed review of features used for HAR applications and belonging to time, frequency and time-frequency domains can be found in [14]. Although the great majority of applications use these kinds of features, three main problems must be addressed: (1) the extraction of frequency-domain and wavelet-domain features could result really hard for a microprocessor [15]; (2) the great majority of these features are not directly related to the acquired signals and, thus, they are difficult to attribute to physical quantities, complicating the interpretation of the results and the understanding of errors; (3) the number of variables proposed in the literature is huge and this is not always associated with high classification accuracy since some of them could be sources of noise [16].

Feature Selection (FS) is a fundamental step when dealing with high-dimensional data, allowing for eliminating those variables that are redundant or irrelevant for the system description. Moreover, it has been proven that FS increases the classification performance [17], due to the removal of those variables introducing noise during the classifier construction and application. Two main categories of FS algorithms have been proposed in the literature and successfully applied in the biomedical field for dataset [18], signal [19] and image [20] processing: filter and wrapper methods [21]. Filter methods perform FS independently of the learning algorithm: variables are examined individually to identify those more relevant for describing the inner structure of the analyzed dataset. Since each variable is considered independently during the selection procedure, groups of features having strong discriminatory power may be ignored. Conversely, in wrapper methods, the selection of the feature subset is performed simultaneously with the estimation of its goodness in the learning task. For this reason, this latter category of FS methods usually can reach better performances than filter methods [21], since it allows for exploring also feature dependencies. On the other hand, wrapper FS could be computationally very intensive and the obtained feature subset optimized only for the specific learning algorithm or classifier.

Moreover, once a feature subset is fixed, different classification results might be obtained changing the classifier parameters, since they strongly influence the classification performance [22]. Several approaches have been developed for parameters tuning, e.g., grid search, random search, heuristic search [23]. However, the simultaneous selection of the optimal feature subset and optimization of the classifier parameters is likely the only way assuring to reach the best performances. Since an exhaustive search of the best couple feature subset-classifier parameters is unfeasible in most real situations, heuristic search represents a convenient way to find a good compromise between reasonable computational time and sub-optimal solutions. In particular, genetic algorithms (GAs) have been applied for solving optimization problems connected to FS [17] and parameter tuning [22], but very scarce applications can be found for the simultaneous optimization of both aspects.

The aim of this study is to compare two sets of features for real-time HAR applications: *FeatSet_A* comprising time, frequency and time-frequency domain parameters presented in the literature and *FeatSet_B* consisting of variables belonging only to the time-domain and derived from the understanding of how a specific activity will affect the sensor signals. The most informative features for each set were identified using a GA that simultaneously performs feature selection and optimization of the classifier parameters. Then, the obtained feature subsets were compared analyzing the performances reached by four different machine learning classifiers.

The rest of the paper is divided as follows: Section 2 describes related works about HAR using wearable sensors. Section 3 presents the protocol and population involved in our experiment, the extracted features and the GA used for simultaneous FS and classifier optimization. Results are presented in Section 4 and discussed in Section 5. Section 6 concludes this study and proposes future directions in this context.

2. Related Work

A huge number of studies was proposed in the literature for HAR by means of wearable sensors. Although an exhaustive analysis of publications dealing with these aspects is beyond the scope of this paper (a recent review can be found in [24]), several aspects can be used to characterize and summarize these studies, such as acquired signals, extracted features and algorithms used for dimensionality reduction and activity recognition.

Accelerometric signals are common to all HAR applications. Some studies used this information alone [25–27], but more often accelerometers were combined with gyroscopes [12,28,29] and magnetometers [30,31]. In few cases other signals were taken into account such as quaternions [32], temperature [1], gravity [33] or data acquired from ambient sensors [1].

Once they were acquired, the raw signals were rarely employed as they are [33,34] but usually some kind of processing was applied to extract a set of informative features. In general, most of extracted features belongs to the time-domain (e.g., mean, standard deviation, minimum value, maximum value, range, ...) and the frequency-domain (such as mean and median frequency, spectral entropy, signal power, entropy) [32,35,36]. However, other different variables can be found in literature, such as time-frequency domain variables used in the studies by Eyobu et al. [12] and Tian et al. [37], or the cepstral features proposed by San-Segundo et al. [26] and Vanrell et al. [38].

Regarding the dimensions of the obtained feature sets, three different approaches were followed in the literature. In some studies no dimensionality reduction was performed and, thus, the whole set of variables was used for the recognition phase [39,40]. The second approach achieves dimensionality reduction by means of a transformation of the original set of variables in a new one with lower dimensionality. The most common method belonging to this category is the principal component analysis (PCA), that was employed for example in ref. [41,42]. Finally, different FS methods were used to reduce the number of variables without any transformation, such as Minimum Redundancy Maximum Relevance [43], recursive feature elimination [34], Information Gain [25], or evolutionary algorithms [44].

Since the aim of a HAR application is to identify the performed activity, a proper learning algorithm must be applied as final step. The great majority of the studies in this fields was based on supervised learning algorithms, ranging from machine learning (support vector machine [33], decision tree [27], random forest [32], multilayer perceptron [44], ...) to the emerging deep learning neural networks [45–47]. However, sporadic applications of unsupervised learning algorithms were proposed [48]. Ensemble learning, that combines different classifiers to improve the final performances, was proposed by Tian et al. [37] and Garcia-Ceja et al. [40].

3. Materials and Methods

3.1. Signal Acquisition and Experimental Setup

Signals were acquired using a MIMU-based device by Medical Technology (Torino, Italy). The sensor unit consisted of a tri-axial accelerometer, a tri-axial gyroscope and a tri-axial magnetometer allowing for acquiring acceleration, rate of turn, and Earth-magnetic field data, for a total of nine signals. The measurement range was ± 4 g for the accelerometers, $\pm 2000°/s$ for the gyroscopes and ± 4 G for the magnetometers. The sampling frequency of all signals was 80 Hz. An example of signals acquired during a walk of a healthy subject is shown in Figure 1. For the purpose of this study, signals were recorded in local data storage devices and transmitted to a laptop for the following analysis.

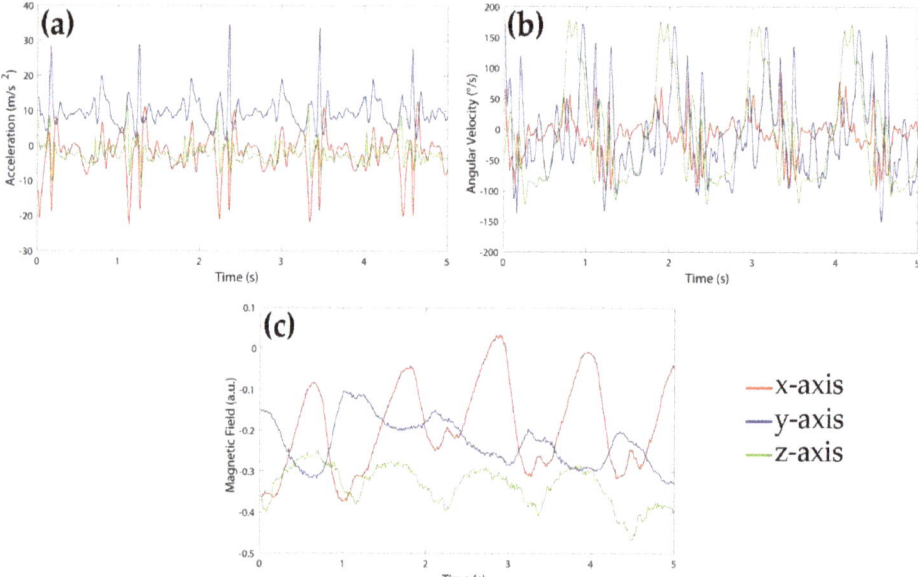

Figure 1. Example of signals acquired by (**a**) accelerometer, (**b**) gyroscope and (**c**) magnetometer during 5 s of walking of a healthy subject.

The MIMU sensor was located on the lateral side of the right thigh. The y-axis was oriented in down-top vertical direction, x-axis was aligned to the antero-posterior direction, and z-axis was aligned to the medio-lateral direction, pointing to lateral side. Sixty-one young and healthy subjects (28 males, 33 females; age: 22 ± 2 years; age range: 20–28 years; height: 169.9 ± 8.3 cm; weight: 64.3 ± 11.0 kg) with no history of physical disabilities or injuries were involved in this study. All subjects were asked to perform seven simple activities: resting (A_1, comprising sitting and laying), upright standing (A_2), level walking (A_3), ascending and descending stairs (A_4 and A_5), uphill and downhill walking (A_6 and A_7). All activities lasted 60 s and were repeated five times by each subject. Activities were executed in indoor and outdoor areas, following a default path, without any speed restriction and style of performing. Each subject signed an informed consent form. Since this was an observational study and subjects were not exposed to any harm, the study protocol was not submitted to an ethical committee nor to an institutional review board.

3.2. Dataset Construction and Feature Extraction

To avoid bias due to the magnetic direction of the performed activities during signals acquisition and magnetic disturbances on the magnetometer, only inertial information (i.e., accelerometer and gyroscope signals) was used for HAR. Each signal was segmented using a 5 s sliding window with an overlap of 3 s between subsequent windows. The total number of processed windows was included in the validation set while the training set was obtained by randomly selecting 10% of windows for each activity of each subject.

For every window, two sets of features were extracted: *FeatSet_A*, comprising features commonly used in literature, and *FeatSet_B*, containing only time-domain features derived from the analysis of the expected biomechanical effect of a given activity on the sensor signals. Since features included in the two sets had different ranges, the min-max scaling method was applied to the training sets to obtain variables between 0 and 1:

$$Var\_norm_i = \frac{Var_i - \min(Var_i)}{\max(Var_i) - \min(Var_i)} \quad (1)$$

where Var_i is the original value of the *i*-th variable.

Even if standardization using mean and variance of each variable is commonly used for machine learning purposes, it is suitable where close-to-Gaussian distribution could be assumed and might be inappropriate for very heterogeneous features [49]. In this study we used features belonging to very different domains, thus we preferred to use the min-max scaling that also preserves the original value distribution of each variable.

Finally, since all machine learning methods tested in this study were supervised methods, each window in the training and validation sets was labeled with the activity performed by the subject in that specific moment. In particular, an integer number was used to codify each activity, ranging from 1 to 7 for activities from A_1 to A_7, respectively.

3.2.1. FeatSet_A

FeatSet_A included 222 features belonging to different domains. In particular, for the six considered signals we calculated:

- 20 time-domain features [14,50,51] (mean value, variance, standard deviation, skewness, kurtosis, minimum and maximum values, 25th and 75th percentiles, interquartile range, 10 samples of the autocorrelation sequence);
- three frequency-domain features [14,50,51] (mean and median frequency of the power spectrum, Shannon spectral entropy);
- 14 time-frequency domain features [14] (norms of approximation and detail coefficients, considering seven levels of decomposition of the discrete wavelet transform).

3.2.2. FeatSet_B

A set of 221 features was extracted based on the time-domain analysis of the signals. First, we defined the positive and negative peaks as the maximum and the minimum values reached between two consecutive zero crossings, respectively. Then, we calculated the following 33 features for the six signals:

- number of zero crossing (one feature);
- number of positive and negative peaks (two features);
- mean value, standard deviation, maximum, minimum, and range of duration for positive, negative, and total peaks (15 features);
- mean value, standard deviation, maximum, minimum, and range of time-to-peak for positive, negative, and total peaks (15 features).

Moreover, we computed single and double integration of the acceleration in the antero-posterior and vertical directions, and the single integration of the rate of turn in medio-lateral direction. These signals represented the velocity and distance traveled by the limb in the corresponding directions. Other 23 features were extracted from these signals:

- mean of the single and double integration of vertical acceleration (two features);
- mean and RMS value of single integration of antero-posterior acceleration (two features);
- RMS value of double integration of antero-posterior acceleration (one feature);
- number of positive, negative and total peaks of the single integration of the rate of turn in medio-lateral direction (three features);
- mean value, standard deviation, maximum, minimum, and range of duration of positive, negative and total peaks of the single integration of the rate of turn in medio-lateral direction (15 features).

3.3. Recognition of Static Activities

Since static (resting and upright standing) and dynamic activities (level walking, ascending and descending stairs, uphill and downhill walking) showed very different types of behavior from the signal point of view, we decided to implement a first recognition step, based on a couple of rules, to discriminate these two classes of movements. Figure 2 shows an example of accelerometer and gyroscope signals acquired during upright standing (panels a and b) and walking (panels c and d) of a healthy subject.

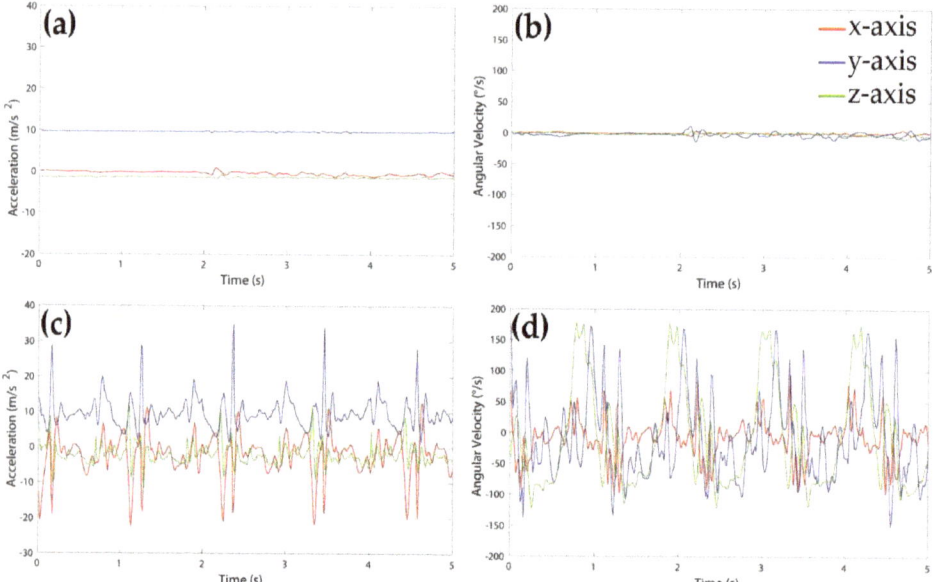

Figure 2. Example of signals acquired by accelerometer (**left panels**) and gyroscope (**right panels**) during 5 s of upright standing (panels (**a,b**)) and walking (panels (**c,d**)) of a healthy subject.

The following rule was used to separate windows representing static activities from those associated to dynamic activities:

if variance of gyroscope signal in z direction *is* below 600 deg·s^{-1}, *then* window represents a static activity, *else* window represents a dynamic activity.

Windows recognized as static activities were further separated between resting and standing windows according to the following rule:

if mean of accelerometer signal in y direction *is* below 8.5 m·s^{-2}, *then* the window is classified as resting, *else* the window is classified as standing.

All windows recognized as dynamic activities were pooled together and used for the following step of HAR based on GA and machine learning classifiers.

3.4. Genetic Algorithm for Simultaneous Feature Selection and Classifier Optimization

GA [52] is a well-known optimization algorithm belonging to the class of metaheuristics, i.e., algorithms designed to search for optimal solutions of a given optimization problem in a reasonable time. A GA is inspired to the Darwin's theory of evolution and, as such, it evolves a population of possible solutions (or individuals) toward better solutions, using the genetic operators of mutation and crossover. The main steps of a generic GA can be summarized as follows:

(1) Generation of an initial population: a random pool of individuals is generated by the algorithm, where an individual is represented by a binary vector, and the fitness value for all of them is calculated. The fitness function is a mathematical function that measures the goodness of a specific individual to solve the optimization problem.

(2) Parents' selection: a subset of individuals is selected to be parents of a new generation of solutions by means of a selection operator. The most used operator is the roulette wheel.

(3) Application of genetic operators: a new generation of individuals is obtained by applying mutation and crossover to the parents. Mutation produces a change in one or more bits of a solution and it is used for maintaining genetic diversity from one generation to the next. The bits to be mutated are randomly selected according to a mutation probability (usually very low, from 0.1 to 0.2). By mutation, a "1" bit in the original solution becomes a "0" bit and vice-versa. Crossover is applied to a couple of individuals with the aim of combining their genetic information. The two individuals are cut in correspondence of one or more random cut-points and the produced substrings are exchanged between them. Each individual has a crossover probability (usually higher than 0.8) to be part of at least one couple.

(4) Termination: if the stopping condition is not reached, a new population of individuals is selected among children and parents and the algorithm restarts from Step 2. The stopping condition is usually based on a given number of iterations or to a plateau in the fitness values of the new generations.

In this study we developed an ad-hoc GA for searching the optimal feature subset and classifier parameters, simultaneously. Four classifiers belonging to machine learning were tested and optimized: K-Nearest Neighbors (KNN), Feedforward Neural Network (FNN), Support Vector Machine (SVM) and Decision Tree (DT). Since all couples classifier-feature set were optimized, a total of 8 GAs were implemented (four classifiers × two feature sets).

Each solution was represented by a binary vector made up of two concatenated substrings: a first substring used for the selection of the most informative features to be input in the classifier and a second substring codifying the classifier parameters. For the first substring, we associated one bit to each available feature, obtaining a number of bits equal to the total number of features included in the considered feature set (*FeatSet_A* or *FeatSet_B*). A bit assuming value equal to "1" identified a feature included in the subset and used by the classifier, while a "0" labelled a not-used feature. The number of bits constituting the second substring was defined for each specific classifier, according to the number of parameters to be optimized and the values we wanted to explore. The details of the codification scheme used for the second substring can be found in the following sections for each classifier tested in this study.

The initial population of possible solutions comprised 400 individuals. The fitness function of each solution was measured according to the following equation:

$$fitness = 1 - acc + 0.3 \times \left(\max_{\forall activity} (acc_{activity}) - \min_{\forall activity} (acc_{activity}) \right) \qquad (2)$$

where the total accuracy (acc) and the accuracy for the *i*-th activity ($acc_{activity}$) were calculated on the validation set for each specific classifier and were expressed in percentage between 0 and 1. The classifiers were trained using the training set, fed with the feature subset defined by the first substring and set up with the parameters codified in the second substring. In Equation (2), the first part of the formula aims at maximizing the classifier performances and the second part is a penalty term introduced to balance the performances among the different classes. Lower fitness values are associated with better solutions.

The parents' selection was based on the roulette wheel algorithm [52], in which the probability of each individual to be selected as parent is proportional to its fitness: individuals with better fitness values have higher probability to become parents of the new generation.

Crossover was implemented with four random cut-points and probability equal to 1. The mutation probability was set to 0.2. Two stopping conditions were implemented: maximum number of iterations (experimentally established as 30) and a plateau in the best fitness value for 15 consecutive iterations. All GAs and classifiers were implemented in Matlab2018a® (The MathWorks, Natick, MA, USA) environment.

3.4.1. K-Nearest Neighbors

KNN algorithm is a simple classification algorithm based on the calculation of the distance (usually the Euclidean distance) between the new element to be classified and the elements in the training set. Firstly, the training elements are sorted in descending order according to their distance from the new element. Then, the most frequent class of the first K elements (called neighbors) is associated to the new element.

For this kind of classifier, only the value of the K neighbors must be decided. A common starting value for K is $K_{in} = \sqrt{N}$ [53], where N was the number of elements in the training set. Beginning from this consideration, we decided to analyze 32 values around K_{in} and, thus, we used five bits for the second substring of each GA solution ($2^5 = 32$): each possible value assumed by the second substring was associated to a specific K value to be set in the classifier.

3.4.2. Feedforward Neural Network

A FNN is made up of a set of neurons, connected by weighted arcs, that process the input information according to the McCulloch and Pitts model [54]:

$$y = f\left(\sum_i w_i \cdot x_i\right) \qquad (3)$$

where y is the output of the neuron, w_i are weights of the incoming connections, x_i are inputs to the neuron, and f is called transfer function and should be selected according to the classification problem.

Neurons in a FNN are organized in layers: in the input layer, one neuron for each input variable is required; the number of neurons in the output layer is decided according to the number of classes to be recognized and the selected transfer function; between input and output layers a certain number of hidden layers can be inserted, whose dimensions are usually decided testing different configurations.

In this study we fixed a basic network structure with input layer and first hidden layer both including one neuron for each feature selected according to the first substring of the GA solution, and an output layer made up of one neuron returning the recognized activity. Then, the number of hidden layers was increased according to the second substring of each solution: three bits were used for adding from one to eight further hidden layers to the basic structure. Each new hidden layer included $1/2$ of the previous layer neurons.

The sigmoid transfer function was used for all hidden layers and the linear transfer function was set for the output neuron. Since the output neuron retuned a real value for each classified element, the round operator was applied to the FNN output and used to assign the final class.

3.4.3. Support Vector Machine

A SVM is a binary classifier (meaning that it is able to distinguish between two classes) that projects the input elements in a new multidimensional space, usually with higher dimensionality than the original one, in which the elements belonging to the two classes are linearly separable. The mapping from the original to the new space is accomplished by means of a function called kernel function, that could be linear or non-linear according to the problem complexity. In the new space, the separation between the classes is obtained with a hyperplane that maximizes its distance from the so-called support vectors. These are the elements of the two classes nearest to the hyperplane and their distance from the hyperplane is called margin.

For this kind of classifier, two different parameters must be set: the kernel function and the penalty term C, that regulates the tradeoff between large margins and small misclassification errors. Thus, we codified in the second substring both information, using two bits for choosing the kernel function and 4 bits for selecting the C value. For the kernel, we examined four different functions: linear, Gaussian, polynomial of order 2 and polynomial of order 3. For the penalty term, the value was set according to the following equation:

$$C = \begin{cases} 0.5 & if\ C_{dec} = 0 \\ 1 & if\ C_{dec} = 1 \\ (C_{dec} - 1) \times 10 & otherwise \end{cases} \quad (4)$$

where C_{dec} is the decimal value of the 4 bits codifying the C term. Using Equation (4) we were able to explore values between 0.5 and 140.

Since the SVM is a binary classifier and, in this study, we would like to identify seven different activities, we implemented a multiclass model for SVM. It combined 21 SVMs using the one vs one strategy in which, for each classifier, only two classes were evaluated, and the rest was ignored. In this way all possible combinations of class pairs were evaluated. The final classification is then obtained using the majority voting.

3.4.4. Decision Tree

A DT is a tree-like classifier belonging to machine learning methods. In general, the tree is constructed top-down by recursively dividing the training set into partitions according to a given splitting rule in the form of "*if variable$_i$ < threshold then partition1, else partition2*". For each splitting rule, a new node is created in the tree. The best splitting rule is identified as that producing two partitions as pure as possible, where pure means that all the elements into a given partition belong to the same class. The construction of a branch stops when the obtained partition is pure or if no more variables can be used for partitioning: in case of pure partitions, the class of the elements is assigned to the leaf node, while in case of no pure partitions, the corresponding leaf node is labeled with the most represented class in the partition. During DT construction it could happen that not all available variables are used, thus a selection of the most discriminant features could be obtained as byproduct of this classifier. Once the tree has been constructed, a new element is classified iteratively applying the splitting rules and following the corresponding branch until a leaf node is reached: the class of the leaf is automatically associated to the new element.

Although several algorithms have been proposed for the tree construction and the identification of the best splitting rule for each node, the CART algorithm [55] and the Gini index [55] are commonly used for the these purposes, respectively, and applied in this study. Once these methods have been selected, no other parameters must be set for DT construction and running. For this reason, in our GA the optimization of the DT did not require bits associated to the second substring.

3.5. Post-Processing

Each couple feature subset-classifier parameters identified by GAs was used for classifying all dynamic windows in the validation set. Furthermore, a post-processing algorithm based on majority voting was implemented on the outputs of each classifier, to reduce isolated classification errors: considering 5 subsequent windows, the most frequently recognized activity was assigned to the entire group of 5 overlapping windows.

3.6. Performance Evaluation

The performances of the eight couples feature subset-classifier parameters were evaluated in terms of accuracy reached for each dynamic activity in every subject involved in the study, after post-processing. The results obtained for *FeatSet_A* and *FeatSet_B* across the 61 subjects were also compared by means of a Student t-test (paired, 2-tail, significance level: $\alpha = 0.05$), for each activity separately. Moreover, the F1-score [56] was calculated for each classifier as:

$$F1 - score = \frac{2 \times precision \times recall}{precision + recall} \quad (5)$$

where *recall* measures the ratio between the number of true positive elements and the total number of positive elements and *precision* measures the ratio between the number of true positive elements and the total number of elements classified as positive.

4. Results

A total of 59780 windows were included in the validation set (61 subjects × 140 windows × 7 activities).

The separation of static activity windows from dynamic activity windows based on rules was able to correctly detect 100% of resting windows and 100% of upright standing windows. Thus, for GA implementation and performance evaluation, 42,700 dynamic windows were used as validation set and 4270 windows were randomly included in the training set.

Table 1 summarizes the GA results for each classifier and for the two feature sets. The following information, related to the best solution found by GAs, are reported: number of features selected by the first substring, classifier parameters codified in the second substring, accuracy obtained on the training set used for the classifier construction, and accuracy reached on the validation set comprising all dynamic windows.

Table 1. GA results for each classifier and for the two feature sets.

Classifier	# of Selected Features		Classifier Parameters		Accuracy on Training Set		Accuracy on Validation Set	
	FeatSet_A	FeatSet_B	FeatSet_A	FeatSet_B	FeatSet_A	FeatSet_B	FeatSet_A	FeatSet_B
KNN	106	132	K = 55	K = 55	87.7%	86.6%	87.7%	86.1%
FNN	114	138	#hidden layers = 6 #hidden neurons = [114, 57, 29, 15, 8, 4]	#hidden layers = 6 #hidden neurons = [138, 69, 35, 18, 9, 5]	91.7%	49.7%	89.7%	48.5%
SVM	118	133	kernel = gaussian scale = 20	kernel = gaussian scale = 10	100.0%	99.9%	98.5%	96.4%
DT	151	103	None	None	97.7%	97.1%	85.9%	82.7%

As it emerges from the table, the GA allowed a substantial reduction of the number of features that was almost halved for both feature sets. Except for DT, a higher number of variables were selected from *FeatSet_B* with respect to *FeatSet_A*, even if this was not associated to substantial differences in the classifiers parameters and this did not produce better performances, neither on training nor on validation set.

Figure 3 shows, for each optimized couple feature subset-classifier parameters, the mean accuracy and the standard error across the 61 subjects involved in the study after post-processing.

Analyzing the behavior of the four classifiers, it emerges that the SVM reached the best performances, allowing to correctly recognize more than 95% of windows for all dynamic activities and for both feature subsets. Comparing the two feature subsets, no significant differences were observed for every dynamic activity using SVM and DT, while FNN fed with *FeatSet_B* was not able to reach acceptable results. This behavior is also evident in Figure 4, where the mean accuracy and F1-score across all seven activities (both static and dynamic) examined in this study is showed for each classifier. Overall, the highest accuracy achieved by the SVM is 97.1% and 96.7% for *FeatSet_A* and *FeatSet_B* respectively, while the worst mean accuracy was 65.5% obtained using FNN fed with *FeatSet_B*. The same behavior can be observed for the F1-score (Figure 4 panel b): the SVM had a score equal to 0.971 and 0.967 for the two sets, meaning that very high values of recall and precision were reached in both cases.

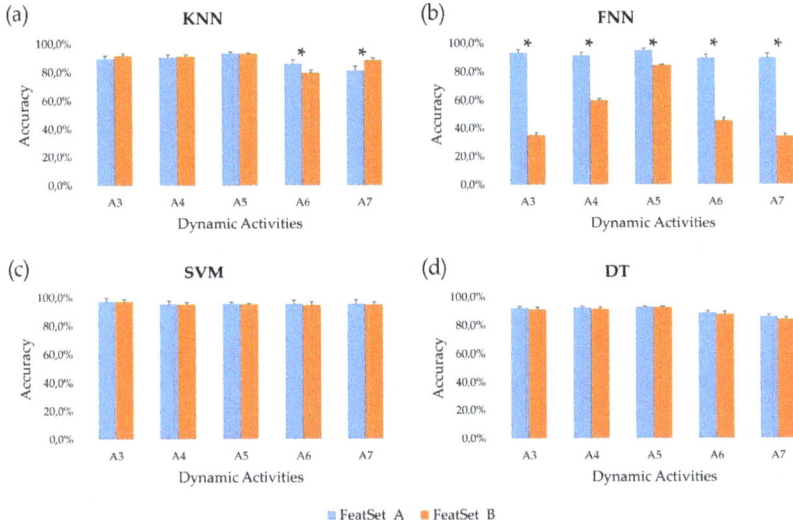

Figure 3. Mean accuracy (bar) and standard error (whisker) across the 61 subjects involved in the study for each dynamic activity (level walking (A_3), ascending and descending stairs (A_4 and A_5), uphill and downhill walking (A_6 and A_7)), after post-processing. Four classifiers are analyzed: (**a**) K-Nearest Neighbors; (**b**) Feedforward Neural Networks; (**c**) Support Vector Machine; (**d**) Decision Tree. Asterisks (*) mark significant differences between accuracies reached by *FeatSet_A* and *FeatSet_B* (p-value < 0.05).

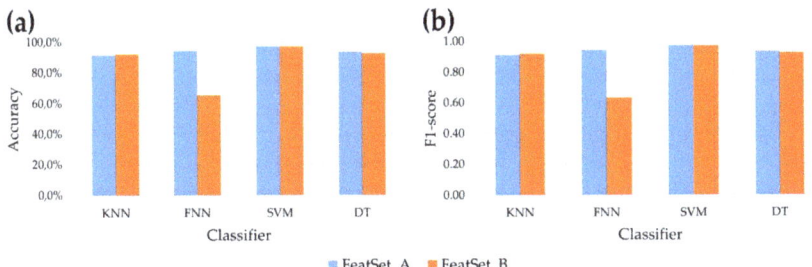

Figure 4. Mean accuracy (panel (**a**)) and F1-score (panel (**b**)) of the four classifiers across the seven activities (both static and dynamic activities), after post-processing, for the two sets of features.

5. Discussion

In this work we compared two sets of features for HAR applications, one comprising features widely used in literature for similar purposes [24] and the second set including variables connected to the expected biomechanical meaning of a given activity on the sensor signals.

With respect to the *FeatSet_A*, our results are in accordance with or better than those obtained by other similar studies. In a recent study by Yurtman et al. [41], the authors compared seven machine learning classifiers using only time- and frequency-domain features. Their results showed that, considering both static and dynamic activities, the best classifier was the SVM, that allowed them to recognize the 86.4% of activities. Similarly, in our study the best results were achieved by the SVM, although our mean accuracy across the seven examined activities was 97.1%. Moreover, our methodology allowed to correctly recognize all windows related to static activities (accuracy = 100%), whereas in ref. [41] better performances were obtained for non-stationary activities with respect to stationary ones (accuracy of 90.7% and 70.6% respectively). Attal et al. [8] analyzed the total accuracy across static and dynamic activities of different classifiers and they found that the best method for HAR was the KNN, that reached 99.3% of correct classification. In our case, the mean accuracy of KNN across the seven examined activities was 91.6% but this was our worst result for *FeatSet_A* (see Figure 4 panel a).

Regarding the second set of variables, sometimes defined as heuristic features [14], it was rarely used for activity classification thus a comparison with previous studies is difficult. Reference [1] used some heuristic variables, such as zero crossing rate and peak-to-peak amplitude, in combination with other time-domain and frequency-domain features. The gyroscope signal integration was used in the study by Najafi et al. [57] for identifying postural transactions and further processed using the discrete wavelet transform. However, to the best of our knowledge, no studies proposed an entire set of features context-based. In our study, these variables were defined with the support of an expert in movement analysis that analyzed in detail the acquired signals during different types of activity and the expected biomechanical effect of a given activity on the sensor signals. From our results it is evident that this kind of variables, associated with the proper classifier, can effectively be used for HAR purposes with very good results (mean accuracy above 96% when used in combination with SVM). From the implementation point of view, the computational complexity of this set of features is lower than the one required by frequency and time-frequency domain features [15], since no transformation of the signals is needed and features are extracted only in time-domain. Moreover, having a direct physical meaning, heuristic features can be useful for supporting the interpretation of results in more complex situations, for example in the monitoring of pathological subjects. In fact, in presence of pathological conditions, the acquired MIMU signals could be altered and consequently some of the extracted features could differ from a "standard" condition. In this case, using *FeatSet_B* and analyzing the physical meaning of these "altered" variables, it could be possible to understand which biomechanical aspect is mostly compromised by a given pathology.

Finally, our study is the first in the HAR field in which the simultaneous optimization of feature subset and classifier parameters was performed. This allows to effectively obtain the optimal combination between input variables and classifier. Moreover, the dimensionality reduction obtained with GA allows for removing redundant and irrelevant features for the initial set of variables, preserving the feature meaning and supporting the results interpretation. On the contrary, other methods widely used in HAR literature, such as PCA [41] or linear discriminant analysis (LDA) [58], produce a transformation of the original variables that could complicates the understanding of the obtained results.

The main advantage of the proposed methodology is that the feature subsets were compared to the best of their performances. In fact, since a wrapper FS method was implemented with GAs, the optimal reduced subset was identified in both situations. Moreover, the simultaneous optimization of the classifiers allowed to find the proper set of parameters suitable for that specific input features.

One limitation of this study lies in the fact that only healthy subjects were involved in our experiment. However, our aim was to compare the two sets of features, thus the most basic and common situation was used, with no introduction of gait variability due to pathological conditions. Nevertheless, we are planning to enlarge our protocol to other neurological pathologies such as Parkinson disease. Moreover, we are implementing the HAR directly on a wearable device composed of three MIMU sensors (accelerometer, gyroscope and magnetometer) and a 32-bit microprocessor equipped with floating point processing unit. The optimized version of the SVM associated with the selected *FeatSet_B* variables was chosen to be implemented on this new device version.

6. Conclusions

This study focused on the emerging field of HAR and aimed at comparing a set of variables commonly used in literature with a completely new one, comprising only time-domain variables associated with the biomechanical meaning of acquired signals. Moreover, we used a methodology for simultaneous feature selection and classifier parameter optimization, based on GA and never used before in similar contexts. From our results it emerged that the two sets of features can both reach very high recognition accuracy, above 96%, if associated with the SVM classifier. However, the newly-proposed set of variables can be easier to be interpreted and their biomechanical meaning could be employed to better understand alterations of the biomechanical behavior in more complex situations, such as when applied to pathological subjects.

Author Contributions: Investigation, S.R.; Methodology, S.R. and G.B.; Supervision, G.B. and M.K.; Writing—original draft, S.R.; Writing—review & editing, G.B. and M.K.

Funding: This research received no external funding.

Conflicts of Interest: The authors declare no conflict of interest.

References

1. Wang, Y.; Cang, S.; Yu, H. A Data Fusion-Based Hybrid Sensory System for Older People's Daily Activity and Daily Routine Recognition. *IEEE Sens. J.* **2018**, *18*, 6874–6888. [CrossRef]
2. Tsinganos, P.; Skodras, A. On the Comparison of Wearable Sensor Data Fusion to a Single Sensor Machine Learning Technique in Fall Detection. *Sensors* **2018**, *18*, 592. [CrossRef] [PubMed]
3. González, S.; Sedano, J.; Villar, J.R.; Corchado, E.; Herrero, Á.; Baruque, B. Features and models for human activity recognition. *Neurocomputing* **2015**, *167*, 52–60. [CrossRef]
4. Roy, S.H.; Cheng, M.S.; Chang, S.-S.; Moore, J.; De Luca, G.; Nawab, S.H.; De Luca, C.J. A Combined sEMG and Accelerometer System for Monitoring Functional Activity in Stroke. *IEEE Trans. Neural Syst. Rehabil. Eng.* **2009**, *17*, 585–594. [CrossRef] [PubMed]
5. De Leonardis, G.; Rosati, S.; Balestra, G.; Agostini, V.; Panero, E.; Gastaldi, L.; Knaflitz, M. Human Activity Recognition by Wearable Sensors: Comparison of different classifiers for real-time applications. In Proceedings of the 2018 IEEE International Symposium on Medical Measurements and Applications (MeMeA), Rome, Italy, 11–13 June 2018; IEEE: Piscataway, NJ, USA, 2018; pp. 1–6.
6. Altun, K.; Barshan, B.; Tunçel, O. Comparative study on classifying human activities with miniature inertial and magnetic sensors. *Pattern Recognit.* **2010**, *43*, 3605–3620. [CrossRef]
7. Torres-Huitzil, C.; Nuno-Maganda, M. Robust smartphone-based human activity recognition using a tri-axial accelerometer. In Proceedings of the 2015 IEEE 6th Latin American Symposium on Circuits & Systems (LASCAS), Montevideo, Uruguay, 24–27 February 2015; IEEE: Piscataway, NJ, USA, 2015; pp. 1–4.
8. Attal, F.; Mohammed, S.; Dedabrishvili, M.; Chamroukhi, F.; Oukhellou, L.; Amirat, Y.; Attal, F.; Mohammed, S.; Dedabrishvili, M.; Chamroukhi, F.; et al. Physical Human Activity Recognition Using Wearable Sensors. *Sensors* **2015**, *15*, 31314–31338. [CrossRef] [PubMed]
9. Bao, L.; Intille, S. Activity recognition from user-annotated acceleration data. *Pervasive Comput.* **2004**, 1–17.
10. Aminian, K.; Rezakhanlou, K.; De Andres, E.; Fritsch, C.; Leyvraz, P.-F.; Robert, P. Temporal feature estimation during walking using miniature accelerometers: An analysis of gait improvement after hip arthroplasty. *Med. Biol. Eng. Comput.* **1999**, *37*, 686–691. [CrossRef] [PubMed]
11. Pirttikangas, S.; Fujinami, K.; Nakajima, T. Feature selection and activity recognition from wearable sensors. *UCS* **2006**, *6*, 516–527.

12. Steven Eyobu, O.; Han, D.; Steven Eyobu, O.; Han, D.S. Feature Representation and Data Augmentation for Human Activity Classification Based on Wearable IMU Sensor Data Using a Deep LSTM Neural Network. *Sensors* **2018**, *18*, 2892. [CrossRef] [PubMed]
13. Preece, S.J.; Goulermas, J.Y.; Kenney, L.P.J.; Howard, D. A Comparison of Feature Extraction Methods for the Classification of Dynamic Activities From Accelerometer Data. *IEEE Trans. Biomed. Eng.* **2009**, *56*, 871–879. [CrossRef] [PubMed]
14. Preece, S.J.; Goulermas, J.Y.; Kenney, L.P.J.; Howard, D.; Meijer, K.; Crompton, R. Activity identification using body-mounted sensors—A review of classification techniques. *Physiol. Meas.* **2009**, *30*, R1–R33. [CrossRef] [PubMed]
15. Figo, D.; Diniz, P.C.; Ferreira, D.R.; Cardoso, J.M.P. Preprocessing techniques for context recognition from accelerometer data. *Pers. Ubiquitous Comput.* **2010**, *14*, 645–662. [CrossRef]
16. Frawley, W.J.; Piatetsky-Shapiro, G.; Matheus, C.J. Knowledge discovery in databases: An overview. *AI Mag.* **1992**, *13*, 57–70. [CrossRef]
17. Giannini, V.; Rosati, S.; Castagneri, C.; Martincich, L.; Regge, D.; Balestra, G. Radiomics for pretreatment prediction of pathological response to neoadjuvant therapy using magnetic resonance imaging: Influence of feature selection. In Proceedings of the 2018 IEEE 15th International Symposium on Biomedical Imaging (ISBI 2018), Washington, DC, USA, 4–7 April 2018; IEEE: Piscataway, NJ, USA, 2018; pp. 285–288.
18. Zaccaria, G.M.; Rosati, S.; Castagneri, C.; Ferrero, S.; Ladetto, M.; Boccadoro, M.; Balestra, G. Data quality improvement of a multicenter clinical trial dataset. In Proceedings of the 39th Annual International Conference of the IEEE Engineering in Medicine and Biology Society (EMBC), Seogwipo, Korea, 11–15 July 2017; IEEE: Piscataway, NJ, USA, 2017; pp. 1190–1193.
19. Rosati, S.; Balestra, G.; Molinari, F. Feature Extraction by QuickReduct Algorithm: Assessment of Migraineurs Neurovascular Pattern. *J. Med. Imaging Heal. Inform.* **2011**, *1*, 184–192. [CrossRef]
20. Rosati, S.; Meiburger, K.M.; Balestra, G.; Acharya, U.R.; Molinari, F. Carotid wall measurement and assessment based on pixel-based and local texture descriptors. *J. Mech. Med. Biol.* **2016**. [CrossRef]
21. Li, J.; Cheng, K.; Wang, S.; Morstatter, F.; Trevino, R.P.; Tang, J.; Liu, H. Feature Selection: A Data Perspective. *ACM Comput. Surv.* **2017**, *50*, 1–45. [CrossRef]
22. Lessmann, S.; Stahlbock, R.; Crone, S.F. Genetic Algorithms for Support Vector Machine Model Selection. In Proceedings of the 2006 IEEE International Joint Conference on Neural Network Proceedings, Vancouver, BC, Canada, 16–21 July 2006; IEEE: Piscataway, NJ, USA, 2006; pp. 3063–3069.
23. Rojas-Dominguez, A.; Padierna, L.C.; Carpio Valadez, J.M.; Puga-Soberanes, H.J.; Fraire, H.J. Optimal Hyper-Parameter Tuning of SVM Classifiers With Application to Medical Diagnosis. *IEEE Access* **2018**, *6*, 7164–7176. [CrossRef]
24. Nweke, H.F.; Teh, Y.W.; Mujtaba, G.; Al-garadi, M.A. Data fusion and multiple classifier systems for human activity detection and health monitoring: Review and open research directions. *Inf. Fusion* **2019**, *46*, 147–170. [CrossRef]
25. Saha, J.; Chowdhury, C.; Biswas, S. Two phase ensemble classifier for smartphone based human activity recognition independent of hardware configuration and usage behaviour. *Microsyst. Technol.* **2018**, *24*, 2737–2752. [CrossRef]
26. San-Segundo, R.; Blunck, H.; Moreno-Pimentel, J.; Stisen, A.; Gil-Martín, M. Robust Human Activity Recognition using smartwatches and smartphones. *Eng. Appl. Artif. Intell.* **2018**, *72*, 190–202. [CrossRef]
27. Yang, F.; Zhang, L. Real-time human activity classification by accelerometer embedded wearable devices. In Proceedings of the 2017 4th International Conference on Systems and Informatics (ICSAI), Hangzhou, China, 11–13 November 2017; IEEE: Piscataway, NJ, USA, 2017; pp. 469–473.
28. Hassan, M.M.; Uddin, M.Z.; Mohamed, A.; Almogren, A. A robust human activity recognition system using smartphone sensors and deep learning. *Futur. Gener. Comput. Syst.* **2018**, *81*, 307–313. [CrossRef]
29. Wang, A.; Chen, G.; Wu, X.; Liu, L.; An, N.; Chang, C.-Y.; Wang, A.; Chen, G.; Wu, X.; Liu, L.; et al. Towards Human Activity Recognition: A Hierarchical Feature Selection Framework. *Sensors* **2018**, *18*, 3629. [CrossRef] [PubMed]
30. Baldominos, A.; Saez, Y.; Isasi, P. Evolutionary Design of Convolutional Neural Networks for Human Activity Recognition in Sensor-Rich Environments. *Sensors* **2018**, *18*, 1288. [CrossRef] [PubMed]

31. Li, F.; Shirahama, K.; Nisar, M.; Köping, L.; Grzegorzek, M.; Li, F.; Shirahama, K.; Nisar, M.A.; Köping, L.; Grzegorzek, M. Comparison of Feature Learning Methods for Human Activity Recognition Using Wearable Sensors. *Sensors* **2018**, *18*, 679. [CrossRef] [PubMed]
32. Zhu, J.; San-Segundo, R.; Pardo, J.M. Feature extraction for robust physical activity recognition. *Human-Centric Comput. Inf. Sci.* **2017**, *7*, 16. [CrossRef]
33. Köping, L.; Shirahama, K.; Grzegorzek, M. A general framework for sensor-based human activity recognition. *Comput. Biol. Med.* **2018**. [CrossRef] [PubMed]
34. Ponce, H.; Martínez-Villaseñor, M.; Miralles-Pechuán, L.; Ponce, H.; Martínez-Villaseñor, M.D.L.; Miralles-Pechuán, L. A Novel Wearable Sensor-Based Human Activity Recognition Approach Using Artificial Hydrocarbon Networks. *Sensors* **2016**, *16*, 1033. [CrossRef] [PubMed]
35. Jansi, R.; Amutha, R. Sparse representation based classification scheme for human activity recognition using smartphones. *Multimed. Tools Appl.* **2018**, 1–19. [CrossRef]
36. Jansi, R.; Amutha, R. A novel chaotic map based compressive classification scheme for human activity recognition using a tri-axial accelerometer. *Multimed. Tools Appl.* **2018**, *77*, 31261–31280. [CrossRef]
37. Tian, Y.; Wang, X.; Chen, W.; Liu, Z.; Li, L. Adaptive multiple classifiers fusion for inertial sensor based human activity recognition. *Cluster Comput.* **2018**, 1–14. [CrossRef]
38. Vanrell, S.R.; Milone, D.H.; Rufiner, H.L. Assessment of Homomorphic Analysis for Human Activity Recognition from Acceleration Signals. *IEEE J. Biomed. Heal. Informatics* **2018**, *22*, 1001–1010. [CrossRef] [PubMed]
39. Cao, J.; Li, W.; Ma, C.; Tao, Z. Optimizing multi-sensor deployment via ensemble pruning for wearable activity recognition. *Inf. Fusion* **2018**, *41*, 68–79. [CrossRef]
40. Garcia-Ceja, E.; Galván-Tejada, C.E.; Brena, R. Multi-view stacking for activity recognition with sound and accelerometer data. *Inf. Fusion* **2018**, *40*, 45–56. [CrossRef]
41. Yurtman, A.; Barshan, B.; Fidan, B.; Yurtman, A.; Barshan, B.; Fidan, B. Activity Recognition Invariant to Wearable Sensor Unit Orientation Using Differential Rotational Transformations Represented by Quaternions. *Sensors* **2018**, *18*, 2725. [CrossRef] [PubMed]
42. Ponce, H.; Miralles-Pechuán, L.; Martínez-Villaseñor, M.; Ponce, H.; Miralles-Pechuán, L.; Martínez-Villaseñor, M.D.L. A Flexible Approach for Human Activity Recognition Using Artificial Hydrocarbon Networks. *Sensors* **2016**, *16*, 1715. [CrossRef] [PubMed]
43. Doewes, A.; Swasono, S.E.; Harjito, B. Feature selection on Human Activity Recognition dataset using Minimum Redundancy Maximum Relevance. In Proceedings of the 2017 IEEE International Conference on Consumer Electronics—Taiwan (ICCE-TW), Taipei, Taiwan, 12–14 June 2017; IEEE: Piscataway, NJ, USA, 2017; pp. 171–172.
44. Wang, H.; Ke, R.; Li, J.; An, Y.; Wang, K.; Yu, L. A correlation-based binary particle swarm optimization method for feature selection in human activity recognition. *Int. J. Distrib. Sens. Networks* **2018**, *14*. [CrossRef]
45. Ignatov, A. Real-time human activity recognition from accelerometer data using Convolutional Neural Networks. *Appl. Soft Comput.* **2018**, *62*, 915–922. [CrossRef]
46. Hassan, M.M.; Huda, S.; Uddin, M.Z.; Almogren, A.; Alrubaian, M. Human Activity Recognition from Body Sensor Data using Deep Learning. *J. Med. Syst.* **2018**, *42*, 99. [CrossRef] [PubMed]
47. Jordao, A.; Torres, L.A.B.; Schwartz, W.R. Novel approaches to human activity recognition based on accelerometer data. *Signal Image Video Process.* **2018**, *12*, 1387–1394. [CrossRef]
48. He, H.; Tan, Y.; Huang, J. Unsupervised classification of smartphone activities signals using wavelet packet transform and half-cosine fuzzy clustering. In Proceedings of the 2017 IEEE International Conference on Fuzzy Systems (FUZZ-IEEE), Naples, Italy, 9–12 July 2017; IEEE: Piscataway, NJ, USA, 2017; pp. 1–6.
49. Stolcke, A.; Kajarekar, S.; Ferrer, L. Nonparametric feature normalization for SVM-based speaker verification. In Proceedings of the 2008 IEEE International Conference on Acoustics, Speech and Signal Processing, Las Vegas, NV, USA, 31 March–4 April 2008; IEEE: Piscataway, NJ, USA, 2008; pp. 1577–1580.
50. Janidarmian, M.; Roshan Fekr, A.; Radecka, K.; Zilic, Z. A Comprehensive Analysis on Wearable Acceleration Sensors in Human Activity Recognition. *Sensors* **2017**, *17*, 529. [CrossRef] [PubMed]
51. Altun, K.; Barshan, B. Human activity recognition using inertial/magnetic sensor units. In Proceedings of the International Workshop on Human Behavior Understanding, Istanbul, Turkey, 22 August 2010; pp. 38–51.
52. Engelbrecht, A.P. *Computational Intelligence: An Introduction*; Wiley Publishing: Hoboken, NJ, USA, 2007; ISBN 0470035617.

53. Rencher, A.C. *Methods of Multivariate Analysis*; J. Wiley: Hoboken, NJ, USA, 2002; ISBN 0471418897.
54. McCulloch, W.S.; Pitts, W. A logical calculus of the ideas immanent in nervous activity. *Bull. Math. Biophys.* **1943**, *5*, 115–133. [CrossRef]
55. Han, J.; Kamber, M.; Pei, J. *(Computer scientist) Data Mining: Concepts and Techniques*; Elsevier/Morgan Kaufmann: Amsterdam, The Netherlands, 2012; ISBN 9780123814791.
56. Sokolova, M.; Lapalme, G. A systematic analysis of performance measures for classification tasks. *Inf. Process. Manag.* **2009**, *45*, 427–437. [CrossRef]
57. Najafi, B.; Aminian, K.; Paraschiv-Ionescu, A.; Loew, F.; Bula, C.J.; Robert, P. Ambulatory system for human motion analysis using a kinematic sensor: Monitoring of daily physical activity in the elderly. *IEEE Trans. Biomed. Eng.* **2003**, *50*, 711–723. [CrossRef] [PubMed]
58. Chen, B.; Zheng, E.; Wang, Q. A locomotion intent prediction system based on multi-sensor fusion. *Sensors (Basel)* **2014**, *14*, 12349–12369. [CrossRef] [PubMed]

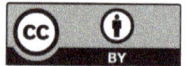

© 2018 by the authors. Licensee MDPI, Basel, Switzerland. This article is an open access article distributed under the terms and conditions of the Creative Commons Attribution (CC BY) license (http://creativecommons.org/licenses/by/4.0/).

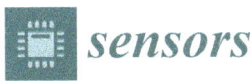

Article

Analysis of the Impact of Interpolation Methods of Missing RR-Intervals Caused by Motion Artifacts on HRV Features Estimations

Davide Morelli [1,2,*], **Alessio Rossi** [3], **Massimo Cairo** [2] **and David A. Clifton** [1]

[1] Institute of Biomedical Engineering, Department of Engineering Science, University of Oxford, Oxford OX2 6DP, UK
[2] Biobeats Group LTD, 3 Fitzhardinge Street, London W1H 6EF, UK
[3] Computer Science Department, University of Pisa, Largo Bruno Pontecorvo 3, 56127 Pisa, Italy
* Correspondence: davide.morelli@eng.ox.ac.uk

Received: 1 June 2019; Accepted: 15 July 2019; Published: 18 July 2019

Abstract: Wearable physiological monitors have become increasingly popular, often worn during people's daily life, collecting data 24 hours a day, 7 days a week. In the last decade, these devices have attracted the attention of the scientific community as they allow us to automatically extract information about user physiology (e.g., heart rate, sleep quality and physical activity) enabling inference on their health. However, the biggest issue about the data recorded by wearable devices is the missing values due to motion and mechanical artifacts induced by external stimuli during data acquisition. This missing data could negatively affect the assessment of heart rate (HR) response and estimation of heart rate variability (HRV), that could in turn provide misleading insights concerning the health status of the individual. In this study, we focus on healthy subjects with normal heart activity and investigate the effects of missing variation of the timing between beats (RR-intervals) caused by motion artifacts on HRV features estimation by randomly introducing missing values within a five min time windows of RR-intervals obtained from the nsr2db PhysioNet dataset by using Gilbert burst method. We then evaluate several strategies for estimating HRV in the presence of missing values by interpolating periods of missing values, covering the range of techniques often deployed in the literature, via linear, quadratic, cubic, and cubic spline functions. We thereby compare the HRV features obtained by handling missing data in RR-interval time series against HRV features obtained from the same data without missing values. Finally, we assess the difference between the use of interpolation methods on time (i.e., the timestamp when the heartbeats happen) and on duration (i.e., the duration of the heartbeats), in order to identify the best methodology to handle the missing RR-intervals. The main novel finding of this study is that the interpolation of missing data on time produces more reliable HRV estimations when compared to interpolation on duration. Hence, we can conclude that interpolation on duration modifies the power spectrum of the RR signal, negatively affecting the estimation of the HRV features as the amount of missing values increases. We can conclude that interpolation in time is the optimal method among those considered for handling data with large amounts of missing values, such as data from wearable sensors.

Keywords: heart rate; IoT wearable monitor; health

1. Introduction

In the last two decades, the interest in the variation of the timing between beats (RR-intervals) of the cardiac cycle, called heart rate variability (HRV), has widely increased in the psycho-physiological research field. Assessment of RR-intervals variability is possible through time and frequency domain analyses that provide parameters able to quantify the amount of fluctuations occurring between consecutive beats, giving therefore an indirect index of autonomic regulation. Actually, the parameters extracted from HRV analysis are useful to provide insight about sympathetic-parasympathetic balance of cardiac vagal tone that was found to be an indicator of cognitive, emotional, social and health status [1].

Thanks to the technological advancements of recent decades, it is now possible to continuously record heart activity during peoples' life via wrist-worn wearable devices equipped with heart rate sensors. This innovation might have a great impact on the medical field because of the low cost of the devices and the possibility to obtain continuous passive measurements performed in an ecological setting, gaining an overview of the users' health status by assessing HRV features during their daily life [2]. These wrist-worn wearable devices, however, produce several inconsistent RR-intervals produced not only by ectopic beats (e.g., atrial fibrillation and premature heart beat), but mainly by motion and mechanical artifacts induced by external stimuli. The number of abnormal RR-intervals increases from 1%—when heart beats are recorded with gold standard technology (i.e., electrocardiography)—[3] to more than 10%—when they are recorded with wrist-worn wearable devices. However, standard methods for calculating HRV features from the time-series of RR-intervals require accurate beat detection. Hence, handling the missing values became a fundamental aspect to correctly evaluate users' physiological response. As a matter of fact, these missing values affect the HRV analysis producing misleading results [4]. In previous studies, the inconsistent RR-interval data were handled by reconstructing the missing values using nearest-neighbour, linear, cubic spline and piecewise cubic Hermite interpolation methods [4,5]. However, these methods can also introduce changes in the reconstructed timeseries that could corrupt the signal spectrum [6], thus reducing the ability to estimate both time or frequency domains HRV features.

In this paper, we focus on healthy subjects with normal heart activity, and investigate the effects of interpolation on time (i.e., the timestamps when the heartbeats happen) and duration (i.e., the duration of the heartbeats) with an increasing amount of missing values (from 0% to 70%) in order to assess which interpolation strategy yields better results when estimating HRV features. In particular, in this paper we show that quadratic interpolation on time is the best approach to reconstruct the missing RR-intervals. Anyway, the main finding of this study is that the interpolation on time produce better HRV feature estimation that the interpolation on Duration suggested by all the previous studies.

1.1. Paper Contribution

To the best of our knowledge, this work is one of the first studies investigating the effect of high percentage of missing values (i.e., 30%, 50% and 70%) on HRV analysis. In previous studies, the inconsistency of RR-intervals was due to a small number of ectopic beats, while wrist-worn wearable devices introduce motion and mechanical artifacts that produce a huge quantity of abnormal heart beats.

Moreover, to the best of our knowledge, this is the first study to analyse the effect on HRV features of interpolation on time versus interpolation on duration. We show the difference among interpolation methods (i.e., no-interpolation, nearest neighbor, linear, quadratic and cubic spline) on both time and duration timeseries in order to detect which interpolation method yields lower error in HRV features estimations. This analysis permits to provide insight about how the interpolation methods work in quantifying the noise introduced into the timeseries.

We conclude by showing that interpolation on time is the best choice for preprocessing RR timeseries with missing values, contradicting the approach traditionally followed, based on durations timeseries.

1.2. Related Work

During the day, approximately 1% of beats are to be expected to be ectopic [3] when they are recorded by using gold standard instrument (i.e., Electrocardiography). An ectopic beat is a disturbance of the cardiac rhythm that induces premature ventricular or atrial contraction. The physiological artifact producing inconsistent beat seriously affects the HRV spectrum, and could result in erroneous results during HRV analysis by introducing non-existing frequencies into the spectrum [7]. In addition to physiological artifact, motion and mechanical artifacts induced by external stimuli introduce a large amount of inconsistent beats when the data are recorded by using wrist-worn wearable device [4–6]. This work is one of the firsts studies that investigate the effect of huge quantities of inconsistent beats that are not only derived from ectopic beats. Since missing data are common in the RR-interval timeseries derived from wrist-worn wearable device, they could complicate the analysis of HRV features making it sometimes impossible. To make reliable HRV analysis, previous studies suggested several preprocessing methods for RR-intervals timeseries (e.g., deletion, interpolations and filtering). However, these preprocessing methods have their own distinct effect on HRV analysis yielding different results [7].

The simplest way of handling the inconsistent RR-intervals provided in literature is to delete them [8]. In this approach, the abnormal RR-intervals are removed and the normal RR-intervals list are merged together. A huge issue of the deletion approach is that it reduces the overall length of the HRV signal. This may significantly influence HRV spectrum [8]. Other interpolation methods maintain the original number of samples, but, by manipulating the duration of RR-intervals, they also change the overall duration by some amount. There are several interpolation approaches useful for handling inconsistent RR-intervals, i.e., zero degree, linear and cubic spline [9]. Zero degree replaces the inconsistent RR-intervals with the mean of the closest normal values. Differently, linear interpolation fits a straight line over the inconsistent RR-intervals to obtain normal values. Finally, the most popular interpolation approach is the spline of order three (i.e., cubic spline). It fits a third degree polynomial smooth curve through a number of data points to obtain new values. This latter approach is recommended when there is only small number of inconsistent RR-intervals [9].

Finally, it was found that the interpolation introduces low frequency components (LF) and reduces high-frequency components (HF) power [6]. This aspect affects frequency domain HRV features [5], while little effect was found in time domain HRV features [4].

We were not able to find any previous work studying the effect of interpolation missing values on the duration versus time, and the propagation of error to HRV features.

2. Materials and Methods

2.1. Dataset

In this paper, we used *nsr2db* (Normal Sinus Rhythm RR Interval Database) PhysioNet dataset [10]. This dataset contains beat annotations of 54 normal sinus rhythm subjects (30 men: 28–76 years; 24 women: 58–73 years) extracted from 23 h long electrocardiogram (ECG) recordings, digitized at 128 samples per second, and beat annotations obtained by automated analysis with manual review and correction.

In order to compute HRV features, the 23 h time series of ECG recording of each user were split into 5 min windows. Moreover, to investigate the effect of missing values on HRV analysis, artificial missing RR-intervals (i.e., 30%, 50% and 70% of missing values) were inserted into the 5 min windows.

The missing values were created in accordance with a burst Gilbert model that simulates burst-error with a two-state Markov chain (i.e., good as 0 and bed as 1) [11]. We define P as the probability of transition form state 0 to the state 1 and p the probability of transition from state 1 to 0. Moreover, Q and q give the probabilities of remaining in the same states 0 or 1 (see Figure 1). Using these parameters, it is possible to represent average bit-error rate P_e as showed in Equation (1) and the average burst length (L_{length}) is set at 10.

$$P_e = \frac{P}{p+P}. \tag{1}$$

Given these equation, we define P, p, Q and q as showed in Equations (2)–(5), respectively.

$$p = 1/L_{burst} \tag{2}$$

$$P = \frac{P_{change}}{1 - P_{change}} * p \tag{3}$$

$$q = 1 - p \tag{4}$$

$$Q = 1 - P, \tag{5}$$

where the P_{change} is set in accordance with the missing values percentage that we want to add in the time series (e.g., if we want 20% of missing values we set P_{change} as 0.3). The missing values were introduced in the time series when the state of the two-state Markov chain is equal to 1. Examples of 30%, 50% and 70% of missing values created by Gilbert model are provided in Figure 2.

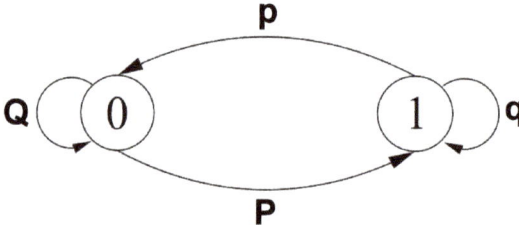

Figure 1. Gilbert model simulates burst-error with a two-state Markov chain (i.e., 0 and 1).

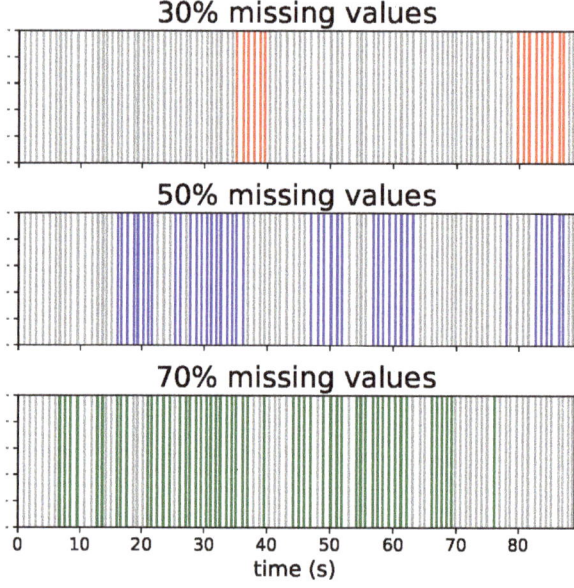

Figure 2. Examples of 30%, 50% and 70% of missing values created by Gilbert model. The colored lines refer to missing beats.

2.2. *Missing Values Interpolation*

The missing values were then handled with six different interpolation methods:

- No interpolation: this approach does not create interpolated values of missing RR-intervals. Differently to the Deletion method that remove missing values merging non-consecutive beats that induce in missing interpretation of HRV features, the no-interpolation method maintains the missing values into the RR-intervals time series.
- Nearest neighbor: the nearest neighbor or proximate interpolation is the easiest interpolation method [12]. This interpolation assigns the value of the closest known (existing) neighbor to the missing- value as shows in Equation (6).

$$X_i = \begin{cases} x_B & \text{if } i < \frac{a+b}{2} \\ x_A & \text{if } i \geq \frac{a+b}{2} \end{cases} \quad (6)$$

where a and b are the indexes of x_A and x_B. Interpolated data by this method are discontinuous and it often yields the worst results [13]
- Linear: this method fits a straight line passing through points x_A and x_B [14]. Interpolated data by the linear model are bound between x_A and x_B as showed in Equation (7).

$$X_i = \frac{x_A - x_B}{a - b}(i - b) + x_B. \quad (7)$$

Gaunck et al. [14] demonstrated that this method is efficient, and most of the time it is better than non-linear interpolations for predicting missing values in environmental phenomena with constant rates. In addition, they also found that in average this interpolation model underestimated the real values but it strongly depends on the distribution of the data.
- Quadratic: differently from the linear interpolation model, the quadratic function needs three points of interest to interpolate missing values in a time series as showed in Equation (8).

$$X_i = x_B \frac{(i-b)(x_C - x_A)}{2(b-a)} + \frac{(i-b)^2(x_A - 2x_B + x_C)}{2(b-a)^2}. \quad (8)$$

Compared to the linear model, quadratic interpolation is found to be in general more accurate [13].
- Spline cubic: fitting datapoints using polynomials of degree higher than one leads to problems of oscillation outside the fitted points, known as Runge's phenomenon [15]. This problem can be avoided by using a spline, a function defined piecewise by polynomials, using datapoints as control points instead of forcing the fitted function to pass through the data points. Cubic spline is a spline composed of piecewise third-order polynomials. By using third degree polynomials is possible to ensure that the resulting curve is smooth [15], avoiding the problem of the straight polynomial interpolation that tends to induce distortions on the edges of the polynomials, given by the fact that, in general, the first and second derivative of the function defined by piecewise polynomials will not be continuous at the edges of polynomials. With cubic spline, it is possible to force the first and second derivatives of consecutive polynomials to be equal, ensuring smoothness of the resulting curve.

We applied each of the interpolation methods listed above to heartbeats expressed as a sequence of durations and as a sequence timestamps, then analyzed the error in HRV features estimations, in order to identify the best approach.

The on-duration approach is the one mostly used in literature to handle missing values. The data used as input to the interpolation methods was the sequence of durations of the heartbeats (the RR-intervals), obtained by subtracting the timestamp of each heartbeat from the timestamp of the subsequent heartbeat in the sequence of heartbeats.

Differently, we propose the the on-time approach whereby interpolation methods are applied to the sequence of timestamps of the heartbeats, postponing the differentiation preprocessing step that transforms timestamps into durations to after the interpolation step.

As shown in Figure 3 the difference between the on-time and on-duration approaches is the order of the processing steps: in the on-duration approach the timestamps are converted to durations as the first processing step; in the on-time approach this step is performed after interpolation is performed.

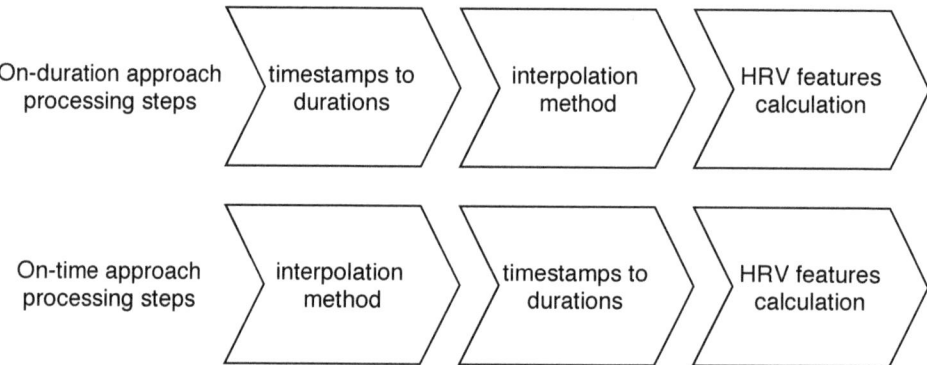

Figure 3. Processing steps in the on-time and in the on-duration approaches.

To better illustrate the differences between interpolation on time and duration, we simulated 100 heartbeats and then we randomly generated 10% of missing RR-intervals in this artificial timeseries by using Gilbert burst approach. The length of the RR-intervals timeseries changes when we interpolate the missing values on duration, while it remains the same when we interpolate on time (Table 1). This result suggests that the interpolation on duration moves beats away from their original position in time, introducing changes to the spectrum, while interpolation on time preserves the position on time of retained heartbeats. In particular, Table 1 shows that the low RR-intervals error (i.e., average difference between heartbeats duration) is obtained with linear interpolation on time. The nearest interpolation on time was not performed because interpolating with this approach is useless, as the interpolated values introduced into the timeseries would have the same time as the closest beat, creating physiologically impossible data.

Table 1. Difference between duration and time interpolation by using different approach (i.e., no-missing values, nearest neighbor, linear, quadratic, and cubic spline).

	Window Time (s)		RMSE (s)		RE (%)	
Interpolation	Time	Duration	Time	Duration	Time	Duration
No-missing values	90.11		—		—	
Nearest	—	91.95	—	0.096	—	5.11
Linear	90.11	91.83	0.075	0.090	3.70	4.86
Quadratic	90.11	92.13	0.084	0.107	4.35	5.83
Cubic spline	90.11	92.24	0.085	0.109	3.46	6.63

Figure 4 provide more detailed analyses of the difference between linear interpolation on both duration and time. The cumulative error when the missing values are interpolated on duration increases as the time series goes by because it creates RR-intervals in accordance with the closest interval values (i.e., the higher is the number of missing values, the higher is the cumulative error) depending on the interpolation type used (e.g., linear, quadratic and cubic spline). Differently, time interpolation did not introduce change in time series length due to the fact that this approach estimates intermediate values between the time when two observed beats happen in accordance with interpolation type.

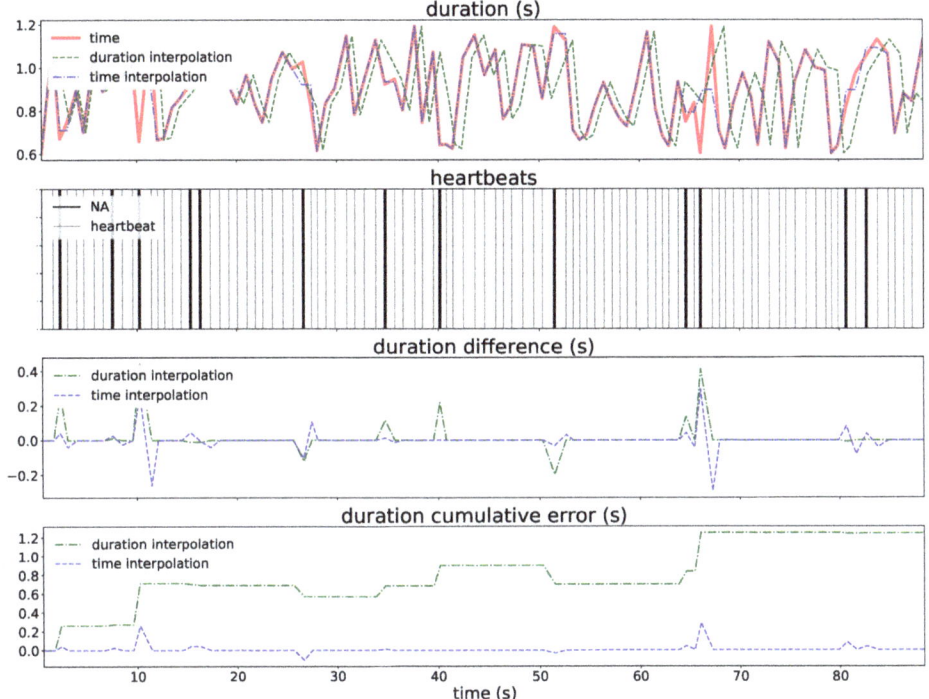

Figure 4. Difference between linear interpolation on time and duration. Red solid line refers to real variation of the timing between beats (RR-intervals) time series, green dashed line refers to the on-duration approach, and green dot dash line refers to the on-time approach.

2.3. Feature Engineering

To obtain HRV features, we analyzed real (i.e., without missing values values), non-interpolated, and interpolated (i.e., with different percentage of artificial missing values values) 5 min ECG time series. We analyze time domain HRV features, frequency, and non-linear domains. Time domain analysis usually contains various statistical variables of the duration time series. The frequency domain analysis investigates the power spectrum of RR-intervals time series in order to assess the cardiac autonomic balance (i.e., sympathetic and parasympathetic nervous systems activity). Additionally, non-linear HRV features try to capture the non-periodic behaviour of the HRV and the complexity that exists inside the RR-interval dynamics. The variables that we incude in our analysis, in both time and frequency domain, are defined as:

- Time domain:
    - HR mean: mean values of heart rate (HR) computed as showed in Equation (9).

$$HR_{mean} = \frac{1}{N-1} \sum_{i=1}^{N-1} 60/(R_{i+1} - R_i), \qquad (9)$$

    where N is the number of beats and R is the time when the beats happened.
    - RMSSD: root mean square of the successive RR-intervals differences (Equation (10)) represents the strength of the autonomic nervous system (specifically the parasympathetic branch) at a given time.

$$RMSSD = \sqrt{\frac{1}{N-1}\sum_{i=1}^{N-1}[(R_{i+1}-R_i)-(R_i-R_{i-1})]^2}, \quad (10)$$

where N is the number of beats and R is the time when the beats happened.
- SDNN: standard deviation of RR-intervals (Equation (11)). It reflects the cyclic components responsible for variability in the RR-intervals time series. The SDNN is the "gold standard" for medical stratification of both morbidity and mortality [16].

$$SDNN = \sqrt{\frac{1}{N-1}\sum_{i=1}^{N}(RR_i - \overline{RR})^2}, \quad (11)$$

where N is the number of beats and RR is the intervals between two consecutive R and $\overline{RR}$ is the mean of RR-intervals in the time series.
- PNN50: the ratio between NN50 (i.e., number of pairs of successive RR intervals that differ by more than 50 ms) and the total number of RR-intervals (Equation (12)).

$$PNN50 = \frac{NN50_{count}}{N_{RR-intervals}} \quad (12)$$

- Frequency domain:
  - Power spectral density (PSD): describes the distribution of power into frequency components composing that signal. The Lomb–Scargle periodogram for PSD estimation was found to be the most appropriate method to analyze RR-interval data [5,6]. VLF (power in very-low-frequency ranges, i.e., ≤ 0.04 Hz), LF (power in low-frequency ranges, i.e., 0.04–0.15 Hz), HF (Power in high-frequency ranges, i.e., 0.15, 0.4 Hz), LF/HF ratio (ratio between LF and HF expressed as ms^2), and total power (Power in all the frequency ranges, i.e., ≤ 0.4) were obtained by the sum of the power in the relevant frequency range in the spectrum.

- Non-linear HRV features:
  - Poincaré plot: it is a type of recurrence plot used to quantify self-similarity in processes. A Poincaré plot is a graph of RR interval (RR_n) against the previous one ($RR_n - 1$). From this scatter plot, it is possible to quantitatively analyze the variance of two consecutive RR-intervals by fitting an ellipse to the plotted shape. $SD1$ is the standard deviation of Poincaré plot perpendicular to the line-of-identity, while $SD2$ is the standard deviation of the Poincaré plot along the line-of-identity.

2.4. Success Metrics

We assessed the difference of HRV variables computed on real time series and the ones with missing values by the root mean squared error (RMSE). Additionally, the relative errors (REs, see Equation (13)) were used to assess the effects of the missing data on the HRV features compared with the parameters calculated from the RR-intervals timeseries without missing data.

$$RE = \frac{|x_{real} - x_k|}{x_{real}} * 100, \quad (13)$$

where x_{real} refers to the HRV features computed from RR-intervals timeseries without missing values, while x_k refers to the values obtained from interpolated timeseries.

3. Results and Discussions

3.1. Results Summary

We analyzed 15,359 RR-intervals timeseries of 5 min in this study. Table 2 shows the descriptive statistic of the HRV features extracted from all users in the dataset. In particular, the users shows an average heart rate of about 75 ± 14 beats per minute.

Table 2. Descriptive statistic of hart rate variability (HRV) features. Mean and 95% coefficient intervals (CI) are provided for all the feature.

HRV Features	Mean	95% CI
IBI (s)	0.78	[0.54, 1.11]
PNN50 (n)	8	[4, 16]
RMSSD (s)	0.039	[0.017, 0.36]
SD1 (s)	0.027	[0.012, 0.26]
SD2 (s)	0.077	[0.040, 0.25]
SDNN (s)	0.059	[0.017, 0.25]
VLF (s^2)	0.87	[0.22, 4.15]
LF (s^2)	0.477	[0.12, 5.57]
HF (s^2)	0.28	[0.050, 3.024]
total power (s^2)	1.91	[0.53, 21.44]
LF/HF (s^2)	2.9	[1.2, 10.2]

Table 3 shows that the on-time approach (i.e., interpolation on the timestamp of heartbeats) produces more reliable HRV feature estimations compared to the on-duration approach (i.e., interpolation on interval duration between two consecutive heartbeats). In this table we provide the results of the best interpolation approach for each HRV feature and for all the percentages of missing values. The RE and RMSE values provided in this table refer to the error induced by missing values when we compare HRV features obtained from the real RR-intervals timeseries versus the ones obtained from interpolated timeseries. The best interpolation methods provided in Table 3 refer to the ones with lower RE. For all of the HRV features, the highest was the percentage of missing RR-intervals, and also the parameters estimation errors. This was due to the fact that the power spectrum of the RR-intervals signal changes with the number of missing values. The choice of the interpolation method also added different types of noise to the signal. As shown in Table 1, the interpolation on time, or not interpolation at all, produces more reliable HRV features compared to interpolating on duration.

Table 3. Best performing interpolation approach (i.e., with low RE) for each HRV feature in each percentage of missing values evaluated. The error in estimating HRV features is reported using RE and root mean squared error (RMSE).

Missing Values (%)	HRV	Interpolation How	Method	RE (%)	RMSE
30	RMSSD (s)	No-interpolation		14.65	0.38
	SDNN (s)	Time	quadratic	9.42	0.34
	PNN50 (n)	No-interpolation		24.37	1.51
	SD1 (s)	No-interpolation		14.68	0.27
	SD2 (s)	Time	quadratic	8.57	0.47
	VLF (s^2)	Time	quadratic	14.50	0.82
	LF (s^2)	Time	quadratic	26.87	2.01
	HF (s^2)	Time	quadratic	32.18	4.48
	LF/HF (s^2)	Time	cubic	41.39	1.73
	total power (s^2)	Time	quadratic	17.16	6.26

Table 3. Cont.

Missing Values (%)	HRV	Interpolation How	Interpolation Method	RE (%)	RMSE
50	RMSSD (ms)	No-interpolation		23.13	0.76
	SDNN (s)	Time	quadratic	15.47	0.41
	PNN50 (n)	No-interpolation		39.01	2.35
	SD1 (s)	No-interpolation		23.18	0.54
	SD2 (s)	Time	quadratic	13.49	0.49
	VLF (s^2)	Time	quadratic	23.72	0.40
	LF (s^2)	Time	quadratic	42.42	1.12
	HF (s^2)	Time	quadratic	52.56	2.48
	LF/HF (s^2)	Time	cubic	58.07	2.26
	total power (s^2)	Time	quadratic	27.59	3.96
70	RMSSD (s)	No-interpolation		34.37	0.91
	SDNN (s)	Time	quadratic	22.76	0.47
	PNN50 (n)	Time	linear	63.90	3.88
	SD1 (s)	No-interpolation		34.46	0.59
	SD2 (s)	Time	quadratic	19.19	0.51
	VLF (s^2)	Time	quadratic	29.73	0.52
	LF (s^2)	Time	quadratic	56.41	1.45
	HF (s^2)	Time	quadratic	72.98	3.34
	LF/HF (s^2)	Time	cubic	72.07	2.80
	total power (s^2)	Time	quadratic	72.07	5.27

The lowest errors on HRV features estimation with missing RR-intervals are obtained using the no-interpolation or the interpolation on time approaches, while the interpolation on duration approach consistently yields the worst results (Table 3). Even if low timeseries difference were detected in simulated linear interpolation on time (Figure 4 and Table 1), Table 3 suggests that the best interpolation method depends of the HRV features that we want to assess. Moreover, this table also shows that, as suspected, the higher is the percentage of missing values, the higher is also the HRV feature estimation error (i.e., RE and RMSE).

3.2. HRV Features

3.2.1. Time Domain

RMSSD and PNN50 do not require any interpolation to obtain reliable estimations for all the percentages of missing values, while SDNN need quadratic interpolation on time (see Table 3). A possible explanation of this result is that RMSSD and PNN50 capture fast changes in heart activity, i.e., high spectrum frequencies, and SDNN captures slow changes, i.e., very low spectrum frequencies. Moreover, interpolation methods, especially interpolation on duration, act as low pass filters, affecting the signal measured by the HRV features (Figure 5). No interpolation changed the spectrum, but did not introduce fictuous durations, thus minimizing the impact on successive differences of durations, that were the first computation step of both RMSSD and PNN50.

3.2.2. Frequency Domain

Figure 5 shows the Lomb–Scargle spectral analysis for different percentages of missing values and for each interpolation method on both time and duration. This figure shows that different interpolation methods introduce different deformations in the resulting power spectra. It is interesting to notice that performing no interpolation results in a flatter spectrum, more similar to a white noise.

In the frequency domain, the interpolation method that produces the least error is the quadratic on time (see Table 3). This figure shows that, as the amount of missing values increases, the no-interpolation approach tends to flatten the HRV spectrum, making it similar to the spectrum of white noise. Figure 5 also shows that cubic spline interpolation on time tends to dampen low frequencies while enhancing high frequencies; that cubic spline interpolation on duration tends to dampen all frequencies; and that quadratic interpolation on duration tends to enhance all frequencies. Finally, Figure 5 also shows that linear and quadratic interpolations on time and that nearest neighbour and linear interpolation on duration have minimal impact on both low and high frequencies, with quadratic interpolation on time having the least effect on all frequencies.

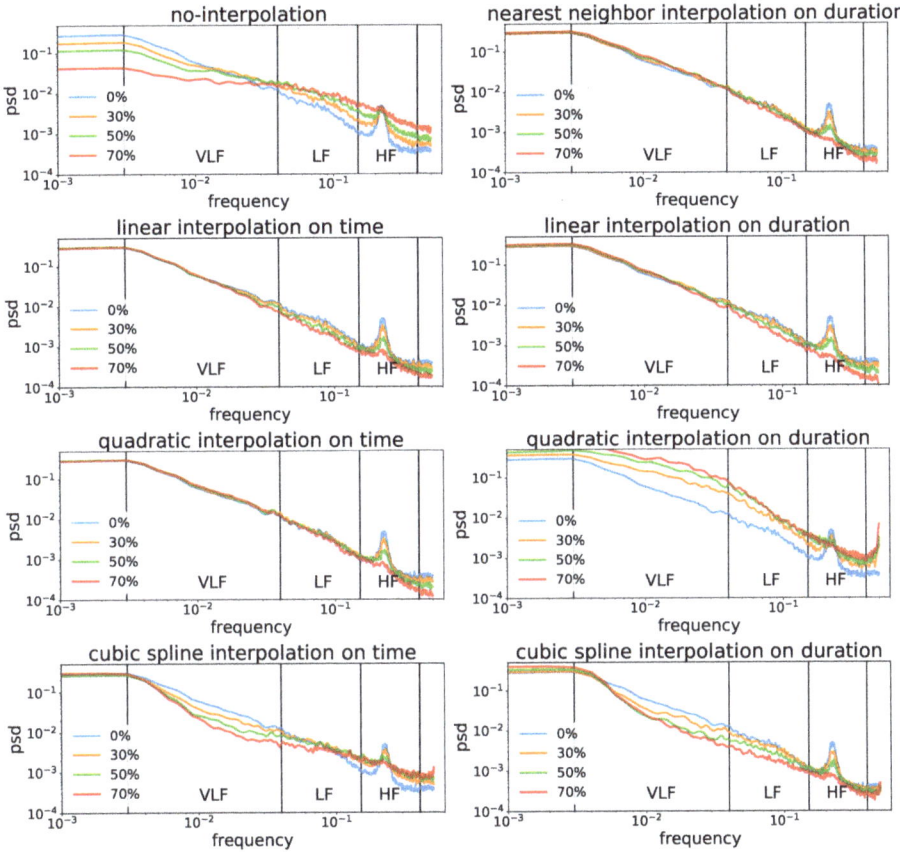

Figure 5. Frequency analysis of a user's RR-intervals timeseries recorded in 5 min with different percentages of missing values (i.e., 0%, 30%, 50% and 70%) handled with different interpolation methods (i.e., nearest neighbor, linear, quadratic and cubic spline) on both time and duration.

3.2.3. Non-Linear Domain

SD1 does not require any interpolation to handle missing values, while SD2 needs quadratic interpolation on time to obtain reliable result (see Table 3). To give an explanation of these results, in Figure 6 we provide an example of the relationship between $RR - interval_n$ and $RR - interval_{n+1}$ (i.e., Poincaré plot) where SD1 and SD2 are extracted. This figure shows Poincaré plots obtained after interpolating missing RR-intervals by using different interpolation method on both time and duration. This figure shows that when the missing values were interpolated on time, the variability of SD1 reduced as the percentage of missing values increased, while the SD2 remain constant. Differently, the interpolation on duration introduce error on both SD1 and SD2 increasing their variability as the missing values increase. Finally, in this figure it can be seen that no-interpolation and quadratic interpolation on time introduced less error compared to the other method on SD1 and SD2, respectively.

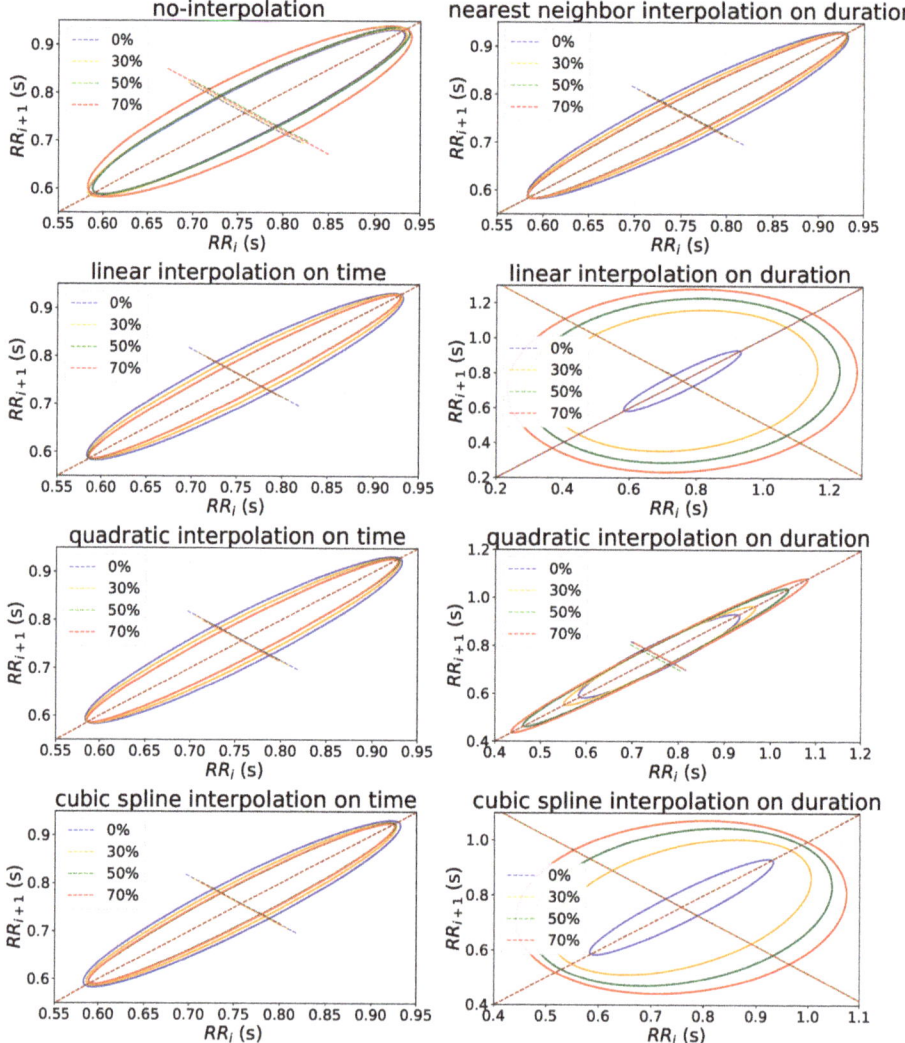

Figure 6. Poincaré plot of a user's RR-intervals timeseries recorded in 5 min with different percentage of missing values (i.e., 0%, 30%, 50% and 70%) handled with different interpolation methods (i.e., nearest neighbor, linear, quadratic and cubic spline) on both time and duration.

4. Conclusions

In this work we quantify the expected error propagation of missing values in RR-intervals timeseries to HRV features, as a function of preprocessing interpolation approach, and amount of missing data. The main findings of this study is that the interpolation of missing values in RR-intervals timeseries on time (i.e., the heartbeats timestamps) produces more reliable HRV features estimations compared to interpolation on duration.

By using this preprocessing approach, the quantification of the expected error on HRV features caused by a huge amount of missing values (e.g., motion artifacts on a wrist-worn wearable device) can support better estimations of users' well-being, by assessing their HRV features. This enables continuous passive monitoring of users' cardiovascular activity in a non-obtrusive way, collecting data during their daily activities that could enable further research on preventative health.

A limitation of this study is the fact that we limited our focus on healthy subjects with normal heart activity, limiting the analysis to large amounts of missing values induced by motion artifacts, ignoring physiological phenomena such as ectopic beats.

Future studies will be useful for researcher and companies, which give insight into heart rate variability recorded by wrist worn IoT wearable devices, in order to better understand the potentiality of the data extracted from these devices to make inference about people heath status. Future work is needed to assess the influence of missing values simulated in accordance with motion and mechanical artifacts induced by external stimuli during data acquisition by using wrist worn IoT wearable devices. Finally, future works will also include the investigating the influence of missing values on HRV features on short timeseries (e.g., 2 min, 1 min and 30 s) and the identification of the shortest time required to obtain accurate estimation of users' HRV features.

Author Contributions: Conceptualization, D.M., A.R. and M.C.; methodology, D.M., A.R. and M.C.; validation, D.M., A.R. and M.C.; formal analysis, D.M., A.R. and M.C.; investigation, D.M., A.R. and M.C.; writing—original draft preparation, D.M., A.R., M.C. and D.A.C.; writing—review and editing, D.M., A.R., M.C. and D.A.C.; visualization, A.R. and M.C.; supervision, D.M. and D.A.C.; project administration, D.M. and D.A.C.; funding acquisition, D.M. and D.A.C.

Funding: This work is partially supported by the European Community's H2020 Program under the funding scheme INFRAIA-1-2014-2015: Research Infrastructures grant agreement 654024, www.sobigdata.eu, SoBigData. The funders had no role in study design, data collection and analysis, decision to publish, or preparation of the manuscript. There was no additional external funding received for this study.

Conflicts of Interest: D.M., M.C. and D.A.C. have a financial and business interests, because they are related to BioBeats Group Ltd, a company that may be affected by the research reported in the enclosed paper. The funders had no role in the design of the study; in the collection, analyses, or interpretation of data; in the writing of the manuscript, or in the decision to publish the results.

References

1. Laborde, S.; Mosley, E.; Thayer, J.F. Heart Rate Variability and Cardiac Vagal Tone in Psychophysiological Research—Recommendations for Experiment Planning, Data Analysis, and Data Reporting. *Front. Psychol.* **2017**, *8*, 213. [CrossRef] [PubMed]
2. Haghi, M.; Thurow, K.; Stoll, R. Wearable Devices in Medical Internet of Things: Scientific Research and Commercially Available Devices. *Healthc. Inform. Res.* **2017**, *23*, 4–15. [CrossRef] [PubMed]
3. Karlsson, M.; Hörnsten, R.; Rydberg, A.; Wiklund, U. Automatic filtering of outliers in RR intervals before analysis of heart rate variability in Holter recordings: A comparison with carefully edited data. *Biomed. Eng.* **2012**, *11*, 2. [CrossRef] [PubMed]
4. Kim, K.K.; Lim, Y.G.; Kim, J.S.; Park, K.S. Effect of missing RR-interval data on heart rate variability analysis in the time domain. *Physiol. Meas.* **2007**, *28*, 1485–1494. [CrossRef] [PubMed]
5. Kim, K.K.; Kim, J.S.; Lim, Y.G.; Park, K.S. The effect of missing RR-interval data on heart rate variability analysis in the frequency domain. *Physiol. Meas.* **2009**, *30*, 1039–1050. [CrossRef] [PubMed]
6. Clifford, G.D.; Tarassenko, L. Quantifying errors in spectral estimates of HRV due to beat replacement and resampling. *IEEE Trans. Biomed. Eng.* **2005**, *52*, 630–638. [CrossRef] [PubMed]
7. Peltola, M.A. Role of editing of R–R intervals in the analysis of heart rate variability. *Front. Physiol.* **2012**, *3*, 148. [CrossRef] [PubMed]
8. Salo, M.; Huikuri, H.; Seppänen, T. Ectopic beats in heart rate variability analysis: Effects of editing on time and frequency domain measures. *Ann. Noninvasive Electrocardiol.* **2001**, *6*, 5–17. [CrossRef] [PubMed]
9. Kamath, M.V.; Fallen, E.L. Correction of the heart rate variability signal for ectopics and missing beats. In *Heart Rate Variability*; Futura Publishing Company: Armonk, NY, USA, 2001; pp. 75–85.
10. Normal Sinus Rhythm RR Interval Database, doi:10.13026/C2S881. Available online: https://physionet.org/physiobank/database/nsr2db/ (accessed on 1 June 2019)

11. Hideki, I. *Essentials of Error-Control Coding Techniques*; Academic Press: Cambridge, MA, USA, 1990.
12. Sibson, R. A brief description of natural neighbor interpolation. In *Interpreting Multivariate Data*; John Wiley & Sons: Sheffield, UK, 1980; pp. 24–27, ISBN 978-0-471-28039-2.
13. Lepot, M.; Aubin, J.B.; Clemens, F.H.L.R. Interpolation in Time Series: An Introductive Overview of Existing Methods, Their Performance Criteria and Uncertainty Assessment. *Water* **2017**, *9*, 796. [CrossRef]
14. Gnauck, A. Interpolation and approximation of water quality time series and process identification. *Anal. Bioanal. Chem.* **2004**, *380*, 484–492. [CrossRef] [PubMed]
15. De Boor, C. *A Practical Guide to Splines*; Springer: Berlin, Germany, 1978.
16. Shaffer, F.; Ginsberg, J.P. An Overview of Heart Rate Variability Metrics and Norms. *Front. Public Health* **2017**, *5*, 258. [CrossRef] [PubMed]

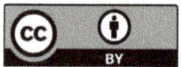

© 2019 by the authors. Licensee MDPI, Basel, Switzerland. This article is an open access article distributed under the terms and conditions of the Creative Commons Attribution (CC BY) license (http://creativecommons.org/licenses/by/4.0/).

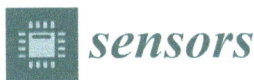

Article

Allumo: Preprocessing and Calibration Software for Wearable Accelerometers Used in Posture Tracking

Alexis Fortin-Côté [1,2], Jean-Sébastien Roy [1,3], Laurent Bouyer [1,3], Philip Jackson [1,2] and Alexandre Campeau-Lecours [1,4,*]

1. Center for Interdisciplinary Research in Rehabilitation and Social Integration, Quebec City, QC G1M 2S8, Canada; alexis.fortin-cote.1@ulaval.ca (A.F.-C.); Jean-Sebastien.Roy@fmed.ulaval.ca (J.-S.R.); Laurent.Bouyer@rea.ulaval.ca (L.B.); Philip.Jackson@psy.ulaval.ca (P.J.)
2. School of Psychology, Université Laval, Quebec City, QC G1V 0A6, Canada
3. Department of Rehabilitation, Université Laval, Quebec City, QC G1V 0A6, Canada
4. Department of Mechanical Engineering, Université Laval, Quebec City, QC G1V 0A6, Canada
* Correspondence: Alexandre.Campeau-Lecours@gmc.ulaval.ca

Received: 13 November 2019; Accepted: 24 December 2019; Published: 31 December 2019

Abstract: Inertial measurement units have recently shown great potential for the accurate measurement of joint angle movements in replacement of motion capture systems. In the race towards long duration tracking, inertial measurement units increasingly aim to ensure portability and long battery life, allowing improved ecological studies. Their main advantage over laboratory grade equipment is their usability in a wider range of environment for greater ecological value. For accurate and useful measurements, these types of sensors require a robust orientation estimation that remains accurate over long periods of time. To this end, we developed the Allumo software for the preprocessing and calibration of the orientation estimate of triaxial accelerometers. This software has an automatic orientation calibration procedure, an automatic erroneous orientation-estimate detection and useful visualization to help process long and short measurement periods. These automatic procedures are detailed in this paper, and two case studies are presented to showcase the usefulness of the software. The Allumo software is open-source and available online.

Keywords: accelerometer; calibration; inertial measurement units; human movement

1. Introduction

Wearable sensors are increasingly being used in research and clinical practice to assess the pose and posture of individuals. For instance, physical rehabilitation may require objective movement measurements over extended periods of time to perform a comprehensive assessment of the patient. Being able to obtain quantitative measurements outside of controlled environments, such as a laboratory, through the use of wearable sensors could help in the diagnosis and treatment of patients. For instance, stride parameters are measured through GPS and inertial measurement unit (IMU) data [1], as well as gait and posture analyzed from pressure-sensitive insoles and IMU data [2]. Navigation estimates using IMUs with [3] and without GPS [4] have also been studied. IMU sensors have proven to be effective in orientation estimation, such as trunk orientation and lower limb kinematics [5] and in measuring the shoulder joint angles [6]. Accelerometers can also be used for impact detection and gait timing [7–9]. They have also been used in harsher conditions such as swimming [10]. As the number of contexts using these types of sensors increases, so does the need to improve orientation estimation accuracy. A static accuracy assessment of the Xsens IMU sensors [11] for 3D orientation positioning has been published [12]. Validation of the Xsens movement measurement [13] reported good correlation (0.96) between Xsens movement and vision-based measurements. Further assessment of accuracy for joint rotation for field-based occupational studies [14] reported measurement errors varying from 4° to 12°. A recent systematic review reported that IMU should be considered as a valid tool to assess the whole body range of motion, and underlined the importance of the calibration step [15] to obtain such levels of accuracy.

Indeed, calibration is an important step to capture accurate pose estimates, especially for joint angle measurement [16]. The published procedure for pose calibration to align an IMU to another motion-capture system, which is presented in [17], and a pose calibration procedure for 3D knee joint angle [18]. Furthermore, Lotter et al. [19] published a procedure for in-use calibration of triaxial accelerometers that shares similarities with our proposed automatic orientation estimation algorithm, such as relying on the fact that the magnitude of the gravity acceleration vector measured with the accelerometer is constant and equals to 1g under quasi-static conditions. They use those assumptions to calibrate the tension readings of the triaxial acceleration (an offset and scaling for each axis). In our proposed automatic orientation algorithm, the same assumptions are leveraged to determine the orientation of the accelerometer reference frame with respect to the fixed, world reference frame. A review of several calibration methods of the former style for motion analysis is available in [20].

In the context of a project to collect mobility data, an important challenge occurs during the assessment of IMU data obtained in the field. Indeed, while the typical use case is a relatively short acquisition duration (minutes to hours long), larger scale mobility projects aim to record data over long periods of time. Corresponding time series data sets are thus quite large and require a tedious and time-consuming manual preprocessing task, during which the accuracy of the pose estimate can decrease. This concern was also raised in [21]. In mobility data, file duration can span over several weeks of continuous recording at 60 Hz (three data channels per accelerometer). While this data file size may not be considered large in a big data context, the amount of manual preprocessing required using the existing commercial tools precludes them from being used at the scale required for many projects. As participants remove and install the equipment, a manual recalibration of the orientation estimate of the devices is required and can be difficult in the field. Whereas some analyses such as automatic activity recognition does not require a known orientation [22], posture monitoring does, and therefore requires this recalibration step. Manual adjustments of the orientation estimate using only the data stream and without direct monitoring from an external observer in the field are impracticable. Furthermore, uncontrolled events such as unwanted shifts of the sensor on the participant may result in erroneous readings stemming from an inaccurate calibration. These also require identification and a subsequent sensor recalibration, which is also manually impracticable using the raw data stream. Identifying such erroneous readings is difficult with the available commercial tools, as they tend to only present time series plots of the data, a counter-intuitive method for detecting erroneous orientation estimate by most observers.

To help in the calibration of the orientation estimate of IMUs used for joint angle measurement, we present a tool for visualization and preprocessing to be used in human posture monitoring and assessment. The development goal of the software presented here was to expedite the identification and recalibration of the orientation estimate of triaxial accelerometer readings by showing an intuitive graphical interface to the observer. An animated humanoid avatar illustrates the estimated posture of the participant along the data stream. It makes it easier to identify erroneous orientation estimates since abnormal postures of the body will be displayed (e.g., wrong limb orientation, walking at a skewed angle).

This paper is structured as follows: first is the presentation and description of the automatic calibration of the orientation estimate, erroneous orientation-estimate detection and activity detection algorithms; second is an overview of the software followed by two case studies to show typical usage of the software.

2. Software Overview

The main software, of which the interface in presented in Figure 1, boasts several features useful for the preprocessing and assessment of IMU data. It features a real-time playback visualization of a humanoid model for easy diagnostics of improbable orientation estimate or wrongly positioned sensors. It helps to identify potential problems by displaying captured motion on an avatar model. For instance, a mis estimated orientation measurement could show a skewed trunk angle or unrealistic leg movement. It can also display a matching video to help with the visual comparison of the movement. Options in the settings are available to synchronize the video playback with the animated human shape motion. There is also a live display of the variables of interest, such as torso and leg joint angles, with respect to the vertical axis. For long duration data acquisitions, the software provides convenient time selection features that allow the definition of a specific working window.

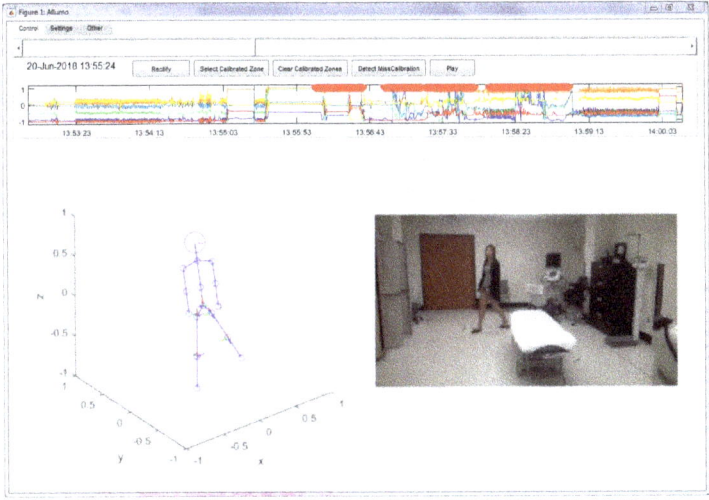

Figure 1. Main interface of the software.

The software also features an interface for manual selection of reference positions that is useful for the initialization of the orientation estimate of short recordings when reference points (neutral position) are known, e.g., a recording that begins with still sensors positioned in a known orientation. To improve the accuracy of the reference point measure, a section (window) of the signal can be marked as the reference orientation so that an averaging can be performed to reduce measurement noise during the reference position in the recording. To further help with this task, an algorithm, used for the automatic detection of erroneous orientation estimates, was implemented and is described in Section 4. Since manual adjustment of the initial orientation estimate can be complex and time-consuming, one of the software's main features is the automatic calibration of the sensor initial orientation through automatic detection of motionless neutral positions (quasi-static), based on filtering and singular value decomposition, all of which are further described in Section 3. A basic automatic activity detection feature, used to distinguish between idling, walking and running, is also available.

Lastly, the software allows the importation of raw accelerometer values from multiple file formats such as Actigraph GT3x, comma-separated values (csv) files, and Excel spreadsheets. It allows the exportation of the calibrated accelerometer values to a convenient csv or Excel file format for uploading to most analytics programs.

3. Automatic Calibration Algorithm

We define the calibration of the orientation estimate of the triaxial accelerometer as "identifying the rotation matrix that aligns the mobile reference frame originating at the accelerometer with the fixed (world) reference frame". In other words, the orientation of the mobile reference frame $\mathscr{R}$, with respect to the fixed reference frame $\mathscr{F}$, is defined by the rotation matrix **R** as seen in Figure 2. This therefore defines the three rotational degrees of freedom (DOF) of the accelerometer. This allows for the full orientation of an arbitrarily placed sensor to be estimated. To this end, the automatic calibration algorithm leverages the gravitational force **g**, which is constant in the fixed reference frame, to constrain two of the three DOF, and a variance analysis to constrain the third DOF, fully defining the matrix **R**. The measured acceleration matrix is defined as

$$\mathbf{A} = \begin{bmatrix} a_{x1} & a_{y1} & a_{z1} \\ \vdots & \vdots & \vdots \\ a_{xm} & a_{ym} & a_{zm} \end{bmatrix} \in \mathbb{R}^{m \times 3}, \tag{1}$$

where a_{xi}, a_{yi}, a_{zi}, are the ith measurements along the $x_{\mathcal{R}}, y_{\mathcal{R}}, z_{\mathcal{R}}$ axes respectively, and m is the index of the last measurement.

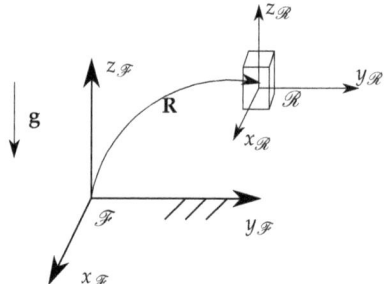

Figure 2. Geometric representation of the accelerometer.

The automatic calibration algorithm works by using three main assumptions. First, when the participant is at rest, he/she is in the neutral position most of the time (e.g., standing upright). Second, the gravity vector can be measured without bias most of the time, meaning that no steady state acceleration should be present outside of gravity, i.e., the system is not in free fall or under centrifugal acceleration. Third, most of the variance in the movement occurs in the plane that is parallel to the gravitational force and in the forward-facing direction $x_{\mathcal{F}}$ (e.g., walking). If these conditions are not met, a manual assisted option is available (see Section 4).

When those assumptions are observed, the algorithm works as follows. The first step is to find the direction of the gravitational force acting on the sensor. To this end, raw accelerometer data are filtered with a bidirectional low-pass filter with a cutoff frequency (COF) of 1/10 Hz to remove impacts, high-frequency noise and human limb movements to keep only low-frequency signals indicative of a steady state acceleration, which should correspond to a large extent to the neutral position. To accurately identify the direction of the gravity vector, the only data points kept for averaging are those where no movement is perceived (quasi-static). Those data points are found using a high-pass filter with the same COF of 1/10 Hz, filtering over the acceleration vector magnitude (l2 norm) instead of over each component, to identify where the signal lies closer to zero. A 2-s Hann window filter is used to further smooth the acceleration magnitude signal and keep only substantially long periods of quasi-static movements. The gravitational acceleration direction is then averaged across these sections with low movements. Knowing the unit vector $\hat{\mathbf{g}}$, which represents the direction of the measured gravitational acceleration, a matrix $\mathbf{R}'$ such as

$$\mathbf{g} = \mathbf{R}' \hat{\mathbf{g}}, \tag{2}$$

that aligns the $z_{\mathcal{R}}$ axis to the $z_{\mathcal{F}}$ axis can be derived, therefore establishing two DOFs. To establish the last DOF, raw acceleration measurements are transformed with matrix $\mathbf{R}'$ so that the measured gravitational acceleration aligns with the negative $z_{\mathcal{F}}$ direction, leaving acceleration on the $x_{\mathcal{R}}, y_{\mathcal{R}}$ planes as the only result of the accelerometer motion. The principal axis of motion is then computed using singular-value decomposition of the acceleration matrix **A** to find the largest singular value, σ_1, and its corresponding singular vector, $\mathbf{v}_1$, such as

$$\mathbf{A} = \mathbf{U\Sigma V}, \tag{3}$$

with $\mathbf{U} \in \mathbb{R}^{m \times m}$, containing the left-singular vectors, $\mathbf{\Sigma} \in \mathbb{R}^{m \times 3}$ containing the singular values $\sigma_1 \ldots \sigma_3$ and $\mathbf{V} \in \mathbb{R}^{3 \times 3}$ containing the right-singular vectors including the vector of interest $\mathbf{v}_1$. The singular vector $\mathbf{v}_1$, which corresponds to the largest singular value, σ_1, is considered to be the forward-facing direction and therefore allows to establish the last DOF which, in turn, allows the full computation of **R**. Note that since the direction of the singular vector can be positive or negative, this leaves the distinction between forward and backward undefined, and is thus a known shortcoming of the method that needs to be corrected manually.

4. Automatic Erroneous-Orientation Detection

When the automatic orientation estimation calibration cannot be used (assumption not met), the automatic erroneous orientation-estimate detection provides an alternative assisted orientation estimation calibration option. It is based on the same assumption as the automatic calibration algorithm, but is only used as a tool for the detection of periods when manual orientation adjustment is necessary. The user can then manually discriminate between erroneous orientation estimates and other movements that may trigger the erroneous orientation-estimate detection, such as lying down for a long period of time. The algorithm operates by checking whether the gravitational acceleration aligns correctly with the negative $z_\mathscr{F}$ direction. Using a bidirectional low-pass filter, it isolates the gravitational measurement, as described in Section 3, and flags sections of the accelerometer measurements in which the angle between the measured direction of gravity and the $z_\mathscr{F}$ direction is larger than a user-defined threshold value. This way, the algorithm can help detect whether or not a sensor has moved since the last adjustment. A visual cue is presented to the user so that he/she can act on the flagged section by manually adding reference orientation point as presented in Section 2, or removing the section altogether.

5. Activity Detection

A basic activity detection algorithm is implemented in the software. It differentiates between three different states: idling, walking or running. Again, using a low-pass filter followed by a Hann window filter over the acceleration vector magnitude (l2 norm) generates an activity intensity signal. By using simple threshold values, the discrimination between idling, walking and running can be achieved.

6. Case Studies

6.1. Demonstration in the Laboratory

A participant wearing two Actigraph GT3X accelerometers, one placed on the left thigh and the other on his back, was asked to perform a 15-min routine with a mix of standing, walking, running and lying down. The activity was captured on video to qualitatively assess the pose estimates of reported by the software. During the routine, the orientation of the sensors on the body was deliberately altered at three different times to test the algorithm's erroneous orientation-estimate detection. This resulted in 5 sections of signal being flagged using the erroneous orientation-estimate detection tool. The three deliberate orientation change and both time the participant lay down for an extended period of time had been correctly flagged. Using the playback of the humanoid visualization, the user can easily identify whether the detection is caused by an erroneous orientation estimate or a real change in steady-state operation such as going from a standing vertical to a horizontal orientation. This demonstration showed good performance in correctly identifying miscalibrated orientation estimates and was able to process the signal by applying the correct orientation adjustment parameters during each segment. With the correct adjustment applied, the user can look at the avatar and easily distinguish certain movements performed by the participant such as sitting, crouching and lying down. The activity detection algorithm was also able to correctly identify the two running events, the six walking events and the corresponding idling sequences between those.

6.2. Demonstration in the Field

In this data collection, the software has been used in the analysis of data from two expeditions lasting 39 and 32 days, respectively. During those expeditions, two participants wore two Actigraph GT3X accelerometers; one of the accelerometers was placed on the pelvis and the other on the left thigh. Both were affixed on shorts so that they moved along with the body. Data acquisition was performed over the 71 days for a total of around 1700 h of recording. Participants wore the sensors for the major part of the days and removed them during most sleep hours. Manual initialization of the orientation estimate for those types of extended periods is impractical. The automatic calibration algorithm was therefore used for each day of acquisition. After automatic calibration is performed, relevant data can be extracted, such as the amount of time walking or running and the trunk angle. The calibrated accelerometer's data can then be exported for further processing. Table 1 shows an example of which data can be obtained for 1 hour segments of a day of recording and the corresponding logbook entries. By comparing the ratio of walking and running detection to corresponding entries, an overall assessment of the activity detection can be made. It can be seen that high trunk angle correlates with nap time and that running detection correlates with high-intensity activities. Walking proportion also varies sensibly with reported activities.

Table 1. Data summary samples for a 1-h expedition segment.

	Walking	Running	Trunk Angle	Logbook Entry
segment 1	7.40%	0.19%	6.28°	Jumping jacks as a warm-up following by work at the computer
segment 2	7.20%	0.00%	71.21°	Lying down for 50 min
segment 3	4.42%	0.00%	3.53°	Work at the computer (mostly siting)
segment 4	12.78%	35.84%	10.61°	30 min jogging followed by work at the laboratory
segment 5	6.89%	0.00%	83.14°	50 min nap (lying down)
segment 6	17.08%	0.83%	6.17°	Helicopter outing and walk ashore
segment 7	9.87%	0.02%	5.47°	Diner and relaxation on board

7. Conclusions

This paper presented a graphical software for preprocessing raw accelerometer data in the context of posture tracking. The software allows the visualization of measured posture on a humanoid form to easily identify errors in measurements or in the orientation estimate of the device in long duration, in the field, experiment. The paper also presented a novel algorithm for automatic calibration of the orientation estimate that can be used when manual initialization of the orientation estimate is impractical. A simple erroneous orientation-estimate detection and basic activity detection algorithms are implemented in the software. Two case studies were used to show typical usage of the software. The software is open-source and available at https://github.com/alexisfcote/allumo.

Author Contributions: Conceptualization, A.F.-C.; Data curation, A.F.-C.; Software, A.F.-C.; Supervision, L.B., P.J. and A.C.-L.;Writing—original draft, A.F.-C.;Writing—review & editing, A.F.-C., J.-S.R., L.B., P.J. and A.C.-L. All authors have read and agreed to the published version of the manuscript.

Funding: This research was funded by Canada Research Excellence Fund -Sentinel North Strategy.

Conflicts of Interest: The authors declare no conflicts of interest.

References

1. Tan, H.; Wilson, A.M.; Lowe, J. Measurement of stride parameters using a wearable GPS and inertial measurement unit. *J. Biomech.* **2008**, *41*, 1398–1406. [CrossRef] [PubMed]
2. Benocci, M.; Rocchi, L.; Farella, E.; Chiari, L.; Benini, L. A wireless system for gait and posture analysis based on pressure insoles and Inertial Measurement Units. In Proceedings of the 2009 3rd International Conference on Pervasive Computing Technologies for Healthcare, London, UK, 1–3 April 2009; pp. 1–6. [CrossRef]
3. Brodie, M.; Walmsley, A.; Page, W. Fusion motion capture: A prototype system using inertial measurement units and GPS for the biomechanical analysis of ski racing. *Sports Technol.* **2008**, *1*, 17–28. [CrossRef]
4. Bebek, O.; Suster, M.A.; Rajgopal, S.; Fu, M.J.; Huang, X.; Cavusoglu, M.C.; Young, D.J.; Mehregany, M.; van den Bogert, A.J.; Mastrangelo, C.H. Personal Navigation via High-Resolution Gait-Corrected Inertial Measurement Units. *IEEE Trans. Instrum. Meas.* **2010**, *59*, 3018–3027. [CrossRef]
5. Bonnet, V.; Mazzà, C.; Fraisse, P.; Cappozzo, A. Real-time Estimate of Body Kinematics During a Planar Squat Task Using a Single Inertial Measurement Unit. *IEEE Trans. Biomed. Eng.* **2013**, *60*, 1920–1926. [CrossRef] [PubMed]
6. Poitras, I.; Bielmann, M.; Campeau-Lecours, A.; Mercier, C.; Bouyer, L.J.; Roy, J.S. Validity of Wearable Sensors at the Shoulder Joint: Combining Wireless Electromyography Sensors and Inertial Measurement Units to Perform Physical Workplace Assessments. *Sensors* **2019**, *19*, 1885. [CrossRef] [PubMed]
7. Peruzzi, A.; Croce, U.D.; Cereatti, A. Estimation of stride length in level walking using an inertial measurement unit attached to the foot: A validation of the zero velocity assumption during stance. *J. Biomech.* **2011**, *44*, 1991–1994. [CrossRef] [PubMed]
8. Bergamini, E.; Picerno, P.; Pillet, H.; Natta, F.; Thoreux, P.; Camomilla, V. Estimation of temporal parameters during sprint running using a trunk-mounted inertial measurement unit. *J. Biomech.* **2012**, *45*, 1123–1126. [CrossRef] [PubMed]
9. Bergamini, E.; Guillon, P.; Camomilla, V.; Pillet, H.; Skalli, W.; Cappozzo, A. Trunk Inclination Estimate During the Sprint Start Using an Inertial Measurement Unit: A Validation Study. *J. Appl. Biomech.* **2013**, *29*, 622–627. [CrossRef] [PubMed]
10. Dadashi, F.; Millet, G.; Aminian, K. Inertial measurement unit and biomechanical analysis of swimming: An update. *Swiss Soc. Sports Med.* **2013**, *61*, 21–26,
11. Roetenberg, D.; Luinge, H.; Slycke, P. *Xsens MVN: Full 6DOF Human Motion Tracking Using Miniature Inertial Sensors*; Xsens Technologies: Enschede, The Netherlands, 2009; pp. 1–7.
12. Brodie, M.; Walmsley, A.; Page, W. The static accuracy and calibration of inertial measurement units for 3D orientation. *Comput. Methods Biomech. Biomed. Eng.* **2008**, *11*, 641–648. [CrossRef] [PubMed]
13. Zhang, J.T.; Novak, A.C.; Brouwer, B.; Li, Q. Concurrent validation of Xsens MVN measurement of lower limb joint angular kinematics. *Physiol. Meas.* **2013**, *34*, N63–N69. [CrossRef] [PubMed]
14. Schal, M.C., Jr.; Fethke, N.B.; Chen, H.; Oyama, S.; Douphrate, D.I. Accuracy and repeatability of an inertial measurement unit system for field-based occupational studies. *Ergonomics* **2016**, *59*, 591–602. [CrossRef] [PubMed]
15. Poitras, I.; Dupuis, F.; Bielmann, M.; Campeau-Lecours, A.; Mercier, C.; Bouyer, L.J.; Roy, J.S. Validity and Reliability of Wearable Sensors for Joint Angle Estimation: A Systematic Review. *Sensors* **2019**, *19*, 1555. [CrossRef] [PubMed]
16. Luinge, H.; Veltink, P.; Baten, C. Ambulatory measurement of arm orientation. *J. Biomech.* **2007**, *40*, 78–85. [CrossRef] [PubMed]
17. Chardonnens, J.; Favre, J.; Aminian, K. An effortless procedure to align the local frame of an inertial measurement unit to the local frame of another motion capture system. *J. Biomech.* **2012**, *45*, 2297–2300. [CrossRef] [PubMed]
18. Favre, J.; Aissaoui, R.; Jolles, B.; de Guise, J.; Aminian, K. Functional calibration procedure for 3D knee joint angle description using inertial sensors. *J. Biomech.* **2009**, *42*, 2330–2335. [CrossRef] [PubMed]
19. Lötters, J.; Schipper, J.; Veltink, P.; Olthuis, W.; Bergveld, P. Procedure for in-use calibration of triaxial accelerometers in medical applications. *Sens. Actuators A Phys.* **1998**, *68*, 221–228. [CrossRef]
20. Nez, A.; Fradet, L.; Laguillaumie, P.; Monnet, T.; Lacouture, P. Comparison of calibration methods for accelerometers used in human motion analysis. *Med. Eng. Phys.* **2016**, *38*, 1289–1299. [CrossRef] [PubMed]

21. Cheung, Y.; Hsueh, P.Y.; Ensari, I.; Willey, J.; Diaz, K. Quantile Coarsening Analysis of High-Volume Wearable Activity Data in a Longitudinal Observational Study. *Sensors* **2018**, *18*, 3056. [CrossRef] [PubMed]
22. Yurtman, A.; Barshan, B.; Fidan, B. Activity Recognition Invariant to Wearable Sensor Unit Orientation Using Differential Rotational Transformations Represented by Quaternions. *Sensors* **2018**, *18*, 2725. [CrossRef] [PubMed]

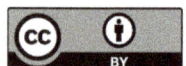 © 2019 by the authors. Licensee MDPI, Basel, Switzerland. This article is an open access article distributed under the terms and conditions of the Creative Commons Attribution (CC BY) license (http://creativecommons.org/licenses/by/4.0/).

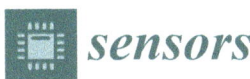

Review

Methods for the Real-World Evaluation of Fall Detection Technology: A Scoping Review

Robert W. Broadley, Jochen Klenk, Sibylle B. Thies, Laurence P. J. Kenney and Malcolm H. Granat

1. School of Health Sciences, University of Salford, Salford, M6 6PU, UK; s.thies@salford.ac.uk (S.B.T.); l.p.j.kenney@salford.ac.uk (L.P.J.K.); m.h.granat@salford.ac.uk (M.H.G.)
2. Department of Clinical Gerontology, Robert-Bosch-Hospital, 70376 Stuttgart, Germany; jochen.klenk@rbk.de
3. Institute of Epidemiology and Medical Biometry, Ulm University, 89081 Ulm, Germany
* Correspondence: r.broadley@edu.salford.ac.uk; Tel.: +44-161-295-2507

Received: 31 May 2018; Accepted: 25 June 2018; Published: 27 June 2018

Abstract: Falls in older adults present a major growing healthcare challenge and reliable detection of falls is crucial to minimise their consequences. The majority of development and testing has used laboratory simulations. As simulations do not cover the wide range of real-world scenarios performance is poor when retested using real-world data. There has been a move from the use of simulated falls towards the use of real-world data. This review aims to assess the current methods for real-world evaluation of fall detection systems, identify their limitations and propose improved robust methods of evaluation. Twenty-two articles met the inclusion criteria and were assessed with regard to the composition of the datasets, data processing methods and the measures of performance. Real-world tests of fall detection technology are inherently challenging and it is clear the field is in its infancy. Most studies used small datasets and studies differed on how to quantify the ability to avoid false alarms and how to identify non-falls, a concept which is virtually impossible to define and standardise. To increase robustness and make results comparable, larger standardised datasets are needed containing data from a range of participant groups. Measures that depend on the definition and identification of non-falls should be avoided. Sensitivity, precision and F-measure emerged as the most suitable robust measures for evaluating the real-world performance of fall detection systems.

Keywords: accidental falls; fall detection; real-world; signal analysis; performance measures; wearable sensors; non-wearable sensors; accelerometers; cameras

1. Introduction

Falls in older adults and their related consequences pose a major healthcare challenge that is set to grow over the coming decades [1]. Approximately 30 percent of those over the age of 65 experience one or more falls each year, which rises to around 45 percent in those over 80 [2]. Roughly six percent of older adult falls result in fractured bones [3,4]. Falls are estimated to cost the UK over one billion pounds each year, with fractures being the most costly fall related injury [5].

Even when the injuries are not so serious, fallers often struggle to get up unaided [6,7], sometimes leading to a 'long-lie' where the faller remains trapped on the floor for an extended period of time. Long-lies can lead to dehydration, pressure sores, pneumonia, hypothermia and death [8–11]. Further to the physical consequences, the fear of falling can impact on older adults' quality of life. A fear of falling is associated with a decline in physical and mental health, and an increased risk of falling [12]. Estimates suggest that between 25 and 50 percent of older adults are fearful of falling and half of these will limit their activities as a result [13,14].

One method used to address the severe consequences associated with falling is the use of a push button alarm system, which can ensure help is received quickly, and reduce the risk of a long-lie. However, studies have shown that 80 percent of fallers do not or cannot activate their alarm following a fall, meaning an alternative approach is needed [6,15]. As a result, there has been extensive research into automatic detection of falls and a broad range of approaches have been developed.

In order to understand the efficacy of the automated fall detection systems, it is important to have a robust method of testing performance. Key to the assessment of these systems is the evaluation of reproducibility and experimental validity [16]. There are two types of experimental validity: internal and external. Internal validity is the extent to which the results truly reflect the capability of the tested system, and were not influenced by other confounding factors or systematic errors. External validity is the extent to which the results can be generalised across people and environments.

External validity has been a central issue in tests of fall detection systems. The poor external validity has been caused by the use of laboratory simulated falls conducted by young healthy adults. The accidental, unexpected and uncontrolled nature of a fall makes it challenging to simulate. When a person simulates a fall the movement is expected, deliberate and carried out in a safe space where injury is highly unlikely. Therefore, reflexes to prevent or lessen the severity of the fall are likely to be suppressed leading to a different pattern of movement. When 13 previously published approaches were tested using real-world fall data, the performance was found to be considerably worse (mean sensitivity and specificity of 0.57 and 0.83, respectively) than had originally been reported from testing using simulations (mean sensitivity and specificity of 0.91 and 0.99, respectively) [17].

Despite the challenge associated with simulating falls, the vast majority of studies have used simulated fall data (for recent reviews see [18,19]). The use of laboratory simulated falls has been an accepted approach due to the challenge associated with recording real-world falls. The rarity of falls means that recording them is both costly and time consuming. Bagala et al. [17] estimated that to collect 100 falls, 100,000 days of activity would need to be recorded, assuming a fall incidence of one fall per person every three years. Despite this challenge, the focus is now moving to real-world fall data due to the external validity issues inherent in simulated fall based testing. Real-world data, by its very nature provides high ecological validity and therefore contributes to higher external validity.

The use of real-world data, while a significant step forward, does not make the test robust. Other factors such as cohort selection and size are important for external validity. In addition, the use of real-world data does not increase the internal validity, in fact, the level of variation and abundance of confounding factors creates a greater risk of systematic errors. Therefore, careful consideration and planning of both the data collection and test procedure is vital to ensure the validity of results.

All methods of testing fall detection systems share the same basic framework which shapes the whole method from data collection through to data processing. Therefore, a basic understanding of this framework is needed to understand the best method to evaluate fall detector performance. Fall detection is a case of binary classification; each movement is classified as either a fall (positive case) or non-fall (negative case). For each movement there are four possible outcomes:

- True Positive (TP)—Correctly detected fall
- True Negative (TN)—Non-fall movement not detected as a fall
- False Positive (FP)—Classified as a fall when none occurred
- False Negative (FN)—A fall which was not detected

These four values can be represented as a table comparing the actual data with the system's predictions, this is known as a confusion matrix (Figure 1). All further measures can be calculated from either a complete confusion matrix or a subset of one. Therefore, studies should aim to collect data and process it in such a way that as many of these four values as possible can be calculated.

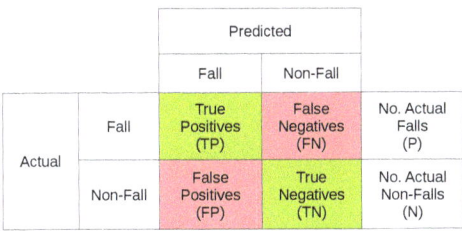

Figure 1. Example confusion matrix.

The aim of this review is to identify the methods which have previously been used to evaluate fall detector performance using real-world data and investigate how the differences in these methods of evaluation effect the results. The review covers the methods of data collection and processing as well as the performance measures which have been used for evaluation. In this review, we aim to identify the strengths and limitations of current approaches and propose a more robust approach of evaluation based on the findings.

2. Methods

A systematic search was conducted in August 2017 and repeated in March 2018, using the following on-line literature databases: Medline, Cinahl, Pubmed, Web of Science and IEEE Xplore. The search aimed to find all records where a fall detection technology (hardware or software) had been tested using real-world falls. The search strategy used is shown in Table 1. Papers were excluded where no fall detection technology was tested, where tests used fall simulations, or the technology was not aimed at older adults. Only articles available in English were included.

Table 1. Example Search Strategy for PubMed.

	fall*-detect*[Title/Abstract] OR fall*-sensor*[Title/Abstract] OR fall*-alarm*[Title/abstract]
AND	real-world[Title/Abstract] OR real-life[Title/Abstract] OR free-living[Title/Abstract] OR community-dwelling[Title/Abstract] OR home-dwelling[Title/Abstract] OR domestic-environment[Title/Abstract] OR long-term-care[Title/Abstract] OR care-home[Title/Abstract] OR nursing-home[Title/Abstract] OR hospital[Title/Abstract]

The studies which met the inclusion criteria were assessed with regard to the method used to test the fall detection system. The focus was to assess the robustness of these tests and we therefore did not assess the systems' design or performance. For a comparison of wearable systems see [17] and for a comparison of non-wearable systems see [20]. All included studies tested fall detection technology using real-world fall data. Where studies reported on both tests using simulated data and tests using real-world data, only the methods used for the real-world portion of the data were considered.

First we reviewed the information studies provided about their participants, how they collected data and the volume of data collected. Next, we examined the methods used to identify fall events and to process the data. Finally, we evaluated the use of each applicable performance measure.

3. Results

The systematic search returned 259 unique records. Following application of the selection criteria, 22 papers were identified for analysis. The full breakdown of the literature identification process, including the reasons for exclusion, is shown in Figure 2. Table 2 provides a breakdown of the 22 included papers with regard to participant groups, devices used, participant numbers, numbers of recorded falls, the quantity and processing of non-fall data and finally, the performance measures reported. The following sections provide further detail to complement Table 2.

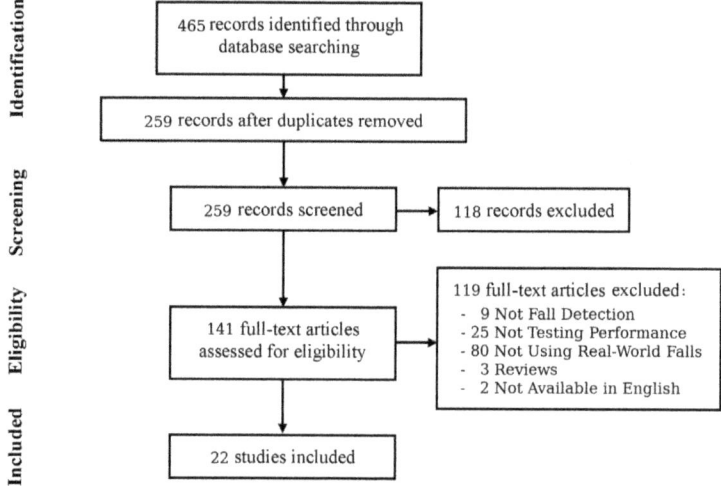

Figure 2. Flow diagram of the systematic search.

Table 2. Summary of papers evaluating fall detection systems using real-world falls.

Author	Participant Group	Additional Information	Device Type	Number of Participants	Number of Falls	Quantity of Non-Fall Data and Method of Preparation		Performance Measures
Aziz [21]	Residents of a long-term care facility who had experienced at least one fall in the previous year	Age, mobility assessment	Accelerometer	9	1	214 h	Data were divided into 2.5 s time windows with a 1.5 s overlap. The 30 s of data following a fall event were ignored.	**Sensitivity, Specificity, FPRT**, TP, FP, FN
	Patients at a hospital geriatrics department with Progressive Supranuclear Palsy	Age	Accelerometer	10	9	178 h		
Bagala [17]	Patients with Progressive Supranuclear Palsy	Age, gender, height, weight	Accelerometer	9	29	A total of 168 h from seven of the participants. Recordings were divided into 60 s windows and only the 1170 windows where max(RSS) − min(RSS) > 1.01 g were included		**Sensitivity, Specificity, FPRT**, Precision NPV, Accuracy
	Community dwelling older adult	None	Accelerometer	1	the number from each group was not provided			

Table 2. Cont.

Author	Participant Group	Additional Information	Device Type	Number of Participants	Number of Falls	Quantity of Non-Fall Data and Method of Preparation	Performance Measures
Bloch [22]	Patients at a geriatric rehabilitation ward with an identified risk of falling	Age	Working alarm composed of an accelerometer and infrared sensor	10	8	A total of 196 days. Data was processed on-line and the analysis compared the alarm times to reported fall times. Assumed 30 fall like events per day to estimate of the number of non-fall events.	**Sensitivity**, **Specificity**, Precision, NPV, TP
Bourke [23]	Patients at a geriatric rehabilitation unit	None	Accelerometer and gyroscope	42	89	A total of 3466 events extracted using a dynamic detection algorithm and further reduced to 367 events where: max(RSS) > 1.05 g Total length of recorded data was not given.	**Sensitivity**, **Specificity**, Accuracy, ROC AUC

Table 2. Cont.

Author	Participant Group	Additional Information	Device Type	Number of Participants	Number of Falls	Quantity of Non-Fall Data and Method of Preparation	Performance Measures
Chaudhuri [24]	Community dwelling older adults	None	Working alarm consisting of an accelerometer, magnetometer, and gyroscope	18	14	A total of 1452.6 days. Details of data preparation not given.	Sensitivity, Specificity, Precision, NPV, Confusion Matrix
Chen [25]	Community dwelling older adults living in geriatric rehabilitation centres	Age, gender, height, weight	Accelerometer	22	22	A total of 22 events. Only data from a 1200 s window around the falls was used, data up to 1 s before each fall were used as non-fall events.	Sensitivity, FPR, Accuracy, Confusion matrix

Table 2. *Cont.*

Author	Participant Group	Additional Information	Device Type	Number of Participants	Number of Falls	Quantity of Non-Fall Data and Method of Preparation	Performance Measures
Debard [26]	Older adults	Age	Camera	4	25	A total of 14,000 h. Only data for the 20 min up to and including the falls were used, this was divided into 2 min windows.	**Sensitivity**, Specificity, **Precision**, Confusion matrix
Debard [27]	Older persons (two community dwelling, one in a nursing home and four in assisted living), two of which did not fall and were excluded	Age, mobility assessment, walking aid use	Camera	7	29	Over 21,000 h recorded. Only data from the 24 h prior to each fall were used which was divided into 1 s windows.	Sensitivity, Precision, PR Curve, PR AUC, TP, FP, FN

Table 2. Cont.

Author	Participant Group	Additional Information	Device Type	Number of Participants	Number of Falls	Quantity of Non-Fall Data and Method of Preparation	Performance Measures
Debard [28]	Older persons (two community dwelling, one in a nursing home and four in assisted living), two of which did not fall and were excluded	Age, mobility assessment, walking aid use	Camera	7	29	Over 21,000 h recorded. Only data from the 24 h prior to each fall were used which was divided into 1 s windows.	Sensitivity, Precision, PR Curve, **PR AUC**, TP, FP, FN, **FPRT**
Feldwieser [29]	Community dwelling older adults	Age, height, weight, mobility assessments, cognitive assessments	Accelerometer	28	12	A total of 1225.7 days (average daily user wear time 8.1 ± 4.8 h). Details of data preparation not given.	**TP**, FP, FPRT
Gietzelt [30]	Older adults with recurrent falls	Age, gender, mobility assessments, cognitive assessments	Accelerometer and camera	3	4	A total of 10 days. Details of data preparation not given.	TP, FPRT

Table 2. Cont.

Author	Participant Group	Additional Information	Device Type	Number of Participants	Number of Falls	Quantity of Non-Fall Data and Method of Preparation	Performance Measures
Godfrey [31]	Older adult with Parkinson's disease	Age, BMI, balance assessment	Accelerometer	1	1	A total of 7 days. No preparatory steps.	TP, FPRT
Hu [32]	Community dwelling older adults with a history of falls	Age, gender, height, weight	Accelerometer and Gyroscope	5	20	A total of 70 days, divided into sliding windows. Window size was varied from 5 to 30 min.	Sensitivity, Specificity
Kangas [33]	Residents of elderly care units	Age, gender, mobility assessments, cognitive assessments	Accelerometer	16	15	A total of 1105 days (average daily user wear time 14.2 ± 6.3 h). Data processed on line, 14 s raw acceleration data where recorded when acceleration of all three axes fell below 0.75 g.	**Sensitivity, FPRT**, TP, FP

Table 2. Cont.

Author	Participant Group	Additional Information	Device Type	Number of Participants	Number of Falls	Quantity of Non-Fall Data and Method of Preparation	Performance Measures
Lipsitz [34]	Residents of a long-term care facility who had at least once in the previous 12 months	Age, gender, height, weight, BMI, prevalence of 21 comorbidities	Working alarm system using an accelerometer	62	89	A total of 9300 days. Working alarm, raw sensor data not stored, analysis compared the alarm times to reported fall times.	Sensitivity, Precision, TP, FP, FN
Liu [35]	Older adult	None	Doppler radar	1	6	A total of 7 days. No preparatory steps.	TP, FPRT

Table 2. Cont.

Author	Participant Group	Additional Information	Device Type	Number of Participants	Number of Falls	Quantity of Non-Fall Data and Method of Preparation	Performance Measures
Palmerini [36]	Patients with Progressive Supranuclear Palsy staying in a geriatric rehabilitation unit	Age, gender	Accelerometer	1	12	A total of 168 h from four of the participants. Recordings were divided into 60 s windows and only the 1170 windows where $\max(RSS) - \min(RSS) > 1.01$ g were included	Sensitivity, Specificity, FPR, FPRT, Informedness, ROC Curve, **ROC AUC**, FP
	Community dwelling patients with Progressive Supranuclear Palsy	Age, gender	Accelerometer	6	16		
	Community dwelling older adult	Age, gender	Accelerometer	1	1		
Rezaee [37]	Nursing home residents	None	Camera	Not given	48	A total of 163 normal movements extracted from video sequences totalling 57,425 frames. Details of identification not given.	Sensitivity, Accuracy, **FPR**, Confusion matrix

Table 2. Cont.

Author	Participant Group	Additional Information	Device Type	Number of Participants	Number of Falls	Quantity of Non-Fall Data and Method of Preparation	Performance Measures
Skubic [20]	Residents of an older adult independent living facility	Age, gender	Doppler radar	1	13	10 days	Sensitivity, FPRT, TP, FP
	Residents of an older adult independent living facility	Age, gender	Kinect	16	9	3,339 days	Details of data preparation not given for any of the datasets.
	Resident of an older adult independent living facility	Age, gender, mobility device use	Kinect	1	142	601 days	
	Residents of assisted living apartments	Gender	Kinect	67	67	10,707 days	
Soaz [38]	Older adult	Age, gender	Accelerometer	1	1	3.5 h	Sensitivity, **FPRT**, FP
	Older adults	Age, gender	Accelerometer	14	0	996 h	No preparatory steps.

471

Table 2. Cont.

Author	Participant Group	Additional Information	Device Type	Number of Participants	Number of Falls	Quantity of Non-Fall Data and Method of Preparation	Performance Measures
Stone [39]	Residents of an older adult independent living facility	Age, gender	Kinect	16	9	A total of 3339 days. Device only stored data for periods where motion was detected.	Sensitivity, FPRT
Yu [40]	FARSEEING data used previously in [17,23] no further details provided	None	Accelerometer	22	22	A total of 2618 normal activities extracted as 1 s windows from the 2 min surrounding the fall signals.	Sensitivity, Precision, Specificity

Notes: Performance measures reported in the articles abstract are shown in bold. Where a working alarm system was tested this is stated in the Device Type column, otherwise the test was carried out off-line, using the collected dataset. Soaz [38] focused on estimating the false alarm rate, however one real fall was recorded by chance and was included. RSS = Root Sum of Squares; FPRT = False Positive Rate Over Time; NPV = Negative Predictive Value; ROC Curve = Receiver Operating Characteristic Curve; ROC AUC = Area Under ROC Curve; PR Curve = Precision Recall Curve; PR AUC = Area Under Precision Recall Curve; TP = True Positives; FP = False Positives; FN = False Negatives; TN = True Negatives.

3.1. Participant Descriptions

The level of detail provided about participants varied considerably. All but three [31,38,40] of the articles stated whether participants were community dwelling, in long-term care or hospital patients. Five articles did not provide any additional descriptive information on the participants [23,24,35,37,40]. The other eighteen articles describe participant's age, twelve also provide gender information and six provide details of height and weight or BMI [17,25,29,31,32,34]. Four articles provided information on specific medical conditions, three recruited participants with Progressive Supranuclear Palsy [17,21,36] and one included a single older adult with Parkinson's disease [31]. Lipsitz et al. [34] provided the most in-depth description with a breakdown of the proportion of participants with a range of 21 comorbidities. Eight articles reported results of mobility assessments [21,27–31,33,38], three articles provided information on walking aid use [20,27,28] and three articles additionally reported results of cognitive assessments [29,30,33]. None of the other 15 articles reported standardised measures of cognitive or mobility status.

3.2. Method of Data Collection

All studies used the same general approach of monitoring participants with one or more sensor devices. Studies can be classified into two main categories, those using wearable technology (e.g. accelerometers or gyroscopes) and those using non-wearable technology (e.g. fixed cameras or Kinect sensors). Both approaches have advantages and disadvantages with regard to fall detection. For example, wearable devices are always with the user, however they may forget to wear the device. In contrast, non-wearable devices have a limited capture area but the user can safely forget about them. For a full discussion on the advantages and disadvantages of different sensor types refer to recent reviews [19,41].

Fifteen studies used wearable technology and ten used non-wearable, Table 2 shows full details of the devices used in each study. Accelerometers are the most common choice of sensor and have been used in 15 of the studies [17,21–25,29–34,36,38,40]. Eight studies tested some form of optical sensor [20,22,26–28,30,37,39], making them the most common choice of non-wearable devices. One additional study deployed an optical sensor as part of their system, but this did not record any falls so they could not test it [29].

Studies can be further classified based on whether the device used was capable of processing data on-line and raising an alarm when it detected a fall. Three studies deployed functioning wearable alarm systems [24,33,34], one study deployed a system combining wearable and non-wearable devices [22], no studies deployed an alarm system solely using non-wearable devices. Two of the studies which tested working alarm systems did not store the raw sensor data, only recording when the alarm went off [22,34], one article did not state if the raw sensor data was stored [24]. The raw sensor data can be used for future development and testing, and therefore the favoured approach is to store this data.

The availability of the collected data is important for future work and the direct comparison of approaches. None of the studies used publicly available datasets nor made their real-world fall data publicly available. Two studies [25,40] made use of a subset of the FARSEEING repository, which is available on request. The FARSEEING project is a real-world fall repository project funded by the European Union. Four studies [17,21,23,36] were conducted by members of the FARSEEING project or in collaboration with members, and also used data from the FARSEEING repository. No other studies provide any information on the availability of their datasets.

3.3. Number of Participants and Falls, and the Volume of Non-Fall Data

There is a large range in the number of participants included, with most studies using small cohorts. One article did not provide any information on the number of participants [37]. Three studies had just a single participant [31,35,38] and one study [20] used data from only one participant in parts of their analysis. The maximum number of participants was 62 [34] and the median was nine (IQR 4–18).

There was an equally large range in the number of fall events recorded. Two studies included just a single real fall [31,38] and in one of the two datasets used by Aziz et al. [21] only one fall was recorded. The maximum number of falls was 89, which was achieved in two separate studies [23,34]. The median number of falls contained in the datasets used was 17.5 (IQR 8.25–29).

Where reported, the length of the monitoring period varied considerably and comparison is made difficult by the inconsistent choice of reported metrics. Thirteen articles provided the total length of the recorded data, but did not provide details of the proportion where the system was recording participant's movement (participant in the capture area or wearing the device) [20–22,24,26–28,30,32,34,35,38,39]. The median length of total recorded data, from studies which provided it, was 592 days (IQR 21–1474). Only three articles provided information on device wear time, in these studies the mean wear times were 8.1 [29], 14.2 [33] and 24 [31] h per day. None of the articles on non-wearable devices provided information on the proportion of time during which participants were in the capture area.

Six articles did not clearly state the time period over which participants were monitored or the amount of data captured, instead they provided the number of extracted non-fall events [17,23,25,36,37,40]. The number of non-fall events used in these studies ranged from 22 [25] to 3466 [23].

3.4. Method of Fall Identification and Validation

One of the main challenges in recording real-world falls is ensuring every fall that occurs is identified accurately. How fall events are identified is influenced by both the choice of device and whether the system is capable of raising alarms in real-time. The device used determines the type and detail of information available for retrospective verification of fall times and types. A camera, for example, provides a greater level of information compared to an accelerometer; assuming the video footage is not highly pre-processed, for privacy reasons, before being stored. Where working alarm systems are deployed, all detected falls can be quickly verified, providing additional robustness over a single reporting method such as staff incident reports.

Four studies [22,24,33,34] deployed a functioning wearable alarm system. As the alarm systems were being validated, a second reporting system was still needed to identify falls which did not trigger an alarm. Three of the studies used staff incident reports in addition to the alarm system [22,33,34]. It was unclear what secondary method of fall identification was used in one of the studies [24]. Of the 18 studies which analysed the data retrospectively, three identified falls using staff reports [17,21,39], five used participant self-report [29–32,38] and ten did not state how falls were identified [20,23,25–28,35–37,40].

Where self-report of falls is used it is important to consider the cognitive ability of participants, especially their memory. Only two of the five studies which used self-report provide results of assessments of cognitive ability [29,30]. Both of these studies used a Mini Mental State Exam [42]. Feldwieser et al. [29] found no signs of cognitive impairment and Gietzelt et al. [30] found that one of their three participants had cognitive impairment, but does not report how they accounted for this.

It is important to consider that reported fall times might not be accurate and that some falls may not be reported, or may be reported by more than one member of staff with different timestamps. This could, for example, be due to delays in completing the report, delays in the faller being discovered, participant recall problems or staff naturally prioritising helping the faller over checking and reporting the time. Only three articles describe methods to check reported fall times [17,21,32]. Two of these [17,21] used datasets from the FARSEEING repository where expert analysis of the sensor signals in combination with fall reports was used to pinpoint the fall signal. Hu et al. [32] reported correlating self-reported fall times with the signals, but provided no details on how this was carried out.

3.5. Methods of Data Processing

There are two approaches for testing real-world fall detection systems, the key difference is how the data is prepared. The first approach is based on simply identifying when falls occur in continuous user movement or a stream of sensor data, we call this the continuous data approach. The second approach is based on a fall detector classifying events as either a fall or not a fall, we call this the event based approach. The following sections explain each of these approaches and review their use. In five studies it was unclear which approach was used [20,24,29,30,39].

3.5.1. Continuous Data Approach

The continuous data approach mirrors real-world usage of fall alarm systems where user movement is the input and fall times or alarms are the output. This approach is therefore the primary way of testing deployed fall alarm systems but can also be used for retrospective testing using existing data. The fall detection systems sensors convert movement into a stream of raw data which is then processed by the software component of the system. In this approach all aspects of data processing are part of the fall detection software and are tested as a single unit. To test performance the systems predictions are compared to the actual verified fall times. This comparison allows quantification of the number of true positives (actual and predicted timestamps match), false positives (predicted fall with no actual fall) and false negatives (fall occurred but none was predicted).

True negatives can be quantified if the times when non-falls occurred were recorded, however, non-falls are not defined. In the strictest sense non-falls are everything which is not a fall, but that does not enable their occurrence to be quantified. It is not possible to count when a fall doesn't occur without arbitrarily dividing the time-series data into events, and counting the events where no fall occurred. Such a method of dividing the data would fall under the event based testing approach. In the continuous data approach any segmenting of the data for processing purposes is part of the fall detection system, not the test procedure.

Six studies used the continuous data approach [22,31,33–35,38]. Bloch et al. [22] processed the data using the continuous data approach, and then used an assumption of thirty 'fall-like' events per day to calculate a number of true negatives (30 × number of days the sensor was in use). The other five studies did not attempt to quantify TN.

3.5.2. Event Based Approach

The event based approach has its roots in tests using laboratory based simulation datasets. When data is collected in the laboratory a predefined set of movements or events is simulated, the times of these events is known and therefore they can be easily extracted. To test performance all the events must first be labelled as either a fall or not a fall using the record of event times. For each event the label is compared to the software's predictions allowing a complete confusion matrix to be generated.

In real-world data, events are less clearly defined than in simulated data since there is no complete record of the movements which occurred. The creation of events from real-world data has been based on arbitrary rules rather than identification of the underlying movements of the users. The events are labelled using reported fall times, where no fall occurred the event is considered a non-fall. As this method always yields non-fall events, true negatives can be quantified, unlike in the continuous approach.

Eleven studies used the event based approach [17,21,23,25–28,32,36,37,40]. The predominant method to create events was based on time windows, where the data is sliced using constant time intervals, for example each 60 seconds of data is one event. However, there is no consensus on what constitutes an event and in practice, a method of reducing the volume of data is often used, for example, to exclude data where no movement was recorded. The time windows can overlap allowing the same data to be processed multiple times, although the rationale for this is not clear.

To create events, one study used 2.5 s windows with a 1.5 s overlap and kept all the events [21]. Two studies divided the data into 60 s windows and used a movement detection algorithm to select events [17,36]. Bourke et al. [23] also used a movement detection algorithm to select events but does not describe the windowing technique. Two studies used the same dataset where the 24 hours prior to each fall was divided into one second windows [27,28]. One study used self-reported wear time to reduce the dataset prior to dividing into windows, but does not provide any details about the windowing technique [32].

Three studies used only a limited section of data from around each fall. Debard et al. [26] divided up the 20 minutes of data prior to a fall into two minute windows. Chen et al. [25] only used data from 20 minutes surrounding each fall and used the section of data up to one second prior to impact as non-fall events. Yu et al. [40] divided the two minutes around each fall into one second windows, removed the one second window where the fall occurred and used the remaining windows as non-fall events.

3.6. Definition of Performance Measures and Review of Their Use

3.6.1. Sensitivity

Sensitivity (also known as recall and true positive rate) is the proportion of falls which are correctly detected (Equation (1)). The inverse of sensitivity is miss rate (false negative rate) which quantifies the proportion of falls not detected (Equation (2)). Sensitivity is by far the most commonly reported statistic; it was reported in 18 of the articles [17,20–28,32–34,36–40] and could be calculated from the information given in the other four [29–31,35].

$$\text{Sensitivity} = \frac{TP}{TP + FN} = \frac{TP}{P} \qquad (1)$$

$$\text{Miss Rate} = \frac{FN}{FN + TP} = \frac{FN}{P} = 1 - \text{Sensitivity} \qquad (2)$$

3.6.2. Specificity

Specificity (also known as true negative rate) is the proportion of non-fall events which are correctly detected (Equation (3)). It quantifies the ability to avoid false positives (false alarms). The inverse of specificity is false positive rate, which is the proportion of non-fall events mistakenly detected as falls (Equation (4)). Nine articles reported specificity [17,21–24,26,32,36,40] and two reported false positive rate [36,37]. It is unclear whether Chen et al. [25] reported specificity or false positive rate, as the reported number of TN and FP suggest that what they report as specificity is in fact false positive rate. Specificity could be calculated from the information provided in a further two of the studies [27,28].

$$\text{Specificity} = \frac{TN}{TN + FP} = \frac{TN}{N} \qquad (3)$$

$$\text{False Positive Rate} = \frac{FP}{FP + TN} = \frac{FP}{N} = 1 - \text{Specificity} \qquad (4)$$

3.6.3. False Positive Rate over Time

False Positive Rate over Time (FPRT) has become a popular measure in real-world tests of fall detection. This measure provides information on the frequency of false alarms. Twelve articles report the number of false positives either per hour or per day [17,20,21,28–31,33,35,36,38,39] and it could be calculated from the information provided in seven others [24–27,32,34,37].

3.6.4. Precision

Precision (also known as positive predictive value) is the proportion of alarms which are true falls (Equation (5)). It therefore provides the probability that an alarm will be an actual fall and not a false alarm. For example, a precision of 0.5 means that half of alarms will be actual falls, and half will be false alarms (1 false positive for every detected fall). Eight articles reported precision [17,22,24,26–28,34,40] and it could be calculated from the information provided in all of the other articles.

$$\text{Precision} = \frac{TP}{TP + FP} \qquad (5)$$

3.6.5. Negative Predictive Value

Negative Predictive Value (NPV) is the proportion of events classified as non-falls which are true non-fall events (Equation (6)). NPV therefore provides information about the ability to correctly classify non-fall events. NPV will be high if a system correctly ignores many times more non-fall events than the number of falls it fails to detect. Therefore, for false negatives to have any notable effect, the number of falls and non-falls must be approximately equal. However, in real-world fall data falls are usually much less frequent than non-fall events, which limits the insights yielded from NPV as systems typically score over 0.99 out of 1 [17,22,24]. Three articles reported NPV in their results [17,22,24]. NPV could also be calculated from the information provided in eleven of the other articles [21,23,25–28,32,34,36,37,40].

$$\text{Negative Predictive Value} = \frac{TN}{TN + FN} \qquad (6)$$

3.6.6. Accuracy

Accuracy is the proportion of predictions which were correct (Equation (7)). Accuracy is a measure which summarises the whole confusion matrix in a single value. Accuracy's major limitation is the inability to handle imbalanced datasets, for example, in real-world fall data where there are many more non-fall events than falls. Similar to NPV, accuracy is dominated by the larger group and the effect is proportional to the size of the imbalance. Therefore, in real-world fall detection studies, accuracy is skewed towards the correct detection of non-fall events over the correct detection of falls. For example, in eight of the algorithms tested by Bagala et al. [17] the accuracies were greater than 0.9 with sensitivities below 0.6, in one case an accuracy of 0.96 with a sensitivity of 0.14. Four articles reported accuracy [17,23,25,37] and it could be calculated from the results provided in seven of the other articles [21,24,26–28,36,40].

$$\text{Accuracy} = \frac{TP + TN}{P + N} \qquad (7)$$

3.6.7. F-Measure

F-measure (also known as F-score) is the harmonic mean of sensitivity and precision (Equation (8)). F-measure, therefore, considers all outcomes except true negatives (non-falls). In fall detection, the priorities are detected falls (TP), missed falls (FN) and false alarms (FP). F-measure considers all of these outcomes and therefore provides a good overview of performance. No articles report a value for F-measure, however it could be easily calculated from their results as eight articles [17,22,24,26–28,34,40] reported both sensitivity and precision and all but two [32,39] reported enough information to calculate both sensitivity and precision.

$$\text{F-measure} = 2 \times \frac{\text{Precision} \times \text{Sensitivity}}{\text{Precision} + \text{Sensitivity}} \qquad (8)$$

3.6.8. Informedness

Informedness (also known as Youden's J Statistics or Youden's Index) is a statistic which combines sensitivity and specificity (Equation (9)). It is the probability that predictions are informed versus a pure guess. Informedness is linked to the proportion of cases classified correctly. However, unlike accuracy, it is robust to an imbalance in the number of fall and non-fall events. This is achieved through equal weighting of sensitivity and specificity which are in turn the proportions of falls detected and non-falls correctly ignored. The value ranges from negative one to positive one. Zero indicates predictions are no better than guessing, positive one indicates perfect predictions and negative one indicates all predictions are the opposite of the true value. In cases where the value is negative, the output classes can simply be swapped over. One study reported informedness [36], however, 12 other articles reported both sensitivity and specificity or false positive rate, or the information necessary to calculate them [17,21–28,37,40], so informedness could be calculated from their results.

$$\text{Informedness} = \text{Sensitivity} + \text{Specificity} - 1 \tag{9}$$

3.6.9. Markedness

Markedness is a statistic which combines precision and NPV (Equation (10)). Markedness is linked with the proportion of predictions which are correct. It combines the proportion of correct positive and negative predictions with equal weighting and is therefore unaffected by imbalance in the number of positive and negative predictions. As with informedness, the result is a value between negative and positive one. No articles reported markedness, but twelve did report enough information for markedness to be calculated [17,21–28,36,37,40].

$$\text{Markedness} = \text{Precision} + \text{NPV} - 1 \tag{10}$$

3.6.10. Matthews Correlation Coefficient

Matthews Correlation Coefficient (MCC) is the geometric mean of informedness and markedness (Equations (11) and (12)). It should be noted that Equation (11) only works if informedness and markedness are both positive, Equation (12) works in all cases. MCC considers both the proportion of events classified correctly and the proportion of correct predictions and is therefore robust to imbalanced datasets. The result is a value between negative and positive one as with both informedness and markedness. None of the articles reported MCC, enough information to calculate MCC was given in 14 articles [17,21–28,32,34,36,37,40].

$$\text{MCC} = \sqrt{\text{Informedness} \times \text{Markedness}} \tag{11}$$

$$\text{MCC} = \frac{TP \times TN - FP \times FN}{\sqrt{(TP + FP)(TP + FN)(TN + FP)(TN + FN)}} \tag{12}$$

3.6.11. Receiver Operating Characteristic Curve

A Receiver Operating Characteristic (ROC) Curve is a plot of sensitivity versus false positive rate as the primary threshold of the classifier is adjusted. ROC curves can therefore be used to understand the trade-off between sensitivity and false positive rate and optimise a primary threshold. There could be debate as to which balance of sensitivity and false positives is optimal, therefore a ROC curve provides useful insight. However, it is difficult to compare systems robustly based on a curve. Consequently, it is in the optimisation where ROC curves are best used, rather than final results, as only the optimised version will be deployed.

ROC curves can be reduced to a single number by calculating the area under the curve (AUC). AUC has been found to be a poor measure for comparing classifiers, particularly where the sample size is small [43–45]. Two studies have used ROC analysis and reported AUC [23,36].

3.6.12. Precision-Recall Curve

A precision-recall (PR) curve is similar to a ROC curve, the difference is that precision is used instead of false positive rate and the term recall is used in place of sensitivity. PR curves are preferred over ROC curves when there is a large imbalance in the data [46]. Calculating AUC for PR curves is more challenging than for ROC curves as precision does not increase linearly, meaning linear interpolation yields incorrect results [46]. Two studies reported PR AUC [27,28], although it is unclear how PR AUC was calculated in these studies.

4. Discussion

This is the first review to be conducted on the methods used to evaluate real-world performance of fall detection systems. Ensuring a sound method is critical for meaningful results, therefore reflecting on the way studies are conducted and seeking improvements to the method is vital in emerging areas of research where no consensus has yet been reached. The real-world testing of fall detection systems is currently in its infancy and this is reflected in our findings. The method is highly variable across studies, which makes comparing the results difficult if not impossible. The following three sections discuss the key issues and make recommendations for future studies.

4.1. Data Collection and Preparation

One major aspect which leads to variation between studies is the participant groups and the differences in the movements and behaviours captured by the sensor systems. If insufficient detail is gathered about participants it is challenging to reproduce the findings as differing results could be due to differing participant characteristics. In addition, one may want to collect new data comparable to that used in a previous study for the purpose of comparing the performance of a new system using different sensors with previously tested systems. Information gathered about participants was both inconsistent and insufficient to allow the data collection to be reproduced.

A comprehensive consensus process has previously been carried out by the FARSEEING consortium [47]. As part of the consensus process the group identified a minimum set of clinical measures which they deemed essential for the interpretation of real-world fall data. The measures included age, height, weight, gender, fall history, assistive device use as well as assessments of mobility, cognitive impairments and visual impairments. None of the reported studies have implemented these recommendations.

Cognitive and mobility tests provide useful information about fall risk and the likelihood of false positives caused by events such as 'falling into a chair' or improper use of the device. Compared to standard metrics such as age, height and weight, assessments of mobility and cognition provide a much deeper insight into participant's fall risk and movement characteristics. Therefore, standardised cognitive and mobility assessments should be prioritised. Deeper insights into participant's movements could be achieved though continuous profiling using activity monitoring software to process the recorded dataset. However, development and validation of activity monitoring software may be a barrier unless an existing activity monitoring system is used for the data collection. Where such profiling is possible details should be reported to enhance the interpretation of results.

Another critical aspect of the test is the size of the dataset. Currently, the datasets used are generally small, have been collected with a low number of participants and contain only a few falls. Small datasets reduce the validity of the test and hinder reproducibility. Where the dataset is small either due to few participants, a low incidence of falls or both, it is possible that only a limited subset of movements and fall types were captured. In such cases comparisons of results to tests of other systems is difficult as the dataset may be the main cause of differences in reported performance. Further, the generalisability of results is questionable where the sample size is small. The small datasets are one factor which makes it difficult to understand which systems perform the best and therefore where future development should focus. The other main factors are the different populations recruited for studies and the limited insights into how this effects the fundamental aspect of the data—the movements captured.

Due to the known challenges in recording fall signals, the only feasible way for most researchers to gain access to a large number of fall signals is through collaboration. In addition, if systems are tested using the same data, the results are directly comparable. Therefore, large shared test datasets are needed to allow the performance of fall detection software to be compared. To facilitate the sharing of datasets, the FARSEEING consortium have established a data repository which currently contains over 300 fall signals [48]. However, more studies are needed to generate datasets that can be added to the repository and used for robust testing of devices and development of improved software.

Even with shared data, there is still an issue of how to ensure all fall signals are accurately identified. We have identified that the method used to identify the fall signals is poorly described in published studies, leaving a large gap in our understanding of how the dataset was prepared. The current prevailing method to identify fall signals is expert signal analysis to verify participant or staff reported fall times. There is a risk that not all falls are reported, leading to real falls being included as non-fall data. Expert signal analysis cannot overcome the issue of under reporting, but does at least give greater confidence that inaccurate reported times were corrected and all included fall signals were real falls.

Expert signal analysis, while clearly better than no verification, could lead to bias. Currently there is an insufficient understanding of fall signals due to a limited number of recorded falls and a lack of research into the profile of the signals. Our limited understanding could lead to atypical falls not being verified and thus excluded. There is a risk that systems are designed to detect certain signal profiles as falls and only these profiles are being verified as falls. Therefore the results could be artificially improved through restricting the test data.

Unless a gold standard fall reporting system is used, such as video analysis, studies will be limited in their ability to verify fall signals, under reporting of falls will remain a concern and there is a risk of bias in the verification process needed to compensate for the inaccuracies of the 'silver standard' reporting system. The current lack of standardised method or gold standard, and the lack of reporting how fall signals were identified and verified, inhibits understanding of results. A consensus is needed on the process for fall signal identification and studies should clearly report their methods.

4.2. Data Processing

Two approaches were identified for preparing sensor signals for fall detection system testing and we named these the continuous data approach and the event based approach. Both approaches have issues surrounding what constitutes a non-fall. In the continuous data approach the issue is centred around the definition and identification of non-falls. In the event based approach non-fall events can be defined as any event which is not a fall. However, events could be defined as anything which is either a fall event or non-fall event, and since falls are defined, the issue returns to what constitutes a non-fall.

The strictest definition of non-falls as everything which is not a fall is not particularly useful. This definition does not allow non-falls to be quantified in the continuous data approach and provides no indication of how the data should be divided into events for the event based approach. A more helpful concept is that of fall-like movements, a subset of non-falls which share characteristics with falls. The FARSEEING consortium defined a fall as "an unexpected event in which the person comes to rest on the ground, floor or lower level" [49]. A fall-like movement could therefore, by removing the unexpected clause, be defined as "any event in which the person comes to rest on the ground, floor or lower level".

With a definition for fall-like events these could be recorded, at least theoretically, in the same manner as falls and therefore, allow true negatives to be quantified robustly. In reality it is not feasible for a researcher to record the times of all fall-like movements in the same way that falls are recorded, due to the vast quantity which would occur. An automated system would be more practical, although it is unlikely to be easier to develop automated fall-like detection than automated fall detection systems. Consequently, researchers must consider if the development of fall-like movement detection systems is worth the investment, simply to extend the testing of fall-detection systems. Given that a robust evaluation of fall detection systems can be achieved without the need for true negatives, and hence non-fall or fall-like movements, we suggest that automated fall-like movement detection is unlikely to bring benefits which outweigh the required investment.

4.3. Performance Measures

It is challenging to compare results across studies or determine the current state-of-the-art due to disparity in the choice of measures reported and challenges calculating unreported measures. The measures used to report and interpret performance vary widely across studies and not all studies report the basic results from which all measures can be calculated (TP, FP, FN and TN). Where TP, FP, FN and TN are not reported these can only be estimated, due to rounding of the reported results. Using one of the tests reported by Bourke et al. [23] as an example, the number of FP could be any value between 18 and 51 based on the reported specificity of 0.99 with 3466 total non-falls. To facilitate the calculation of additional measures, future studies should report TP, FP, FN and TN if these can be calculated robustly and are used in the calculation of the reported performance measures.

In addition to reporting enough information to allow further measures to be calculated, it is important that the headline measures give a true reflection of performance and allow robust comparisons to be made with other systems. Sensitivity has been a mainstay in previous studies, it is an important aspect of system performance. Sensitivity only quantifies the ability to detect falls, it does not consider false positives. The question is therefore which measure to pair sensitivity with to provide understanding of the ability to avoid false positives. In addition, a single combined measure which considers both aspects is important in order to understand the overall level of performance.

Specificity has been the most common choice of measure to quantify the ability to avoid false alarms in laboratory based testing [19] and it has remained a common choice in real-world tests. Specificity considers how well non-fall events are classified, it could therefore be considered sensitivity's natural counterpart. The weakness of specificity in the context of real-world fall detection is the reliance on non-falls, which are poorly defined and troublesome to identify.

The need for researchers to design or select methods for non-fall identification opens up a considerable possibility of bias. A method could be used which suits the specific system and dataset causing distortion of the results and hindering comparisons with other systems. In the case of specificity, the difficulty of the test is very much determined by the definition of a non-fall; the more inclusive the definition, the more non-fall events and therefore the higher the score for the same number of false positives. This effect can be seen in the study of Bourke et al. [23], where tests were conducted twice using different definitions of non-falls. With the most restrictive definition of non-falls, specificity ranged from 0.83 to 0.91. With the more open definition, specificity was consistently 0.98 or greater. Expanding the definition includes more movements which are less fall-like, thus it creates an easier test.

It is hard to prevent bias in selecting a definition of non-falls as it is likely unintentional. One solution is to remove the need to select a method on a study by study basis, however, standardising the method is challenging. Since there is currently no clear way to standardise non-fall identification, the best option may simply be to avoid them altogether. A solution might be standard publicly available datasets, with an agreed method to identify non-fall events. In such a case, the results are comparable to each other, but not to other studies using other datasets or methods.

Using standard data is challenging due to the vast array of sensors which could be used and the huge number of combinations. It is simply not possible to have a single dataset used to test all systems. Furthermore, it seems impossible to identify all types of relevant non-fall movements needed for a universal standard dataset. Any measures which rely on non-falls (specificity, NPV, accuracy, informedness, markedness, MCC and ROC AUC) are subject to the above problems and therefore should not be used as a primary measure. Where measures reliant on non-falls are used the methods should be described in detail and their limitations should be made clear to avoid confusion and misinterpretation.

The issues surrounding non-falls substantially reduces the options for quantifying the ability to avoid false positives and gauge overall performance. There are four possible measures which do not rely on non-falls, these are FPRT, precision, F-measure and PR AUC.

FPRT is a useful measure to understand the frequency of false alarms, however differences in the datasets affect the calculation. Wear time or time in the capture area must be considered, as false positives will, most likely, be far lower when the device is not in use. Another consideration is which hours of the day the device is in use; false positive rate during night time hours would be very different to day time hours. Reporting of times when the device was monitoring participants was found to be inadequate. Of the 11 articles which reported FPRT only two clearly reported wear time or time in the capture area [29,33] and none reported any details on the distribution of this time throughout the day.

Our findings suggest that there is a lack of an agreed and clearly defined method to calculate FPRT. Only one study clearly states that FPRT was calculated using solely the time a participant was being monitored by the device [33]. None of the other studies appear to have taken usage time into account when calculating FPRT. If usage time is not considered or reported it is unclear what extent device usage, or lack thereof affected the result. An unused system is unlikely to produce false positives. The issues in identifying wear time or time in the capture area could make FPRT an unreliable measure to compare across studies. Although users and clinicians may find the rate of false positives over time useful, it might be better to use a rate of something other than time.

Precision is an alternative to specificity and FPRT, it quantifies the false positives (FP) in relation to detected falls (TP). TP and FP should, for any reasonable level of performance, be in the same order of magnitude, therefore precision is resilient to the imbalance in the data. Further, the ratio between TP and FP is unlikely to be notably affected by usage time, if a device is used half of the time, TP and FP would be expected to be half compared to full device usage. Therefore, compared to FPRT, precision is far less affected by device usage, or lack thereof. The proportion of fall predictions which were true falls could be more useful than FPRT since frequent false positives may be acceptable to a frequent faller, assuming the falls are detected. Precision should be the primary measure of the ability to avoid false positives.

Sensitivity and precision together quantify the ability to detect falls and avoid false alarms, therefore providing a complete portrayal of performance. In addition to sensitivity and precision it is important to have a single measure which can quantify the trade-off between them. PR AUC is one possible option, however it considers the performance of multiple sub-optimum versions of the system as the system's parameters are adjusted. Since only the optimised system can be deployed, it is the optimised version which should be the focal point of the evaluation. F-measure, the harmonic mean of sensitivity and precision, appears to be the most suitable single measure for objective comparison. This trio of measures has two major advantages in robustness: (1) it does not rely on non-falls and (2) it is resistant to issues surrounding wear time and time in the capture area. Future studies should report sensitivity, precision and F-measure, and F-measure should be used as the standard for comparing systems.

5. Summary and Conclusions

As focus in fall detection performance evaluation shifts from simulated to real-world fall data, one must consider if the approach used for evaluating on simulations is optimum for real-world data.

Through examining the published articles on evaluation of real-world fall detection, two issues have become apparent:

1. The approaches to quantifying performance are inconsistent and many studies use measures which provide limited representation of performance.
2. The number of falls is generally small and study populations are diverse, making comparison between the datasets and results difficult.

It is critical that a consensus is reached on the most appropriate method to evaluate real-world performance of fall detection systems.

To address the issues with the datasets there needs to be greater collaboration and sharing of data. The FARSEEING consortium have made substantial steps to facilitate data sharing and have recorded over 300 falls through collaboration between six institutions [48]. Six of the 22 studies published to date have used parts of this data to develop or test approaches to fall detection [17,21,23,25,36,40], highlighting the importance of this data. However, further work is still needed to grow the volume of available data, record more falls, improve standardisation and further develop fall detection technology. Only through collaboration will the collection of a dataset large enough for robust development and testing become possible.

To address the issues surrounding how performance is quantified studies should avoid the need for non-falls. The concept is poorly defined and standardisation seems to be extremely problematic. The concept of non-falls is only needed to allow the calculation of measures such as specificity and accuracy, both of which are common in simulation based studies [19]. However, quantification of the difference in false alarm rate between simulated and real-world tests is not possible due to the disparity of the data. Therefore, traditional measures such as specificity and accuracy are of little value. Continued use of these traditional measures may lead to confusion and improper interpretation of performance. Measures which do not depend on non-falls should be used instead of these traditional measures. Sensitivity and precision should be the cornerstones of the evaluation with F-measure used for the objective comparison of systems.

Author Contributions: Conceptualization, R.W.B.; Methodology, R.W.B.; Formal Analysis, R.W.B.; Investigation, R.W.B.; Data Curation, R.W.B.; Writing-Original Draft Preparation, R.W.B.; Writing-Review & Editing, J.K., M.H.G., L.P.J.K., S.B.T.; Supervision, M.H.G., L.P.J.K., S.B.T.; Funding Acquisition, M.H.G., L.P.J.K., S.B.T.

Funding: This research was funded by the Dowager Countess Eleanor Peel Trust.

Conflicts of Interest: The authors declare no conflict of interest. The funding sponsors had no role in the design of the study; in the collection, analyses, or interpretation of data; in the writing of the manuscript, and in the decision to publish the results.

Abbreviations

The following abbreviations are used in this manuscript:

P	Positive cases
N	Negative cases
TP	True Positives
FP	False Positives
FN	False Negatives
TP	True Positives
NPV	Negative Predictive Value
FPRT	False Positive Rate over Time
MCC	Mathews Correlation Coefficient
ROC	Receiver Operating Characteristic
PR	Precision-Recall
AUC	Area Under Curve
RSS	Root Sum of Squares
IQR	InterQuartile Range

References

1. World Health Organisation. *WHO Global Report on Falls Prevention in Older Age*; World Health Organization: Geneva, Switzerland, 2007.
2. Department of Health (UK). *Falls and Fractures: Effective Interventions in Health and Social Care*; Technical Report; Department of Health (UK): London, UK, 2009.
3. Luukinen, H.; Koski, K.; Honkanen, R.; Kivelä, S.L. Incidence of Injury-Causing Falls among Older Adults by Place of Residence: A Population-Based Study. *J. Am. Geriatr. Soc.* **1995**, *43*, 871–876, doi:10.1111/j.1532-5415.1995.tb05529.x.
4. Tinetti, M.E.; Speechley, M.; Ginter, S.F. Risk Factors for Falls among Elderly Persons Living in the Community. *N. Engl. J. Med.* **1988**, *319*, 1701–1707, doi:10.1056/NEJM198812293192604.
5. Heinrich, S.; Rapp, K.; Rissmann, U.; Becker, C.; König, H.H. Cost of Falls in Old Age: A Systematic Review. *Osteoporos. Int.* **2010**, *21*, 891–902, doi:10.1007/s00198-009-1100-1.
6. Fleming, J.; Brayne, C. Inability to Get up after Falling, Subsequent Time on Floor, and Summoning Help: Prospective Cohort Study in People over 90. *BMJ* **2008**, *337*, a2227, doi:10.1136/bmj.a2227.
7. Treml, J.; Husk, J.; Lowe, D.; Vasilakis, N. *Falling Standards, Broken Promises: Report of the National Audit of Falls and Bone Health in Older People 2010*; Technical Report; Royal College of Physicians: London, UK, 2010.
8. King, M.B.; Tinetti, M.E. Falls in Community-Dwelling Older Persons. *J. Am. Geriatr. Soc.* **1995**, *43*, 1146–1154, doi:10.1111/j.1532-5415.1995.tb07017.x.
9. Lord, S.R.; Sherrington, C.; Menz, H.B. *Falls in Older People : Risk Factors and Strategies for Prevention*; Cambridge University Press: Cambridge, UK, 2001.
10. Nevitt, M.C.; Cummings, S.R.; Kidd, S.; Black, D. Risk Factors for Recurrent Nonsyncopal Falls: A Prospective Study. *JAMA* **1989**, *261*, 2663–2668.
11. Wild, D.; Nayak, U.S.; Isaacs, B. How Dangerous Are Falls in Old People at Home? *Br. Med. J. (Clin. Res. Ed.)* **1981**, *282*, 266–268, doi:10.1136/bmj.282.6260.266.
12. Scheffer, A.C.; Schuurmans, M.J.; Van Dijk, N.; Van Der Hooft, T.; De Rooij, S.E. Fear of Falling: Measurement Strategy, Prevalence, Risk Factors and Consequences among Older Persons. *Age Ageing* **2008**, *37*, 19–24, doi:10.1093/ageing/afm169.
13. Howland, J.; Lachman, M.E.; Peterson, E.W.; Cote, J.; Kasten, L.; Jette, A. Covariates of Fear of Falling and Associated Activity Curtailment. *Gerontologist* **1998**, *38*, 549–555, doi:10.1093/geront/38.5.549.
14. Murphy, S.L.; Williams, C.S.; Gill, T.M. Characteristics Associated with Fear of Falling and Activity Restriction in Community-Living Older Persons. *J. Am. Geriatr. Soc.* **2002**, *50*, 516–520, doi:10.1046/j.1532-5415.2002.50119.x.
15. Heinbüchner, B.; Hautzinger, M.; Becker, C.; Pfeiffer, K. Satisfaction and Use of Personal Emergency Response Systems. *Z. Gerontol. Geriatr.* **2010**, *43*, 219–223, doi:10.1007/s00391-010-0127-4.
16. Baker, M. 1,500 Scientists Lift the Lid on Reproducibility. *Nature* **2016**, *533*, 452–454, doi:10.1038/533452a.
17. Bagala, F.; Becker, C.; Cappello, A.; Chiari, L.; Aminian, K.; Hausdorff, J.M.; Zijlstra, W.; Klenk, J. Evaluation of Accelerometer-Based Fall Detection Algorithms on Real-World Falls. *PLoS ONE* **2012**, *7*, e37062, doi:10.1371/journal.pone.0037062.
18. Schwickert, L.; Becker, C.; Lindemann, U.; Marechal, C.; Bourke, A.; Chiari, L.; Helbostad, J.L.; Zijlstra, W.; Aminian, K.; Todd, C.; et al. Fall Detection with Body-Worn Sensors : A Systematic Review. *Z. Gerontol. Geriatr.* **2013**, *46*, 706–719, doi:10.1007/s00391-013-0559-8.
19. Chaudhuri, S.; Thompson, H.; Demiris, G. Fall Detection Devices and Their Use with Older Adults: A Systematic Review. *J. Geriatr. Phys. Ther.* **2014**, *37*, 178–196, doi:10.1519/JPT.0b013e3182abe779.
20. Skubic, M.; Harris, B.H.; Stone, E.; Ho, K.C.; Su, B.Y.; Rantz, M. Testing Non-Wearable Fall Detection Methods in the Homes of Older Adults. In Proceedings of the 2016 38th Annual International Conference of the IEEE Engineering in Medicine and Biology Society (EMBC), Orlando, FL, USA, 16–20 August 2016; pp. 557–560, doi:10.1109/EMBC.2016.7590763.
21. Aziz, O.; Klenk, J.; Schwickert, L.; Chiari, L.; Becker, C.; Park, E.J.; Mori, G.; Robinovitch, S.N. Validation of Accuracy of SVM-Based Fall Detection System Using Real-World Fall and Non-Fall Datasets. *PLoS ONE* **2017**, *12*, e0180318, doi:10.1371/journal.pone.0180318.

22. Bloch, F.; Gautier, V.; Noury, N.; Lundy, J.E.; Poujaud, J.; Claessens, Y.E.; Rigaud, A.S. Evaluation under Real-Life Conditions of a Stand-Alone Fall Detector for the Elderly Subjects. *Ann. Phys. Rehabil. Med.* **2011**, *54*, 391–398, doi:10.1016/j.rehab.2011.07.962.
23. Bourke, A.K.; Klenk, J.; Schwickert, L.; Aminian, K.; Ihlen, E.A.F.; Mellone, S.; Helbostad, J.L.; Chiari, L.; Becker, C. Fall Detection Algorithms for Real-World Falls Harvested from Lumbar Sensors in the Elderly Population: A Machine Learning Approach. In Proceedings of the 2016 38th Annual International Conference of the IEEE Engineering in Medicine and Biology Society (EMBC), Orlando, FL, USA, 16–20 August 2016; pp. 3712–3715, doi:10.1109/EMBC.2016.7591534.
24. Chaudhuri, S.; Oudejans, D.; Thompson, H.J.; Demiris, G. Real World Accuracy and Use of a Wearable Fall Detection Device by Older Adults. *J. Am. Geriatr. Soc.* **2015**, *63*, 2415–2416, doi:10.1111/jgs.13804.
25. Chen, K.H.; Hsu, Y.W.; Yang, J.J.; Jaw, F.S. Enhanced Characterization of an Accelerometer-Based Fall Detection Algorithm Using a Repository. *Instrum. Sci. Technol.* **2017**, *45*, 382–391, doi:10.1080/10739149.2016.1268155.
26. Debard, G.; Karsmakers, P.; Deschodt, M.; Vlaeyen, E.; Van Den Bergh, J.; Dejaeger, E.; Milisen, K.; Goedeme, T.; Tuytelaars, T.; Vanrumste, B. Camera Based Fall Detection Using Multiple Features Validated with Real Life Video. In Workshop Proceedings of the 7th International Conference on Intelligent Environments, The Netherlands, 2011; Volume 10, pp. 441–450, doi:10.3233/978-1-60750-795-6-441.
27. Debard, G.; Mertens, M.; Deschodt, M.; Vlaeyen, E.; Devriendt, E.; Dejaeger, E.; Milisen, K.; Tournoy, J.; Croonenborghs, T.; Goedeme, T.; et al. Camera-Based Fall Detection Using Real-World versus Simulated Data: How Far Are We from the Solution? *J. Ambient Intell. Smart Environ.* **2016**, *8*, 149–168, doi:10.3233/AIS-160369.
28. Debard, G.; Mertens, M.; Goedeme, T.; Tuytelaars, T.; Vanrumste, B. Three Ways to Improve the Performance of Real-Life Camera-Based Fall Detection Systems. *J. Sens.* **2017**, doi:10.1155/2017/8241910.
29. Feldwieser, F.; Gietzelt, M.; Goevercin, M.; Marschollek, M.; Meis, M.; Winkelbach, S.; Wolf, K.H.; Spehr, J.; Steinhagen-Thiessen, E. Multimodal Sensor-Based Fall Detection within the Domestic Environment of Elderly People. *Z. Gerontol. Geriatr.* **2014**, *47*, 661–665, doi:10.1007/s00391-014-0805-8.
30. Gietzelt, M.; Spehr, J.; Ehmen, Y.; Wegel, S.; Feldwieser, F.; Meis, M.; Marschollek, M.; Wolf, K.H.; Steinhagen-Thiessen, E.; Govercin, M. GAL@Home: A Feasibility Study of Sensor-Based in-Home Fall Detection. *Z. Gerontol. Geriatr.* **2012**, *45*, 716–721, doi:10.1007/s00391-012-0400-9.
31. Godfrey, A.; Bourke, A.; Del Din, S.; Morris, R.; Hickey, A.; Helbostad, J.L.; Rochester, L.; Godfrey, A.; Bourke, A.; Del Din, S.; et al. Towards Holistic Free-Living Assessment in Parkinson's Disease: Unification of Gait and Fall Algorithms with a Single Accelerometer. In Proceedings of the Annual International Conference of the IEEE Engineering in Medicine And Biology Society, Orlando, FL, USA , 16–20 August 2016; pp. 651–654, doi:10.1109/EMBC.2016.7590786.
32. Hu, X.; Dor, R.; Bosch, S.; Khoong, A.; Li, J.; Stark, S.; Lu, C. Challenges in Studying Falls of Community-Dwelling Older Adults in the Real World. In Proceedings of the 2017 IEEE International Conference on Smart Computing (SMARTCOMP), Hong Kong, China, 29–31 May 2017; pp. 1–7, doi:10.1109/SMARTCOMP.2017.7946993.
33. Kangas, M.; Korpelainen, R.; Vikman, I.; Nyberg, L.; Jamsa, T. Sensitivity and False Alarm Rate of a Fall Sensor in Long-Term Fall Detection in the Elderly. *Gerontology* **2015**, *61*, 61–68, doi:10.1159/000362720.
34. Lipsitz, L.A.; Tchalla, A.E.; Iloputaife, I.; Gagnon, M.; Dole, K.; Su, Z.Z.; Klickstein, L. Evaluation of an Automated Falls Detection Device in Nursing Home Residents. *J. Am. Geriatr. Soc.* **2016**, *64*, 365–368, doi:10.1111/jgs.13708.
35. Liu, L.; Popescu, M.; Skubic, M.; Rantz, M. An Automatic Fall Detection Framework Using Data Fusion of Doppler Radar and Motion Sensor Network. In Proceedings of the Annual International Conference of the IEEE Engineering in Medicine and Biology Society, Chicago, IL, USA, 26–30 August 2014; pp. 5940–5943, doi:10.1109/EMBC.2014.6944981.
36. Palmerini, L.; Bagala, F.; Zanetti, A.; Klenk, J.; Becker, C.; Cappello, A. A Wavelet-Based Approach to Fall Detection. *Sensors* **2015**, *15*, 11575–11586, doi:10.3390/s150511575.
37. Rezaee, K.; Haddadnia, J.; Delbari, A. Intelligent Detection of the Falls in the Elderly Using Fuzzy Inference System and Video-Based Motion Estimation Method. In Proceedings of the 2013 8th Iranian Conference on Machine Vision and Image Processing (MVIP), Zanjan, Iran, 10–12 September 2013; pp. 284–288, doi:10.1109/IranianMVIP.2013.6779996.

38. Soaz, C.; Lederer, C.; Daumer, M. A New Method to Estimate the Real Upper Limit of the False Alarm Rate in a 3 Accelerometry-Based Fall Detector for the Elderly. In Proceedings of the 2012 Annual International Conference of the IEEE Engineering in Medicine and Biology Society, San Diego, CA, USA, 28 August–1 September 2012; pp. 244–247, doi:10.1109/EMBC.2012.6345915.
39. Stone, E.E.; Skubic, M. Fall Detection in Homes of Older Adults Using the Microsoft Kinect. *IEEE J. Biomed. Health Inform.* **2015**, *19*, 290–301, doi:10.1109/JBHI.2014.2312180.
40. Yu, S.; Chen, H.; Brown, R.A. Hidden Markov Model-Based Fall Detection with Motion Sensor Orientation Calibration: A Case for Real-Life Home Monitoring. *IEEE J. Biomed. Health Inform.* **2017**, doi:10.1109/JBHI.2017.2782079.
41. Delahoz, Y.S.; Labrador, M.A. Survey on Fall Detection and Fall Prevention Using Wearable and External Sensors. *Sensors* **2014**, *14*, 19806–19842, doi:10.3390/s141019806.
42. Folstein, M.F.; Folstein, S.E.; McHugh, P.R. "Mini-Mental State": A Practical Method for Grading the Cognitive State of Patients for the Clinician. *J. Psychiatr. Res.* **1975**, *12*, 189–198, doi:10.1016/0022-3956(75)90026-6.
43. Hand, D.J. Measuring Classifier Performance: A Coherent Alternative to the Area under the ROC Curve. *Mach. Learn.* **2009**, *77*, 103–123, doi:10.1007/s10994-009-5119-5.
44. Hanczar, B.; Hua, J.; Sima, C.; Weinstein, J.; Bittner, M.; Dougherty, E.R. Small-Sample Precision of ROC-Related Estimates. *Bioinformatics* **2010**, *26*, 822–830, doi:10.1093/bioinformatics/btq037.
45. Lobo, J.M.; Jiménez-Valverde, A.; Real, R. AUC: A Misleading Measure of the Performance of Predictive Distribution Models. *Glob. Ecol. Biogeogr.* **2008**, *17*, 145–151, doi:10.1111/j.1466-8238.2007.00358.x.
46. Davis, J.; Goadrich, M. The Relationship between Precision-Recall and ROC Curves. In Proceedings of the 23rd International Conference on Machine Learning, Pittsburgh, PA, USA, 25–29 June 2006; pp. 233–240.
47. Klenk, J.; Chiari, L.; Helbostad, J.; Zijlstra, W.; Aminian, K.; Todd, C.; Bandinelli, S.; Kerse, N.; Schwickert, L.; Mellone, S. Development of a Standard Fall Data Format for Signals from Body-Worn Sensors. *Z. Gerontol. Geriatr.* **2013**, *46*, 720–726.
48. Klenk, J.; Schwickert, L.; Palmerini, L.; Mellone, S.; Bourke, A.; Ihlen, E.A.F.; Kerse, N.; Hauer, K.; Pijnappels, M.; Synofzik, M.; et al. The FARSEEING Real-World Fall Repository: A Large-Scale Collaborative Database to Collect and Share Sensor Signals from Real-World Falls. *Eur. Rev. Aging Phys. Act.* **2016**, *13*, 8, doi:10.1186/s11556-016-0168-9.
49. Becker, C.; Schwickert, L.; Mellone, S.; Bagala, F.; Chiari, L.; Helbostad, J.L.; Zijlstra, W.; Aminian, K.; Bourke, A.; Todd, C.; et al. Proposal for a Multiphase Fall Model Based on Real-World Fall Recordings with Body-Fixed Sensors. *Z. Gerontol. Geriatr.* **2012**, *45*, 707–715, doi:10.1007/s00391-012-0403-6.

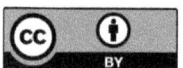

© 2018 by the authors. Licensee MDPI, Basel, Switzerland. This article is an open access article distributed under the terms and conditions of the Creative Commons Attribution (CC BY) license (http://creativecommons.org/licenses/by/4.0/).

MDPI
St. Alban-Anlage 66
4052 Basel
Switzerland
Tel. +41 61 683 77 34
Fax +41 61 302 89 18
www.mdpi.com

Sensors Editorial Office
E-mail: sensors@mdpi.com
www.mdpi.com/journal/sensors

www.ingramcontent.com/pod-product-compliance
Lightning Source LLC
LaVergne TN
LVHW070128100526
838202LV00016B/2244